APPLIED
BIOPHARMACEUTICS
& PHARMACOKINETICS

FIFTH EDITION

APPLIED
BIOPHARMACEUTICS
& PHARMACOKINETICS

FIFTH EDITION

LEON SHARGEL, PhD, RPh
Vice President, Biopharmaceutics
Eon Labs, Inc.
Wilson, North Carolina

Adjunct Associate Professor
School of Pharmacy
University of Maryland
Baltimore, Maryland

SUSANNA WU–PONG PhD, RPh
Associate Professor
Department of Pharmaceutics
Medical College of Virginia Campus
Virginia Commonwealth University
Richmond, Virginia

ANDREW B.C. YU PhD, RPh
Registered Pharmacist
Gaithersburg, MD
Formerly Associate Professor of Pharmaceutics
Albany College of Pharmacy
Present Affiliation: HFD–520, CDER, FDA*

*The content of this book represents the personal views of the authors and not that of the FDA.

McGraw-Hill
Medical Publishing Division

New York Chicago San Francisco Lisbon London Madrid Mexico City Milan
New Delhi San Juan Seoul Singapore Sydney Toronto

Applied Biopharmaceutics and Pharmacokinetics, Fifth Edition

1 2 3 4 5 6 7 8 9 0   DOC/DOC 0 9 8 7 6 5 4

ISBN 0-07-137550-3

This book was set in New Baskerville by TechBooks.
The editors were Michael Brown and Christie Naglieri.
The production service was TechBooks.
The production supervisor was Phil Galea.
The cover designer was Kelly Parr.
RR Donnelley was printer and binder.

This book is printed on acid-free paper.

Library of Congress Cataloging-in-Publication Data
Shargel, Leon, 1941–
    Applied biopharmaceutics & pharmacokinetics/Leon Shargel, Susanna Wu, Andrew B.C. Yu. —5th ed.
        p. ; cm.
    Includes bibliographical references and index.
    ISBN 0-07-137550-3
    1. Biopharmaceutics.   2. Pharmacokinetics.   I. Title: Applied biopharmaceutics and pharmacokinetics.   II. Wu-Pong, Susanna.   III. Yu, Andrew B. C.,
    1945- IV. Title.
        [DNLM: 1. Biopharmaceutics.   2. Models, Chemical.   3. Pharmacokinetics.
    QV 38 S531a 2004] RM301.4.S52 2004
    615'.7—dc22
                                                                    2004044993

Please tell the authors and publisher what you think of this book by sending your comments to pharmacy@mcgraw-hill.com. Please put the author and title of the book in the subject line.

CONTENTS

PREFACE

The fifth edition of *Applied Biopharmaceutics and Pharmacokinetics* continues to maintain the scope and objectives of the previous editions. The major objective is to provide the reader with a basic understanding of the principles of biopharmaceutics and pharmacokinetics that can be applied to drug product development and drug therapy. This revised and updated edition of the popular text remains unique in teaching the student the basic concepts that may be applied to understanding the complex issues associated with the processes of drug delivery and the essentials of safe and effective drug therapy.

This text integrates basic scientific principles with clinical pharmacy practice and drug product development. Practical examples and questions are included to encourage students to apply the principles in patient care and drug consultation situations. Active learning and outcome-based objectives are highlighted.

The primary audience is pharmacy students enrolled in pharmaceutical science courses in pharmacokinetics and biopharmaceutics. This text fulfills course work offered in separate or combined courses in these subjects. A secondary audience for this textbook is research and development scientists in the pharmaceutical industry, particularly those in pharmaceutics, biopharmaceutics, and pharmacokinetics.

Some of the improvements in this edition include the re-ordering of the chapters and content to reflect the current curriculum in pharmaceutical sciences and the addition of two new chapters including *Pharmacogenetics* and *Impact of Drug Product Quality and Biopharmaceutics on Clinical Efficacy*. Each chapter has been revised to include the latest concepts in biopharmaceutics and pharmacokinetics with new practice problems and clinical examples that can be applied to pharmacy practice and research.

Susanna Wu-Pong, PhD, RPh, Associate Professor, Department of Pharmaceutics, Virginia Commonwealth University, Richmond, Virginia, has collaborated with the original authors. Her expertise adds to the quality of this edition.

Leon Shargel
Susanna Wu-Pong
Andrew B.C. Yu
August 2004

GLOSSARY

A, B, C	Preexponential constants for three-compartment model equation	BA	Bioavailability
		BCS	Biopharmaceutics classification system
a, b, c	Exponents for three-compartment model equation	BE	Bioequivalence
		BMI	Body mass index
α, β, γ	Exponents for three-compartment model equation (equivalent to a, b, c above)	C	Concentration (mass/volume)
		C_a	Drug concentration in arterial plasma
$\lambda_1, \lambda_2, \lambda_3$	Exponents for three-compartment-type exponential equation (equivalent to a, b, c above; more terms may be added and indexed numerically with λ subscripts for multiexponential models)	C_{av}^{∞}	Average steady-state plasma drug concentration
		C_c or C_p	Concentration of drug in the central compartment or in plasma
		C_{Cr}	Serum creatinine concentration, usually expressed as mg%
		C_{eff}	Minimum effective drug concentration
Ab	Amount of drug in the body of time t; *see also* D_B	C_{GI}	Concentration of drug in gastrointestinal tract
Ab^{∞}	Total amount of drug in the body		
ANDA	Abbreviated New Drug Application; *see also* NDA	CI	Confidence interval
		C_m	Metabolite plasma concentration
ANOVA	Analysis of variance	C_{max}	Maximum concentration of drug
AUC	Area under the plasma level–time curve	C_{max}^{∞}	Maximum steady-state drug concentration
$[AUC]_0^{\infty}$	Area under the plasma level–time curve extrapolated to infinite time	C_{min}	Minimum concentration of drug
$[AUC]_0^t$	Area under the plasma level–time curve from $t = 0$ to last measurable plasma drug concentration at time t	C_{min}^{∞}	Minimum steady-state drug concentration
		C_p	Concentration of drug in plasma
AUMC	Area under the (first) moment–time curve	C_p^0	Concentration of drug in plasma at zero time ($t = 0$)

C_p^∞	Steady-state plasma drug concentration (equivalent to C_{SS})
C_{p_n}	Last measured plasma drug concentration
C_{SS}	Concentration of drug at steady state
C_t	Concentration of drug in tissue
Cl_{Cr}	Creatinine clearance
Cl_D	Dialysis clearance
Cl_h	Hepatic clearance
Cl_{int}	Intrinsic clearance
Cl'_{int}	Intrinsic clearance (unbound or free drug)
Cl_{nr}	Nonrenal clearance
Cl_R	Renal clearance
Cl_R^u	Renal clearance of uremic patient
Cl_T	Total body clearance
CRFA	Cumulative relative fraction absorbed
C_v	Drug concentration in venous plasma
D	Amount of drug (mass, eg, mg)
D_A	Amount of drug absorbed
D_B	Amount of drug in body
D_E	Drug eliminated
D_{GI}	Amount of drug in gastrointestinal tract
D_L	Loading (initial) dose
D_m	Maintenance dose
D_μ	Total amount of metabolite excreted in the urine
D_N	Normal dose
D_P	Drug in central compartment
D_t	Amount of drug in tissue
D_u	Amount of drug in urine
D_0	Dose of drug
D^0	Amount of drug at zero time ($t = 0$)
E	Pharmacologic effect
e	Intercept on y axis of graph relating

	pharmacologic response to log drug concentration
E_{max}	Maximum pharmacologic effect
E_0	Pharmacologic effect at zero drug concentration
EC_{50}	Drug concentration that produces 50% maximum pharmacologic effect
ELS	Extended least square
ER	Extraction constant (equivalent to E_h); extraction ratio
F	Fraction of dose absorbed (bioavailability factor)
f	Fraction of dose remaining in body
f_e	Fraction of unchanged drug excreted unchanged in urine
f_u	unbound fraction of drug
FDA	U.S. Food and Drug Administration
$f(t)$	Function representing drug elimination over time (time is the independent variable)
$f'(t)$	Derivative of $f(t)$
GFR	Glomerular filtration rate
GI	Gastrointestinal tract
GMP	Good Manufacturing Practice
IBW	Ideal body weight
IVIVC	*In-vitro–in-vivo* correlation
k	Overall drug elimination rate constant ($k = k_e + k_m$); first-order rate constant, similar to k_{el}
K_a	Association binding constant
k_a	First-order absorption rate constant
K_d	Dissociation binding constant

k_e	Excretion rate constant (first order)	MRT_c	Mean residence time from the central compartment
k_{e0}	Transfer rate constant out of the effect compartment	MRT_p	Mean residence time from the peripheral compartment
K_M	Michaelis–Menten constant	MRT_t	Mean residence time from the tissue compartment (same as MRT_p)
k_m	Metabolism rate constant (first order)		
k_N	Normal elimination rate constant (first order)	MTC	Minimum toxic concentration
k_{NR}^N	Nonrenal elimination constant of normal patient	μ_0	Area under the zero moment curve (same as AUC)
k_{NR}^U	Renal elimination constant of uremic patient	μ_1	Area under the first moment curve (same as AUMC)
k_u	Uremic elimination rate constant (first order)	NDA	New Drug Application
k_0	Zero-order absorption rate constant	NONMEN	Nonlinear mixed effect model
k_{1e}	Transfer rate constant from the central to the effect compartment	P	Amount of protein
		PD	Pharmacodynamics
		PK	Pharmacokinetics
k_{12}	Transfer rate constant (from the central to the tissue compartment); first-order transfer rate constant from compartment 1 to compartment 2	Q	Blood flow
		R	infusion rate; ratio of C_{max} after N dose to C_{max} after one dose (Chapter 8) (accumulation ratio); pharmacologic response (Chapter 19)
k_{21}	Transfer rate constant (from the tissue to the central compartment); first-order transfer rate constant from compartment 2 to compartment 1	r	Ratio of mole of drug bound to total moles of protein
		R_{max}	Maximum pharmacologic response
LBW	Lean body weight	SD	Standard deviation
m	Slope (also slope of E versus log C)	t	Time (hours or minutes); denotes tissue when used as a subscript
M_u	Amount of metabolite excreted in urine	t_{eff}	Duration of pharmacologic response to drug
MAT	Mean absorption time		
MDT	Mean dissolution time	t_{inf}	Infusion period
MEC	Minimum effective concentration	t_{lag}	Lag time
		t_{max}	Time of occurrence for maximum (peak) drug concentration
MLP	Maximum life-span potential		
MRT	Mean residence time	t_0	Initial or zero time

$t_{1/2}$	Half-life	V_e	Volume of the effect compartment
τ	Time interval between doses	V_{max}	Maximum metabolic rate
USP	*United States Pharmacopeia*	V_p	Volume of plasma (central compartment)
V	Volume (L or mL)		
v	Velocity	V_t	Volume of tissue compartment
V_{app}	Apparent volume of distribution (binding)	$(V_D)_{exp}$	Extrapolated volume of distribution
V_C	Volume of central compartment	$(V_D)_{SS}$ or V_{DSS}	Steady-state volume of distribution
V_D	Volume of distribution		

1

INTRODUCTION TO BIOPHARMACEUTICS AND PHARMACOKINETICS

BIOPHARMACEUTICS

All pharmaceuticals, from the generic analgesic tablet in the community pharmacy to the state-of-the-art immunotherapy in specialized hospitals, undergo extensive research and development prior to approval by the U.S. Food and Drug Administration (FDA). The physicochemical characteristics of the active pharmaceutical ingredient (API, or drug substance), the dosage form or the drug, and the route of administration are critical determinants of the *in-vivo* performance, safety and efficacy of the drug product. The properties of the drug and its dosage form are carefully engineered and tested to produce a stable drug product that upon administration provides the desired therapeutic response in the patient. Both the pharmacist and the pharmaceutical scientist must understand these complex relationships to comprehend the proper use and development of pharmaceuticals.

To illustrate the importance of the drug substance and the drug formulation on absorption, and distribution of the drug to the site of action, one must first consider the sequence of events that precede elicitation of a drug's therapeutic effect. First, the drug in its dosage form is taken by the patient either by an oral, intravenous, subcutaneous, transdermal, etc., route of administration. Next, the drug is released from the dosage form in a predictable and characterizable manner. Then, some fraction of the drug is absorbed from the site of administration into either the surrounding tissue, into the body (as with oral dosage forms), or both. Finally, the drug reaches the site of action. If the drug concentration at the site of action exceeds the *minimum effective concentration* (MEC), a pharmacologic response results. The actual dosing regimen (dose, dosage form, dosing interval) was carefully determined in clinical trials to provide the correct drug concentrations at the site of action. This sequence of events is profoundly affected—in fact, sometimes orchestrated—by the design of the dosage form, the drug itself, or both.

Historically, pharmaceutical scientists have evaluated the relative drug availability to the body *in vivo* after giving a drug product to an animal or human, and then comparing specific pharmacologic, clinical, or possible toxic responses. For example, a drug such as isoproterenol causes an increase in heart rate when given intravenously but has no observable effect on the heart when given orally at the same dose level. In addition, the *bioavailability* (a measure of systemic availability of a drug) may differ from one drug product to another containing the same drug, even for the same route of administration. This difference in drug bioavailability may be manifested by observing the difference in the therapeutic effectiveness of the drug products. In other words, the nature of the drug molecule, the route of delivery, and the formulation of the dosage form can determine whether an administered drug is therapeutically effective, toxic, or has no apparent effect at all.

Biopharmaceutics is the science that examines this interrelationship of the physicochemical properties of the drug, the dosage form in which the drug is given, and the route of administration on the rate and extent of systemic drug absorption. Thus, biopharmaceutics involves factors that influence (1) the stability of the drug within the drug product, (2) the release of the drug from the drug product, (3) the rate of dissolution/release of the drug at the absorption site, and (4) the systemic absorption of the drug. A general scheme describing this dynamic relationship is described in Figure 1-1.

The study of biopharmaceutics is based on fundamental scientific principles and experimental methodology. Studies in biopharmaceutics use both *in-vitro* and *in-vivo* methods. *In-vitro* methods are procedures employing test apparatus and equipment without involving laboratory animals or humans. *In-vivo* methods are more complex studies involving human subjects or laboratory animals. Some of these methods will be discussed in Chapter 14. These methods must be able to assess the impact of the physical and chemical properties of the drug, drug stability, and large-scale production of the drug and drug product on the biologic performance of the drug. Moreover, biopharmaceutics considers the properties of the drug and dosage form in a physiologic environment, the drug's intended therapeutic use, and the route of administration.

Figure 1-1. Scheme demonstrating the dynamic relationship between the drug, the drug product, and the pharmacologic effect.

PHARMACOKINETICS

After a drug is released from its dosage form, the drug is absorbed into the surrounding tissue, the body, or both. The distribution through and elimination of the drug in the body varies for each patient but can be characterized using mathematical models and statistics. *Pharmacokinetics* is the science of the kinetics of drug absorption, distribution, and elimination (ie, excretion and metabolism). The description of drug distribution and elimination is often termed *drug disposition*. Characterization of drug disposition is an important prerequisite for determination or modification of dosing regimens for individuals and groups of patients.

The study of pharmacokinetics involves both experimental and theoretical approaches. The experimental aspect of pharmacokinetics involves the development of biologic sampling techniques, analytical methods for the measurement of drugs and metabolites, and procedures that facilitate data collection and manipulation. The theoretical aspect of pharmacokinetics involves the development of pharmacokinetic models that predict drug disposition after drug administration. The application of statistics is an integral part of pharmacokinetic studies. Statistical methods are used for pharmacokinetic parameter estimation and data interpretation ultimately for the purpose of designing and predicting optimal dosing regimens for individuals or groups of patients. Statistical methods are applied to pharmacokinetic models to determine data error and structural model deviations. Mathematics and computer techniques form the theoretical basis of many pharmacokinetic methods. Classical pharmacokinetics is a study of theoretical models focusing mostly on model development and parameterization.

CLINICAL PHARMACOKINETICS

During the drug development process, large numbers of patients are tested to determine optimum dosing regimens, which are then recommended by the manufacturer to produce the desired pharmacologic response in the majority of the anticipated patient population. However, intra- and interindividual variations will frequently result in either a subtherapeutic (drug concentration below the MEC) or toxic response (drug concentrations above the *minimum toxic concentration,* MTC), which may then require adjustment to the dosing regimen. *Clinical pharmacokinetics* is the application of pharmacokinetic methods to drug therapy. Clinical pharmacokinetics involves a multidisciplinary approach to individually optimized dosing strategies based on the patient's disease state and patient-specific considerations.

The study of clinical pharmacokinetics of drugs in disease states requires input from medical and pharmaceutical research. Table 1.1 is a list of 10 age-adjusted rates of death from 10 leading causes of death in the United States, 2003. The influence of many diseases on drug disposition is not adequately studied. Age, gender, genetic, and ethnic differences can also result in pharmacokinetic differences that may affect the outcome of drug therapy. The study of pharmacokinetic differences of drugs in various population groups is termed *population pharmacokinetics* (Sheiner and Ludden, 1992).

TABLE 1.1   Ratio of Age-Adjusted Death Rates, by Male/Female Ratio from the 10 Leading Causes of Death in the USA, 2003

DISEASE	RANK	MALE:FEMALE
Disease of heart	1	1.5
Malignant neoplasms	2	1.5
Cerebrovascular diseases	3	4.0
Chronic lower respiration diseases	4	1.4
Accidents and others*	5	2.2
Diabetes mellitus	6	1.2
Pneumonia and influenza	7	1.4
Alzheimers	8	0.8
Nephrotis, nephrotic syndrome and nephrosis	9	1.5
Septicemia	10	1.2

*Death due to adverse effects suffered as defined by CDC.

Source: National Vital Statistics Report Vol 52, No. 3, 2003

Pharmacokinetics is also applied to *therapeutic drug monitoring* (TDM) for very potent drugs such as those with a narrow therapeutic range, in order to optimize efficacy and to prevent any adverse toxicity. For these drugs, it is necessary to monitor the patient, either by monitoring plasma drug concentrations (eg, theophylline) or by monitoring a specific pharmacodynamic endpoint such as prothrombin clotting time (eg, warfarin). Pharmacokinetic and drug analysis services necessary for safe drug monitoring are generally provided by the *clinical pharmacokinetic service* (CPKS). Some drugs frequently monitored are the aminoglycosides and anticonvulsants. Other drugs closely monitored are those used in cancer chemotherapy, in order to minimize adverse side effects (Rodman and Evans, 1991).

PHARMACODYNAMICS

Pharmacodynamics refers to the relationship between the drug concentration at the site of action (receptor) and pharmacologic response, including biochemical and physiologic effects that influence the interaction of drug with the receptor. The interaction of a drug molecule with a receptor causes the initiation of a sequence of molecular events resulting in a pharmacologic or toxic response. Pharmacokinetic-pharmacodynamic models are constructed to relate plasma drug level to drug concentration in the site of action and establish the intensity and time course of the drug. Pharmacodynamics and pharmacokinetic-pharmacodynamic models are discussed more fully in Chapter 19.

TOXICOKINETICS AND CLINICAL TOXICOLOGY

Toxicokinetics is the application of pharmacokinetic principles to the design, conduct, and interpretation of drug safety evaluation studies (Leal et al, 1993) and in validating dose-related exposure in animals. Toxicokinetic data aids in the interpretation of toxicologic findings in animals and extrapolation of the resulting data to humans. Toxicokinetic studies are performed in animals during preclinical drug development and may continue after the drug has been tested in clinical trials.

Clinical toxicology is the study of adverse effects of drugs and toxic substances (poisons) in the body. The pharmacokinetics of a drug in an overmedicated (intoxicated) patient may be very different from the pharmacokinetics of the same drug given in lower therapeutic doses. At very high doses, the drug concentration in the body may saturate enzymes involved in the absorption, biotransformation, or active renal secretion mechanisms, thereby changing the pharmacokinetics from linear to nonlinear pharmacokinetics. Nonlinear pharmacokinetics is discussed in Chapter 9. Drugs frequently involved in toxicity cases include acetaminophen, salicylates, morphine, and the tricylic antidepressants (TCAs). Many of these drugs can be assayed conveniently by fluorescence immunoassay (FIA) kits.

MEASUREMENT OF DRUG CONCENTRATIONS

Because drug concentrations are an important element in determining individual or population pharmacokinetics, drug concentrations are measured in biologic samples, such as milk, saliva, plasma, and urine. Sensitive, accurate, and precise analytical methods are available for the direct measurement of drugs in biologic matrices. Such measurements are generally validated so that accurate information is generated for pharmacokinetic and clinical monitoring. In general, chromatographic methods are most frequently employed for drug concentration measurement, because chromatography separates the drug from other related materials that may cause assay interference.

Sampling of Biologic Specimens

Only a few biologic specimens may be obtained safely from the patient to gain information as to the drug concentration in the body. *Invasive methods* include sampling blood, spinal fluid, synovial fluid, tissue biopsy, or any biologic material that requires parenteral or surgical intervention in the patient. In contrast, *noninvasive methods* include sampling of urine, saliva, feces, expired air, or any biologic material that can be obtained without parenteral or surgical intervention. The measurement of drug and metabolite concentration in each of these biologic materials yields important information, such as the amount of drug retained in, or transported into, that region of the tissue or fluid, the likely pharmacologic or toxicologic outcome of drug dosing, and drug metabolite formation or transport.

Drug Concentrations in Blood, Plasma, or Serum

Measurement of drug concentration (levels) in the blood, serum, or plasma is the most direct approach to assessing the pharmacokinetics of the drug in the body. Whole blood contains cellular elements including red blood cells, white blood cells, platelets, and various other proteins, such as albumin and globulins. In general, serum or plasma is most commonly used for drug measurement. To obtain serum, whole blood is allowed to clot and the serum is collected from the supernatant after centrifugation. Plasma is obtained from the supernatant of centrifuged whole blood to which an anticoagulant, such as heparin, has been added. Therefore, the protein content of serum and plasma is not the same. Plasma perfuses all the tissues of the body, including the cellular elements in the blood. Assuming that a drug in the plasma is in dynamic equilibrium with the tissues, then changes in the drug concentration in plasma will reflect changes in tissue drug concentrations.

Plasma Level–Time Curve

The plasma level–time curve is generated by obtaining the drug concentration in plasma samples taken at various time intervals after a drug product is administered. The concentration of drug in each plasma sample is plotted on rectangular-coordinate graph paper against the corresponding time at which the plasma sample was removed. As the drug reaches the general (systemic) circulation, plasma drug concentrations will rise up to a maximum. Usually, absorption of a drug is more rapid than elimination. As the drug is being absorbed into the systemic circulation, the drug is distributed to all the tissues in the body and is also *simultaneously* being eliminated. Elimination of a drug can proceed by excretion, biotransformation, or a combination of both.

The relationship of the drug level–time curve and various pharmacologic parameters for the drug is shown in Figure 1-2. MEC and MTC represent the *minimum effective concentration* and *minimum toxic concentration* of drug, respectively. For some drugs, such as those acting on the autonomic nervous system, it is useful to know the concentration of drug that will just barely produce a pharmacologic effect (ie, MEC). Assuming the drug concentration in the plasma is in equilibrium with the tissues, the MEC reflects the minimum concentration of drug needed at the receptors to produce the desired pharmacologic effect. Similarly, the MTC represents the drug concentration needed to just barely produce a toxic effect. The *onset time* corresponds to the time required for the drug to reach the MEC. The

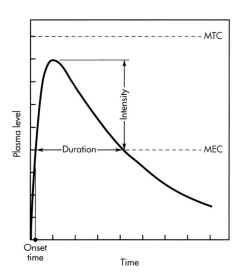

Figure 1-2. Generalized plasma level–time curve after oral administration of a drug.

intensity of the pharmacologic effect is proportional to the number of drug receptors occupied, which is reflected in the observation that higher plasma drug concentrations produce a greater pharmacologic response, up to a maximum. The *duration of drug action* is the difference between the onset time and the time for the drug to decline back to the MEC.

In contrast, the pharmacokineticist can also describe the plasma level–time curve in terms of such pharmacokinetic terms as *peak plasma level, time for peak plasma level,* and *area under the curve,* or AUC (Fig. 1-3). The time of peak plasma level is the time of maximum drug concentration in the plasma and is a rough marker of average rate of drug absorption. The peak plasma level or maximum drug concentration is related to the dose, the rate constant for absorption, and the elimination constant of the drug. The AUC is related to the amount of drug absorbed systemically. These and other pharmacokinetic parameters are discussed in succeeding chapters.

Drug Concentrations in Tissues

Tissue biopsies are occasionally removed for diagnostic purposes, such as the verification of a malignancy. Usually, only a small sample of tissue is removed, making drug concentration measurement difficult. Drug concentrations in tissue biopsies may not reflect drug concentration in other tissues nor the drug concentration in all parts of the tissue from which the biopsy material was removed. For example, if the tissue biopsy was for the diagnosis of a tumor within the tissue, the blood flow to the tumor cells may not be the same as the blood flow to other cells in this tissue. In fact, for many tissues, blood flow to one part of the tissues need not be the same as the blood flow to another part of the same tissue. The measurement of the drug concentration in tissue biopsy material may be used to ascertain if the drug reached the tissues and reached the proper concentration within the tissue.

Figure 1-3. Plasma level–time curve showing peak time and concentration. The shaded portion represents the AUC (area under the curve).

Drug Concentrations in Urine and Feces

Measurement of drug in urine is an indirect method to ascertain the bioavailability of a drug. The rate and extent of drug excreted in the urine reflects the rate and extent of systemic drug absorption. The use of urinary drug excretion measurements to establish various pharmacokinetic parameters is discussed in Chapter 15.

Measurement of drug in feces may reflect drug that has not been absorbed after an oral dose or may reflect drug that has been expelled by biliary secretion after systemic absorption. Fecal drug excretion is often performed in mass balance studies, in which the investigator attempts to account for the entire dose given to the patient. For a mass balance study, both urine and feces are collected and their drug content measured. For certain solid oral dosage forms that do not dissolve in the gastrointestinal tract but slowly leach out drug, fecal collection is performed to recover the dosage form. The undissolved dosage form is then assayed for residual drug.

Drug Concentrations in Saliva

Saliva drug concentrations have been reviewed for many drugs for therapeutic drug monitoring (Pippenger and Massoud, 1984). Because only free drug diffuses into the saliva, saliva drug levels tend to approximate free drug rather than total plasma drug concentration. The saliva/plasma drug concentration ratio is less than 1 for many drugs. The saliva/plasma drug concentration ratio is mostly influenced by the pKa of the drug and the pH of the saliva. Weak acid drugs and weak base drugs with pKa significantly different than pH 7.4 (plasma pH) generally have better correlation to plasma drug levels. The saliva drug concentrations taken after equilibrium with the plasma drug concentration generally provide more stable indication of drug levels in the body. The use of salivary drug concentrations as a therapeutic indicator should be used with caution and preferably as a secondary indicator.

Forensic Drug Measurements

Forensic science is the application of science to personal injury, murder, and other legal proceedings. Drug measurements in tissues obtained at autopsy or in other bodily fluids such as saliva, urine, and blood may be useful if a suspect or victim has taken an overdose of a legal medication, has been poisoned, or has been using drugs of abuse such as opiates (eg, heroin), cocaine, or marijuana. The appearance of social drugs in blood, urine, and saliva drug analysis shows short-term drug abuse. These drugs may be eliminated rapidly, making it more difficult to prove that the subject has been using drugs of abuse. The analysis for drugs of abuse in hair samples by very sensitive assay methods, such as gas chromatography coupled with mass spectrometry, provides information regarding past drug exposure. A study by Cone et al (1993) showed that the hair samples from subjects who were known drug abusers contained cocaine and 6-acetylmorphine, a metabolite of heroine (diacetylmorphine).

Significance of Measuring Plasma Drug Concentrations

The intensity of the pharmacologic or toxic effect of a drug is often related to the concentration of the drug at the receptor site, usually located in the tissue cells.

Because most of the tissue cells are richly perfused with tissue fluids or plasma, measuring the plasma drug level is a responsive method of monitoring the course of therapy.

Clinically, individual variations in the pharmacokinetics of drugs are quite common. Monitoring the concentration of drugs in the blood or plasma ascertains that the calculated dose actually delivers the plasma level required for therapeutic effect. With some drugs, receptor expression and/or sensitivity in individuals varies, so monitoring of plasma levels is needed to distinguish the patient who is receiving too much of a drug from the patient who is supersensitive to the drug. Moreover, the patient's physiologic functions may be affected by disease, nutrition, environment, concurrent drug therapy, and other factors. Pharmacokinetic models allow more accurate interpretation of the relationship between plasma drug levels and pharmacologic response.

In the absence of pharmacokinetic information, plasma drug levels are relatively useless for dosage adjustment. For example, suppose a single blood sample from a patient was assayed and found to contain 10 mg/mL. According to the literature, the maximum safe concentration of this drug is 15 mg/mL. In order to apply this information properly, it is important to know when the blood sample was drawn, what dose of the drug was given, and the route of administration. If the proper information is available, the use of pharmacokinetic equations and models may describe the blood level–time curve accurately.

Monitoring of plasma drug concentrations allows for the adjustment of the drug dosage in order to individualize and optimize therapeutic drug regimens. In the presence of alteration in physiologic functions due to disease, monitoring plasma drug concentrations may provide a guide to the progress of the disease state and enable the investigator to modify the drug dosage accordingly. Clinically, sound medical judgment and observation are most important. Therapeutic decisions should not be based solely on plasma drug concentrations.

In many cases, the *pharmacodynamic response* to the drug may be more important to measure than just the plasma drug concentration. For example, the electrophysiology of the heart, including an electrocardiogram (ECG), is important to assess in patients medicated with cardiotonic drugs such as digoxin. For an anticoagulant drug, such as dicumarol, prothrombin clotting time may indicate whether proper dosage was achieved. Most diabetic patients taking insulin will monitor their own blood or urine glucose levels.

For drugs that act irreversibly at the receptor site, plasma drug concentrations may not accurately predict pharmacodynamic response. Drugs used in cancer chemotherapy often interfere with nucleic acid or protein biosynthesis to destroy tumor cells. For these drugs, the plasma drug concentration does not relate directly to the pharmacodynamic response. In this case, other pathophysiologic parameters and side effects are monitored in the patient to prevent adverse toxicity.

BASIC PHARMACOKINETICS AND PHARMACOKINETIC MODELS

Drugs are in a dynamic state within the body as they move between tissues and fluids, bind with plasma or cellular components, or are metabolized. The biologic nature of drug distribution and disposition is complex, and drug events often happen simultaneously. Yet such factors must be considered when designing drug therapy regimens. The inherent and infinite complexity of these events require the use of mathematical models and statistics to estimate drug dosing and to predict the time course of drug efficacy for a given dose.

A *model* is a hypothesis using mathematical terms to describe quantitative relationships concisely. The predictive capability of a model lies in the proper selection and development of mathematical function(s) that parameterize the essential factors governing the kinetic process. The key parameters in a process are commonly estimated by fitting the model to the experimental data, known as *variables*. A *pharmacokinetic parameter* is a constant for the drug that is estimated from the experimental data. For example, estimated pharmacokinetic parameters such as k depend on the method of tissue sampling, the timing of the sample, drug analysis, and the predictive model selected.

A pharmacokinetic function relates an *independent variable* to a *dependent variable*, often through the use of parameters. For example, a pharmacokinetic model may predict the drug concentration in the liver 1 hour after an oral administration of a 20-mg dose. The independent variable is time and the dependent variable is the drug concentration in the liver. Based on a set of time-versus-drug concentration data, a model equation is derived to predict the liver drug concentration with respect to time. In this case, the drug concentration depends on the time after the administration of the dose, where the time:concentration relationship is defined by a pharmacokinetic parameter, k, the elimination rate constant.

Such mathematical models can be devised to simulate the rate processes of drug absorption, distribution, and elimination to describe and *predict* drug concentrations in the body as a function of time. Pharmacokinetic models are used to:

1. Predict plasma, tissue, and urine drug levels with any dosage regimen
2. Calculate the optimum dosage regimen for each patient individually
3. Estimate the possible accumulation of drugs and/or metabolites
4. Correlate drug concentrations with pharmacologic or toxicologic activity
5. Evaluate differences in the rate or extent of availability between formulations (bioequivalence)
6. Describe how changes in physiology or disease affect the absorption, distribution, or elimination of the drug
7. Explain drug interactions

Simplifying assumptions are made in pharmacokinetic models to describe a complex biologic system concerning the movement of drugs within the body. For example, most pharmacokinetic models assume that the plasma drug concentration reflects drug concentrations globally within the body.

A model may be empirically, physiologically, or compartmentally based. The model that simply interpolates the data and allows an empirical formula to estimate drug level over time is justified when limited information is available. *Empirical models* are practical but not very useful in explaining the mechanism of the actual process by which the drug is absorbed, distributed, and eliminated in the body. Examples of empirical models used in pharmacokinetics are described in Chapter 22.

Physiologically based models also have limitations. Using the example above, and apart from the necessity to sample tissue and monitor blood flow to the liver *in vivo*, the investigator needs to understand the following questions. What does liver drug concentration mean? Should the drug concentration in the blood within the tissue be determined and subtracted from the drug in the liver tissue? What type of cell is representative of the liver if a selective biopsy liver tissue sample can be collected without contamination from its surroundings? Indeed, depending on the spatial location of the liver tissue from the hepatic blood vessels, tissue drug concentrations can differ depending on distance to the blood vessel or even on the type of cell in the liver. Moreover, changes in the liver blood perfusion will alter the tissue drug concentration. If heterogeneous liver tissue is homogenized and assayed, the homogenized tissue represents only a hypothetical concentration that is an *average* of all the cells and blood in the liver at the time of collection. Since tissue homogenization is not practical for human subjects, the drug concentration in the liver may be estimated by knowing the liver extraction ratio for the drug based on knowledge of the physiologic and biochemical composition of the body organs.

A great number of models have been developed to estimate regional and global information about drug disposition in the body. Some physiologic pharmacokinetic models are also discussed in Chapter 22. Individual pharmacokinetic processes are discussed in separate chapters under the topics of drug absorption, drug distribution, drug elimination, and pharmacokinetic drug interactions involving one or all the above processes. Theoretically, an unlimited number of models may be constructed to describe the kinetic processes of drug absorption, distribution, and elimination in the body, depending on the degree of detailed information considered. Practical considerations have limited the growth of new pharmacokinetic models.

A very simple and useful tool in pharmacokinetics is *compartmentally based models*. For example, assume a drug is given by intravenous injection and that the drug dissolves (distributes) rapidly in the body fluids. One pharmacokinetic model that can describe this situation is a tank containing a volume of fluid that is rapidly equilibrated with the drug. The concentration of the drug in the tank after a given dose is governed by two parameters: (1) the fluid volume of the tank that will dilute the drug, and (2) the elimination rate of drug per unit of time. Though this model is perhaps an overly simplistic view of drug disposition in the human body, a drug's pharmacokinetic properties can frequently be described using a fluid-filled tank model called the *one-compartment open model* (see below). In both the tank and the one-compartment body model, a fraction of the drug would be continually eliminated as a function of time (Fig. 1-4). In pharmacokinetics, these parameters are assumed to be constant for a given drug. If drug concentrations in the tank are determined at various time intervals following administration of a known dose, then the volume of fluid in the tank or compartment (V_D, volume of distribution) and the rate of drug elimination can be estimated.

In practice, pharmacokinetic parameters such as k and V_D are determined experimentally from a set of drug concentrations collected over various times and known as *data*. The number of parameters needed to describe the model depends on the complexity of the process and on the route of drug administration. In

Figure 1-4. Tank with a constant volume of fluid equilibrated with drug. The volume of the fluid is 1.0 L. The fluid outlet is 10 mL/min. The fraction of drug removed per unit of time is 10/1000, or 0.01 min^{-1}.

general, as the number of parameters required to model the data increases, accurate estimation of these parameters becomes increasingly more difficult. With complex pharmacokinetic models, computer programs are used to facilitate parameter estimation. However, for the parameters to be valid, the number of data points should always exceed the number of parameters in the model.

Because a model is based on a hypothesis and simplifying assumptions, a certain degree of caution is necessary when relying totally on the pharmacokinetic model to predict drug action. For some drugs, plasma drug concentrations are not useful in predicting drug activity. For other drugs, an individual's genetic differences, disease state, and the compensatory response of the body may modify the response of a drug. If a simple model does not fit all the experimental observations accurately, a new, more elaborate model may be proposed and subsequently tested. Since limited data are generally available in most clinical situations, pharmacokinetic data should be interpreted along with clinical observations rather than replacing sound judgment by the clinician. Development of pharmacometric statistical models may help to improve prediction of drug levels among patients in the population (Sheiner and Beal, 1982; Mallet et al, 1988). However, it will be some time before these methods become generally accepted.

Compartment Models

If the tissue drug concentrations and binding are known, physiologic pharmacokinetic models, which are based on actual tissues and their respective blood flow, describe the data realistically. Physiologic pharmacokinetic models are frequently used in describing drug distribution in animals, because tissue samples are easily available for assay. On the other hand, tissue samples are often not available for human subjects, so most physiological models assume an average set of blood flow for individual subjects.

In contrast, because of the vast complexity of the body, drug kinetics in the body are frequently simplified to be represented by one or more tanks, or compartments, that communicate reversibly with each other. A compartment is not a real physiologic or anatomic region but is considered as a tissue or group of tissues that have similar blood flow and drug affinity. Within each compartment, the drug is considered to be uniformly distributed. Mixing of the drug within a compartment is rapid and homogeneous and is considered to be "well stirred," so that the drug concentration represents an average concentration, and each drug molecule has an equal probability of leaving the compartment. Rate constants are used to represent the overall rate processes of drug entry into and exit from the compartment. The model is an *open system* because drug can be eliminated from the system. Compartment models are based on linear assumptions using linear differential equations.

Mammillary Model

A compartmental model provides a simple way of grouping all the tissues into one or more compartments where drugs move to and from the central or plasma compartment. The *mammillary model* is the most common compartment model used in pharmacokinetics. The mammillary model is a strongly connected system, because one can estimate the amount of drug in any compartment of the system after drug is introduced into a given compartment. In the one-compartment model, drug is both added to and eliminated from a central compartment. The central compartment is assigned to represent plasma and highly perfused tissues that rapidly equilibrate with drug. When an intravenous dose of drug is given, the drug enters directly into the central compartment. Elimination of drug occurs from the central compartment because the organs involved in drug elimination, primarily kidney and liver, are well-perfused tissues.

In a two-compartment model, drug can move between the central or plasma compartment to and from the tissue compartment. Although the tissue compartment does not represent a specific tissue, the mass balance accounts for the drug present in all the tissues. In this model, the total amount of drug in the body is simply the sum of drug present in the central compartment plus the drug present in the tissue compartment. Knowing the parameters of either the one- or two-compartment model, one can estimate the amount of drug left in the body and the amount of drug eliminated from the body at any time. The compartmental models are particularly useful when little information is known about the tissues.

Several types of compartment models are described in Figure 1-5. The pharmacokinetic rate constants are represented by the letter k. Compartment 1 represents the plasma or central compartment, and compartment 2 represents the tissue compartment. The drawing of models has three functions. The model (1) enables the pharmacokineticist to write differential equations to describe drug concentration changes in each compartment, (2) gives a visual representation of the rate processes, and (3) shows how many pharmacokinetic constants are necessary to describe the process adequately.

MODEL 1. One-compartment open model, IV injection.

MODEL 2. One-compartment open model with first-order absorption.

MODEL 3. Two-compartment open model, IV injection.

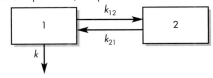

MODEL 4. Two-compartment open model with first-order absorption.

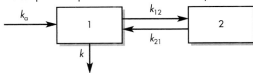

Figure 1-5. *Various compartment models.*

EXAMPLE

Two parameters are needed to describe model 1 (Fig. 1-5): the volume of the compartment and the elimination rate constant, k. In the case of model 4, the pharmacokinetic parameters consist of the volumes of compartments 1 and 2 and the rate constants—k_a, k, k_{12}, and k_{21}—for a total of six parameters.

In studying these models, it is important to know whether drug concentration data may be sampled directly from each compartment. For models 3 and 4 (Fig. 1-5), data concerning compartment 2 cannot be obtained easily because tissues are not easily sampled and may not contain homogeneous concentrations of drug. If the amount of drug absorbed and eliminated per unit time is obtained by sampling compartment 1, then the amount of drug contained in the tissue compartment 2 can be estimated mathematically. The appropriate mathematical equations for describing these models and evaluating the various pharmacokinetic parameters are given in the succeeding chapters.

Catenary Model

In pharmacokinetics, the mammillary model must be distinguished from another type of compartmental model called the catenary model. The *catenary model* consists of compartments joined to one another like the compartments of a train (Fig. 1-6). In contrast, the mammillary model consists of one or more compartments around a central compartment like satellites. Because the catenary model does not apply to the way most functional organs in the body are directly connected to the plasma, it is not used as often as the mammillary model.

Physiologic Pharmacokinetic Model (Flow Model)

Physiologic pharmacokinetic models, also known as blood flow or perfusion models, are pharmacokinetic models based on known anatomic and physiologic data. The models describe the data kinetically, with the consideration that blood flow is responsible for distributing drug to various parts of the body. Uptake of drug into organs is determined by the binding of drug in these tissues. In contrast to an estimated tissue volume of distribution, the actual tissue volume is used. Because there are many tissue organs in the body, each tissue volume must be obtained and its drug concentration described. The model would potentially predict realistic tissue drug concentrations, which the two-compartment model fails to do. Unfortunately, much of the information required for adequately describing a physiologic pharmacokinetic model are experimentally difficult to obtain. In spite of this limitation, the physiologic pharmacokinetic model does provide much better insight into how

Figure 1-6.   Example of caternary model.

physiologic factors may change drug distribution from one animal species to another. Other major differences are described below.

First, no data fitting is required in the perfusion model. Drug concentrations in the various tissues are predicted by organ tissue size, blood flow, and experimentally determined drug tissue–blood ratios (ie, partition of drug between tissue and blood).

Second, blood flow, tissue size, and the drug tissue–blood ratios may vary due to certain pathophysiologic conditions. Thus, the effect of these variations on drug distribution must be taken into account in physiologic pharmacokinetic models.

Third, and most important of all, physiologically based pharmacokinetic models can be applied to several species, and, for some drugs, human data may be extrapolated. Extrapolation from animal data is not possible with the compartment models, because the volume of distribution in such models is a mathematical concept that does not relate simply to blood volume and blood flow. To date, numerous drugs (including digoxin, lidocaine, methotrexate, and thiopental) have been described with perfusion models. Tissue levels of some of these drugs cannot be predicted successfully with compartment models, although they generally describe blood levels well. An example of a perfusion model is shown in Figure 1-7.

The number of tissue compartments in a perfusion model varies with the drug. Typically, the tissues or organs that have no drug penetration are excluded from consideration. Thus, such organs as the brain, the bones, and other parts of the central nervous system are often excluded, as most drugs have little penetration into these organs. To describe each organ separately with a differential equation would make the model very complex and mathematically difficult. A simpler but equally good approach is to group all the tissues with similar blood perfusion properties into a single compartment.

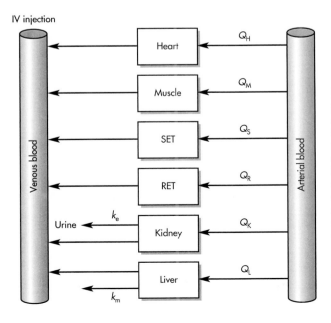

Figure 1-7. Pharmacokinetic model of drug perfusion. The k's represent kinetic constants: k_e is the first-order rate constant for urinary drug excretion and k_m is the rate constant for hepatic elimination. Each "box" represents a tissue compartment. Organs of major importance in drug absorption are considered separately, while other tissues are grouped as RET (rapidly equilibrating tissue) and SET (slowly equilibrating tissue). The size or mass of each tissue compartment is determined physiologically rather than by mathematical estimation. The concentration of drug in the tissue is determined by the ability of the tissue to accumulate drug as well as by the rate of blood perfusion to the tissue, represented by Q.

A perfusion model has been used successfully to describe the distribution of lidocaine in blood and various organs. In this case, organs such as lung, liver, brain, and muscle were individually described by differential equations, whereas other tissues were grouped as RET (rapidly equilibrating tissue) and SET (slowly equilibrating tissue), as shown in Figure 1-7. Figure 1-8 shows that the blood concentration of lidocaine declines biexponentially and was well predicted by the physiologic model based on blood flow. The tissue lidocaine level in the lung, muscle, and adipose and other organs is shown in Figure 1-9. The model shows that adipose tissue accumulates drugs slowly because of low blood supply. In contrast, vascular tissues, like the lung, equilibrate rapidly with the blood and start to decline as soon as drug level in the blood starts to fall. The physiologic pharmacokinetic model provides a realistic means of modeling tissue drug levels. Unfortunately, the simulated tissues levels in Figure 1-9 cannot be verified in humans because drug levels in tissues are not available. A criticism of physiologic pharmacokinetic models in general has been that there are fewer data points than parameters that one tries to fit. Consequently, the projected data are not well *constrained.*

The real significance of the physiologically based model is the potential application of this model in the prediction of human pharmacokinetics from animal data (Sawada et al, 1985). The mass of various body organs or tissues, extent of protein binding, drug metabolism capacity, and blood flow in humans and other species are often known or can be determined. Thus, physiologic and anatomic parameters can be used to predict the effects of drugs on humans from the effects on animals in cases where human experimentation is difficult or restricted.

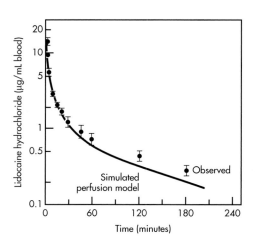

Figure 1-8. Observed mean (●) and simulated (—) arterial lidocaine blood concentrations in normal volunteers receiving 1 mg/kg per min constant infusion for 3 minutes.
(From Benowitz et al 1974, with permission; data from Tucker GT, Boas RA: *Anesthesiology* **34:**538, 1971.)

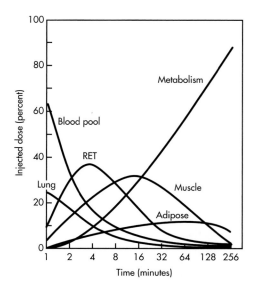

Figure 1-9. *Perfusion model simulation of the distribution of lidocaine in various tissues and its elimination from humans following an intravenous infusion for 1 minute.*
(From Benowitz et al 1974, with permission.)

FREQUENTLY ASKED QUESTIONS

1. Why is plasma or serum drug concentration, rather than blood concentration, used to monitor drug concentration in the body?

2. What are reasons to use a multicompartment model instead of a physiologic model?

3. At what time should plasma drug concentration be taken in order to best predict drug response and side effects?

LEARNING QUESTIONS

1. What is the significance of the plasma level–time curve? How does the curve relate to the pharmacologic activity of a drug?

2. What is the purpose of pharmacokinetic models?

3. Draw a diagram describing a three-compartment model with first-order absorption and drug elimination from compartment 1.

4. The pharmacokinetic model presented in Figure 1-10 represents a drug that is eliminated by renal excretion, biliary excretion, and drug metabolism. The metabolite distribution is described by a one-compartment open model. The following questions pertain to Figure 1-10.

    a. How many parameters are needed to describe the model if the drug is injected intravenously (ie, the rate of drug absorption may be neglected)?

    b. Which compartment(s) can be sampled?

    c. What would be the overall elimination rate constant for elimination of drug from compartment 1?

    d. Write an expression describing the rate of change of drug concentration in compartment 1 (dC_1/dt).

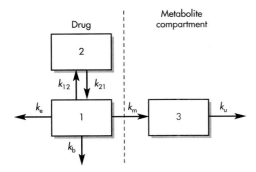

Figure 1-10. Pharmacokinetic model for a drug eliminated by renal and biliary excretion and drug metabolism. k_m = rate constant for metabolism of drug: k_u = rate constant for urinary excretion of metabolites; k_b = rate constant for biliary excretion of drug; and k_e = rate constant for urinary drug excretion.

5. Give two reasons for the measurement of the plasma drug concentration, C_p assuming (a) the C_p relates directly to the pharmacodynamic activity of the drug and (b) the C_p does not relate to the pharmacodynamic activity of the drug.

6. Consider two biologic compartments separated by a biologic membrane. Drug A is found in compartment 1 and in compartment 2 in a concentration of c_1 and c_2, respectively.

   a. What possible conditions or situations would result in concentration $c_1 > c_2$ at equilibrium?

   b. How would you experimentally demonstrate these conditions given above?

   c. Under what conditions would $c_1 = c_2$ at equilibrium?

   d. The total amount of Drug A in each biologic compartment is A_1 and A_2, respectively. Describe a condition in which $A_1 > A_2$, but $c_1 = c_2$ at equilibrium.

Include in your discussion, how the physicochemical properties of Drug A or the biologic properties of each compartment might influence equilibrium conditions.

REFERENCES

Benowitz N, Forsyth R, Melmon K, Rowland M: Lidocaine disposition kinetics in monkey and man. *Clin Pharmacol Ther* **15:**87–98, 1974

Cone EJ, Darwin WD, Wang W-L: The occurrence of cocaine, heroin and metabolites in hair of drug abusers. *Forensic Sci Int* **63:**55–68, 1993

Leal M, Yacobi A, Batra VJ: Use of toxicokinetic principles in drug development: Bridging preclinical and clinical studies. In Yacobi A, Skelly JP, Shah VP, Benet LZ (eds), *Integration of Pharmacokinetics, Pharmacodynamics and Toxicokinetics in Rational Drug Development.* New York, Plenum Press, 1993, pp 55–67

Mallet A, Mentre F, Steimer JL, Lokiec F: Pharmacometrics: Nonparametric maximum likelihood estimation for population pharmacokinetics, with application to cyclosporine. *J Pharm Biopharm* **16:**311–327, 1988

Pippenger CE and Massoud N: Therapeutic drug monitoring. In Benet LZ, et al (eds). *Pharmacokinetic Basis for Drug Treatment.* New York, Raven, 1984, chap 21

Rodman JH and Evans WE: Targeted systemic exposure for pediatric cancer therapy. In D'Argenio DZ (ed), *Advanced Methods of Pharmacokinetic and Pharmacodynamic Systems Analysis.* New York, Plenum Press, 1991, pp 177–183

Sawada Y, Hanano M, Sugiyama Y, Iga T: Prediction of the disposition of nine weakly acidic and six weekly basic drugs in humans from pharmacokinetic parameters in rats. *J Pharmacokinet Biopharm* **13:**477–492, 1985

Sheiner LB and Beal SL: Bayesian individualization of pharmacokinetics. Simple implementation and comparison with nonBayesian methods. *J Pharm Sci* **71:**1344–1348, 1982

Sheiner LB and Ludden TM: Population pharmacokinetics/dynamics. *Annu Rev Pharmacol Toxicol* **32:**185–201, 1992

BIBLIOGRAPHY

Benet LZ: General treatment of linear mammillary models with elimination from any compartment as used in pharmacokinetics. *J Pharm Sci* **61:**536–541, 1972

Bischoff K and Brown R: Drug distribution in mammals. *Chem Eng Med* **62:**33–45, 1966

Bischoff K, Dedrick R, Zaharko D, Longstreth T: Methotrexate pharmacokinetics. *J Pharm Sci* **60:**1128–1133, 1971

Chiou W: Quantitation of hepatic and pulmonary first-pass effect and its implications in pharmacokinetic study, I: Pharmacokinetics of chloroform in man. *J Pharm Biopharm* **3**:193–201, 1975

Colburn WA: Controversy III: To model or not to model. *J Clin Pharmacol* **28**:879–888, 1988

Cowles A, Borgstedt H, Gilles A: Tissue weights and rates of blood flow in man for the prediction of anesthetic uptake and distribution. *Anesthesiology* **35**:523–526, 1971

Dedrick R, Forrester D, Cannon T, et al: Pharmacokinetics of 1-β-d-arabinofurinosulcytosine (ARA-C) deamination in several species. *Biochem Pharmacol* **22**:2405–2417, 1972

Gerlowski LE and Jain RK: Physiologically based pharmacokinetic modeling: Principles and applications. *J Pharm Sci* **72**:1103–1127, 1983

Gibaldi M: *Biopharmaceutics and Clinical Pharmacokinetics*, 3rd ed. Philadelphia, Lea & Febiger, 1984

Gibaldi M: Estimation of the pharmacokinetic parameters of the two-compartment open model from post-infusion plasma concentration data. *J Pharm Sci* **58**:1133–1135, 1969

Himmelstein KJ and Lutz RJ: A review of the applications of physiologically based pharmacokinetic modeling. *J Pharm Biopharm* **7**:127–145, 1979

Lutz R and Dedrick RL: Physiologic pharmacokinetics: Relevance to human risk assessment. In Li AP (ed), *Toxicity Testing: New Applications and Applications in Human Risk Assessment*. New York, Raven, 1985, pp 129–149

Lutz R, Dedrick R, Straw J, et al: The kinetics of methotrexate distribution in spontaneous canine lymphosarcoma. *J Pharm Biopharm* **3**:77–97, 1975

Metzler CM: Estimation of pharmacokinetic parameters: Statistical considerations. *Pharmacol Ther* **13**:543–556, 1981

Montandon B, Roberts R, Fischer L: Computer simulation of sulfobromophthalein kinetics in the rat using flow-limited models with extrapolation to man. *J Pharm Biopharm* **3**:277–290, 1975

Rescigno A and Beck JS: The use and abuse of models. *J Pharm Biopharm* **15**:327–344, 1987

Ritschel WA and Banerjee PS: Physiologic pharmacokinetic models: Applications, limitations and outlook. *Meth Exp Clin Pharmacol* **8**:603–614, 1986

Rowland M, Thomson P, Guichard A, Melmon K: Disposition kinetics of lidocaine in normal subjects. *Ann N Y Acad Sci* **179**:383–398, 1971

Rowland M and Tozer T: *Clinical Pharmacokinetics—Concepts and Applications*, 3rd ed. Philadelphia, Lea & Febiger, 1995

Segre G: Pharmacokinetics: Compartmental representation. *Pharm Ther* **17**:111–127, 1982

Tozer TN: Pharmacokinetic principles relevant to bioavailability studies. In Blanchard J, Sawchuk RJ, Brodie BB (eds), *Principles and Perspectives in Drug Bioavailability*. New York, S Karger, 1979, pp 120–155

Wagner JG: Do you need a pharmacokinetic model, and, if so, which one? *J Pharm Biopharm* **3**:457–478, 1975

Welling P and Tse F: *Pharmacokinetics*. New York, Marcel Dekker, 1993

Winters ME: *Basic Clinical Pharmacokinetics*, 3rd ed. Vancouver, WA, Applied Therapeutics, 1994

2

MATHEMATICAL FUNDAMENTALS IN PHARMACOKINETICS

Because pharmacokinetics and biopharmaceutics have a strong mathematical basis, a solid foundation in mathematical principles in algebra, calculus, exponentials, logarithms, and unit analysis are critical for students in these disciples. A self-exam is included in this chapter to provide a self-assessment of possible weaknesses in one's basic math skills. Difficulties with questions in the self-exam indicate that a review of mathematical essentials is necessary. Mathematical fundamentals are summarized here for review purposes only. For a more complete discussion of fundamental principles, a suitable textbook in mathematics should be consulted.

MATH SELF-EXAM

1. What are the units for concentration?
2. A drug solution has a concentration of 50 mg/mL. What amount of drug is contained within 20.5 mL of the solution? In 0.4 L? What volume of the solution will contain 30 mg of drug?
3. Convert the units in the above solution from mg/mL to g/L and μg/uL. If the molecular weight of the drug is 325 Da, what are the units in M?
4. If 20 mg of drug are added to a container of water and result in a concentration of 0.55 mg/L, what volume of water was in the container?
5. For the following equation:

   $y = 0.5x + 2$

   a. Sketch a plot of the equation.
   b. Describe the relevance of each part of this equation.
   c. If $x = 0.6$, what is y?
   d. If $y = 4.1$, what is x?

6.   Solve the following equations for x:
   a. $\log x = 0.95$
   b. $e^x = 0.44$
   c. $\ln x = 1.22$

7.   What is the slope of the line that connects the following two points?
   Point 1: $x = 2$ $y = 5.6$
   Point 2: $x = 0.6$ $y = 2.38$

8.   For the following graph, determine C if $x = 2$. If $x = 12$.

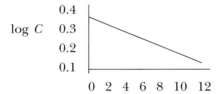

ESTIMATION AND THE USE OF CALCULATORS AND COMPUTERS

Most of the mathematics needed for pharmacokinetics and other calculations presented in this book may be performed with pencil, graph paper, and logical thought processes. A scientific calculator with logarithmic and exponential functions will make the calculations less tedious. Special computer software (see Appendix B) are available for disease state calculations in clinical pharmacokinetics.

Whenever a calculation affecting drug dose is made, one should mentally approximate whether the answer is correct given the set of information. For example, for a given problem, consider whether the number in the answer has the correct magnitude and units; eg, if the correct answer should be between 100 and 200 mg, then answers such as 12.5 mg or 1250 mg have to be wrong.

The units for the answer to a problem should be checked carefully; eg, if the expected answer is a concentration unit, then mg/L or μg/mL are acceptable; and units such as L or mg/hr are definitely wrong. Wrong units may be caused by an incorrect substitution or by the selection of an incorrect formula. In pharmacokinetic calculation, the answer is correct only if both the number and the units are correct.

Approximation

Approximation is a useful process for checking whether the answer to a given set of calculations is probably correct. Approximation can be performed with pencil and paper and sometimes with a pencil, graph paper, and ruler. The procedure is especially useful in a busy environment when answers must be checked quickly.

To estimate a series of computations, round the numbers and write the numbers using scientific notation. Then perform the series of calculations, remembering the laws of exponents. For example, estimate the answer to the following problem:

$$\frac{58 \times 489}{2114 \times 0.04} \approx \frac{6 \times 10 \times 5 \times 10^2}{2 \times 10^3 \times 4 \times 10^{-2}} \approx \frac{30 \times 10^3}{8 \times 10} \approx 400$$

The precise answer to the above calculation is 335.4. Notice, the approximated answer should be somewhat less than 400, since $30 \div 8$ is between 3 and 4.

For some pharmacokinetic problems, data, such as time versus drug concentration, may be placed on either regular or semilog graph paper. The approximated answer to the problem may be obtained by inspection of the line that is fitted to all the data points. Graphical methods for solving pharmacokinetic problems are given later in this chapter.

Calculators

A scientific handheld calculator is essential for calculations. Most scientific calculators include exponential and logarithmic functions, which are frequently used in pharmacokinetics. Additional functions such as mean, standard deviation, and linear regression analysis are used to determine the half-life of drugs. Statistical parameters, such as correlation coefficient, are used to determine how well the model agrees with the observed data.

Exponents and Logarithms

Exponents
In the expression

$$N = b^x \tag{2.1}$$

x is the exponent, b is the base, and N represents the number when b is raised to the xth power, ie, b^x. For example,

$$1000 = 10^3$$

where 3 is the exponent, 10 is the base, and 10^3 is the third power of the base, 10. The numeric value, N in equation 2.1, is 1000. In this example, it can be reversely stated that the log of N to the base 10 is 3. Thus, taking the log of the number N has the effect of "compressing" the number; some numbers are easier to handle when "compressed" or transformed to base 10. Transformation simplifies many mathematical operations.

Laws of Exponents	Example
$a^x \cdot a^y = a^{x+y}$	$10^2 \cdot 10^3 = 10^5$
$(a^x)^y = a^{xy}$	$(10^2)^3 = 10^6$
$\dfrac{a^x}{a^y} = a^{x-y}$	$\dfrac{10^2}{10^4} = 10^{-2}$
$\dfrac{1}{a^x} = a^{-x}$	$\dfrac{1}{10^2} = 10^{-2}$
$\sqrt[y]{a} = a^{1/y}$	$\sqrt[3]{a} = a^{1/3}$

Logarithms
The logarithm of a positive number N to a given base b is the exponent (or the power) x to which the base must be raised to equal the number N. Therefore, if

$$N = b^x \tag{2.2}$$

then

$$\log_b N = x \tag{2.3}$$

For example, with common logarithms (log), or logarithms using base 10,

$$100 = 10^2$$

$$\log 100 = 2$$

The number 100 is considered the *antilogarithm* of 2.

Natural logarithms (ln) use the base e, whose value is 2.718282. To relate natural logarithms to common logarithms, the following equation is used:

$$2.303 \log N = \ln N \tag{2.4}$$

Exponential Expression	Logarithmic Statement
$10^3 = 1000$	$\log 1000 = 3$
$10^2 = 100$	$\log 100 = 2$
$10^1 = 10$	$\log 10 = 1$
$10^0 = 1$	$\log 1 = 0$
$10^{-1} = 0.1$	$\log 0.1 = -1$
$10^{-2} = 0.01$	$\log 0.01 = -2$
$10^{-3} = 0.001$	$\log 0.001 = -3$

Laws of Logarithms

$$\log ab = \log a + \log b$$

$$\log \frac{a}{b} = \log a - \log b$$

$$\log a^x = x \log a$$

$$-\log \frac{a}{b} = + \log \frac{a}{b}$$

Of special interest is the following relationship:

$$\ln e^{-x} = -x \tag{2.5}$$

Equation 2.5 can be compared with the following example:

$$\log 10^{-2} = -2$$

A logarithm does not have units. A logarithm is dimensionless and is considered a real number. The logarithm of 1 is zero; the logarithm of a number less than 1 is a negative number, and the logarithm of a number greater than 1 is a positive number.

 # PRACTICE PROBLEMS

Many calculators and computers have logarithmic and exponential functions. The following problems review methods for calculations involving logarithmic or exponential functions using a calculator. Earlier editions of this text demonstrate the use of logarithmic and exponential tables to perform these problems. Before starting any new calculations, be sure to clear the calculator of any previous numbers.

1. Find the log of 35.

Solution
Enter the number 35 into your calculator.
Press the LOG function key.
Answer = 1.5441
(For some calculators, the LOG function key is pressed first, followed by the number; the answer is obtained by pressing the = key).
Notice that the correct answer for log 35 is the same as calculating the exponent of 10, which will equal 35 as shown below.

$$35 = 10^{1.5441}$$

Estimation—Since the number 35 is between 10 and 100 (ie, 10^1 and 10^2), then the log of 35 must be between 1.0 and 2.0.

2. Find the log of 0.028
Estimation—Since the number 0.028 is between 10^{-1} and 10^{-2}, then the log of 0.028 must be between -1.0 and -2.0.

Solution
Use the same procedure above.
Enter the number 0.028 into your calculator.
Press the LOG function key.
Answer = -1.553

3. Find the antilog of 0.028.
The process for finding an antilog is the reverse of finding a log. The antilog is the number that corresponds to the logarithm, such that the antilog for 3 (in base 10) is 1000 (or 10^3). This problem is the inverse of Practice Problem 2, above. In this case, the calculation determines what the number is when 10 is raised to 0.028 (ie, $10^{0.028}$).

Solution
The following methods may be used, depending on the type of calculator being used.

Method 1
If your calculator has a function key marked 10^x, then do the following:
Enter 0.028.
Press 10^x.
Answer = 1.0666

Method 2
Some calculators assume that the user knows that 10^x is the inverse of log x. For this calculation:
Enter 0.028.
Press the key marked INV.

Then press the key marked LOG.
Answer = 1.0666

4. Evaluate $e^{-1.3}$

Solution
The following methods may be used, depending on the type of calculator being used.

Method 1
If your calculator has a function key marked e^x, then do the following:
Enter 1.3.
Change the sign to minus by pressing the key marked $\pm$.
Press e^x.
Answer = 0.2725

Method 2
Some calculators assume that the user knows that e^x is the inverse of ln x. For this calculation:
Enter 1.3.
Change the sign to minus by pressing the key marked $\pm$.
Press the key marked INV.
Then press the key marked LN.
Answer = 0.2725
Thus, $e^{-1.3} = 0.2725$

5. Find the value of k in the following expression:
$25 = 50e^{-4k}$

Solution

$$e^{-4k} = \frac{25}{50} = 0.50$$

Take the natural logarithm, ln, for both sides of the equation:

$$\ln e^{-4k} = \ln 0.50$$

From Equation 2.5, ln $e^{-x} = -x$. Therefore, ln $e^{-4k} = -4k$ and ln $0.50 = -0.693$. (Calculator: Enter 0.5, then press LN function key.)

$$-4k = -0.693$$

$$k = \frac{-0.693}{-4} = 0.173$$

6. A very common problem in pharmacokinetics is to evaluate an expression such as

$$C_p = C_p^0 e^{-kt}$$

For example, find the value of C_p in the following equation when $t = 2$:

$$C_p = 35e^{-0.15t}$$

Solution
Using a calculator:
Enter 0.15.

Press $\pm$ key $\qquad = -0.15$
Multiply by 2 $\qquad\qquad = -0.30$
Press e^x function key $\quad = 0.7408$
Multiply by 35 $\qquad\quad = 25.93$
$\qquad C_p = 35e^{-0.15t} = 35(0.7408) = 25.93$

Because $e^{-x} = 1/e^x$, as the value for x becomes larger, the value for e^{-x} becomes smaller.

Spreadsheets for Performing Calculations

Spreadsheet software, such as LOTUS 123, QUATRO PRO, and EXCEL, is available on many personal computers, including both the MAC and IBM-compatible PCs. These spreadsheets are composed of a grid as shown in Figure B-2 of Appendix B. Detailed spreadsheet operation examples are found in Appendix B.

CALCULUS

Since pharmacokinetics considers drugs in the body to be in a dynamic state, calculus is an important mathematic tool for analyzing drug movement quantitatively. Differential equations are used to relate the concentrations of drugs in various body organs over time. Integrated equations are frequently used to model the cumulative therapeutic or toxic responses of drugs in the body.

Differential Calculus

Differential calculus is a branch of calculus that involves finding the rate at which a variable quantity is changing. For example, a specific amount of drug X is placed in a beaker of water to dissolve. The rate at which the drug dissolves is determined by the rate of drug diffusing away from the surface of the solid drug and is expressed by the *Noyes-Whitney equation*:

$$\text{Dissolution rate} = \frac{dX}{dt} = \frac{DA}{l}(C_1 - C_2)$$

where d = denotes a very small change; X = drug X; t = time; D = diffusion coefficient; A = effective surface area of drug; l = length of diffusion layer; C_1 = surface concentration of drug in the diffusion layer; and C_2 = concentration of drug in the bulk solution.

The derivative dX/dt may be interpreted as a change in X (or a derivative of X) with respect to a change in t.

In pharmacokinetics, the amount of drug in the body is a variable quantity (dependent variable), and time is considered to be an independent variable. Thus, we consider the amount of drug to vary with respect to time.

EXAMPLE

The concentration C of a drug changes as a function of time t:

$$C = f(t) \qquad\qquad (2.6)$$

Consider the following data:

Time (hr)	Plasma Concentration of Drug C (μg/mL)
0	12
1	10
2	8
3	6
4	4
5	2

The concentration of drug C in the plasma is declining by 2 μg/mL for each hour of time. The rate of change in the concentration of the drug with respect to time (ie, the derivative of C) may be expressed as

$$\frac{dC}{dt} = 2\,\mu\text{g/mL/hr}$$

Here, $f(t)$ is a mathematical equation that describes how C changes, expressed as

$$C = 12 - 2t \qquad\qquad (2.7)$$

Integral Calculus

Integration is the reverse of differentiation and is considered the summation of $f(x) \cdot dx$; the integral sign $\int$ implies summation. For example, given the function $y = ax$, plotted in Figure 2-1, the integration is $\int ax \cdot dx$. Figure 2-2 is a graph of the function $y = Ae^{-x}$, commonly observed after an intravenous bolus drug injection. The integration process is actually a summing up of the small individual pieces under the graph. When x is specified and is given boundaries from a to b, then the expression becomes a definite integral, ie, the summing up of the area from $x = a$ to $x = b$.

A *definite integral* of a mathematical function is the sum of individual areas under the graph of that function. There are several reasonably accurate numerical methods for approximating an area. These methods can be programmed into a computer for rapid calculation. The *trapezoidal rule* is a numerical method frequently used in pharmacokinetics to calculate the area under the plasma drug concentration-versus-time curve, called the area under the curve (AUC). For example, Figure 2-2 shows a curve depicting the elimination of a drug from the plasma after a single intravenous injection. The drug plasma levels and the corresponding time intervals plotted in Figure 2-2 are as follows:

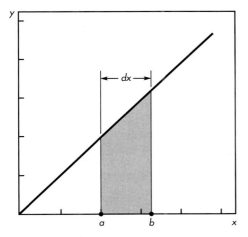

Figure 2-1. Integration of $y = ax$ or $\int ax \cdot dx$.

Time (hr)	Plasma Drug Level (μg/mL)
0.5	38.9
1.0	30.3
2.0	18.4
3.0	11.1
4.0	6.77
5.0	4.10

The area between time intervals is the area of a trapezoid and can be calculated with the following formula:

$$[\text{AUC}]_{t_{n-1}}^{t_n} = \frac{C_{n-1} + C_n}{2}(t_n - t_{n-1}) \tag{2.8}$$

where [AUC] = area under the curve, t_n = time of observation of drug concentration C_n, and t_{n-1} = time of prior observation of drug concentration corresponding to C_{n-1}.

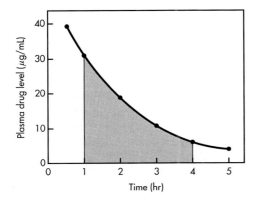

Figure 2-2. Graph of the elimination of drug from the plasma after a single IV injection.

To obtain the AUC from 1 to 4 hours in Figure 2-2, each portion of this area must be summed. The AUC between 1 and 2 hours is calculated by proper substitution into Equation 2.8:

$$[\text{AUC}]_{t1}^{t2} = \frac{30.3 + 18.4}{2} (2-1) = 24.35 \ \mu\text{g hr/mL}$$

Similarly, the AUC between 2 and 3 hours is calculated as 14.75 μg hr/mL, and the AUC between 3 and 4 hours is calculated as 8.94 μg hr/mL. The total AUC between 1 and 4 hours is obtained by adding the three smaller AUC values together.

$$[\text{AUC}]_{t1}^{t4} = [\text{AUC}]_{t1}^{t2} + [\text{AUC}]_{t2}^{t3} + [\text{AUC}]_{t3}^{t4}$$

$$= 24.35 + 14.75 + 8.94$$

$$= 48.04 \ \mu\text{g hr/mL}$$

The total area under the plasma drug level-versus-time curve (Fig. 2-2) is obtained by summation of each individual area between two consecutive time intervals using the trapezoidal rule. The value on the y axis when time equals zero is estimated by back extrapolation of the data points using a log linear plot (ie, log y versus x).

This numerical method of obtaining the AUC is fairly accurate if sufficient data points are available. As the number of data points increases, the trapezoidal method of approximating the area becomes more accurate.

The trapezoidal rule assumes a linear or straight-line function between data points. If the data points are spaced widely, then the normal curvature of the line will cause a greater error in the area estimate.

At times, the area under the plasma level time curve is extrapolated to $t = \infty$. In this case the residual area $[\text{AUC}]_{tn}^{t\infty}$ is calculated as follows:

$$[\text{AUC}]_{tn}^{t\infty} = \frac{C_{pn}}{k} \tag{2.9}$$

where C_{pn} = last observed plasma concentration at t_n and k = slope obtained from the terminal portion of the curve.

The trapezoidal rule written in its full form to calculate the AUC from $t = 0$ to $t = \infty$ is as follows:

$$[\text{AUC}]_{0}^{\infty} = \Sigma[\text{AUC}]_{tn-1}^{tn} + \frac{C_{pn}}{k}$$

GRAPHS

The construction of a curve or straight line by plotting observed or experimental data on a graph is an important method of visualizing relationships between variables. By general custom, the values of the independent variable (x) are placed on the horizontal line in a plane, or on the abscissa (x axis), whereas the values of the dependent variable are placed on the vertical line in the plane, or on the ordinate (y axis), as demonstrated in Figure 2-3. The values are usually arranged so that they increase from left to right and from bottom to top. The values may be spaced arbitrarily along each axis to optimize any observable relationships between the two variables.

Figure 2-3. *Standard arrangement of independent (x) and dependent (y) variables on a graph.*

In pharmacokinetics, time is the independent variable and is plotted on the abscissa (*x* axis), whereas drug concentration is the dependent variable and is plotted on the ordinate (*y* axis).

Two types of graph paper are usually used in pharmacokinetics. These are Cartesian or rectangular coordinate graph paper (Fig. 2-4) and semilog graph paper (Fig. 2-5).

Semilog paper is available with one, two, three, or more cycles per sheet, each cycle representing a 10-fold increase in the numbers, or a single log10 unit. This paper allows placement of the data at logarithmic intervals so that the numbers need not be converted to their corresponding log values prior to plotting on the graph.

Curve Fitting

Fitting a curve to the points on a graph implies that there is some sort of relationship between the variables *x* and *y*, such as dose of drug versus pharmacologic effect (eg, lowering of blood pressure). Moreover, the relationship is not confined to isolated points but is a continuous function of *x* and *y*. In many cases, a hypothesis is made concerning the relationship between the variables *x* and *y*. Then, an empirical equation is formed that best describes the hypothesis. This empirical equation must satisfactorily fit the experimental or observed data.

Physiological variables are not always linearly related. However, the data may be arranged or transformed to express the relationship between the variables as a straight line. Straight lines are very useful for accurately predicting values for which there are no experimental observations. The general equation of a straight line is

$$y = mx + b \qquad\qquad\qquad (2.10)$$

where m = slope and b = y intercept. Equation 2.10 could yield any one of the graphs shown in Figure 2-6, depending on the value of m. The absolute magnitude of m gives some idea of the steepness of the curve. For example, as the value of m

Figure 2-4.   Rectangular coordinates.

Figure 2-5.   Semilog coordinates.

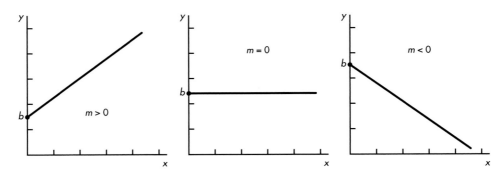

Figure 2-6. Graphic demonstration of variations in slope (*m*).

approaches 0, the line becomes more horizontal. As the absolute value of *m* becomes larger, the line slopes farther upward or downward, depending on whether *m* is positive or negative, respectively. For example, the equation

$$y = -15x + 7$$

indicates a slope of -15 and a *y* intercept at $+7$. The negative sign indicates that the curve is sloping downward from left to right.

Determination of the Slope

Slope of a Straight Line on a Rectangular Coordinate Graph
The value of the slope may be determined from any two points on the curve (Fig. 2-7). The slope of the curve is equal to $\Delta y/\Delta x$, as shown in the following equation:

$$\text{Slope} = \frac{y_2 - y_1}{x_2 - x_1} \tag{2.11}$$

The slope of the line plotted in Figure 2-7 is

$$m = \frac{2 - 3}{3 - 1} = \frac{-1}{2}$$

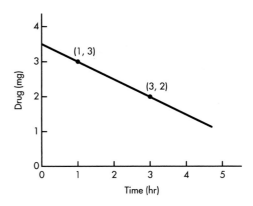

Figure 2-7. Graphic representation of a line with a slope value of $m = -\frac{1}{2}$.

Because the y intercept is equal to 3.5, the equation for the curve by substitution into Equation 2.10 is

$$y = -\frac{1}{2}x + 3.5$$

Slope of a Straight Line on a Semilog Graph

When using semilog paper, the y values are plotted on a logarithmic scale without performing actual logarithmic conversions, whereas the corresponding x values are plotted on a linear scale. Therefore, to determine the slope of a straight line on semilog paper graph, the y values must be converted to logarithms, as shown in the following equation:

$$\text{Slope} = 2.3 \frac{(\log y_2 - \log y_1)}{x_2 - x_1} = \frac{\ln y_2 - \ln y_1}{x_2 - x_1} \tag{2.12}$$

The slope value is often used to calculate k, a constant that determines the rate of drug decline:

$$k = 2.3 \text{ slope}$$

Least-Squares Method

Very often an empirical equation is calculated to show the relationship between two variables. Experimentally, data may be obtained that suggest a linear relationship between an independent variable x and a dependent variable y. The straight line that characterizes the relationship between the two variables is called a *regression line*. In many cases, the experimental data may have some error and therefore show a certain amount of scatter or deviations from linearity. The *least-squares method* is a useful procedure for obtaining the line of best fit through a set of data points by minimizing the deviation between the experimental and the theoretical line. In using this method, it is often assumed, for simplicity, that there is a linear relationship between the variables. If a linear line deviates substantially from the data, it may suggest the need for a nonlinear regression model, although several variables (multiple linear regression) may be involved. Nonlinear regression models are complex mathematical procedures that are best performed with a computer program (see Appendix B).

When the equation of a linear model is examined, the dependent variables can be expressed as the sum of products of the independent variables and parameters. In nonlinear models, at least one of the parameters appears as other than a coefficient. For example,

Linear model: $y = ax$, $y = ax + bx + cx^2$, $y = ax + bx_1 + cx^2$
Nonlinear model: $y = ax/(b + cx)$, $y = 10e^{-3x}$
(a, b, and c are parameters and x and x_1 are variables)

The second nonlinear example as written is nonlinear, but may be transformed to a linear equation by taking the natural log on both sides:

$$\ln y = -3x$$

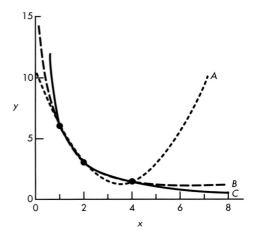

Figure 2-8. Three points equally well fitted by different curves. The parabola, $y = 10.5 - 5.25x + 0.75x^2$ (*curve A*); the exponential, $y = 12.93e^{-1.005x} + 1.27$ (*curve B*); and the rectangular hyperbola, $y = 6/x$ (*curve C*) all fit the three points (1, 6), (2, 3), and (4, 1.5) perfectly, as would an infinite number of other curves.
(From Riggs, 1963, with permission.)

Problems of Fitting Points to a Graph

When x and y data points are plotted on a graph, a relationship between the x and y variables is sought. Linear relationships are useful for predicting values for the dependent variable y, given values for the independent variable x.

The *linear regression* calculation using the least-squares method is used for calculation of a straight line through a given set of points. However, it is important to realize that, when using this method, one has already assumed that the data points are related linearly. Indeed, for three points, this linear relationship may not always be true. As shown in Figure 2-8, Riggs (1963) calculated three different curves that fit the data accurately. Generally, one should consider the *law of parsimony*, which broadly means "keep it simple"; that is, if a choice between two hypotheses is available, choose the more simple relationship.

If a linear relationship exists between the x and y variables, one must be careful as to the estimated value for the dependent variable y, assuming a value for the independent variable x. *Interpolation*, which means filling the gap between the observed data on a graph, is usually safe and assumes that the trend between the observed data points is consistent and predictable. In contrast, the process of *extrapolation* means predicting new data beyond the observed data, and assumes that the same trend obtained between two data points will extend in either direction beyond the last observed data points. The use of extrapolation may be erroneous if the regression line no longer follows the same trend beyond the measured points.

PRACTICE PROBLEMS

1. Plot the following data and obtain the equation for the line that best fits the data by (a) using a ruler and (b) using the method of least squares.

x (mg)	y (hr)	x (mg)	y (hr)
1	3.1	5	15.3
2	6.0	6	17.9
3	8.7	7	22.0
4	12.9	8	23.0

Solution

a. *Ruler*

Place a ruler on a straight edge over the data points and draw the best line that can be observed. Take any two points and determine the slope by the slope formula given in Equation 2.11 and the *y* intercept. This method can give a reasonably quick approximation if there is very little scatter in the data.

b. *Least-Squares Method*

In the least-squares method the slope *m* and the *y* intercept *b* (Eq. 2.13) are calculated so that the average sum of the deviations squared is minimized. The deviation, *d*, is defined by

$$b + mx - y = d \tag{2.13}$$

If there are no deviations from linearity, then $d = 0$ and the exact form of Equation 2.13 is as follows:

$$b + mx - y = 0$$

To find the slope, *m*, and the intercept, *y*, the following equations are used:

$$m = \frac{\Sigma(x)\,\Sigma(y) - n\Sigma(xy)}{[\Sigma(x)]^2 - n\Sigma(x^2)} \tag{2.14}$$

where n = number of data points.

$$b = \frac{\Sigma(x)\,\Sigma(xy) - \Sigma(x^2)\,\Sigma y}{[\Sigma(x)]^2 - n\Sigma(x^2)} \tag{2.15}$$

where Σ is the sum of *n* data points.

Using the data above, tabulate values for *x*, *y*, x^2, and *xy* as shown below:

x	y	x^2	xy
1	3.1	1	3.1
2	6.0	4	12.0
3	8.7	9	26.1
4	12.9	16	51.6
5	15.3	25	76.5
6	17.9	36	107.4
7	22.0	49	154.0
8	23.0	64	184.0
$\Sigma x = 36$	$\Sigma y = 108.9$	$\Sigma x^2 = 204$	$\Sigma xy = 614.7$

Now substitute the values into Equations 2.14 and 2.15.

$$b = \frac{(36)(614.7) - (204)(108.9)}{(36)^2 - (8)(204)} = 0.257 \text{ mg}$$

$$m = \frac{(36)(108.9) - (8)(614.7)}{(36)^2 - (8)(204)} = 2.97 \text{ mg/hr}$$

Therefore, the linear equation that best fits the data is

$$y = 2.97x + 0.257$$

Although an equation for a straight line is obtained by the least-squares procedure, the reliability of the values should be ascertained. A correlation coefficient, r, is a useful statistical term that indicates the relationship of the x, y data to a straight line. For a perfect linear relationship between x and y, $r = +1$ if the slope is ascending and -1 if the slope is descending. If $r = 0$, then no linear relationship exists between x and y. Usually, $r \geq 0.95$ demonstrates good evidence or a strong correlation that there is a linear relationship between x and y.

2. *Determination of slope can be carried out using a calculator.* Many calculators have a statistical linear regression program to determine the slope of the regression line and the coefficient of correlation. The calculator must be cleared and the statistical routine initiated. For regular linear regression, the data may be entered directly in pairs as follows:

   a. *Linear Regression*

Enter Time	Enter Concentration
0	0
2	20
4	40

   In this case, the slope should be 10 if linear regression is performed correctly, and the process is zero order. This slope value should be close to the slope determined by graphic method on regular graph paper.

   b. *Log Linear Regression*

   In this case, the data below is not a linear relationship but can be transformed (take the log of concentration) to make the data linear. Use the same linear regression program above, except, each time after concentration is entered, press LOG as shown below:

Enter Time	Enter Concentration	Key Stroke
0	10	LOG
2	5	LOG
4	2.5	LOG

The slope obtained should approximate the value determined by graphic method on the semilog paper. The slope value is -0.151.

If the LN key is pressed each time instead of LOG in all the steps above, the slope will be -0.346, or equal to $-k$, the elimination constant. This is a shortcut method sometimes used to determine k of a first-order process. The regression involves regressing ln concentration versus time directly, ie, ln C versus t, because ln $C = -kt +$ intercept, the slope m is $-k$ (see later section of this chapter).

UNITS IN PHARMACOKINETICS

For an equation to be valid, the units or dimensions must be constant on both sides of the equation. Many different units are used in pharmacokinetics, as listed in Table 2.1. For an accurate equation, both the integers and the units must balance. For example, a common expression for total body clearance is

$$Cl_T = kV_d \tag{2.16}$$

After insertion of the proper units for each term in the above equation from Table 2.1,

$$\frac{mL}{hr} = \frac{1}{hr} mL$$

Thus, the above equation is valid, as shown by the equality mL/hr = mL/hr.

An important rule in using equations with different units is that the units may be added, subtracted, divided, or multiplied as long as the final units are consistent

TABLE 2.1   Common Units Used in Pharmacokinetics

PARAMETER	SYMBOL	UNIT	EXAMPLE
Rate	$\dfrac{dD}{dt}$	$\dfrac{Mass}{Time}$	mg/hr
	$\dfrac{dc}{dt}$	$\dfrac{Concentration}{Time}$	μg/mL hr
Zero-order rate constant	k_0	$\dfrac{Concentration}{Time}$	μg/mL hr
		$\dfrac{Mass}{Time}$	mg/hr
First-order rate constant	k	$\dfrac{1}{Time}$	1/hr or hr^{-1}
Drug dose	D_0	Mass	mg
Concentration	C	$\dfrac{Mass}{Volume}$	μg/mL
Plasma drug concentration	C_p	$\dfrac{Drug}{Volume}$	μg/mL
Volume	V	Volume	mL or L
Area under the curve	AUC	Concentration $\times$ time	μg hr/mL
Fraction of drug absorbed	F	No units	0 to 1
Clearance	Cl	$\dfrac{Volume}{Time}$	mL/hr
Half-life	$t_{1/2}$	Time	hr

and valid. When in doubt, check the equation by inserting the proper units. For example,

$$\text{AUC} = \frac{FD_0}{kV_D} = \text{concentration} \times \text{time} \tag{2.17}$$

$$\frac{\mu g}{mL} \, hr = \frac{1 \, mg}{hr^{-1} \, liter} = \frac{\mu g \, hr}{mL}$$

Certain terms have no units. These terms include logarithms and ratios. Percent may have no units and is expressed mathematically as a decimal between 0 and 1 or as 0 to 100%, respectively. On occasion, percent may indicate mass/volume, volume/volume, or mass/mass. Table 2.1 lists common pharmacokinetic parameters with their symbols and units.

A constant is often inserted in an equation to quantitate the relationship of the dependent variable to the independent variable. For example, *Fick's law of diffusion* relates the rate of drug diffusion, dQ/dt, to the change in drug concentration, C, the surface area of the membrane, A, and the thickness of the membrane h. In order to make this relationship an equation, a diffusion constant D is inserted:

$$\frac{dQ}{dt} = \frac{DA}{h} \times \triangle C \tag{2.18}$$

To obtain the proper units for D, the units for each of the other terms must be inserted:

$$\frac{mg}{hr} = \frac{D \, (cm^2)}{cm} \times \frac{mg}{cm^3}$$

$$D = cm^2/hr$$

The diffusion constant D must have the units of area/time or cm^2/hr if the rate of diffusion is in mg/hr.

Graphs should always have the axes (abscissa and ordinate) properly labeled with units. For example, in Figure 2-7 the amount of drug on the ordinate (y axis) is given in milligrams and the time on the abscissa (x axis) is given in hours. The equation that best fits the points on this curve is the equation for a straight line, or $y = mx + b$. Because the slope $m = \Delta y/\Delta x$, the units for the slope should be milligrams per hour (mg/hr). Similarly, the units for the y intercept b should be the same units as those for y, namely, milligrams (mg).

MEASUREMENT AND USE OF SIGNIFICANT FIGURES

Every measurement is performed within a certain degree of accuracy, which is limited by the instrument used for the measurement. For example, the weight of freight on a truck may be measured accurately to the nearest 0.5 kg, whereas the mass of drug in a tablet may be measured to 0.001 g (1 mg). Measuring the weight of freight on a truck to the nearest milligram is not necessary and would require a very costly balance or scale to detect a change in a milligram quantity.

Significant figures are the number of accurate digits in a measurement. If a balance measures the mass of a drug to the nearest milligram, measurements containing digits representing less than 1 mg are inaccurate. For example, in reading the weight or mass of a drug of 123.8 mg from this balance, the 0.8 mg is only approximate; the number is therefore rounded to 124 mg and reported as the observed mass.

For practical calculation purposes, all figures may be used until the final number (answer) is obtained. However, the answer should retain only the number of significant figures in the least accurate initial measurement.

UNITS FOR EXPRESSING BLOOD CONCENTRATIONS

Various units have been used in pharmacology, toxicology, and the clinical laboratory to express drug concentrations in blood, plasma, or serum. Drug concentrations or drug levels should be expressed as mass/volume. The expressions mcg/mL, μg/mL, and mg/L are equivalent and are commonly reported in the literature. Drug concentrations may also be reported as mg% or mg/dL, both of which indicate milligrams of drug per 100 mL (deciliter). Two older expressions for drug concentration occasionally used in veterinary medicine are the terms ppm and ppb, which indicate the number of parts of drug per million parts of blood (ppm) or per billion parts of blood (ppb). One ppm is equivalent to 1.0 μg/mL. The accurate interconversion of units is often necessary to prevent confusion and misinterpretation.

STATISTICS

All measurements have some degree of error. An *error* is the difference between the true or absolute value and the observed value. Errors in measurement may be *determinate* (constant) or *indeterminate* (random, accidental). Determinate errors may be minimized in analytical procedures by using properly calibrated instrumentation, standardized chemicals, and appropriate blanks and control samples. Indeterminate errors are random and occur due to chance. For practical purposes, several measurements of a given sample are usually performed, and the result averaged. The mean $\pm$ SD is often reported. SD or *standard deviation* (see Appendix A) is a statistical way of expressing the spread between the individual measurements from the mean. A small SD relative to the mean value is indicative of good consistency and reproducibility of the measurements. A large SD indicates poor consistency and data fluctuations. Frequently, the variability of the measurements may be expressed as RSD or *relative standard deviation*, which is calculated as the SD divided as the mean of the data. RSD allows variability to be expressed on a percent basis and is useful in comparing the variability of two sets of measurements when the means are different.

In measurements involving a single subject or sample, only measuring error is involved. On the other hand, when two or more samples or subjects in a group are measured, there is usually variation due to individual differences. For example, the weight of each student in a class is likely different from that of the others because of individual physical differences such as height and sex. Therefore, in determining the weight of a group of students, we deal with variations due to biologic differences as well as weighing errors. A major error in group measurement is *sampling error,* an error due to nonuniform sampling. Sampling is essential be-cause the measurement of all members in the group is not practical.

We use statistics to obtain a valid interpretation of the experimental data. *Statistics* is the logical use of mathematics, which includes (1) experimental design, (2) col-lection of data, (3) analysis of data, (4) interpretation of data, and (5) hypothesis testing. A more complete discussion of statistics is found in Appendix A.

PRACTICAL FOCUS

In pharmacokinetics and therapeutics, plasma or tissue samples are often moni-tored to determine if a prescribed dose needs to be adjusted. Comparisons of lit-erature data from several medical centers are often made. The pharmacist should to be familiar with all units involving dosing and be able to make conversions. Some physicians prescribe a drug dose based on body weight, whereas others prefer the body surface area method. Significant differences in plasma drug concentrations may result if the dose is based on a different method. Drug concentrations may also be different if a dose is injected rapidly versus infused over a period of time. Table 2.2 lists some of the common methods of dosing.

Most potent drugs are dosed precisely for the individual patient, and the body weight of the patient should be known. For example, theophylline is dosed at 5 mg/kg. Since the body weight (BW) of individuals may vary with age, sex, disease, and nutritional state, an individualized dose based on body weight will more ac-curately reflect the appropriate therapy needed for the patient. For drugs with a narrow therapeutic index and potential for side effects, dosing based on body sur-face is common. During chemotherapy with antitumor drugs, many drugs are dosed according to the body surface area (BSA) of the patient. The body surface area may be determined from the weight of the patient using the empirical equation

$$\text{BSA} = \left(\frac{\text{BW}}{70 \text{ kg}}\right)^{0.73} \times 1.73 \text{ m}^2$$

where BSA = body surface area in m^2, and BW = body weight in kg. Some common units and conversions used in pharmacokinetics and toxicology are listed in Table 2.3.

TABLE 2.2 Dosing Unit Based on Body Weight or Body Surface Area[a]

METHOD	ORAL DRUG UNIT	INFUSION UNIT	REMARKS
General	mg	mg/hr	BW not used
BW	mg/kg	mg/kg/hr	Known BW
BSA	mg/1.73 m^2	mg/1.73 m^2/hr	Estimated BSA

[a]BW, body weight; BSA, body surface area.

TABLE 2.3   Pharmacokinetic Units and Conversions

UNITS IN VOLUME	VOLUME (BASED ON BODY WEIGHT)
mL	mL/kg
dL	dL/kg
L	L/kg

CONCENTRATION	WEIGHT CONVERSION
gm/L	1 kg = 1000 g
mg/L	1 g = 1000 mg
mg/dL	1 mg = 1000 μg
mg/mL	1 μg = 1000 ng
ng/mL	1 ng = 1000 pg
pg/mL	

Examples of Concentration Conversion Used in Toxicology and Therapeutics
1 mg% = 1 mg/dL
1 mg/L = 1 μg/mL
1 μg/L = 1 ng/mL
1 ng/L = 1 pg/mL

EXAMPLE

The rate of ethanol elimination in four alcoholics undergoing detoxification was reported to be 17 to 33 mg/dL/hr (Jones, 1992). (1) What is the rate of elimination in μg/mL/hr? (2) The peak blood concentration in one subject (SP) is 90 μg/dL. What is his peak blood concentration in μg/mL? (3) To which category would SP belong according to the following classification for blood alcohol (where values are in mg%)?

a. >0.55 mg%—fatal

b. 0.50–0.55 mg%—dead drunk

c. 0.10–0.50 mg%—illegal

d. 0.05–0.10 mg%—questionable

e. <0.05 mg%—safe

Solution

1. 17 μg/dL/hr = 17,000 μg/100 mL/hr = 170 μg/mL/hr

   33 μg/dL/hr = 33,000 μg/100 mL/hr = 330 μg/mL/hr

2. 90 mg/dL = 90 μg/100 mL = 0.9 μg/mL

3. 90 mg/dL = 0.090 mg/100 dL = 0.090 mg%

   Subject SP is questionable.

PRACTICE PROBLEM

The volume of distribution of theophylline is 0.7 L/kg. In most patients, the optimal benefits of theophylline therapy are seen at serum concentration of >10 mg/L; setting a plasma drug concentration of 5 mg/L lower therapeutic limit may result in reduced clinical efficacy (Eder and Bryan, 1996). (1) What is the volume of distribution in a 20-year-old male patient weighing 70 kg? (2) What is the total dose for the patient if he is dosed at 5 mg/kg?

Solution

(1) (5 mg/L is an alternative way to express 5 μg/mL)

Volume of patient = 0.7 L/kg $\times$ 70 kg = 49 L

(2) Dose for patient = 5 mg/kg $\times$ 70 kg = 350 mg

RATES AND ORDERS OF REACTIONS

Rate

The rate of a chemical reaction of process is the velocity with which the reaction occurs. Consider the following chemical reaction:

drug A → drug B

If the amount of drug A is decreasing with respect to time (that is, the reaction is going in a forward direction), then the rate of this reaction can be expressed as

$$-\frac{dA}{dt}$$

Since the amount of drug B is increasing with respect to time, the rate of the reaction can also be expressed as

$$+\frac{dB}{dt}$$

Usually only the parent (or pharmacologically active) drug is measured experimentally. The metabolites of the drug or the products of the decomposition of the drug may not be known or may be very difficult to quantitate. The rate of a reaction is determined experimentally by measuring the disappearance of drug A at given time intervals.

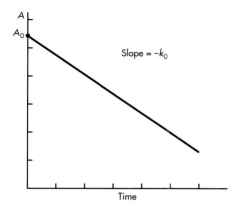

Figure 2-9. Graph of Equation 2.20.

Rate Constant

The order of a reaction refers to the way in which the concentration of drug or reactants influences the rate of a chemical reaction or process.

Zero-Order Reactions

If the amount of drug A is decreasing at a constant time interval t, then the rate of disappearance of drug A is expressed as

$$\frac{dA}{dt} = -k_0 \qquad\qquad (2.19)$$

The term k_0 is the zero-order rate constant and is expressed in units of mass/time (eg, mg/min). Integration of Equation 2.19 yields the following expression:

$$A = -k_0 t + A_0 \qquad\qquad (2.20)$$

where A_0 is the amount of drug at $t = 0$. Based on this expression (Eq. 2.20), a graph of A versus t yields a straight line (Fig. 2-9). The y intercept is equal to A_0, and the slope of the line is equal to k_0.

Equation 2.20 may be expressed in terms of drug concentration, which can be measured directly.

$$C = -k_0 t + C_0 \qquad\qquad (2.21)$$

C_0 is the drug concentration at time 0, C is the drug concentration at time t, and k_0 is the zero-order decomposition constant.

 ## EXAMPLE

A pharmacist weighs exactly 10 g of a drug and dissolves it in 100 mL of water. The solution is kept at room temperature, and samples are removed periodically and assayed for the drug. The pharmacist obtains the following data:

Drug Concentration (mg/mL)	Time (hr)
100	0
95	2
90	4
85	6
80	8
75	10
70	12

From these data, a graph constructed by plotting the concentration of drug versus time will yield a straight line. Therefore, the rate of decline in drug concentration is of zero order.

The zero-order rate constant k_0 may be obtained from the slope of the line or by proper substitution into Equation 2.21.

If

C_0 = concentration of 100 mg/mL at $t = 0$

and

C = concentration of 90 mg/mL at $t = 4$ hr

then

$$90 = -k_0(4) + 100$$

and

$$k_0 = 2.5 \text{ mg/mL hr}$$

Careful examination of the data will also show that the concentration of drug declines 5 mg/mL for each 2-hour interval. Therefore, the zero-order rate constant may be obtained by dividing 5 mg/mL by 2 hours:

$$k_0 = \frac{5 \text{ mg/ml}}{2 \text{ hr}} = 2.5 \text{ mg/mL hr}$$

First-Order Reactions

If the amount of drug A is decreasing at a rate that is proportional to the amount of drug A remaining, then the rate of disappearance of drug A is expressed as

$$\frac{dA}{dt} = -kA \tag{2.22}$$

where k is the first-order rate constant and is expressed in units of time^{-1} (eg, hr^{-1}). Integration of Equation 2.22 yields the following expression:

$$\ln A = -kt + \ln A_0 \tag{2.23}$$

Equation 2.23 may also be expressed as

$$A = A_0 e^{-kt} \tag{2.24}$$

Because $\ln = 2.3 \log$, Equation 2.23 becomes

$$\log A = \frac{-kt}{2.3} + \log A_0 \tag{2.25}$$

When drug decomposition involves a solution, starting with initial concentration C_0, it is often convenient to express the rate of change in drug decomposition, dC/dt, in terms of drug concentration, C, rather than amount because drug concentration is assayed. Hence,

$$\frac{dC}{dt} = -kC \tag{2.26}$$

$$\ln C = -kt + \ln C_0 \tag{2.27}$$

Equation 2.27 may be expressed as

$$C = C_0 e^{-kt} \tag{2.28}$$

Because $\ln = 2.3 \log$, Equation 2.27 becomes

$$log\ C = \frac{-kt}{2.3} + log\ C_0 \tag{2.29}$$

According to Equation 2.25, a graph of $\log A$ versus t will yield a straight line (Fig. 2-10), the y intercept will be $\log A_0$, and the slope of the line will be $-k/2.3$ (Fig. 2-10). Similarly, a graph of $\log C$ versus t will yield a straight line according to Equation 2.29. The y intercept will be $\log C_0$, and the slope of the line will be $-k/2.3$. For convenience, C versus t may be plotted on semilog paper without the need to convert C to $\log C$. An example is shown in Figure 2-11.

Half-Life

Half-life ($t_{1/2}$) expresses the period of time required for the amount or concentration of a drug to decrease by one-half.

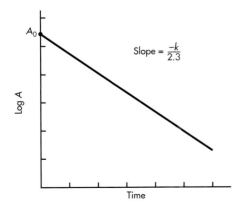

Figure 2-10.   Graph of Equation 2.25.

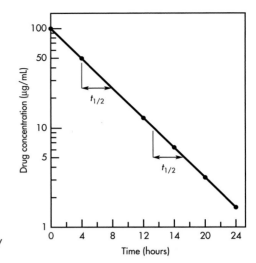

Figure 2-11.   This graph demonstrates the constancy of the $t_{1/2}$ in a first-order reaction.

First-Order Half-Life

The $t_{1/2}$ for a first-order reaction may be found by means of the following equation:

$$t_{1/2} = \frac{0.693}{k} \tag{2.30}$$

It is apparent from this equation that, for a first-order reaction, $t_{1/2}$ is a constant. No matter what the initial amount or concentration of drug is, the time required for the amount to decrease by one-half is a constant (Fig. 2-11).

Zero-Order Half-Life

In contrast to the first-order $t_{1/2}$, the $t_{1/2}$ for a zero-order process is not constant. The zero-order $t_{1/2}$ is proportional to the initial amount or concentration of the drug and is inversely proportional to the zero-order rate constant k_0:

$$t_{1/2} = \frac{0.5A_0}{k_0} \tag{2.31}$$

Because the $t_{1/2}$ changes as drug concentrations decline, the zero-order $t_{1/2}$ has little practical value.

 EXAMPLE

A pharmacist dissolves exactly 10 g of a drug into 100 mL of water. The solution is kept at room temperature, and samples are removed periodically and assayed for the drug. The pharmacist obtains the following data:

Drug Concentration (mg/mL)	Time (hr)	Log Drug Concentration
100.00	0	2.00
50.00	4	1.70
25.00	8	1.40
12.50	12	1.10
6.25	16	0.80
3.13	20	0.50
1.56	24	0.20

With these data, a graph constructed by plotting the logarithm of the drug concentrations versus time will yield a straight line on rectangular coordinates. More conveniently, the drug concentration values can be plotted directly at a logarithmic axis on semilog paper against time, and a straight line will be obtained (Fig. 2-11). The relationship of time versus drug concentration in Figure 2-11 indicates a first-order reaction.

The $t_{1/2}$ for a first-order process is constant and may be obtained from any two points on the graph that show a 50% decline in drug concentration. In this example, the $t_{1/2}$ is 4 hours. The first-order rate constant may be found by (1) obtaining the product of 2.3 times the slope or (2) by dividing 0.693 by the $t_{1/2}$, as follows:

$$\text{Slope} = -\frac{k}{2.3} = \frac{\log y_2 - \log y_1}{x_2 - x_1}$$

$$-k = \frac{2.3\,(\log 50 - \log 100)}{4 - 0} \qquad k = 0.173 \text{ hr}^{-1}$$

$$k = \frac{0.693}{t_{1/2}}$$

$$k = \frac{0.693}{4} = 0.173 \text{ hr}^{-1}$$

 # FREQUENTLY ASKED QUESTIONS

1. How do I know my graph is first order when plotted on semilog paper?
2. I plotted the plasma drug concentration versus time data on semilog paper, and got a slope with an incorrect k. Why?
3. I performed linear regression on t versus ln C_p. How do I determine the C_p^0 from the intercept?

LEARNING QUESTIONS

1. Plot the following data on both semilog graph paper and standard rectangular coordinates.

Time (min)	Drug A (mg)
10	96.0
20	89.0
40	73.0
60	57.0
90	34.0
120	10.0
130	2.5

    a. Does the decrease in the amount of drug A appear to be a zero-order or a first-order process?

    b. What is the rate constant k?

    c. What is the half-life $t_{1/2}$?

    d. Does the amount of drug A extrapolate to zero on the x axis?

    e. What is the equation for the line produced on the graph?

2. Plot the following data on both semilog graph paper and standard rectangular coordinates.

Time (min)	Drug A (mg)
4	70.0
10	58.0
20	42.0
30	31.0
60	12.0
90	4.5
120	1.7

Answer questions **a, b, c, d,** and **e** as stated in Question 1.

3. A pharmacist dissolved a few milligrams of a new antibiotic drug into exactly 100 mL of distilled water and placed the solution in a refrigerator (5°C). At various time intervals, the pharmacist removed a 10-mL aliquot from the solution and measured the amount of drug contained in each aliquot. The following data were obtained.

Time (hr)	Antibiotic (μg/mL)
0.5	84.5
1.0	81.2
2.0	74.5
4.0	61.0
6.0	48.0
8.0	35.0
12.0	8.7

a. Is the decomposition of this antibiotic a first-order or a zero-order process?

b. What is the rate of decomposition of this antibiotic?

c. How many milligrams of antibiotics were in the original solution prepared by the pharmacist?

d. Give the equation for the line that best fits the experimental data.

4. A solution of a drug was freshly prepared at a concentration of 300 mg/mL. After 30 days at 25°C, the drug concentration in the solution was 75 mg/mL.

a. Assuming first-order kinetics, when will the drug decline to one-half of the original concentration?

b. Assuming zero-order kinetics, when will the drug decline to one-half of the original concentration?

5. How many half-lives $(t_{1/2})$ would it take for 99.9% of any initial concentration of a drug to decompose? Assume first-order kinetics.

6. If the half-life for decomposition of a drug is 12 hours, how long will it take for 125 mg of the drug to decompose by 30%? Assume first-order kinetics and constant temperature.

7. Exactly 300 mg of a drug are dissolved into an unknown volume of distilled water. After complete dissolution of the drug, 1.0-mL samples were removed and assayed for the drug. The following results were obtained:

Time (hr)	Concentration (mg/mL)
0.5	0.45
2.0	0.3

Assuming zero-order decomposition of the drug, what was the original volume of water in which the drug was dissolved?

8. For most drugs, the overall rate of drug elimination is proportional to the amount of drug remaining in the body. What does this imply about the kinetic order of drug elimination?

9. A single cell is placed into a culture tube containing nutrient agar. If the number of cells doubles every 2 minutes and the culture tube is completely filled in 8 hours, how long does it take for the culture tube to be only half full of cells?

10. The volume of distribution of warfarin is 9.8 ± 4.2 L. Assuming normal distribution, this would mean that 95% of the subjects would have a volume of distribution ranging from _____ L to _____ L.

11. Which of the following functions has the steepest declining slope? (t is the independent variable and y is the dependent variable.)

a. $y = 2e^{-3t}$

b. $y = 3e^{-2t}$

c. $y = 2e^{t}$

12. Which of the following equations predicts y increasing as t increases? (t is a positive number.)

a. $y = 2e^{-3t}$

b. $y = 3e^{-2t}$

c. $y = 2e^{t}$

13. Which of the following would result in an error message if you took the log of *x* using a calculator?

   a. $x = 2.5$

   b. $x = 0.024$

   c. $x = 10^{-2}$

   d. $x = -0.2$

14. Which of the following equation(s) would have the greatest value at *t* equal to zero assuming that *t* is not negative.

   a. e^{-3t}

   b. $3e^{-2t}$

   c. $2/e^t$

REFERENCES

Eder AF, Bryan WA: Theophylline: Recent consensus and current controversy. *Am Assoc Clin Chem* TDX/Tox, **17:** Jan, p 1051, 1996

Jones AW: Disappearance rate of ethanol from the blood of human subjects: Implications in forensic toxicology. *J Forensic Sci* May, 104–118, 1992

Riggs DS: *The Mathematical Approach to Physiological Problems.* Baltimore, Williams & Wilkins, 1963, p 51

BIBLIOGRAPHY

Bolton S: *Pharmaceutical Statistics.* New York, Marcel Dekker, 1984

Randolph LK, Cuminera JL: Statistics. In Gennaro AR (ed), *Remington's Pharmaceutical Sciences,* 17th ed. Easton, PA, Mack, 1985, pp 104–139

3

ONE-COMPARTMENT OPEN MODEL: INTRAVENOUS BOLUS ADMINISTRATION

The most common and most desirable route of drug administration is orally—by mouth—using tablets, capsules, or oral solutions. In developing pharmacokinetic models to describe and predict drug disposition kinetically, the model must account for both the route of administration and the kinetic behavior of the drug in the body.

The *one-compartment open model* offers the simplest way to describe the process of drug distribution and elimination in the body. This model assumes that the drug can enter or leave the body (ie, the model is "open"), and the body acts like a single, uniform compartment. The simplest route of drug administration from a modeling perspective is a rapid intravenous injection (IV bolus). The simplest kinetic model that describes drug disposition in the body is to consider that the drug is injected all at once into a box, or compartment, and that the drug distributes instantaneously and homogenously throughout the compartment. Drug elimination also occurs from the compartment immediately after injection.

Of course, this model is a simplistic view of drug disposition in the body, which in reality is infinitely more complex than a single compartment. In the body, when a drug is given in the form of an IV bolus, the entire dose of drug enters the bloodstream immediately, and the drug absorption process is considered to be instantaneous. In most cases, the drug distributes via the circulatory system to potentially all the tissues in the body. Uptake of drugs by various tissue organs will occur at varying rates, depending on the blood flow to the tissue, the lipophilicity of the drug, the molecular weight of the drug, and the binding affinity of the drug for the tissue mass. Most drugs are eliminated from the body either through the kidney and/or by being metabolized in the liver. Because of rapid drug equilibration between the blood and tissue, drug elimination occurs as if the dose is all dissolved in a tank of uniform fluid (a single compartment) from which the drug is eliminated. The volume in which the drug is distributed is termed the *apparent volume of distribution*, V_D. The apparent volume of distribution assumes that the drug is uniformly distributed in the body. The V_D is determined from the preinjected amount of the dose in the syringe and the plasma drug concentration resulting immediately after the dose is injected.

The apparent volume of distribution is a parameter of the one-compartment model and governs the plasma concentration of the drug after a given dose. A second pharmacokinetic parameter is the *elimination rate constant, k*, which governs the rate at which the drug concentration in the body declines over time. The one-compartment model that describes the distribution and elimination after an IV bolus dose is given in Figure 3-1.

The one-compartment open model does not predict actual drug levels in the tissues. However, the model assumes that changes in the plasma levels of a drug will result in proportional changes in tissue drug levels, since their kinetic profile is consistent with inclusion within the vascular compartment and the various drug concentrations within the compartment are in equilibrium. The *drug in the body*, D_B, cannot be measured directly; however, accessible body fluids (such as blood) can be sampled to determine drug concentrations.

ELIMINATION RATE CONSTANT

The rate of elimination for most drugs from a tissue or from the body is a first-order process, in which the rate of elimination is dependent on the amount or concentration of drug present. The elimination rate constant, k, is a first-order elimination rate constant with units of time^{-1} (eg, hr^{-1} or $1/\text{hr}$). Generally, the parent or active drug is measured in the vascular compartment. Total removal or elimination of the parent drug from this compartment is effected by metabolism (biotransformation) and excretion. The elimination rate constant represents the sum of each of these processes:

$$k = k_m + k_e \tag{3.1}$$

where k_m = first-order rate process of metabolism and k_e = first-order rate process of excretion. There may be several routes of elimination of drug by metabolism or excretion. In such a case, each of these processes has its own first-order rate constant.

A rate expression for Figure 3-1 is

$$\frac{dD_B}{dt} = -kD_B \tag{3.2}$$

This expression shows that the rate of elimination of drug in the body is a first-order process, depending on the overall elimination rate constant, k, and the

Figure 3-1. Pharmacokinetic model for a drug administered by rapid intravenous injection. D_B = drug in body; V_D = apparent volume of distribution; k = elimination rate constant.

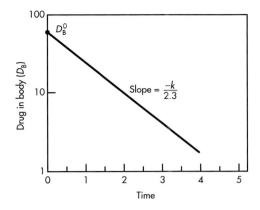

Figure 3-2. Semilog graph of the rate of drug elimination in a one-compartment model.

amount of drug in the body, D_B, remaining at any given time, t. Integration of Equation 3.2 gives the following expression:

$$\log D_B = \frac{-kt}{2.3} + \log D_B^0 \tag{3.3}$$

where D_B = drug in the body at time t and D_B^0 = drug in the body at $t = 0$. When $\log D_B$ is plotted against t for this equation, a straight line is obtained (Fig. 3-2). In practice, instead of transforming values of D_B to their corresponding logarithms, each value of D_B is placed at logarithmic intervals on semilog paper.

Equation 3.3 can also be expressed as

$$D_B = D_B^0 e^{-kt} \tag{3.4}$$

APPARENT VOLUME OF DISTRIBUTION

In general, drug equilibrates rapidly in the body. When plasma or any other biologic compartment is sampled and analyzed for drug content, the results are usually reported in units of concentration instead of amount. Each individual tissue in the body may contain a different concentration of drug due to differences in drug affinity for that tissue. Therefore, the amount of drug in a given location can be related to its concentration by a proportionality constant that reflects the volume of fluid the drug is dissolved in. The *volume of distribution* represents a volume that must be considered in estimating the amount of drug in the body from the concentration of drug found in the sampling compartment. The volume of distribution is also the apparent volume (V_D) in which the drug is dissolved (Eq. 3.5). Because the value of the volume of distribution does not have a true physiologic meaning in terms of an anatomic space, the term *apparent* volume of distribution is used.

The amount of drug in the body is not determined directly. Instead, a blood sample is removed at periodic intervals and analyzed for its concentration of drug. The V_D relates the concentration of drug in plasma (C_p) and the amount of drug in the body (D_B), as in the following equation:

$$D_B = V_D C_p \tag{3.5}$$

By substituting Equation 3.5 into Equation 3.3, a similar expression based on drug concentration in plasma is obtained for the first-order decline of drug plasma levels:

$$\log C_{p} = \frac{-kt}{2.3} + \log C_{p}^{0} \qquad (3.6)$$

where C_{p} = concentration of drug in plasma at time t and C_{p}^{0} = concentration of drug in plasma at $t = 0$. Equation 3.6 can also be expressed as

$$C_{p} = C_{p}^{0} e^{-kt} \qquad (3.7)$$

The relationship between apparent volume, drug concentration, and total amount of drug may be better understood by the following example.

 # EXAMPLE

Exactly 1 g of a drug is dissolved in an unknown volume of water. Upon assay, the concentration of this solution is 1 mg/mL. What is the original volume of this solution?

The original volume of the solution may be obtained by the following proportion, remembering that 1 g = 1000 mg:

$$\frac{1000 \text{ mg}}{x \text{ mL}} = \frac{1 \text{ mg}}{\text{mL}} \qquad x = 1000 \text{ mL}$$

Therefore, the original volume was 1000 mL or 1 L.

If, in the above example, the volume of the solution is known to be 1 L, and the concentration of the solution is 1 mg/mL, then, to calculate the total amount of drug present,

$$\frac{x \text{ mg}}{1000 \text{ mL}} = \frac{1 \text{ mg}}{\text{mL}} \qquad x = 1000 \text{ mg}$$

Therefore, the total amount of drug in the solution is 1000 mg, or 1 g.

From the preceding example, if the volume of solution in which the drug is dissolved and the drug concentration of the solution are known, then the total amount of drug present in the solution may be calculated. This relationship between drug concentration, volume in which the drug is dissolved, and total amount of drug present is given in the following equation:

$$V_{D} = \frac{\text{Dose}}{C_{p}^{0}} = \frac{D_{B}^{0}}{C_{p}^{0}} \qquad (3.8)$$

where D = total amount of drug, V = total volume, and C = drug concentration. From Equation 3.8, which is similar to Equation 3.5, if any two parameters are known, then the third term may be calculated.

The body may be considered as a constant-volume system or compartment. Therefore, the apparent volume of distribution for any given drug is generally a constant. If both the concentration of drug in the plasma and the apparent volume of distribution for the drug are known, then the total amount of drug in the body (at the time in which the plasma sample was obtained) may be calculated from Equation 3.5.

Calculation of Volume of Distribution

In a one-compartment model (IV administration), the V_D is calculated with the following equation:

$$V_D = \frac{\text{Dose}}{C_p^0} = \frac{D_B^0}{C_p^0} \tag{3.9}$$

When C_p^0 is determined by extrapolation, it represents the instantaneous drug concentration (concentration of drug at $t = 0$) after drug equilibration in the body (Fig. 3-3). The dose of drug given by IV bolus (rapid IV injection) represents the amount of drug in the body, D_B^0, at $t = 0$. Because both D_B^0 and C_p^0 are known at $t = 0$, then the apparent volume of distribution, V_D, may be calculated from Equation 3.9.

From Equation 3.2 (repeated here), the rate of drug elimination is

$$\frac{dD_B}{dt} = -kD_B$$

By substitution of Equation 3.5, $D_B = V_D C_p$, into Equation 3.2, the following expression is obtained:

$$\frac{dD_B}{dt} = -kV_D C_p \tag{3.10}$$

Rearrangement of Equation 3.10 gives

$$dD_B = -kV_D C_p dt \tag{3.11}$$

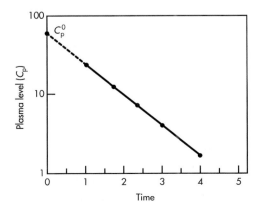

Figure 3-3. Semilog graph giving the value of C_p^0 by extrapolation.

As both k and V_D are constants, Equation 3.10 may be integrated as follows:

$$\int_0^{D_0} dD_B = -kV_D \int_0^{\infty} C_p dt \qquad (3.12)$$

Equation 3.12 shows that a small change in time (dt) results in a small change in the amount of drug in the body, D_B.

The integral $\int_0^{\infty} C_p dt$ represents the AUC_0^{∞}, which is the summation of the area under the curve from $t = 0$ to $t = \infty$. Thus, the apparent V_D may also be calculated from knowledge of the dose, elimination rate constant, and the area under the curve (AUC) from $t = 0$ to $t = \infty$. The AUC_0^{∞} is usually estimated by the trapezoidal rule (see Chapter 2). After integration, Equation 3.12 becomes

$$D_0 = kV_D[\text{AUC}]_0^{\infty}$$

which upon rearrangement yields the following equation:

$$V_D = \frac{D_0}{k[\text{AUC}]_0^{\infty}} \qquad (3.13)$$

The calculation of the apparent V_D by means of Equation 3.13 is a *model-independent* method, because no pharmacokinetic model is considered and the AUC is determined directly by the trapezoidal rule.

Significance of the Apparent Volume of Distribution

The apparent volume of distribution is not a true physiologic volume. Most drugs have an apparent volume of distribution smaller than, or equal to, the body mass. For some drugs, the volume of distribution may be several times the body mass. Equation 3.9 shows that the apparent V_D is dependent on C_p^0. For a given dose, a very small C_p^0 may occur in the body due to concentration of the drug in peripheral tissues and organs. For this dose, the small C_p^0 will result in a large V_D.

Drugs with a large apparent V_D are more concentrated in extravascular tissues and less concentrated intravascularly. If a drug is highly bound to plasma proteins or remains in the vascular region, then C_p^0 will be higher, resulting in a smaller apparent V_D. Consequently, binding of a drug to peripheral tissues or to plasma proteins will significantly affect V_D.

The apparent V_D is a volume term that can be expressed as a simple volume or in terms of percent of body weight. In expressing the apparent V_D in terms of percent body weight, a 1-L volume is assumed to be equal to the weight of 1 kg. For example, if the V_D is 3500 mL for a subject weighing 70 kg, the V_D expressed as percent of body weight is

$$\frac{3.5 \text{ kg}}{70 \text{ kg}} \times 100 = 5\% \text{ of body weight}$$

If V_D is a very large number—ie, >100% of body weight—then it may be assumed that the drug is concentrated in certain tissue compartments. Thus, the apparent V_D is a useful parameter in considering the relative amounts of drug in the vascular and in the extravascular tissues.

TABLE 3.1   Fluid in the Body

WATER COMPARTMENT	PERCENT OF BODY WEIGHT	PERCENT OF TOTAL BODY WATER
Plasma	4.5	7.5
Total extracellular water	27.0	45.0
Total intracellular water	33.0	55.0
Total body water	60.0	100.0

Pharmacologists often attempt to conceptualize the apparent V_D as a true physiologic or anatomic fluid compartment. By expressing the V_D in terms of percent of body weight, values for the V_D may be found that appear to correspond to true anatomic volumes (Table 3.1). However, it may be only fortuitous that the value for the apparent V_D of a drug has the same value as a real anatomic volume. If a drug is to be considered to be distributed in a true physiologic volume, then an investigation is needed to test this hypothesis.

Given the apparent V_D for a particular drug, the total amount of drug in the body at any time after administration of the drug may be determined by the measurement of the drug concentration in the plasma (Eq. 3.5). Because the magnitude of the apparent V_D is a useful indicator for the amount of drug outside the sampling compartment (usually the blood), the larger the apparent V_D, the greater the amount of drug in the extravascular tissues.

For each drug, the apparent V_D is a constant. In certain pathologic cases, the apparent V_D for the drug may be altered if the distribution of the drug is changed. For example, in edematous conditions, the total body water and total extracellular water increase; this is reflected in a larger apparent V_D value for a drug that is highly water soluble. Similarly, changes in total body weight and lean body mass (which normally occur with age) may also affect the apparent V_D.

CLEARANCE

Clearance is a measure of drug elimination from the body without identifying the mechanism or process. Clearance is also discussed in subsequent chapters. Clearance (*drug clearance, systemic clearance, total body clearance, Cl_T*) considers the entire body as a drug-eliminating system from which many elimination processes may occur.

Drug Clearance in the One-Compartment Model

The body is considered as a system of organs perfused by plasma and body fluids. Drug elimination from the body is an ongoing process due to both metabolism (biotransformation) and drug excretion through the kidney and other routes. The mechanisms of drug elimination are complex, but collectively drug elimination from the body may be quantitated using the concept of drug clearance. Drug clearance refers to the volume of plasma fluid that is cleared of drug per unit time. Clearance may also be considered as the fraction of drug removed per unit time. The rate of drug elimination may be expressed in several ways, each of which essentially describes the same process, but with different levels of insight and application in pharmacokinetics.

Drug Elimination Expressed as Amount per Time Unit

The expression of drug elimination from the body in terms of mass per unit time (eg, mg/min, or mg/hr) is simple, absolute, and unambiguous. For a zero-order elimination process, expressing the rate of drug elimination as mass per unit time is convenient because the rate is constant (Fig. 3-4A). In contrast, the rate of drug elimination for a first-order elimination process is not constant and changes with respect to the drug concentration in the body. For a first-order elimination, drug clearance expressed as volume per unit time (eg, L/hr or mL/min) is convenient because it is a constant.

Drug Elimination Expressed as Volume per Time Unit

The concept of expressing a rate in terms of volume per unit time is common in pharmacy. For example, a patient may be dosed at the rate of 2 teaspoonsful (10 mL) of a liquid medicine (10 mg/mL) daily, or alternatively, a dose (weight) of 100 mg of the drug daily.

Clearance is a concept that expresses "the rate of drug removal" in terms of volume of drug solution removed per unit time (at whatever drug concentration in the body prevailing at that time) (Fig. 3-4B). In contrast to a solution in a bottle, the drug concentration in the body will gradually decline by a first-order process such that the mass of drug removed over time is not constant. The plasma volume in the healthy state is relatively constant because water lost through the kidney is rapidly replaced with fluid absorbed from the gastrointestinal tract.

Since a constant volume of plasma (about 120 mL/min in humans) is filtered through the glomeruli of the kidneys, the rate of drug removal is dependent on the plasma drug concentration at all times. This observation is based on a first-order process governing drug elimination. For many drugs, the rate of drug elimination is dependent on the plasma drug concentration, multiplied by a constant

Figure 3-4. Diagram illustrating three different ways of describing drug elimination after a dose of 100 mg injected IV into a volume of 10 mL (a mouse, for example).

factor ($dC/dt = kC$). When the plasma drug concentration is high, the rate of drug removal is high, and vice versa.

Clearance (volume of fluid removed of drug) for a first-order process is constant regardless of the drug concentration because clearance is expressed in volume per unit time rather than drug amount per unit time. Mathematically, the rate of drug elimination is similar to Equation 3.10:

$$\frac{dD_{B}}{dt} = -kC_{p}V_{D} \tag{3.2a}$$

Dividing this expression on both sides by C_{p} yields Equation 3.14:

$$\frac{dD_{B}/dt}{C_{p}} = \frac{-kC_{p}V_{D}}{C_{p}} \tag{3.14}$$

$$\frac{dD_{B}/dt}{C_{p}} = -kV_{D} = -Cl \tag{3.15}$$

where dD_{B}/dt is the rate of drug elimination from the body (mg/hr), C_{p} is the plasma drug concentration (mg/L), k is a first-order rate constant (hr^{-1} or 1/hr), and V_{D} is the apparent volume of distribution (L). Cl is clearance and has the units L/hr in this example. In the example in Fig. 3-4B, Cl is in mL/min.

Clearance, Cl, is expressed as volume/time. Equation 3.15 shows that clearance is a constant because V_{D} and k are both constants. D_{B} is the amount of drug in the body, and dD_{B}/dt is the rate of change (of amount) of drug in the body with respect to time. The negative sign refers to the drug exiting from the body.

Drug Elimination Expressed as Fraction Eliminated per Time Unit

Consider a compartment volume, containing V_{D} liters. If Cl is expressed in liters per minute (L/min), then the fraction of drug cleared per minute in the body is equal to Cl/V_{D}.

Expressing drug elimination as the fraction of total drug eliminated is applicable regardless or whether one is dealing with an amount or a volume (Fig. 3-4C). This approach is most flexible and convenient because of its dimensionless nature. Thus, it is valid to express drug elimination as a fraction (eg, one-tenth of the amount of drug in the body is eliminated or one-tenth of the drug volume is eliminated). Pharmacokineticists have incorporated this concept into the first-order equation (ie, k) that describes drug elimination from the one-compartment model. Indeed, the universal nature of many processes forms the basis of the first-order equation of drug elimination (eg, a fraction of the total drug molecules in the body will perfuse the glomeruli, a fraction of the filtered drug molecules will be reabsorbed at the renal tubules, and a fraction of the filtered drug molecules will be excreted from the body giving an overall first-order drug elimination rate constant, k). The rate of drug elimination is the product of k and the drug concentration (Eq. 3.2a). The first-order equation of drug elimination can be also based on probability and a consideration of the statistical moment theory (Chapter 20).

Clearance and Volume of Distribution Ratio, Cl/V_D

 EXAMPLE

Consider that 100 mg of drug is dissolved in 10 mL of fluid and 10 mg of drug is removed in the first minute. The drug elimination process could be described as:

a. Number of mg of drug eliminated per minute (mg/min)

b. Number of mL of fluid cleared of drug per minute

c. Fraction of drug eliminated per minute

The relationship of the three drug elimination processes is illustrated in Figure 3-4A–C. Note that in Figure 3-4C, the fraction Cl/V_D is dependent on both the volume of distribution and the rate of drug clearance from the body. This clearance concept forms the basis of classical pharmacokinetics and is later extended to flow models in pharmacokinetic modeling. If the drug concentration is C_p, the rate of drug elimination (in terms of rate of change in concentration, dC_p/dt) is:

$$\frac{dC_p}{dt} = -(Cl/V_D) \times C_p \tag{3.16}$$

For a first-order process,

$$\frac{dC_p}{dt} = -kC_p = \text{rate of drug administration} \tag{3.17}$$

Equating the two expressions yields:

$$kC_p = Cl/V_D \times C_p \tag{3.18}$$

$$k = \frac{Cl}{V_D} \tag{3.19}$$

Thus, a first-order rate constant is the fractional constant Cl/V_D. Some pharmacokineticists regard drug clearance and the volume of distribution as independent parameters that are necessary to describe the time course of drug elimination. Equation 3.19 is a rearrangement of Equation 3.15 given earlier.

One-Compartment Model Equation in Terms of *Cl* and V_D

Equation 3.20 may be rewritten in terms of clearance and volume of distribution by substituting Cl/V_D for k. The clearance concept may also be applied a biologic system in physiologic modeling without the need of a theoretical compartment.

$$C_p = C_p^{0-kt} \tag{3.20}$$

$$C_p = D_0/V_D e^{-(Cl/V_D)t} \tag{3.21}$$

Equation 3.21 is applied directly in clinical pharmacy to determine clearance and volume of distribution in patients. When only one sample is available, ie, C_p is known at one sample time point, t after a given dose, the equation cannot be determined unambiguously because two unknown parameters must be solved, ie, Cl and V_D. In practice, the mean values for Cl and V_D of a drug are obtained from the population values (derived from a large population of subjects or patients) in the literature. The values of Cl and V_D for the patient are adjusted using a computer program. Ultimately, a new pair of Cl and V_D values that better fit the observed plasma drug concentration is found. The process is repeated through iterations until the "best" parameters are obtained. Since many mathematical techniques (algorithms) are available for iteration, different results may be obtained using different iterative programs. An objective test to determine the accuracy of the estimated clearance and V_D values is to monitor how accurately those parameters will predict the plasma level of the drug after a new dose is given to the patient. In subsequent chapters, mean predictive error will be discussed and calculated in order to determine the performance of various drug monitoring methods in practice.

The ratio of Cl/V_D may be calculated regardless of compartment model type using minimal plasma samples. Clinical pharmacists have applied many variations of this approach to therapeutic drug monitoring and drug dosage adjustments in patients.

 # PRACTICAL FOCUS

The most accurate kinetic method to determine the volume of distribution and the distribution kinetic of a drug in a patient is to give the drug by a single IV bolus dose. An IV bolus dose avoids many variables such as delayed, irregular, and/or incomplete absorption compared to other routes of administration.

The IV single dose Equation 3.22 may be modified to calculate the elimination rate constant or half-life of a drug in a patient when two plasma samples and their time of collection are known:

$$\ln C_p = \ln C_p^0 - kt \tag{3.22}$$

If the first plasma sample is taken at t_1 instead of at zero and corresponds to plasma drug concentration, then C_2 is the concentration at time t_2 and t is set to $(t_2 - t_1)$.

$$C_2 = C_1 e^{-k(t_2 - t_1)}$$
$$\ln C_2 = \ln C_1 - k(t_2 - t_1) \tag{3.23}$$

Rearranging:

$$\ln C_2 - \ln C_1 = -k(t_2 - t_1)$$
$$k = \frac{\ln C_1 - \ln C_2}{(t_2 - t_1)} \tag{3.24}$$

$$t_{1/2} = \frac{0.693(t_2 - t_1)}{\ln C_1 - \ln C_2} \tag{3.25}$$

where

t_1 = time of first sample collection
C_1 = plasma drug concentration at t_1
t_2 = time of second sample collection
C_2 = plasma drug concentration at t_2

In a clinical practice, several drug doses may have been given to the patient and the prior dosing times may not be accurately known. If the pharmacist judges that the drug in the body is in a declining phase (ie, absorption is completed), this equation may be used to determine the half-life of the drug in the patient by taking two plasma samples far apart and recording the times of sampling.

Clearance from Drug-Eliminating Tissues

Clearance may be applied to any organ that is involved in drug elimination from the body. As long as first-order elimination processes are involved, clearance represents the sum of the clearances for each drug-eliminating organ as shown in Equation 3.26:

$$Cl_T = Cl_R + Cl_{NR} \tag{3.26}$$

where Cl_R is renal clearance or drug clearance through the kidney, and Cl_{NR} is non-renal clearance through other organs. Generally, clearance is considered as the sum of renal, Cl_R, and nonrenal drug clearance, Cl_{NR}. Cl_{NR} is assumed to be due primarily to hepatic clearance (Cl_H) in the absence of other significant drug clearances, such as elimination through the lung or the bile, as shown in Equation 3.27:

$$Cl_T = Cl_R + Cl_H \tag{3.27}$$

Drug clearance considers that the drug in the body is uniformly dissolved in a volume of fluid (apparent volume of distribution, V_D) from which drug concentrations can be measured easily. Typically, plasma fluid concentration is measured and drug clearance is then calculated as the fixed volume of plasma fluid (containing the drug) cleared of drug per unit of time. The units for clearance are volume/time (eg, mL/min, L/hr).

Alternatively, Cl_T may be defined as the rate of drug elimination divided by the plasma drug concentration. Thus, clearance is expressed in terms of the volume of plasma containing drug that is eliminated per unit time. This clearance definition is equivalent to the previous definition and provides a practical way to calculate clearance based on plasma drug concentration data.

$$Cl_T = \frac{\text{elimination rate}}{\text{plasma concentration } (C_p)} \tag{3.28}$$

$$Cl_T = \frac{(dD_E/dt)}{C_p} = (\mu g/min)/(\mu g/mL) = mL/min \tag{3.29}$$

where D_E is the amount of drug eliminated and dD_E/dt is the rate of drug elimination.

Rearrangement of Equation 3.29 gives Equation 3.30:

$$\text{Drug elimination rate} = \frac{dD_E}{dt} = C_p \, Cl_T \tag{3.30}$$

Therefore Cl_T is a constant for a specific drug and represents the slope of the line obtained by plotting dD_E/dt versus C_p, as shown in Equation 3.30.

For drugs that follow first-order elimination, the rate of drug elimination is dependent on the amount of drug remaining in the body.

$$\frac{dD_E}{dt} = kD_B = kC_p V_D \tag{3.31}$$

Substituting the elimination rate in Equation 3.30 for $kC_p V_D$ in Equation 3.31 and solving for Cl_T gives Equation 3.32:

$$Cl_T = \frac{kC_p V_D}{C_p} = kV_D \tag{3.32}$$

Equation 3.32 shows that clearance, Cl_T, is the product of V_D and k, both of which are constant. This Equation 3.32 is similar to Equation 3.19 shown earlier. As the plasma drug concentration decreases during elimination, the rate of drug elimination, dD_E/dt, will decrease accordingly, but clearance will remain constant. Clearance will be constant as long as the rate of drug elimination is a first-order process.

For some drugs, the elimination rate process is more complex and a noncompartment method may be used to calculate certain pharmacokinetic parameters such as clearance. In this case, clearance can be determined directly from the plasma drug concentration-versus-time curve by

$$Cl_T = \frac{D_0}{[\text{AUC}]_0^\infty} \tag{3.33}$$

where D_0 is the dose and $[\text{AUC}]_0^\infty = \int_0^\infty C_p dt$.

Because $[\text{AUC}]_0^\infty$ is calculated from the plasma drug concentration-versus-time curve from 0 to infinity (∞) using the trapezoidal rule, no compartmental model is assumed. However, to extrapolate the data to infinity to obtain the residual $[\text{AUC}]_0^\infty$ or $(C_p t/k)$, first-order elimination is usually assumed. In this case, if the drug follows the kinetics of a one-compartment model, the Cl_T is numerically similar to the product of V_D and k obtained by fitting the data to a one-compartment model.

CALCULATION OF K FROM URINARY EXCRETION DATA

The elimination rate constant k may be calculated from urinary excretion data. In this calculation the excretion rate of the drug is assumed to be first order. The term

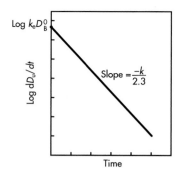

Figure 3-5.   Graph of Equation 3.36: log rate of drug excretion versus t on regular paper.

k_e is the renal excretion rate constant, and D_u is the amount of drug excreted in the urine.

$$\frac{dD_u}{dt} = k_e D_B \tag{3.34}$$

From Equation 3.4, D_B can be substituted for $D_B^0 e^{-kt}$:

$$\frac{dD_u}{dt} = k_e D_B^0 e^{-kt} \tag{3.35}$$

Taking the natural logarithm of both sides and then transforming to common logarithms, the following expression is obtained:

$$\log \frac{dD_u}{dt} = \frac{-kt}{2.3} + \log k_e D_B^0 \tag{3.36}$$

A straight line is obtained from this equation by plotting log dD_u/dt vs time on regular paper or on semilog paper dD_u/dt against time (Figs. 3-5 and 3-6). The slope of this curve is equal to $-k/2.3$ and the y intercept is equal to $k_e D_B^0$. For rapid intravenous administration, D_B^0 is equal to the dose D_0. Therefore, if D_B^0 is known, the renal excretion rate constant (k_e) can be obtained. Because both k_e and k can be determined by this method, the nonrenal rate constant (k_{nr}) for any route of elimination other than renal excretion can be found as follows:

$$k - k_e = k_{nr} \tag{3.37}$$

Figure 3-6.   Semilog graph of rate of drug excretion versus time according to Equation 3.36 on semilog paper (intercept = $k_e D_B^0$).

Substitution of k_m for k_{nr} in Equation 3.37 gives Equation 3.1. Because the major routes of elimination for most drugs are renal excretion and metabolism (biotransformation), k_{nr} is approximately equal to k_m.

$$k_{nr} = k_m \tag{3.38}$$

The drug urinary excretion rate (dD_u/dt) cannot be determined experimentally for any given instant. Therefore, the average rate of urinary drug excretion, D_u/t is plotted against the average time, t^*, for the collection of the urine sample. In practice, urine is collected over a specified time interval, and the urine specimen is analyzed for drug. An average urinary excretion rate is then calculated for that collection period. The average value of dD_u/dt is plotted on a semilogarithmic scale against the time that corresponds to the midpoint (average time) of the collection period.

PRACTICE PROBLEM

A single IV dose of an antibiotic was given to a 50-kg woman at a dose level of 20 mg/kg. Urine and blood samples were removed periodically and assayed for parent drug. The following data were obtained:

Time (hr)	C_p (µg/mL)	D_u (mg)
0.25	4.2	160
0.50	3.5	140
1.0	2.5	200
2.0	1.25	250
4.0	0.31	188
6.0	0.08	46

Solution

Set up the following table:

Time (hr)	D_u (mg)	D_u/t	mg/hr	t^* (hr)
0.25	160	160/0.25	640	0.125
0.50	140	140/0.25	560	0.375
1.0	200	200/0.5	400	0.750
2.0	250	250/1	250	1.50
4.0	188	188/2	94	3.0
6.0	46	46/2	23	5.0

Here t^* = midpoint of collection period; and t = time interval for collection of urine sample.

Construct a graph on a semilogarithmic scale of D_u/t versus t^*. The slope of this line should equal $-k/2.3$. It is usually easier to determine the elimination $t_{1/2}$ directly from the curve and then calculate k from

$$k = \frac{0.693}{t_{1/2}}$$

In this problem, $t_{1/2} = 1.0$ hr and $k = 0.693$ hr^{-1}. A similar graph of the C_p values versus t should yield a curve with a slope having the same value as that derived from the previous curve. Note that the slope of the log excretion rate constant is a function of elimination rate constant k and not of the urinary excretion rate constant k_e (Fig. 3-6).

An alternative method for the calculation of the elimination rate constant k from urinary excretion data is the *sigma-minus method,* or *the amount of drug remaining to be excreted method.* The sigma-minus method is sometimes preferred over the previous method because fluctuations in the rate of elimination are minimized.

The amount of unchanged drug in the urine can be expressed as a function of time through the following equation:

$$D_u = \frac{k_e D_0}{k}(1 - e^{-kt}) \tag{3.39}$$

where D_u is the cumulative amount of unchanged drug excreted in the urine.

The amount of unchanged drug that is ultimately excreted in the urine, D_u^∞, can be determined by making time t equal to ∞. Thus, the term e^{-kt} becomes negligible and the following expression is obtained:

$$D_u^\infty = \frac{k_e D_0}{k} \tag{3.40}$$

Substitution of D_u^∞ for $k_e D_0/k$ in Equation 3.39 and rearrangement yields

$$D_u^\infty - D_u = D_u^\infty e^{-kt} \tag{3.41}$$

Equation 3.41 can be written in logarithmic form to obtain a linear equation:

$$\log(D_u^\infty - D_u) = \frac{-kt}{2.3} + \log D_u^\infty \tag{3.42}$$

Equation 3.42 describes the relationship for the amount of drug remaining to be excreted $(D_u^\infty - D_u)$ versus time.

A linear curve is obtained by graphing the logarithm scale of the amount of unchanged drug yet to be eliminated, $\log(D_u^\infty - D_u)$ versus time. On semilog paper, the slope of this curve is $-k/2.3$ and the y intercept is D_u^∞ (Fig. 3-7).

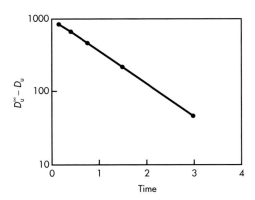

Figure 3-7. Sigma-minus method, or the amount of drug remaining to be excreted method, for the calculation of the elimination rate constant according to Equation 3.42.

PRACTICE PROBLEM

Using the data in the preceding problem, determine the elimination rate constant.

Solution

Construct the following table:

Time (hr)	D_u (mg)	Cumulative D_u	$D_u^\infty - D_u$
0.25	160	160	824
0.50	140	300	684
1.0	200	500	484
2.0	250	750	234
4.0	188	938	46
6.0	46	984	0

Plot $\log(D_u^\infty - D_u)$ versus time. Use a semilogarithmic scale for $(D_u^\infty - D_u)$. Evaluate k and $t_{1/2}$ from the slope.

Comparison of the Rate and the Sigma-Minus Methods

The rate method does not require knowledge of D_u^∞, and the loss of one urine specimen does not invalidate the entire urinary drug excretion study. The sigma-minus method requires an accurate determination of D_u^∞, which requires the collection of urine until urinary drug excretion is complete. A small error in the assessment of D_u^∞ introduces an error in terms of curvature of the plot, because each point is based on $\log(D_u^\infty - D_u)$ versus time. Fluctuations in the rate of drug elimination and experimental errors including incomplete bladder emptying for a collection period cause appreciable departure from linearity using the rate method, whereas the accuracy of the sigma-minus method is less affected. The rate method is applicable to zero-order drug elimination process, while the sigma-minus method is not. Lastly, the renal drug excretion rate constant may be obtained from the rate method but not from the sigma-minus method.

CLINICAL APPLICATION

The sigma-minus method and the excretion rate method was applied to the urinary drug excretion in subjects following the smoking of a single marijuana cigarette (Huestis et al, 1996). The urinary excretion curves of 11-nor-carboxy 9-tetrahydrocannabinol (THCCOOH), a metabolite of marijuana, in one subject from 24 to 144 hours after smoking one marijuana cigarette are shown in Figures 3-8 and 3-9. A total of 199.7 mg of THCCOOH was excreted in the urine over 7 days, which represents 0.54% of the total 9-tetrahydrocannabinol available in the cigarette. Using either urinary drug excretion method, the elimination half-life was determined to be about 30 hours. However, the urinary drug excretion rate method data

Figure 3-8. Amount remaining to be excreted method. The half-life of THCCOOH was calculated to be 29.9 hr from the slope of this curve; the correlation coefficient *r* was equal to 0.992. (Adapted from Huestis et al., 1996, with permission.)

were more scattered (variable) and the correlation coefficient *r* was equal to 0.744 (Fig. 3-9), compared to the correlation coefficient *r* of 0.992 using the sigma-minus method (Fig. 3-8).

Problems in Obtaining Valid Urinary Excretion Data

Certain factors can make it difficult to obtain valid urinary excretion data. Some of these factors are as follows:

1. A significant fraction of the unchanged drug must be excreted in the urine.
2. The assay technique must be specific for the unchanged drug and must not include interference due to drug metabolites that have similar chemical structures.
3. Frequent sampling is necessary for a good curve description.
4. Urine samples should be collected periodically until almost all of the drug is excreted. A graph of the cumulative drug excreted versus time will yield a curve that approaches an asymptote at "infinite" time (Fig. 3-10). In practice, approximately seven elimination half-lives are needed for 99% of the drug to be eliminated.

Figure 3-9. Excretion rate method. The half-life of THCCOOH was calculated to be 30.7 hr from the slope of this curve; the correlation coefficient *r* was equal to 0.744. (Adapted from Huestis et al., 1996, with permission.)

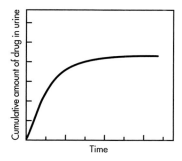

Figure 3-10. *Graph showing the cumulative urinary excretion of drug as a function of time.*

5. Variations in urinary pH and volume may cause significant variation in urinary excretion rates.
6. Subjects should be carefully instructed as to the necessity of giving a complete urine specimen (ie, completely emptying the bladder).

FREQUENTLY ASKED QUESTIONS

1. What is the difference between a rate and a rate constant?
2. Why does k always have the unit 1/time (eg, hr^{-1}), regardless of what concentration unit is plotted?
3. If a drug is distributed in the one-compartment model, does it mean that there is no drug in the tissue?
4. How is clearance related to the volume of distribution and k?
5. If we use a physiologic model, are we dealing with actual volumes of blood and tissues? Why do we still use volumes of distribution that often are greater than the real physical volume?

LEARNING QUESTIONS

1. A 70-kg volunteer is given an intravenous dose of an antibiotic, and serum drug concentrations were determined at 2 hours and 5 hours after administration. The drug concentrations were 1.2 and 0.3 μg/mL, respectively. What is the biologic half-life for this drug, assuming first-order elimination kinetics?
2. A 50-kg woman was given a single IV dose of an antibacterial drug at a dose level of 6 mg/kg. Blood samples were taken at various time intervals. The

concentration of the drug (C_p) was determined in the plasma fraction of each blood sample and the following data were obtained:

t (hr)	C_p ($\mu g/mL$)
0.25	8.21
0.50	7.87
1.00	7.23
3.00	5.15
6.00	3.09
12.0	1.11
18.0	0.40

a. What are the values for V_D, k, and $t_{1/2}$ for this drug?

b. This antibacterial agent is not effective at a plasma concentration of less than 2 $\mu g/mL$. What is the duration of activity for this drug?

c. How long would it take for 99.9% of this drug to be eliminated?

d. If the dose of the antibiotic were doubled exactly, what would be the increase in duration of activity?

3. A new drug was given in a single intravenous dose of 200 mg to an 80-kg adult male patient. After 6 hours, the plasma drug concentration of drug was 1.5 mg/100 mL of plasma. Assuming that the apparent V_D is 10% of body weight, compute the total amount of drug in the body fluids after 6 hours. What is the half-life of this drug?

4. A new antibiotic drug was given in a single intravenous bolus of 4 mg/kg to five healthy male adults ranging in age from 23 to 38 years (average weight 75 kg). The pharmacokinetics of the plasma drug concentration–time curve for this drug fits a one-compartment model. The equation of the curve that best fits the data is

$$C_p = 78e^{-0.46t}$$

Determine the following (assume units of $\mu g/mL$ for C_p and hr for t):

a. What is the $t_{1/2}$?

b. What is the V_D?

c. What is the plasma level of the drug after 4 hours?

d. How much drug is left in the body after 4 hours?

e. Predict what body water compartment this drug might occupy and explain why you made this prediction.

f. Assuming the drug is no longer effective when levels decline to less than 2 $\mu g/mL$, when should you administer the next dose?

5. Define the term *apparent volume of distribution*. What criteria are necessary for the measurement of the apparent volume of distribution to be useful in pharmacokinetic calculations?

6. A drug has an elimination $t_{1/2}$ of 6 hours and follows first-order kinetics. If a single 200-mg dose is given to an adult male patient (68 kg) by IV bolus injection, what percent of the dose is lost in 24 hours?

7. A rather intoxicated young man (75 kg, age 21) was admitted to a rehabilitation center. His blood alcohol content was found to be 210 mg%. Assuming the average elimination rate of alcohol is 10 mL of ethanol per hour, how long would it take for his blood alcohol concentration to decline to less than the legal blood alcohol concentration of 100 mg%? (*Hint:* Alcohol is eliminated by zero-order kinetics.) The specific gravity of alcohol is 0.8. The apparent volume of distribution for alcohol is 60% of body weight.

8. A single IV bolus injection containing 500 mg of cefamandole nafate (Mandol, Lilly) is given to an adult female patient (63 years, 55 kg) for a septicemic infection. The apparent volume of distribution is 0.1 L/kg and the elimination half-life is 0.75 hour. Assuming the drug is eliminated by first-order kinetics and may be described by a one-compartment model, calculate the following:

   a. The C_p^0

   b. The amount of drug in the body 4 hours after the dose is given

   c. The time for the drug to decline to 0.5 μg/mL, the minimum inhibitory concentration for streptococci

9. If the amount of drug in the body declines from 100% of the dose (IV bolus injection) to 25% of the dose in 8 hours, what is the elimination half-life for this drug? (Assume first-order kinetics.)

10. A drug has an elimination half-life of 8 hours and follows first-order elimination kinetics. If a single 600-mg dose is given to an adult female patient (62 kg) by rapid IV injection, what percent of the dose is eliminated (lost) in 24 hours assuming the apparent V_D is 400 mL/kg? What is the expected plasma drug concentration (C_p) at 24 hours postdose?

11. For drugs that follow the kinetics of a one-compartment open model, must the tissues and plasma have the same drug concentration? Why?

12. An adult male patient (age 35 years, weight 72 kg) with a urinary tract infection was given a single intravenous bolus of an antibiotic (dose = 300 mg). The patient was instructed to empty his bladder prior to being medicated. After dose administration, the patient saved his urine specimens for drug analysis. The urine specimens were analyzed for both drug content and sterility (lack of bacteriuria). The drug assays gave the following results:

t (hr)	Amount of Drug in Urine (mg)
0	0
4	100
8	26

   a. Assuming first-order elimination, calculate the elimination half-life for the antibiotic in this patient.

   b. What are the practical problems in obtaining valid urinary drug excretion data for the determination of the drug elimination half-life?

REFERENCE

Huestis MA, Mitchell J, Cone EJ: Prolonged urinary excretion of marijuana metabolite (abstract). Committee on Problems of Drug Dependence, San Juan, PR, June 25, 1996.

BIBLIOGRAPHY

Gibaldi M, Nagashima R, Levy G: Relationship between drug concentration in plasma or serum and amount of drug in the body. *J Pharm Sci* **58:**193–197, 1969

Riegelman S, Loo JCK, Rowland M: Shortcomings in pharmacokinetic analysis by conceiving the body to exhibit properties of a single compartment. *J Pharm Sci* **57:**117–123, 1968

Riegelman S, Loo J, Rowland M: Concepts of volume of distribution and possible errors in evaluation of this parameter. *Science* **57:**128–133, 1968

Wagner JG, Northam JI: Estimation of volume of distribution and half-life of a compound after rapid intravenous injection. *J Pharm Sci* **58:**529–531, 1975

4

MULTICOMPARTMENT MODELS: INTRAVENOUS BOLUS ADMINISTRATION

Pharmacokinetic models may be used to represent drug distribution and elimination in the body. Ideally, a model should mimic closely the physiologic processes in the body. In practice, models seldom consider all the rate processes ongoing in the body and are therefore simplified mathematical expressions. The inability to measure all the rate processes in the body, including the lack of access to biological samples from the interior of the body, limits the sophistication of a model. Compartmental models are classical pharmacokinetic models that simulate the kinetic processes of drug absorption, distribution, and elimination with little physiologic detail. In contrast, the more sophisticated physiologic model is discussed in Chapter 22. In compartmental models, drug tissue concentration is assumed to be uniform within a given hypothetical compartment. Hence, all muscle mass and connective tissues may be lumped into one hypothetical tissue compartment that equilibrates with drug from the central (or plasma) compartment. Since no data is collected on the tissue mass, the theoretical tissue concentration is unconstrained and cannot be used to forecast actual tissue drug levels. However, tissue drug uptake and tissue drug binding from the plasma fluid is kinetically simulated by considering the presence of a tissue compartment. Indeed, most drugs given by IV bolus dose decline rapidly soon after injection, and then decline moderately as some of the drug initially distributes into the tissue moves back into the plasma.

Multicompartment models were developed to explain this observation that, after a rapid IV injection, the plasma level–time curve does not decline linearly as a single, first-order rate process. The plasma level–time curve reflects first-order elimination of the drug from the body only after distribution equilibrium, or plasma drug equilibrium with peripheral tissues occurs. Drug kinetics after distribution is characterized by the first-order rate constant, b (or beta, β).

Nonlinear plasma level–time curves occur because some drugs distribute at various rates into different tissue groups. Multicompartment models were developed to explain and predict plasma and tissue concentrations for the behavior of these drugs. In contrast, a one-compartment model is used when the drug appears to distribute into tissues instantaneously and uniformly. For both one- and multicompartment models, the drug in the tissues that have the highest blood perfusion equilibrates rapidly with the drug in the plasma. These highly perfused tissues and blood make up the *central compartment*. While this initial drug distribution is taking place, multicompartment drugs are delivered concurrently to one or more *peripheral compartments* composed of groups of tissues with lower blood perfusion and different affinity for the drug. A drug will concentrate in a tissue in accordance with the affinity of the drug for that particular tissue. For example, lipid-soluble drugs tend to accumulate in fat tissues. Drugs that bind plasma proteins may be more concentrated in the plasma, because protein-bound drugs do not diffuse easily into the tissues. Drugs may also bind with tissue proteins and other macromolecules, such as DNA and melanin. Tissue sampling is invasive, and the drug concentration in the tissue sample may not represent the drug concentration in the entire organ. Occasionally, tissue samples may be collected after a drug-overdose episode. For example, the two-compartment model has been used to describe the distribution of colchicine, even though the drug's toxic tissue levels after fatal overdoses has only been recently described (Rochdi et al, 1992). The drug isotretinoin has a long half-life because of substantial distribution into lipid tissues.

Kinetic analysis of a multicompartment model assumes that all transfer rate processes for the passage of drug into or out of individual compartments are first-order processes. On the basis of this assumption, the plasma level–time curve for a drug that follows a multicompartment model is best described by the summation of a series of exponential terms, each corresponding to first-order rate processes associated with a given compartment.

Because of these distribution factors, drugs will generally concentrate unevenly in the tissues, and different groups of tissues will accumulate the drug at different rates. A summary of the approximate blood flow to major human tissues is presented in Table 4.1. Many different tissues and rate processes are involved in the distribution of any drug. However, limited physiologic significance has been assigned to a few groups of tissues (Table 4.2).

The nonlinear profile of plasma drug concentration versus time is the result of many factors interacting together, including blood flow to the tissues, the permeability of the drug into the tissues, the capacity of the tissues to accumulate drug, and the effect of disease factors on these processes (see Chapter 10). Impaired cardiac function may produce a change in blood flow and in the drug distributive phase, whereas impairment of the kidney or the liver may decrease drug elimination as shown by a prolonged elimination half-life and corresponding reduction in the slope of the terminal elimination phase of the curve. Frequently, multiple factors can complicate the distribution profile in such a way that the profile can only be described clearly with the assistance of a simulation model.

TABLE 4.1 Blood Flow to Human Tissues

TISSUE	PERCENT BODY WEIGHT	PERCENT CARDIAC OUTPUT	BLOOD FLOW (mL/100 g tissue per min)
Adrenals	0.02	1	550
Kidneys	0.4	24	450
Thyroid	0.04	2	400
Liver			
Hepatic	2.0	5	20
Portal		20	75
Portal-drained viscera	2.0	20	75
Heart (basal)	0.4	4	70
Brain	2.0	15	55
Skin	7.0	5	5
Muscle (basal)	40.0	15	3
Connective tissue	7.0	1	1
Fat	15.0	2	1

Adapted with permission from Butler (1972).

TWO-COMPARTMENT OPEN MODEL

Many drugs given in a single intravenous bolus dose demonstrate a plasma level–time curve that does not decline as a single exponential (first-order) process. The plasma level–time curve for a drug that follows a two-compartment model (Fig. 4-1) shows that the plasma drug concentration declines *biexponentially* as the sum of two first-order processes—distribution and elimination. A drug that follows the pharmaco-kinetics of a two-compartment model does not equilibrate rapidly throughout the body, as is assumed for a one-compartment model. In this model, the drug distributes into two compartments, the central compartment and the tissue, or peripheral compartment. The *central compartment* represents the blood, extracellular fluid, and highly perfused tissues. The drug distributes rapidly and uniformly in the central compartment. A second compartment, known as the *tissue* or *peripheral compartment,* contains tissues in which the drug equilibrates more slowly. Drug transfer between the two compartments is assumed to take place by first-order processes.

TABLE 4.2 General Grouping of Tissues According to Blood Supply[a]

BLOOD SUPPLY	TISSUE GROUP	PERCENT BODY WEIGHT
Highly perfused	Heart, brain, hepatic-portal system, kidney, and endocrine glands	9
	Skin and muscle	50
	Adipose (fat) tissue and marrow	19
Slowly perfused	Bone, ligaments, tendons, cartilage, teeth, and hair	22

[a]Tissue uptake will also depend on such factors as fat solubility, degree of ionization, partitioning, and protein binding of the drug.

Adapted from Eger (1963).

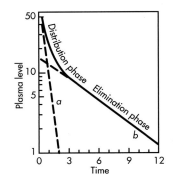

Figure 4-1. *Plasma level–time curve for the two-compartment open model (single IV dose) described in Figure 4-2 (model A).*

There are several possible two-compartment models (Fig. 4-2). Model A is used most often and describes the plasma level–time curve observed in Figure 4-1. By convention, compartment 1 is the central compartment and compartment 2 is the tissue compartment. The rate constants k_{12} and k_{21} represent the first-order rate transfer constants for the movement of drug from compartment 1 to compartment 2 (k_{12}) and from compartment 2 to compartment 1 (k_{21}). The transfer constants are sometimes termed *microconstants*, and their values cannot be estimated directly. Most two-compartment models assume that elimination occurs from the central compartment model, as shown in Figure 4-2 (model A), unless other information about the drug is known. Drug elimination is presumed to occur from the central compartment, because the major sites of drug elimination (renal excretion and hepatic drug metabolism) occur in organs, such as the kidney and liver, which are highly perfused with blood.

The plasma level–time curve for a drug that follows a two-compartment model may be divided into two parts, (*a*) a distribution phase and (*b*) an elimination phase. The two-compartment model assumes that, at $t = 0$, no drug is in the tissue compartment. After an IV bolus injection, drug equilibrates rapidly in the central compartment. The *distribution phase* of the curve represents the initial, more rapid decline of drug from the central compartment into the tissue compartment (Fig. 4-1, line *a*). Although drug elimination and distribution occur *concurrently* during the distribution phase, there is a net transfer of drug from the central compartment

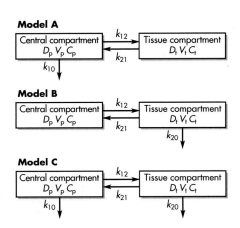

Figure 4-2. *Two-compartment open models, intravenous injection.*

to the tissue compartment. The fraction of drug in the tissue compartment during the distribution phase increases up to a maximum in a given tissue, whose value may be greater or less than the plasma drug concentration. At maximum tissue concentrations, the rate of drug entry into the tissue equals the rate of drug exit from the tissue. The fraction of drug in the tissue compartment is now in equilibrium (*distribution equilibrium*) with the fraction of drug in the central compartment (Fig. 4-3), and the drug concentrations in both the central and tissue compartments decline in parallel and more slowly compared to the distribution phase. This decline is a first-order process and is called the *elimination phase* or the *beta* (β) phase (Fig. 4-1, line *b*). Since plasma and tissue concentrations decline in parallel, plasma drug concentrations provide some indication of the concentration of drug in the tissue. At this point, drug kinetics appear to follow a one-compartment model in which drug elimination is a first-order process described by *b* (also known as beta). A typical tissue drug level curve after a single intravenous dose is shown in Figure 4-3.

Tissue drug concentrations are theoretical only. The drug level in the theoretical tissue compartment can be calculated once the parameters for the model are determined. However, the drug concentration in the tissue compartment represents the average drug concentration in a group of tissues rather than any real anatomic tissue drug concentration. In reality, drug concentrations may vary among different tissues and possibly within an individual tissue. These varying tissue drug concentrations are due to differences in the partitioning of drug into the tissues, as discussed in Chapter 10. In terms of the pharmacokinetic model, the differences in tissue drug concentration is reflected in the k_{12}/k_{21} ratio. Thus, tissue drug concentration may be higher or lower than the plasma drug concentrations, depending on the properties of the individual tissue. Moreover, the elimination of drug from the tissue compartment may not be the same as the elimination from the central compartment. For example, if $k_{12} \cdot C_p$ is greater than $k_{21} \cdot C_t$ (rate into tissue > rate out of tissue), the tissue drug concentrations will increase and plasma drug concentrations will decrease. Real tissue drug concentration can sometimes be calculated by the addition of compartments to the model until a compartment that mimics the experimental tissue concentrations is found.

In spite of the hypothetical nature of the tissue compartment, the theoretical tissue level is still valuable information for clinicians. The theoretical tissue concentration, together with the blood concentration, gives an accurate method of calculating the total amount of drug remaining in the body at any time (see digoxin example later, Table 4.5). This information would not be available without pharmacokinetic models.

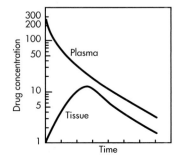

Figure 4-3. Relationship between tissue and plasma drug concentrations for a two-compartment open model. The maximum tissue drug concentration may be greater or less than the plasma drug concentration.

In practice, a blood sample is removed periodically from the central compartment and the plasma is analyzed for the presence of drug. The drug plasma level–time curve represents a phase of initial rapid equilibration with the central compartment (the distribution phase) followed by an elimination phase after the tissue compartment has also been equilibrated with drug. The distribution phase may take minutes or hours and may be missed entirely if the blood is sampled too late or at wide intervals after drug administration.

In the model depicted above, k_{12} and k_{21} are first-order rate constants that govern the rate of drug change in and out of the tissues:

$$\frac{dC_t}{dt} = k_{12}C_p - k_{21}C_t \tag{4.1}$$

The relationship between the amount of drug in each compartment and the concentration of drug in that compartment is shown by Equations 4.2 and 4.3:

$$C_p = \frac{D_p}{V_p} \tag{4.2}$$

$$C_t = \frac{D_t}{V_t} \tag{4.3}$$

where D_p = amount of drug in the central compartment, D_t = amount of drug in the tissue compartment, V_p = volume of drug in the central compartment, and V_t = volume of drug in the tissue compartment.

$$\frac{dC_p}{dt} = k_{21}\frac{D_t}{V_t} - k_{12}\frac{D_p}{V_p} - k\frac{D_p}{V_p} \tag{4.4}$$

$$\frac{dC_t}{dt} = k_{12}\frac{D_p}{V_p} - k_{21}\frac{D_t}{V_t} \tag{4.5}$$

Solving Equations 4.4 and 4.5 will give Equations 4.6 and 4.7, which describe the change in drug concentration in the blood and in the tissue with respect to time:

$$C_p = \frac{D_P^0}{V_P}\left(\frac{k_{21} - a}{b - a}e^{-at} + \frac{k_{21} - b}{a - b}e^{-bt}\right) \tag{4.6}$$

$$C_t = \frac{D_P^0}{V_t}\left(\frac{k_{12}}{b - a}e^{-at} + \frac{k_{12}}{a - b}e^{-bt}\right) \tag{4.7}$$

$$D_p = D_P^0\left(\frac{k_{21} - a}{b - a}e^{-at} + \frac{k_{21} - b}{a - b}e^{-bt}\right) \tag{4.8}$$

$$D_t = D_P^0\left(\frac{k_{12}}{b - a}e^{-at} + \frac{k_{12}}{a - b}e^{-bt}\right) \tag{4.9}$$

where D_P^0 = dose given intravenously, t = time after administration of dose, and a and b are constants that depend solely on k_{12}, k_{21}, and k. The amount of drug remaining in the plasma and tissue compartment at any time may be described realistically by Equations 4.8 and 4.9.

The rate constants for the transfer of drug between compartments are referred to as *microconstants* or *transfer constants,* and relate the amount of drug being transferred per unit time from one compartment to the other. The values for these microconstants cannot be determined by direct measurement but can be estimated by a graphic method.

$$a + b = k_{12} + k_{21} + k \tag{4.10}$$
$$ab = k_{21}k \tag{4.11}$$

The constants a and b are hybrid first-order rate constants for the distribution phase and elimination phase, respectively. The mathematical relationship of a and b to the rate constants are given by Equations 4.10 and 4.11, which are derived after integration of Equations 4.4 and 4.5. Equation 4.6 can be transformed into the following expression:

$$C_p = Ae^{-at} + Be^{-bt} \tag{4.12}$$

The constants a and b are rate constants for the distribution phase and elimination phase, respectively. The constants A and B are intercepts on the y axis for each exponential segment of the curve in Equation 4.12. These values may be obtained graphically by the method of residuals or by computer. Intercepts A and B are actually hybrid constants, as shown in Equations 4.13 and 4.14, and do not have actual physiologic significance.

$$A = \frac{D_0(a - k_{21})}{V_p(a - b)} \tag{4.13}$$

$$B = \frac{D_0(k_{21} - b)}{V_p(a - b)} \tag{4.14}$$

Method of Residuals

The *method of residuals* (also known as *feathering* or *peeling*) is a useful procedure for fitting a curve to the experimental data of a drug when the drug does not clearly follow a one-compartment model. For example, 100 mg of a drug was administered by rapid IV injection to a 70-kg, healthy adult male. Blood samples were taken periodically after the administration of drug, and the plasma fraction of each sample was assayed for drug. The following data were obtained:

Time (hr)	Plasma Concentration (μg/mL)
0.25	43.00
0.5	32.00
1.0	20.00
1.5	14.00
2.0	11.00
4.0	6.50
8.0	2.80
12.0	1.20
16.0	0.52

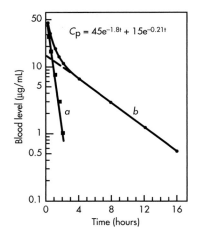

Figure 4-4. Plasma level–time curve for a two-compartment open model. The rate constants and intercepts were calculated by the method of residuals.

When these data are plotted on semilogarithmic graph paper, a curved line is observed (Fig. 4-4). The curved-line relationship between the logarithm of the plasma concentration and time indicates that the drug is distributed in more than one compartment. From these data a biexponential equation, Equation 4.12, may be derived, either by computer or by the method of residuals.

As shown in the biexponential curve in Figure 4-4, the decline in the initial distribution phase is more rapid than the elimination phase. The rapid distribution phase is confirmed with the constant a being larger than the rate constant b. Therefore, at some later time the term Ae^{-at} will approach zero, while Be^{-bt} will still have a value. At this later time Equation 4.12 will reduce to

$$C_p = Be^{-bt} \tag{4.15}$$

which, in common logarithms, is

$$\log C_p = \frac{-bt}{2.3} + \log B \tag{4.16}$$

From Equation 4.16, the rate constant can be obtained from the slope ($-b/2.3$) of a straight line representing the terminal exponential phase (Fig. 4-4). The $t_{1/2}$ for the elimination phase (beta half-life) can be derived from the following relationship:

$$t_{1/2_b} = \frac{0.693}{b} \tag{4.17}$$

In the sample case considered here, b was found to be 0.21 hr^{-1}. From this information the regression line for the terminal exponential or b phase is extrapolated to the y axis; the y intercept is equal to B, or 15 μg/mL. Values from the extrapolated line are then subtracted from the original experimental data points (Table 4.3) and a straight line is obtained. This line represents the rapidly distributed a phase (Fig. 4-4).

The new line obtained by graphing the logarithm of the residual plasma concentration ($C_p - C'_p$) against time represents the a phase. The value for a is 1.8 hr^{-1},

TABLE 4.3 Application of the Method of Residuals

TIME (hr)	C_p OBSERVED PLASMA LEVEL	C_p' EXTRAPOLATED PLASMA CONCENTRATION	$C_p - C_p'$ RESIDUAL PLASMA CONCENTRATION
0.25	43.0	14.5	28.5
0.5	32.0	13.5	18.5
1.0	20.0	12.3	7.7
1.5	14.0	11.0	3.0
2.0	11.0	10.0	1.0
4.0	6.5		
8.0	2.8		
12.0	1.2		
16.0	0.52		

and the y intercept is 45 μg/mL. The elimination $t_{1/2b}$ is computed from b by use of Equation 4.17 and has the value of 3.3 hr.

A number of pharmacokinetic parameters may be derived by proper substitution of rate constants a and b and y intercepts A and B into the following equations:

$$k = \frac{ab(A + B)}{Ab + Ba} \tag{4.18}$$

$$k_{12} = \frac{AB(b - a)^2}{(A + B)(Ab + Ba)} \tag{4.19}$$

$$k_{21} = \frac{Ab + Ba}{A + B} \tag{4.20}$$

Simulation of Plasma and Tissue Level of a Two-Compartment Model Drug—Digoxin in a Normal Patient and in a Renal-Failure Patient

Once the pharmacokinetic parameters are determined for an individual, the amount of drug remaining in the plasma and tissue compartment may be calculated using Equations 4.8 and 4.9. The pharmacokinetic data for digoxin was calculated in a normal and in a renal-impaired, 70-kg subject using the parameters in Table 4.4 as reported in the literature. The amount of digoxin remaining in the plasma and tissue compartment are tabulated in Table 4.5 and plotted in Figure 4-5.

TABLE 4.4 Two-Compartment Model Pharmacokinetic Parameters of Digoxin

PARAMETER	UNIT	NORMAL	RENAL IMPAIRED
k_{12}	hr^{-1}	1.02	0.45
k_{21}	hr^{-1}	0.15	0.11
k	hr^{-1}	0.18	0.04
V_p	L/kg	0.78	0.73
D	μg/kg	3.6	3.6
a	1/hr	1.331	0.593
b	1/hr	0.019	0.007

It can be seen that digoxin stored in the plasma declines rapidly during the initial distributive phase, while drug amount in the tissue compartment take 3–4 hours ($5t_{1/2} = 5 \times 35$ min) to accumulate. It is interesting that clinicians have recommended that digoxin plasma samples be taken at least several hours after IV bolus dosing (3−4+ hr, Winters, 1994, and 4–8 hr, Schumacher, 1995), since the equilibrated level is more representative of myocardium digoxin level. In the simulation below, the amount of the drug in the plasma compartment at any time divided by V_p (54.6 L for the normal subject) will yield the plasma digoxin level. At 4 hours after an IV dose of 0.25 mg, $C_p = D_p/V_p = 24.43$ μg/54.6 L = 0.45 ng/mL, corresponding to 3×0.45 ng/mL = 1.35 ng/mL if a full loading dose of 0.75 mg is given in a single dose. Although the initial plasma drug levels were much higher than after equilibration, the digoxin plasma concentrations are generally regarded as not toxic, since drug distribution is occurring rapidly. The tissue drug levels were not calculated. The tissue drug concentration represents the hypothetical tissue pool, which may not represent actual drug concentrations in the myocardium. In contrast, the amount of drug remaining in the tissue pool is real, since the amount of drug is calculated using mass balance. The rate of drug entry into the tissue in micrograms per hour at any time is $k_{12}D_p$, while the rate of drug leaving the tissue is $k_{21}D_t$ in the same units. Both of these rates may be calculated from Table 4.5 using k_{12} and k_{21} values listed in Table 4.4.

Although some clinicians assume that tissue and plasma concentrations are equal when at full equilibration, tissue and plasma drug ratios are determined by

TABLE 4.5 Amount of Digoxin in Plasma and Tissue Compartment after an IV Dose of 0.252 mg in a Normal and a Renal-Failure Patient Weighing 70 kg[a]

	DIGOXIN AMOUNT			
	NORMAL RENAL FUNCTION		RENAL FAILURE (RF)	
Time (hr)	D_p (μg)	D_t (μg)	D_p (μg)	D_t (μg)
0.00	252.00	0.00	252.00	0.00
0.10	223.68	24.04	240.01	11.01
0.60	126.94	105.54	189.63	57.12
1.00	84.62	140.46	158.78	85.22
2.00	40.06	174.93	107.12	131.72
3.00	27.95	181.45	78.44	156.83
4.00	24.43	180.62	62.45	170.12
5.00	23.17	177.91	53.48	176.88
6.00	22.53	174.74	48.39	180.04
7.00	22.05	171.50	45.45	181.21
8.00	21.62	168.28	43.69	181.29
9.00	21.21	165.12	42.59	180.77
10.00	20.81	162.01	41.85	179.92
11.00	20.42	158.96	41.32	178.89
12.00	20.03	155.97	40.89	177.77
13.00	19.65	153.04	40.53	176.60
16.00	18.57	144.56	39.62	173.00
24.00	15.95	124.17	37.44	163.59

[a]D_p, drug in plasma compartment; D_t, drug in tissue compartment.

Source: Data generated from parameters published by Harron (1989).

Figure 4-5. Amount of digoxin (simulated) in plasma and tissue compartment after an IV dose to a normal and a renal-failure (RF) patient.

the partition coefficient (a drug-specific physical ratio that measures the lipid/water affinity of a drug) and the extent of protein binding of the drug. Figure 4-5 shows that the time for the RF (renal failure or renal impaired) patient to reach stable tissue drug levels is longer than the time for the normal subject due to changes in the elimination and transfer rate constants. As expected, a significantly higher amount of digoxin remains in both the plasma and tissue compartment in the renally impaired subject compared to the normal subject.

PRACTICE PROBLEM

From Figure 4-5 or Table 4.4, how many hours does it take for maximum tissue concentration to be reached in the normal and the renal-impaired patient?

Solution

At maximum tissue concentration, the rate of drug entering the tissue compartment is equal to the rate leaving (ie, at the peak of the tissue curve, where the slope = 0 or not changing). This occurs at about 3–4 hours for the normal patient and at 7–8 hours for the renal-impaired patient. This may be verified by examining at what time $D_p k_{12} = D_t k_{21}$ using the data from Tables 4.4 and 4.5. Before maximum C_t is reached, there is a net flux of drug into the tissue, ie, $D_p k_{12} > D_t k_{21}$, and beyond this point, there is a net flux of drug out the tissue compartment, ie, $D_t k_{12} > D_p k_{12}$.

Apparent Volumes of Distribution

As discussed in Chapter 3, the apparent V_D is a useful parameter that relates plasma concentration to the amount of drug in the body. For drugs with large extravascular distribution, the apparent volume of distribution is generally large. Conversely, for polar drugs with low lipid solubility, the apparent V_D is generally small. Drugs with high peripheral tissue binding also contribute to a large apparent V_D. In multiple-compartment kinetics, such as the two-compartment model, several volumes of distribution can be calculated. Volumes of distribution generally reflect the extent of drug distribution in the body on a relative basis, and the calculations depend on the availability of data. In general, it is important to refer to the same volume parameter when comparing kinetic changes in disease states. Unfortunately, values of apparent volumes of distribution of drugs from tables in the clinical literature are often listed without specifying the underlying kinetic processes, model parameter, or method of calculation.

Volume of the Central Compartment

The volume of the central compartment is useful for determining the drug concentration directly after an IV injection into the body. In clinical pharmacy, this volume is also referred to as V_i or the initial volume of distribution as the drug distributes within the plasma and other accessible body fluids. This volume is generally smaller than the terminal volume of distribution after drug distribution to tissue is completed. The volume of the central compartment is generally greater than 3 L, which is the volume of the plasma fluid for an average adult. For many polar drugs, an initial volume of 7–10 L may be interpreted as rapid drug distribution within the plasma and some extracellular fluids. For example, the V_p of moxalactam ranges from 0.12 to 0.15 L/kg, corresponding to about 8.4 to 10.5 L for a typical 70-kg patient (Table 4.6). In contrast, V_p of hydromorphone is about 24 L, possibly because of its rapid exit from the plasma into tissues even during the initial phase.

As in the case of the one-compartment model, V_p may be determined from the dose and the instantaneous plasma–drug concentration, C_p^0. V_p is also useful in the determination of drug clearance if k is known, as in Chapter 3.

In the two-compartment model, V_p may also be considered as a mass balance factor governed by the mass balance between dose and concentration, ie, drug concentration multiplied by the volume of the fluid must equal the dose at time zero. At time zero, no drug is eliminated, $D_0 = V_p C_p$. The basic model assumption

TABLE 4.6   *Pharmacokinetic Parameters (mean ± SD) of Moxalactam in Three Groups of Patients*

GROUP	A μg/mL	B μg/mL	a hr^{-1}	b hr^{-1}	k hr^{-1}
1	138.9 ± 114.9	157.8 ± 87.1	6.8 ± 4.5	0.20 ± 0.12	0.38 ± 0.26
2	115.4 ± 65.9	115.0 ± 40.8	5.3 ± 3.5	0.27 ± 0.08	0.50 ± 0.17
3	102.9 ± 39.4	89.0 ± 36.7	5.6 ± 3.8	0.37 ± 0.09	0.71 ± 0.16

GROUP	CL mL/min	V_p L/kg	V_t L/kg	$(V_D)_{ss}$ L/kg	$(V_D)_\beta$ L/kg
1	40.5 ± 14.5	0.12 ± 0.05	0.08 ± 0.04	0.20 ± 0.09	0.21 ± 0.09
2	73.7 ± 13.1	0.14 ± 0.06	0.09 ± 0.04	0.23 ± 0.10	0.24 ± 0.12
3	125.9 ± 28.0	0.15 ± 0.05	0.10 ± 0.05	0.25 ± 0.08	0.29 ± 0.09

is that plasma–drug concentration is representative of drug concentration within the distribution fluid. If this statement is true, then the volume of distribution will be 3 L; if it is not, then distribution of drug may also occur outside the vascular pool.

$$V_p = \frac{D_0}{C_p^0} \tag{4.21}$$

At zero time $(t = 0)$, all of the drug in the body is in the central compartment. C_p^0 can be shown to be equal to $A + B$ by the following equation.

$$C_p = Ae^{-at} + Be^{-bt} \tag{4.22}$$

At $t = 0$, $e^0 = 1$. Therefore,

$$C_p^0 = A + B \tag{4.23}$$

V_p is determined from Equation 4.24 by measuring A and B after feathering the curve, as discussed previously:

$$V_p = \frac{D_0}{A + B} \tag{4.24}$$

Alternatively, the volume of the central compartment may be calculated from the $[\text{AUC}]_0^\infty$ in a manner similar to the calculation for the apparent V_D in the one-compartment model. For a one-compartment model,

$$[\text{AUC}]_0^\infty = \frac{D_0}{kV_D} \tag{4.25}$$

In contrast, $[\text{AUC}]_0^\infty$ for the two-compartment model is

$$[\text{AUC}]_0^\infty = \frac{D_0}{kV_p} \tag{4.26}$$

Rearrangement of this equation yields

$$V_p = \frac{D_0}{k[\text{AUC}]_0^\infty} \tag{4.27}$$

Apparent Volume of Distribution at Steady State

At steady-state conditions, the rate of drug entry into the tissue compartment from the central compartment is equal to the rate of drug exit from the tissue compartment into the central compartment. These rates of drug transfer are described by the following expressions:

$$D_t k_{21} = D_p k_{12} \tag{4.28}$$

$$D_t = \frac{k_{12} D_p}{k_{21}} \tag{4.29}$$

Because the amount of drug in the central compartment, D_p, is equal to $V_p C_p$, by substitution in the above equation,

$$D_t = \frac{k_{12} C_p V_p}{k_{21}} \tag{4.30}$$

The total amount of drug in the body at steady state is equal to the sum of the amount of drug in the tissue compartment, D_t, and the amount of drug in the central compartment, D_p. Therefore, the apparent volume of drug at steady state $(V_D)_{ss}$ may be calculated by dividing the total amount of drug in the body by the concentration of drug in the central compartment at steady state:

$$(V_D)_{ss} = \frac{D_p + D_t}{C_p} \tag{4.31}$$

By substitution of Equation 4.30 into Equation 4.31, and by expressing D_p as $V_p C_p$, a more useful equation for the calculation of $(V_D)_{ss}$ is obtained:

$$(V_D)_{ss} = \frac{C_p V_p + k_{12} V_p C_p / k_{21}}{C_p} \tag{4.32}$$

which reduces to

$$(V_D)_{ss} = V_p + \frac{k_{12}}{k_{21}} V_p \tag{4.33}$$

In practice, Equation 4.33 is used to calculate $(V_D)_{ss}$. The $(V_D)_{ss}$ is a function of the transfer constants, k_{12} and k_{21}, which represent the rate constants of drug going into and out of the tissue compartment, respectively. The magnitude of $(V_D)_{ss}$ is dependent on the hemodynamic factors responsible for drug distribution and on the physical properties of the drug, properties which, in turn, determine the relative amount of intra- and extravascular drug remaining in the body.

Extrapolated Volume of Distribution

The extrapolated volume of distribution $(V_D)_{exp}$ is calculated by the following equation:

$$(V_D)_{exp} = \frac{D_0}{B} \tag{4.34}$$

where B is the y intercept obtained by extrapolation of the b phase of the plasma level curve to the y axis (Fig. 4-4). Because the y intercept is a hybrid constant, as shown by Equation 4.14, $(V_D)_{exp}$ may also be calculated by the following expression:

$$(V_D)_{exp} = V_p \left(\frac{a - b}{k_{21} - b} \right) \tag{4.35}$$

This equation shows that a change in the distribution of a drug, which is observed by a change in the value for V_p, will be reflected in a change in $(V_D)_{exp}$.

Volume of Distribution by Area

The volume of distribution by area $(V_D)_{area}$, also known as $(V_D)_\beta$, is obtained through calculations similar to those used to find V_p, except that the rate constant b is used instead of the overall elimination rate constant k. $(V_D)_\beta$ is often calculated from total body clearance divided by b and is influenced by drug elimination in the beta, or b phase. Reduced drug clearance from the body may increase AUC, such that $(V_D)_\beta$ is either reduced or unchanged depending on the value of b, as shown by Equation 4.35.

$$(V_D)_\beta = (V_D)_{area} = \frac{D_0}{b[\text{AUC}]_0^\infty} \tag{4.36}$$

Generally, reduced drug clearance is accompanied by a decrease in the constant b (ie, an increase in the b elimination half-life). For example, in patients with renal dysfunction, the elimination half-life of the antibiotic amoxacillin is longer because renal clearance is reduced.

Because total body clearance is equal to $D_0/[\text{AUC}]_0^\infty$, $(V_D)_\beta$ may be expressed in terms of clearance and the rate constant b:

$$(V_D)_\beta = \frac{\text{clearance}}{b} \tag{4.37}$$

By substitution of kV_p for clearance in Equation 4.37, one obtains:

$$(V_D)_\beta = \frac{kV_p}{b} \tag{4.38}$$

Theoretically, the value for b may remain unchanged in patients showing various degrees of moderate renal impairment. In this case, a reduction in $(V_D)_\beta$ may account for all the decrease in Cl, while b is unchanged in Equation 4.38. Within the body, a redistribution of drug between the plasma and the tissue will mask the expected decline in b. The following example in two patients shows that the b elimination rate constant remains the same, while the distributional rate constants change. Interestingly, V_p is unchanged, while $(V_D)_\beta$ would be greatly changed in the simulated example. An example of a drug showing constant b slope while the renal function as measured by Cl_{cr} decreases from 107 to 56, 34, and 6 mL/min (chapter 6) has been observed with the aminoglycoside drug gentamicin in various patients after IV bolus dose (Schentag et al, 1977). Gentamicin follows polyexponential decline with a significant distributive phase. The following simulation problem may help to clarify the situation by changing k and clearance while keeping b constant.

PRACTICE PROBLEM

Simulated plasma drug concentration after an IV bolus dose (100 mg) of an antibiotic in two patients, Patient 1 with a normal k, and Patient 2 with a reduced k, is shown in Figure 4-6. The data in the two patients were simulated with parameters using the two-compartment model equation. The parameters used are as follows:

Normal subject, $k = 0.3$ hr^{-1}, $V_p = 10$ L, $Cl = 3$ L/hr
$k_{12} = 5$ hr^{-1}, $k_{21} = 0.2$ hr^{-1}

Subject with moderate renal impairment, $k = 0.1$ hr^{-1}, $V_p = 10$ L, $Cl = 1$ L/hr
$k_{12} = 2$ hr^{-1}, $k_{21} = 0.25$ hr^{-1}

Questions

1. Is a reduction in drug clearance generally accompanied by increase in plasma drug concentration, regardless of which compartment model the drug follows?

2. Is a reduction in drug clearance generally accompanied by an increase in the b elimination half-life of a drug? [Find $(V_D)_\beta$ using Eq. 4.37, then b using Eq. 4.38.]

3. Many antibiotics follow multiexponential plasma drug concentration profiles showing drug distribution into tissue compartments. In clinical pharmacokinetics, the terminal half-life is often determined with limited early data. Which patient has a greater terminal half-life based on the simulated data?

Solution

1. A reduction in drug clearance results in less drug being removed from the body per unit time. Drug clearance is model independent. Therefore, the plasma drug

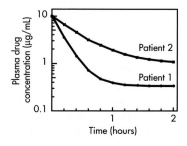

Figure 4-6.   *Simulation of plasma drug concentration after an IV bolus dose (100 mg) of an antibiotic in two patients, one with a normal k (patient 1) and the other, reduced k (patient 2).*

concentration should be higher in subjects with decreased drug clearance compared to subjects with normal drug clearance, regardless of which compartment model is used (see Fig. 4-6).

2. Clearance in the two-compartment model is affected by the elimination rate constant, b, and the volume of distribution in the b phase, which reflects the data. A decrease in the $(V_D)_\beta$ with b unchanged is possible, although this is not the common case. When this happens, the terminal data (see Fig. 4-6) concludes that the beta elimination half-life of patients 1 and 2 are the same due to a similar b. Actually, the real elimination half-life of the drug derived from k is a much better parameter, since k reflects the changes in renal function, but not b, which remains unchanged since it is masked by the changes in $(V_D)_\beta$.

3. Both patients have the same b value ($b = 0.011$ hr^{-1}); the terminal slopes are identical. Ignoring early points by only taking terminal data would lead to an erroneous conclusion that the renal elimination process is unchanged, while the volume of distribution of the renally impaired patient is smaller. In this case, the renally impaired patient has a clearance of 1 L/hr compared with 3 L/hr for the normal subject, and yet the terminal slopes are the same. The rapid distribution of drug into the tissue in the normal subject causes a longer and steeper distribution phase. Later, redistribution of drug out of tissues masks the effect of rapid drug elimination through the kidney. In the renally impaired patient, distribution to tissue is reduced; as a result, little drug is redistributed out from the tissue in the b phase. Hence, it appears that the beta phases are identical in the two patients.

Significance of the Volumes of Distribution

From Equations 4.31 and 4.32 we can observe that $(V_D)_\beta$ is affected by changes in the overall elimination rate (ie, change in k) and by change in total body clearance of the drug. After the drug is distributed, the total amount of drug in the body during the elimination of b phase is calculated by using $(V_D)_\beta$.

V_p is sometimes called the initial volume of distribution and is useful in the calculation of drug clearance. The magnitudes of the various apparent volumes of distribution have the following relationships to each other:

$$(V_D)_{exp} > (V_D)_\beta > V_p$$

Calculation of another V_D, $(V_D)_{ss}$, is possible in multiple dosing or infusion (see Chapters 5 and 8). $(V_D)_{ss}$ is much larger than V_p; it approximates $(V_D)_\beta$ but differs somewhat in value, depending on the transfer constants.

In a study involving a cardiotonic drug given intravenously to a group of normal and congestive heart failure (CHF) patients, the average AUC for CHF was 40% higher than in the normal subjects. The b elimination constant was 40% less in CHF patients, whereas the average $(V_D)_\beta$ remained essentially the same. In spite of the edematous conditions of these patients, the volume of distribution apparently remained constant. No change was found in the V_p or $(V_D)_\beta$. In this study, a 40%

increase in AUC in the CHF subjects was offset by a 40% smaller b elimination constant estimated by using computer methods. Because the dose was the same, the $(V_D)_\beta$ would not change unless the increase in AUC is not accompanied by a change in b elimination constant.

From Equation 4.31, the clearance of the drug in CHF patients was reduced by 40% and accompanied by a corresponding decrease in the b elimination constant, possibly due to a reduction in renal blood flow as a result of reduced cardiac output in CHF patients. In physiologic pharmacokinetics, clearance (Cl) and volume of distribution (V_D) are assumed to be independent parameters that explain the impact of disease factors on drug disposition. Thus, an increase in AUC of a cardiotonic in a CHF patient was assumed to be due to a reduction in drug clearance, since the volume of distribution was unchanged. The elimination half-life was reduced due to reduction in drug clearance. In reality, pharmacokinetic changes in a complex system are dependent on many factors that interact within the system. Clearance is affected by drug uptake, metabolism, binding, and more; all of these factors can also influence the drug distribution volume. Many parameters are assumed to be constant and independent for simplification of the model. Blood flow is an independent parameter that will affect both clearance and distribution. However, blood flow is, in turn, affected and regulated by many physiologic compensatory factors.

For drugs that follow two-compartment model kinetics, changes in disease states may not result in different pharmacokinetic parameters. Conversely, changes in pharmacokinetic parameters should not be attributed to physiologic changes without careful consideration of method of curve fitting and intersubject differences. Equation 4.38 shows that, unlike a simple one-compartment open model, $(V_D)_\beta$ may be estimated from k, b, and V_p. Errors in fitting are easily carried over to the other parameter estimates even if the calculations are performed by computer. The terms k_{12} and k_{21} often fluctuate due to minor fitting and experimental difference and may affect calculation of other parameters.

Drug in the Tissue Compartment

The apparent volume of the tissue compartment (V_t) is a conceptual volume only and does not represent true anatomic volumes. The V_t may be calculated from knowledge of the transfer rate constants and V_p:

$$V_t = \frac{V_p k_{12}}{k_{21}} \qquad (4.39)$$

The calculation of the amount of drug in the tissue compartment does not entail the use of V_t. Calculation of the amount of drug in the tissue compartment provides an estimate for drug accumulation in the tissues of the body. This information is vital in estimating chronic toxicity and relating the duration of pharmacologic activity to dose. Tissue compartment drug concentration is an average estimate of the tissue pool and does not mean that all tissues have this concentration. The drug concentration in a tissue biopsy will provide an estimate for drug in that tissue sample. Due to differences in blood flow and drug partitioning into the tissue, and heterogenicity, even a biopsy from the same tissue may have different drug concentrations. Together with V_p and C_p, which calculate the amount of drug in the plasma, the compartment model provides mass balance information. Moreover, the pharmacodynamic activity may correlate better with the tissue drug concentration–time curve. To calculate the amount of drug in the tissue compartment D_t, the following expression is used:

$$D_t = \frac{k_{12} D_p^0}{a - b}\left(e^{-bt} - e^{-at}\right) \tag{4.40}$$

PRACTICAL FOCUS

The therapeutic plasma concentration of digoxin is between 1 and 2 ng/mL; because digoxin has a long elimination half-life, digoxin takes a long time to reach a stable, constant (steady-state) level in the body. A loading dose is usually given with the initiation of digoxin therapy. Consider the implications of the loading dose of 1 mg suggested for a 70-kg subject. The clinical source cited an apparent volume of distribution of 7.3 L/kg for digoxin in determining the loading dose of digoxin. Use the pharmacokinetic parameters for digoxin in Table 4.4.

Solution

The loading dose was calculated by considering the body as a one-compartment during steady state, at which time the drug well penetrates the tissue compartment. The volume of distribution $(V_D)_\beta$ of digoxin is much larger than V_p, or the volume of the plasma compartment.

Using Equation (4.38),

$$(V_D)_\beta = \frac{kV_p}{b}$$

$$= \frac{0.18/\text{hr} \times 0.78\ \text{L/kg}}{0.19/\text{hr}} = 7.39\ \text{L/kg}$$

$$D_L = 7390\ \frac{\text{mL}}{\text{kg}} \times 70\ \text{kg} \times 1.5\ \frac{\text{ng}}{\text{mL}}$$

The loading dose is generally divided into two or three doses or is administered as 50% in the first dose and the remaining drug given in two divided doses 6–8 hours apart to minimize potential side effects from overdigitization. If the entire loading dose were administered intravenously, the plasma level would be about 4–5 ng/mL after 1 hour, while the level would drop to about 1.5 ng/mL at about 4 hours. The exact level after a given IV dose may be calculated using Equation 4.6 at any time desired. The pharmacokinetic parameters for digoxin are available in Table 4.4.

Drug Clearance

The definition of clearance of a drug that follows a two-compartment model is similar to that of the one-compartment model. *Clearance* is the volume of plasma that is cleared of drug per unit time. Clearance may be calculated without consideration of the compartment model. Thus, clearance may be viewed as a physiologic concept for drug removal, even though the development of clearance is rooted in classical pharmacokinetics.

Clearance is often calculated by a noncompartmental approach, as in Equation 4.35, in which the bolus IV dose is divided by the area under the plasma–time concentration curve from zero to infinity, $[\text{AUC}]_0^\infty$. In evaluating the $[\text{AUC}]_0^\infty$, early time points must be collected frequently to observe the rapid decline in drug concentrations (distribution phase) for drugs with multicompartment pharmacokinetics. In the calculation of clearance using the noncompartmental approach, underestimating the area can inflate the calculated value of clearance.

$$Cl = \frac{D_0}{[\text{AUC}]_0^\infty} \tag{4.41}$$

Equation 4.41 may be rearranged to Equation 4.42 to show that Cl in the two-compartment model is the product of $(V_D)_\beta$ and b.

$$Cl = (V_D)_\beta b \tag{4.42}$$

If both parameters are known, then calculation of clearance is simple and more accurate than using the trapezoidal rule to obtain area. Clearance calculations that use the two-compartment model are viewed as model dependent because more assumptions are required, and such calculations cannot be regarded as noncompartmental. However, the assumptions provide additional information and, in some sense, specifically describe the drug concentration–time profile as biphasic.

Clearance is a term that is useful in calculating average drug concentrations. With many drugs, a biphasic profile suggests a rapid tissue distribution phase followed by a slower elimination phase. Multicompartment pharmacokinetics is an important consideration in understanding drug permeation and toxicity. For example, the plasma–time profiles of aminoglycosides, such as gentamicin, are more useful in explaining toxicity than average plasma or drug concentration taken at peak or trough time.

Elimination Rate Constant

In the two-compartment model (IV administration), the elimination rate constant, k, represents the elimination of drug from the central compartment, whereas b represents drug elimination during the beta or elimination phase, when distribution is mostly complete. Because of redistribution of drug out of the tissue compartment, the plasma–drug level curve declines more slowly in the b phase. Hence b is smaller than k; thus k is a true elimination constant, whereas b is a hybrid elimination rate constant that is influenced by the rate of transfer of drug in and out of the tissue compartment. When it is impractical to determine k, b is calculated from the b slope. The $t_{1/2\beta}$ is often used to calculate the drug dose.

THREE-COMPARTMENT OPEN MODEL

The three-compartment model is an extension of the two-compartment model, with an additional deep tissue compartment. A drug that demonstrates the necessity of a three-compartment open model is distributed most rapidly to a highly perfused central compartment, less rapidly to the second or tissue compartment, and very slowly to the third or deep tissue compartment, containing such poorly perfused tissue as bone and fat. The deep tissue compartment may also represent tightly bound drug in the tissues. The three-compartment open model is shown in Figure 4-7.

A solution of the differential equation describing the rates of flow of drug into and out of the central compartment gives the following equation:

$$C_p = Ae^{-at} + Be^{-bt} + Ce^{-ct} \tag{4.43}$$

where A, B, and C are the y intercepts of extrapolated lines for the central, tissue, and deep tissue compartments, respectively, and a, b, and c are first-order rate constants for the central, tissue, and deep tissue compartments, respectively.

A three-compartment equation may be written by statisticians in the literature as

$$C_p = Ae^{-\lambda_1 t} + Be^{-\lambda_2 t} + Ce^{-\lambda_3 t} \tag{4.43a}$$

instead of a, b, c, etc., $\lambda_1, \lambda_2, \lambda_3$ are substituted to express the triexponential feature of the equation. Similarly, the n-compartment model may be expressed with $\lambda_1, \lambda_2, \ldots, \lambda_n$. In classical pharmacokinetics, the symbols a, b, c that we have adopted are actually Greek symbols, α, β, χ. The preexponential terms are sometimes expressed as C_1, C_2, and C_3.

The parameters in Equation 4.43 may be solved graphically by the method of residuals (Fig. 4-8) or by computer. The calculations for the elimination rate constant k, volume of the central compartment, and area are shown in the following equations:

$$k = \frac{(A + B + C)abc}{Abc + Bac + Cab} \tag{4.44}$$

$$V_p = \frac{D_0}{A + B + C} \tag{4.45}$$

$$[\text{AUC}] = \frac{A}{a} + \frac{B}{b} + \frac{C}{c} \tag{4.46}$$

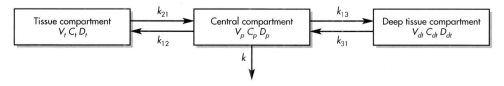

Figure 4-7. Three-compartment open model. This model, as with the previous two-compartment models, assumes that all drug elimination occurs via the central compartment.

$$C_p = 70e^{-1.5t} + 20e^{-0.2t} + 24e^{-0.03t}$$

Figure 4-8.   *Plasma level–time curve for a three-compartment open model. The rate constants and intercepts were calculated by the method of residuals.*

 PRACTICAL FOCUS

Hydromorphone (Dilaudid)

Three independent studies on the pharmacokinetics of hydromorphone after a bolus intravenous injection reported that hydromorphone followed the pharmacokinetics of a one-compartment model (Vallner et al, 1981), a two-compartment model (Parab et al, 1988) or a three-compartment model (Hill et al, 1991), respectively. A comparison of these studies is listed in Table 4.7.

Comments

The adequacy of the pharmacokinetic model will depend on the sampling intervals and the drug assay. The first two studies showed a similar elimination half-life. However, both Vallner et al (1981) and Parab et al (1988) did not observe a three-compartment pharmacokinetic model due to lack of appropriate description of the early distribution phases for hydromorphone. After an IV bolus injection, hydromorphone is very rapidly distributed into the tissues. Hill et al (1991) obtained a triexponential function by closely sampling early time periods after the dose. Average distribution half-lives were 1.27 and 14.7 min, and the average terminal elimination was 184 min ($t_{1/2\beta}$). The average values for systemic clearance (Cl) was 1.66 L/min; the initial dilution volume was 24.4 L. If distribution is rapid, the drug becomes distributed during absorption. Thus, hydromorphone pharmacokinetics follow a one-compartment model after a single oral dose.

TABLE 4.7 *Comparison of Hydromorphone Pharmacokinetics*

STUDY	TIMING OF BLOOD SAMPLES	PHARMACOKINETIC PARAMETERS
6 Males, 25–29 yrs; mean weight, 76.8 kg Dose, 2-mg IV bolus Vallner et al, 1981	0, 15, 30, 45 min 1, 1.5, 2, 3, 4, 6, 8, 10, 12 hr	One-compartment model Terminal $t_{1/2}$ = 2.64 (± 0.88) hr
8 Males, 20–30 yrs; weight, 50–86 kg Dose, 2-mg IV bolus Parab et al, 1988	0, 3, 7, 15, 30, 45 min 1, 1.5, 2, 3, 4, 6, 8, 10, 12 hr	Two-compartment model Terminal $t_{1/2}$ = 2.36 (± 0.58) hr
10 Males, 21–38 yrs; mean weight, 72.7 kg Dose, 10, 20, and 40 μg/kg, IV bolus Hill et al, 1991	1, 2, 3, 4, 5, 7, 10, 15, 20, 30, 45 min 1, 1.5, 2, 2.5, 3, 4, 5 hr	Three-compartment model Terminal $t_{1/2}$ = 3.07 (± 0.25) hr

Hydromorphone is administered to relieve acute pain in cancer or postoperative patients. Rapid pain relief is obtained by IV injection. Although the drug is effective orally, about 50–60% of the drug is cleared by the liver through first-pass effects. The pharmacokinetics of hydromorphone after IV injection suggest a multicompartment model. The site of action is probably within the central nervous system, as part of the tissue compartment. The initial volume or initial dilution volume, V_p, is the volume into which IV injections are injected and diluted. Hydromorphone follows linear kinetics, ie, drug concentration is proportional to dose. Hydromorphone systemic clearance is much larger than the glomerular filtration rate (GFR) of 120 mL/min (see chapter 6), hence the drug is probably metabolized significantly by the hepatic route. A clearance of 1.66 L/min is faster than the blood flow of 1.2–1.5 L/min to the liver. The drug must be rapidly extracted or, in addition, must have extrahepatic elimination. When the distribution phase is short, the distribution phase may be disregarded, provided that the targeted plasma concentration is sufficiently low and the terminal elimination phase is relatively long. If the drug has a sufficiently high target plasma drug concentration and the elimination half-life is short, the distributive phase must not be ignored. For example, lidocaine target effective concentration often lies close to the distributive phase, since its beta elimination half-life is very short; and ignoring the alpha phase will result in a large error in dosing projection.

DETERMINATION OF COMPARTMENT MODELS

Models based on compartmental analysis should always use the fewest number of compartments necessary to describe the experimental data adequately. Once an empirical equation is derived from the experimental observations, it becomes necessary to examine how well the theoretical values that are calculated from the derived equation fit the experimental data.

The observed number of compartments or exponential phases will depend on (1) the route of drug administration, (2) the rate of drug absorption, (3) the total time for blood sampling, (4) the number of samples taken within the collection period, and (5) the assay sensitivity. If drug distribution is rapid, then, after oral administration, the drug will become distributed during absorption, and the distribution phase will not be observed. For example, theophylline follows the kinetics of a one-compartment model after oral absorption, but after intravenous bolus (given as aminophylline), theophylline follows the kinetics of a two-compartment model. Furthermore, if theophylline is given by a slow intravenous infusion rather than by intravenous bolus, the distribution phase will not be observed. Hydromorphone (Dilaudid), which follows a three-compartment model, also follows a one-compartment model after oral administration, since the first two distribution phases are rapid.

Depending on the sampling intervals, a compartment may be missed because samples may be taken too late after administration of the dose to observe a possible distributive phase. For example, the data plotted in Figure 4-9 could easily be mistaken for those of a one-compartment model, because the distributive phase has been missed and extrapolation of the data to C_p^0 will give a lower value than was actually the case. Slower drug elimination compartments may also be missed if sampling is not performed at later sampling times, when the dose or the assay for the drug cannot measure very low plasma drug concentrations.

The total time for collection of blood samples is usually estimated from the terminal elimination half-life of the drug. However, lower drug concentrations may not be measured if the sensitivity of the assay is not adequate. As the assay for the drug becomes more sensitive in its ability to measure lower drug concentrations, then another compartment with a smaller first-order rate constant may be observed.

In describing compartments, each new compartment requires an additional first-order plot. Compartment models having more than three compartments are rarely of pharmacologic significance. In certain cases, it is possible to "lump" a few compartments together to get a smaller number of compartments, which, together, will describe the data adequately.

An adequate description of several tissue compartments can be difficult. When the addition of a compartment to the model seems necessary, it is important to realize that the drug may be retained or slowly concentrated in a deep tissue compartment.

Figure 4-9. *The samples from which data were obtained for this graph were taken too late to show the distributive phase; therefore, the value of C_p^0 obtained by extrapolation (straight broken line) is deceptively low.*

PRACTICAL FOCUS

**Two-Compartment Model: Relation between Distribution
and Apparent (Beta) Half-Life**

The distribution half-life of a drug is dependent on the type of tissues the drug penetrates as well as by blood supply to those tissues. In addition, the capacity of the tissue to store drug is also a factor. Distribution half-life is generally short for many drugs because of the rapid blood supply and drug equilibration in the tissue compartment. However, there is some supporting evidence that a drug with a long elimination half-life is often associated with a longer distribution phase. It is conceivable that a tissue with little blood supply may not attain a sufficiently high drug concentration to exert its impact and influence the overall plasma drug concentration profile in the presence of rapid elimination. In contrast, drugs such as digoxin have a long elimination half-life, and drug concentration declines slowly to allow more time for distribution to tissues. Human follicle-stimulating hormone (hFSH) injected intravenously has a very long elimination half-life, and its distribution half-life is also quite long. Drugs such as lidocaine, theophylline, and milrinone have short elimination half-lives and generally relatively short distributional half-lives.

In order to examine the effect of changing k (from 0.6 to 0.2 hr^{-1}) on the distributional (alpha phase) and elimination (beta phase) half-lives of various drugs, four simulations based on a two-compartment model were generated (Table 4.8). The simulations show that a drug with a smaller k has a longer beta elimination half-life. Keeping all other parameters (k_{12}, k_{21}, V_p) constant, a smaller k will result

TABLE 4.8 Comparison of Beta Half-Life and Distributional Half-Life of Selected Drugs

DRUG	BETA HALF-LIFE	DISTRIBUTIONAL HALF-LIFE
Lidocaine	1.8 hr	8 min
Cocaine	1 hr	18 min
Theophylline	4.33 hr	7.2 min
Ergometrine	2 hr	11 min
Hydromorphone	3 hr	14.7 min
Milrinone	3.6 hr	4.6 min
Procainamide	2.5–4.7 hr	6 min
Quinidine	6–8 hr	7 min
Lithium	21.39 hr	5 hr
Digoxin	1.6 days	35 min
Human FSH	1 day	60 min
IgG1 kappa MAB	9.6 days (monkey)	6.7 hr
Simulation 1	13.26 hr	36.24 min
Simulation 2	16.60 hr	43.38 min
Simulation 3	26.83 hr	53.70 min
Simulation 4	213.7 hr	1.12 hr

Simulation was performed using V_p of 10 L; dose = 100 mg; $k_{12} = 0.5$ hr^{-1}; $k_{21} = 0.1$ hr^{-1}; $k = 0.6$, 0.4, 0.2, and 0.02 hr for simulations 1–4, respectively (using Eqs. 4.10 and 4.11).

Source: From manufacturer and Schumacher (1995), with permission.

in a smaller *a*, or a slower distributional phase. Examples of drugs with various distribution and elimination half-lives are shown in Table 4.8.

Clinical Example: Moxalactam, Effect of Changing Renal Function in Patients with Sepsis

The pharmacokinetics of moxalactam (see Table 4.6) was examined in 40 patients with abdominal sepsis (Swanson et al, 1983). The patients were grouped according to creatinine clearances into three groups:

Group 1: Average creatinine clearance = 35.5 mL/min/1.73 m^2
Group 2: Average creatinine clearance = 67.1 ± 6.7 mL/min/1.73 m^2
Group 3: Average creatinine clearance = 117.2 ± 29.9 mL/min/1.73 m^2

After intravenous bolus administration, the serum drug concentrations followed a biexponential decline (Fig. 4-10). The pharmacokinetics at steady state (2 g every 8 hr) was also examined in these patients. Mean steady-state serum concentrations ranged from 27.0 to 211.0 μg/mL and correlated inversely with creatinine clearance ($r = 0.91$, $p < 0.0001$). The terminal half-life ranged from 1.27 to 8.27 hours and reflected the varying renal function of the patients. Moxalactam total body clearance (*Cl*) had excellent correlation with creatinine clearance ($r^2 = 0.92$). *Cl* determined by noncompartmental data analysis was in agreement with *Cl* determined by nonlinear least-squares regression ($r = 0.99$, $p < 0.0001$). Moxalactam total body clearance was best predicted from creatinine clearance corrected for body surface area.

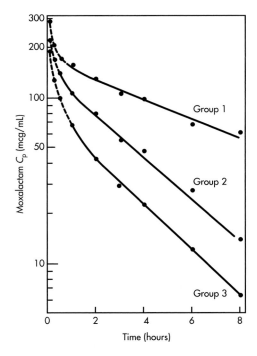

Figure 4-10. Moxalactam serum concentration in three groups of patients: group 1, average creatinine concentration = 35.5 mL/min/1.73 m^2; group 2, average creatinine concentration = 67.1 ± 6.7 mL/min/1.73 m^2; group 3, average creatinine concentration = 117.2 ± 29.9 mL/min/1.73 m^2.

Questions (Refer to Table 4.6)

1. Calculate the beta half-life of moxalactam in the most renally impaired group.

2. What indicator is used to predict moxalactam clearance in the body?

3. What is the beta volume of distribution of patients in group 3 with normal renal function?

4. What is the initial volume (V_i) of moxalactam?

Solutions

1. Mean beta half-life is $0.693/0.20 = 3.47$ hours in the most renally impaired group.

2. Creatinine is mainly filtered through the kidney, and creatinine clearance is used as an indicator of renal glomerular filtration rate. Group 3 has normal renal function (average creatinine clearance $= 117.2$ mL/min/1.73 m^2) (see chapter 6).

3. Beta volume of distribution: Moxalactam clearance in group 3 subjects is 125.9 mL/min. From Equation 4.31,

$$(V_D)_\beta = \frac{\text{clearance}}{b}$$
$$= \frac{125.9 \text{ mL/min} \times 60 \text{ min/hr}}{0.37 \text{ hr}^{-1}}$$
$$= 20,416 \text{ mL} \quad \text{or} \quad 20.4 \text{ L}$$

4. The volume of the plasma compartment, V_p, is sometimes referred to as the initial volume. V_p ranges from 0.12 to 0.15 L/kg among the three groups and is considerably smaller than the steady-state volume of distribution.

Clinical Example: Azithromycin Pharmacokinetics

Following oral administration, azithromycin is rapidly absorbed and widely distributed throughout the body. Azithromycin is rapidly distributed into tissues, with high drug concentrations within cells, resulting in significantly higher azithromycin concentrations in tissue than in plasma. The high values for plasma clearance (630 mL/min) suggest that the prolonged half-life is due to extensive uptake and subsequent release of drug from tissues.

Plasma concentrations of azithromycin decline in a polyphasic pattern, resulting in an average terminal half-life of 68 hours. With this regimen, C_{min} and C_{max} remained essentially unchanged from day 2 through day 5 of therapy. However, without a loading dose, azithromycin C_{min} levels required 5–7 days to reach desirable plasma levels.

The pharmacokinetic parameters of azithromycin in healthy elderly male subjects (65–85 years) were similar to those in young adults. Although higher peak drug concentrations (increased by 30–50%) were observed in elderly women, no significant accumulation occurred.

Questions

1. Do you agree with the following statements for a drug that is described by a two-compartment pharmacokinetic model? At peak C_t, the drug is well equilibrated between the plasma and the tissue compartment, $C_p = C_t$, and the rates of drug diffusion into and from the plasma compartment are equal.

2. What happens after peak C_t?

3. Why is a loading dose used?

4. What is V_i? How is this volume related to V_p?

5. What population factors could affect the concentration of azithromycin?

Solutions

1. For a drug that follows a multicompartment model, the rates of drug diffusion into the tissues from the plasma and from the tissues into the plasma are equal at peak tissue concentrations. However, the tissue drug concentration is generally not equal to the plasma drug concentration.

2. After peak C_t, the rate out of the tissue exceeds the rate into the tissue, and C_t falls. The decline of C_t parallels that of C_p, and occurs because distribution equilibrium has occurred.

3. When drugs are given in a multiple-dose regimen, a loading dose may be given to achieve desired therapeutic drug concentrations more rapidly (see Chapter 8).

4. The volume of the plasma compartment, V_p, is sometimes referred to as the initial volume.

5. Age and gender may affect the C_{max} level of the drug.

Clinical Example: Etoposide

Etoposide is a drug used for the treatment of lung cancer. Understanding the distribution of etoposide in normal and metastatic tissues is important to avoid drug toxicity. Etoposide follows a two-compartment model. The $(V_D)_\beta$ is 0.28 L/kg, and the beta elimination half-life is 12.9 hours. Total body clearance is 0.25 mL/min/kg.

Questions

1. What is the $(V_D)_\beta$ in a 70-kg subject?

2. How is the $(V_D)_\beta$ different than the volume of the plasma fluid, V_p?

3. Why is the $(V_D)_\beta$ useful if it does not represent a real tissue volume?

4. How is $(V_D)_\beta$ calculated from plasma time–concentration profile data for etoposide? Is $(V_D)_\beta$ related to total body clearance?

Solutions

1. $(V_D)_\beta$ of etoposide in a 70-kg subject is 0.28 L/kg $\times$ 70 kg = 19.6 L.

2. The plasma fluid volume is about 3 L in a 70-kg subject and is much smaller than $(V_D)_\beta$. The apparent volume of distribution, $(V_D)_\beta$, is also considerably larger than the volume of the plasma compartment (also referred to as the initial volume by some clinicians), which includes some extracellular fluid.

3. Etoposide is a drug that follows a two-compartment model with a beta elimination phase. Within the first few minutes after an intravenous bolus dose, most of the drug is distributed in the plasma fluid. Subsequently, the drug will diffuse into tissues and drug uptake may occur. Eventually, plasma drug levels will decline due to elimination, and some redistribution as etoposide in tissue diffuses back into the plasma fluid.

The real tissue drug level will differ from the plasma drug concentration, depending on the partitioning of drug in tissues and plasma. This volume of distribution, $(V_D)_\beta$, allows the area under the curve to be calculated, an area that has been related to toxicities associated with many cancer chemotherapy agents.

The two-compartment model allows continuous monitoring of the amount of the drug present in and out of the vascular system, including the amount of drug eliminated. This information is important in pharmacotherapy.

4. $(V_D)_\beta$ may be determined from the total drug clearance and beta:

$$Cl = b \times (V_D)_\beta$$

$(V_D)_\beta$ is also calculated from Equation 4.36 where

$$(V_D)_\beta = (V_D)_{area} = \frac{D_0}{b[\text{AUC}]_0^\infty}$$

This method for $(V_D)_\beta$ determination $[\text{AUC}]_0^\infty$ is popular because $[\text{AUC}]_0^\infty$ is easily calculated using the trapezoidal rule. Many values for apparent volumes of distribution reported in the clinical literature are obtained using the area equation. In general, both volume terms reflect extravascular drug distribution. $(V_D)_\beta$ appears to be affected by the dynamics of drug disposition in the beta phase. In clinical practice, many potent drugs are not injected by bolus dose. Instead, these drugs are infused over a short interval, making it difficult to obtain accurate information on the distributive phase. As a result, many drugs that follow a two-compartment model are approximated using a single compartment. It should be cautioned that there are substantial deviations in some cases. When in doubt, the full equation with all parameters should be applied for comparison. A small bolus (test) dose may be injected to obtain the necessary data if a therapeutic dose injected rapidly causes side effects or discomfort to the subject.

FREQUENTLY ASKED QUESTIONS

1. My preceptors and I both agree that the "hypothetical" or "mathematical" compartment models are just about useless in helping me with dosing in the clinical setting. Does "hypothetical" mean "not real"?

2. What is the apparent volume of distribution, and why are there so many different volumes of distribution?

3. If physiologic models are better than compartment models, why not just use physiologic models?

4. Can I just learn clearance and forget about the other pharmacokinetic parameters, because clearance is the term most often used in clinical pharmacy?

5. What is the error if I assume a one-compartment model instead of a two-compartment or multicompartment model?

6. What kind of improvement in terms of patient care or drug therapy was made using the compartment model?

LEARNING QUESTIONS

1. A drug was administered by rapid IV injection into a 70-kg adult male. Blood samples were withdrawn over a 7-hour period and assayed for intact drug. The results are tabulated below. Using the method of residuals, calculate the values for intercepts A and B and slopes a, b, k, k_{12}, and k_{21}.

Time (hr)	C_p (μg/mL)	Time (hr)	C_p (μg/mL)
0.00	70.0	2.5	14.3
0.25	53.8	3.0	12.6
0.50	43.3	4.0	10.5
0.75	35.0	5.0	9.0
1.00	29.1	6.0	8.0
1.50	21.2	7.0	7.0
2.00	17.0		

2. A 70-kg male subject was given 150 mg of a drug by IV injection. Blood samples were removed and assayed for intact drug. Calculate the slopes and intercepts of the three phases of the plasma level–time plot from the results tabulated below. Give the equation for the curve.

Time (hr)	C_p (μg/mL)	Time (hr)	C_p (μg/mL)
0.17	36.2	3.0	13.9
0.33	34.0	4.0	12.0
0.50	27.0	6.0	8.7
0.67	23.0	7.0	7.7
1.00	20.8	18.0	3.2
1.50	17.8	23.0	2.4
2.00	16.5		

3. Mitenko and Ogilvie (1973) demonstrated that theophylline followed a two-compartment pharmacokinetic model in human subjects. After administering a single intravenous dose (5.6 mg/kg) in nine normal volunteers, these investigators

demonstrated that the equation best describing theophylline kinetics in humans was as follows:

$$C_p = 12e^{-5.8t} + 18e^{-0.16t}$$

What is the plasma level of the drug 3 hours after the IV dose?

4. A drug has a distribution that can be described by a two-compartment open model. If the drug is given by IV bolus, what is the cause of the initial or rapid decline in blood levels (a phase)? What is the cause of the slower decline in blood levels (b phase)?

5. What does it mean when a drug demonstrates a plasma level–time curve that indicates a three-compartment open model? Can this curve be described by a two-compartment model?

6. A drug that follows a multicompartment pharmacokinetic model is given to a patient by rapid intravenous injection. Would the drug concentration in each tissue be the same after the drug equilibrates with the plasma and all the tissues in the body? Explain.

7. Park and associates (1983) studied the pharmacokinetics of amrinone after a single IV bolus injection (75 mg) in 14 healthy adult male volunteers. The pharmacokinetics of this drug followed a two-compartment open model and fit the following equation:

$$C_p - Ae^{-at} + Be^{-at}$$

where

$$A = 4.62 \pm 12.0\,\mu g/mL$$
$$B = 0.64 \pm 0.17\,\mu g/mL$$
$$a = 8.94 \pm 13\ hr^{-1}$$
$$b = 0.19 \pm 0.06\ hr^{-1}$$

From these data, calculate:

a. The volume of the central compartment
b. The volume of the tissue compartment
c. The transfer constants k_{12} and k_{21}
d. The elimination rate constant from the central compartment
e. The elimination half-life of amrinone after the drug has equilibrated with the tissue compartment

8. A drug may be described by a three-compartment model involving a central compartment and two peripheral tissue compartments. If you could sample the tissue compartments (organs), in which organs would you expect to find a drug level corresponding to the two theoretical peripheral tissue compartments?

9. A drug was administered to a patient at 20 mg by IV bolus dose and the time–plasma drug concentration is listed below. Use a suitable compartment model to describe the data and list the fitted equation and parameters. What are the statistical criteria used to describe your fit?

Hour	mg/L
0.20	3.42
0.40	2.25
0.60	1.92
0.80	1.80
1.00	1.73
2.00	1.48
3.00	1.28
4.00	1.10
6.00	0.81
8.00	0.60
10.00	0.45
12.00	0.33
14.00	0.24
18.00	0.13
20.00	0.10

10. The toxicokinetics of colchicine in seven cases of acute human poisoning was studied by Rochdi et al (1992). In three further cases, postmortem tissue concentrations of colchicine were measured. Colchicine follows the two-compartment model with wide distribution in various tissues. Depending on the time of patient admission, two disposition processes were observed. The first, in three patients, admitted early, showed a biexponential plasma colchicine decrease, with distribution half-lives of 30, 45, and 90 minutes. The second, in four patients, admitted late, showed a monoexponential decrease. Plasma terminal half-lives ranged from 10.6 to 31.7 hours for both groups.

11. Postmortem tissue analysis of colchicine showed that colchicine accumulated at high concentrations in the bone marrow (more than 600 ng/g), testicle (400 ng/g), spleen (250 ng/g), kidney (200 ng/g), lung (200 ng/g), heart (95 ng/g), and brain (125 ng/g). The pharmacokinetic parameters of colchicine are:

Fraction of unchanged colchicine in urine = 30%
Renal clearance = 13 L/hr
Total body clearance = 39 L/hr
Apparent volume of distribution = 21 L/kg

   a. Why is colchicine described by a monoexponential profile in some subjects and a biexponential in others?
   b. What is the range of distribution of half-life of colchicine in the subjects?
   c. Which parameter is useful in estimating tissue drug level at any time?
   d. Some clinical pharmacists assumed that, at steady state when equilibration is reached between the plasma and the tissue, the tissue drug concentration would be the same as the plasma. Do you agree?
   e. Which tissues may be predicted by the tissue compartment?

REFERENCES

Butler TC: The distribution of drugs. In LaDu BN et al (eds), *Fundamentals of Drug Metabolism and Disposition.* Baltimore, Williams & Wilkins, 1972

Eger E: In EM Papper and JR Kitz (eds), *Uptake and Distribution of Anesthetic Agents.* New York, McGraw Hill, 1963, p. 76

Harron DWG: Digoxin pharmacokinetic modelling—10 years later. *Int J Pharm* **53:**181–188, 1989

Hill HF, Coda BA, Tanaka A, Schaffer R: Multiple-dose evaluation of intravenous hydromorphone pharmacokinetics in normal human subjects. *Anesth Analg* **72:**330–336, 1991

Mitenko PA, Ogilvie RI: Pharmacokinetics of intravenous theophylline. *Clin Pharmacol Ther* **14:**509, 1973

Parab PV, Ritschel WA, Coyle DE, Gree RV, Denson DD: Pharmacokinetics of hydromorphone after intravenous, peroral and rectal administration to human subjects. *Biopharm Drug Dispos* **9:**187–199, 1988

Park GP, Kershner RP, Angellotti J, et al: Oral bioavailability and intravenous pharmacokinetics of amrinone in humans. *J Pharm Sci* **72:**817, 1983

Rochdi M, Sabouraud A, Baud FJ, Bismuth C, Scherrmann JM: Toxicokinetics of colchicine in humans: Analysis of tissue, plasma and urine data in ten cases. *Hum Exp Toxicol* **11**(6):510–516, 1992

Schentag JJ, Jusko WJ, Plaut ME, Cumbo TJ, Vance JW, and Abutyn E: Tissue persistence of gentamicin in man. *JAMA* **238:**327–329, 1977

Schumacher GE: *Therapeutic Drug Monitoring.* Norwalk, CT, Appleton & Lange, 1995

Swanson DJ, Reitberg DP, Smith IL, Wels PB, Schentag JJ: Steady-state moxalactam pharmacokinetics in patients: Noncompartmental versus two-compartmental analysis. *J Pharmacokinet-Biopharm* **11**(4):337–353, 1983

Vallner JJ, Stewart JT, Kotzan JA, Kirsten EB, Honiger IL: Pharmacokinetics and bioavailability of hydromorphone following intravenous and oral administration to human subjects. *J Clin Pharmacol* **21:**152–156, 1981

Winters ME: *Basic Clinical Pharmacokinetics,* 3rd ed. Vancouver, WA, Applied Therapeutics, 1994, p. 23

BIBLIOGRAPHY

Dvorchick BH, Vessell ES: Significance of error associated with use of the one-compartment formula to calculate clearance of 38 drugs. *Clin Pharmacol Ther* **23:**617–623, 1978

Jusko WJ, Gibaldi M: Effects of change in elimination on various parameters of the two-compartment open model. *J Pharm Sci* **61:**1270–1273, 1972

Loughman PM, Sitar DS, Oglivie RI, Neims AH: The two-compartment open-system kinetic model: A review of its clinical implications and applications. *J Pediatr* **88:**869–873, 1976

Mayersohn M, Gibaldi M: Mathematical methods in pharmacokinetics, II: Solution of the two-compartment open model. *Am J Pharm Ed* **35:**19–28, 1971

Riegelman S, Loo JCK, Rowland M: Concept of a volume of distribution and possible errors in evaluation of this parameter. *J Pharm Sci* **57:**128–133, 1968

Riegelman S, Loo JCK, Rowland M: Shortcomings in pharmacokinetics analysis by conceiving the body to exhibit properties of a single compartment. *J Pharm Sci* **57:**117–123, 1968

INTRAVENOUS INFUSION

Drugs may be administered to patients by one of several routes, including oral, topical, or parenteral routes of administration. Examples of parenteral routes of administration include intravenous, subcutaneous, and intramuscular. Intravenous (IV) drug solutions may be given either as a bolus dose (injected all at once) or infused slowly through a vein into the plasma at a constant or zero-order rate. The main advantage for giving a drug by IV infusion is that IV infusion allows precise control of plasma drug concentrations to fit the individual needs of the patient. For drugs with a narrow therapeutic window (eg, heparin), IV infusion maintains an effective constant plasma drug concentration by eliminating wide fluctuations between the peak (maximum) and trough (minimum) plasma drug concentration. Moreover, the IV infusion of drugs, such as antibiotics, may be given with IV fluids that include electrolytes and nutrients. Furthermore, the duration of drug therapy may be maintained or terminated as needed using IV infusion.

The plasma drug concentration-versus-time curve of a drug given by constant IV infusion is shown in Figure 5-1. Because no drug was present in the body at zero time, drug level rises from zero drug concentration and gradually becomes constant when a *plateau* or *steady-state* drug concentration is reached. At steady state, the rate of drug leaving the body is equal to the rate of drug (infusion rate) entering the body. Therefore, at steady state, the rate of change in the plasma drug concentration, $dC_p/dt = 0$, and

Rate of drug input = rate of drug output
   (infusion rate)   (elimination rate)

Based on this simple mass balance relationship, a pharmacokinetic equation for infusion may be derived depending on whether the drug follows one- or two-compartment kinetics.

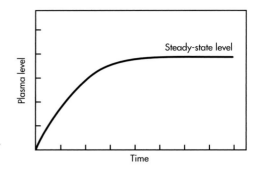

Figure 5-1. Plasma level–time curve for constant IV infusion.

ONE-COMPARTMENT MODEL DRUGS

The pharmacokinetics of a drug given by constant IV infusion follows a zero-order input process in which the drug is infused directly into the systemic blood circulation. Equation 5.2, below, gives the plasma drug concentration at any time during the IV infusion, where t is the time for infusion. The graph of Equation 5.2 appears in Figures 5-1 and 5-2. For most drugs, elimination of drug from the plasma is a first-order process. Therefore, in this one-compartment model, the infused drug follows zero-order input and first-order output. The change in the amount of drug in the body at any time (dD_B/dt) during the infusion is the rate of input minus the rate of output.

$$\frac{dD_B}{dt} = R - kD_B \tag{5.1}$$

where D_B is the amount of drug in the body, R is the infusion rate (zero order), and k is the elimination rate constant (first order).

Integration of Equation 5.1 and substitution of $D_B = C_p V_D$ gives

$$C_p = \frac{R}{V_D k}(1 - e^{-kt}) \tag{5.2}$$

As the drug is infused, the value for time (t) increases in Equation 5.2. At infinite time, $t = \infty$, e^{-kt} approaches zero, and Equation 5.2 reduces to Equation 5.4.

$$C_p = \frac{R}{V_D k}(1 - e^{-\infty}) \tag{5.3}$$

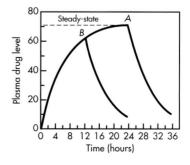

Figure 5-2. Plasma drug concentrations versus time profiles after IV infusion. IV infusion is stopped at steady state (A) or prior to steady state (B). In both cases, plasma drug concentrations decline exponentially (first order) according to a similar slope.

$$C_{SS} = \frac{R}{V_D k} \tag{5.4}$$

$$C_{SS} = \frac{R}{V_D k} = \frac{R}{Cl} \tag{5.5}$$

Steady-State Drug Concentration (C_{SS}) and Time Needed to Reach C_{SS}

As stated earlier, the rate of drug leaving the body is equal to the rate of drug entering the body (infusion rate) at steady state (Fig. 5-2). In other words, there is no *net* change in the amount of drug in the body, D_B, as a function of time during steady state. Drug elimination occurs according to first-order elimination rate. Whenever the infusion stops either at steady state or before steady state is reached, the log drug concentration declines according to first-order kinetics with the slope of the elimination curve equal to $-k/2.3$. If the infusion is stopped before steady state is reached, the slope of the elimination curve remains the same (Fig. 5-2B).

Mathematically, the time to reach true steady-state drug concentration, C_{SS}, would take an infinite time. The time required to reach the steady-state drug concentration in the plasma is dependent on the elimination rate constant of the drug for a constant volume of distribution, as shown in Equation 5.4. Because drug elimination is exponential (first order), the plasma drug concentration becomes asymptotic to the theoretical steady-state plasma drug concentration. For a zero-order elimination process, if the rate of input is greater than the rate of elimination, plasma drug concentration will keep increasing and no steady state will be reached. This is a potentially dangerous situation that will occur when saturation of metabolic process occurs.

In clinical practice, a plasma drug concentration prior to, but asymptotically approaching, the theoretical steady state is considered the steady-state plasma drug concentration (C_{SS}). In a constant IV infusion, drug solution is infused at a constant or zero-order rate, R. During the IV infusion, the drug concentration increases in the plasma and the rate of drug elimination increases because rate of elimination is concentration dependent (ie, rate of drug elimination = kC_p). C_p keeps increasing until steady state is reached, at which time the rate of drug input (IV infusion rate) equals the rate of drug output (elimination rate). The resulting plasma drug concentration at steady state (C_{SS}) is related to the rate of infusion and inversely related to the body clearance of the drug, as shown in Equation 5.5.

In clinical practice, the activity of the drug will be observed when the drug concentration is close to the desired plasma drug concentration, which is usually the *target* or *desired* steady-state drug concentration. The time to reach 90%, 95%, and 99% of the steady-state drug concentration, C_{SS}, may be calculated (Table 5.1). For therapeutic purposes, the time for the plasma drug concentration to reach more than 95% of the steady-state drug concentration in the plasma is often estimated. As detailed in Table 5.1, after IV infusion of the drug for 5 half-lives, the plasma drug concentration will be between 95% ($4.32t_{1/2}$) and 99% ($6.65t_{1/2}$) of the steady-state drug concentration. Thus, the time for a drug whose $t_{1/2}$ is 6 hours to reach at least 95% of the steady-state plasma drug concentration will be $5t_{1/2}$,

TABLE 5.1   Number of $t_{1/2}$ to Reach a Fraction of C_{ss}

PERCENT OF C_{ss} REACHED[a]	NUMBER OF HALF-LIVES
90	3.32
95	4.32
99	6.65

[a]C_{ss} is the steady-state drug concentration in plasma.

or 5×6 hours = 30 hours. The calculation of the values in Table 5.1 is given in the example that follows.

An increase in the infusion rate will not shorten the time to reach the steady-state drug concentration. If the drug is given at a more rapid infusion rate, a higher steady-state drug level will be obtained, but the time to reach steady state is the same (Fig. 5-3). This equation may also be obtained with the following approach. At steady state, the rate of infusion equals the rate of elimination. Therefore, the rate of change in the plasma drug concentration is equal to zero.

$$\frac{dC_p}{dt} = 0$$

$$\frac{dC_p}{dt} = \frac{R}{V_D} - kC_p = 0$$

$$(Rate_{in}) - (rate_{out}) = 0$$

$$\frac{R}{V_D} = kC_p$$

$$C_{ss} = \frac{R}{V_D k} \tag{5.6}$$

Equation 5.6 shows that the steady-state concentration (C_{ss}) is dependent on the volume of distribution, the elimination rate constant, and the infusion rate. Altering any one of these factors can affect steady-state concentration.

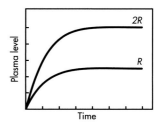

Figure 5-3.   Plasma level–time curve for IV infusions given at rates of R and $2R$, respectively.

EXAMPLES

1. An antibiotic has a volume of distribution of 10 L and a k of 0.2 hr^{-1}. A steady-state plasma concentration of 10 μg/mL is desired. The infusion rate needed to maintain this concentration can be determined as follows.

   Equation 5.6 can be rewritten as

   $$R = C_{SS}\, V_D\, k$$

   $$R = (10\ \mu g/mL)\,(10)\,(1000\ mL)\,(0.2\ hr^{-1})$$

   $$R = 20\ mg/hr$$

   Assume the patient has a uremic condition and the elimination rate constant has decreased to 0.1 hr^{-1}. To maintain the steady-state concentration of 10 μg/mL, we must determine a new rate of infusion as follows.

   $$R = (10\ \mu g/mL)\,(10)\,(1000\ mL)\,(0.1\ hr^{-1}) = 10\ mg/hr$$

   When the elimination rate constant decreases, the infusion rate must decrease proportionately to maintain the same C_{SS}. However, because the elimination rate constant is smaller (ie, the elimination $t_{1/2}$ is longer), the time to reach C_{SS} will be longer.

2. An infinitely long period of time is needed to reach steady-state drug levels. However, in practice it is quite acceptable to reach 99% C_{SS} (ie, 99% steady-state level). Using Equation 5.6, we know that the steady state level is

   $$C_{SS} = \frac{R}{V_D k}$$

   and 99% steady-state level is

   $$99\%\ \frac{R}{V_D k}$$

   Substituting into Equation 5.2 for C_p, we can find the time needed to reach steady state by solving for t.

   $$99\%\ \frac{R}{V_D k} = \frac{R}{V_D k}\,(1 - e^{-kt})$$

   $$99\% = 1 - e^{-kt}$$

   $$e^{-kt} = 1\%$$

   Take the natural logarithm on both sides:

   $$-kt = \ln 0.01$$

$$t_{99\%SS} = \frac{\ln 0.01}{-k} = \frac{-4.61}{-k} = \frac{4.61}{k}$$

substituting $(0.693/t_{1/2})$ for k,

$$t_{99\%SS} = \frac{4.61}{(0.693/t_{1/2})} = \frac{4.61}{0.693} t_{1/2}$$

$$t_{99\%SS} = 6.65 t_{1/2}$$

Notice that in the equation directly above, the time needed to reach steady state is not dependent on the rate of infusion, but only on the elimination half-life. Using similar calculations, the time needed to reach any percentage of the steady-state drug concentration may be obtained (Table 5.1).

Intravenous infusion may be used to determine total body clearance if the infusion rate and steady-state level are known, as with Equation 5.6 repeated here:

$$C_{SS} = \frac{R}{V_D k} \qquad (5.6)$$

$$V_D k = \frac{R}{C_{SS}}$$

because total body clearance, Cl_T, is equal to $V_D k$,

$$Cl_T = \frac{R}{C_{SS}} \qquad (5.7)$$

3. A patient was given an antibiotic ($t_{1/2} = 6$ hr) by constant IV infusion at a rate of 2 mg/hr. At the end of 2 days, the serum drug concentration was 10 mg/L. Calculate the total body clearance Cl_T for this antibiotic.

The total body clearance may be estimated from Equation 5.7. The serum sample was taken after 2 days or 48 hours of infusion, which time represents $8 \times t_{1/2}$, therefore, this serum drug concentration approximates the C_{SS}.

$$Cl_T = \frac{R}{C_{SS}} = \frac{2\,\text{mg/hr}}{10\,\text{mg/L}} = 200 \text{ mL/hr}$$

INFUSION METHOD FOR CALCULATING PATIENT ELIMINATION HALF-LIFE

The C_p-versus-time relationship that occurs during an IV infusion (Eq. 5.2) may be used to calculate k, or indirectly the elimination half-life of the drug in a patient. Some information about the elimination half-life of the drug in the population must be known, and one or two plasma samples must be taken at a known time after infusion. Knowing the half-life in the general population helps to determine if the sample is taken at steady state in the patient. To simplify calculation, Equation 5.2 is arranged to solve for k:

$$C_p = \frac{R}{V_D k} (1 - e^{-kt})$$ (5.2)

Since

$$C_{SS} = \frac{R}{V_D K}$$

Substituting into Equation 5.2;

$$C_p = C_{SS} (1 - e^{-kt})$$

Rearranging and taking the log on both sides,

$$\log\left(\frac{C_{SS} - C_p}{C_{SS}}\right) = -\frac{kt}{2.3} \quad \text{and} \quad k = \frac{-2.3}{t} \log\left(\frac{C_{SS} - C_p}{C_{SS}}\right)$$ (5.8)

where C_p is the plasma drug concentration taken at time t; C_{SS} is the approximate steady-state plasma drug concentration in the patient.

 # EXAMPLE 1

An antibiotic has an elimination half-life of 3–6 hours in the general population. A patient was given an IV infusion of an antibiotic at an infusion rate of 15 mg/hr. Blood samples were taken at 8 and at 24 hours and plasma drug concentrations were 5.5 and 6.5 mg/L, respectively. Estimate the elimination half-life of the drug in this patient.

Solution

Because the second plasma sample was taken at 24 hours, or $24/6 = 4$ half-lives after infusion, the plasma drug concentration in this sample is approaching 95% of the true plasma steady-state drug concentration assuming the extreme case of $t_{1/2} = 6$ hours.
By substitution into Equation 5.8,

$$\log\left(\frac{6.5 - 5.5}{6.5}\right) = -\frac{k(8)}{2.3}$$

$$k = 0.234 \text{ hr}^{-1}$$

$$t_{1/2} = \frac{0.693}{0.234} = 2.96 \text{ hr}$$

The elimination half-life calculated in this manner is not as accurate as the calculation of $t_{1/2}$ using multiple plasma drug concentration time points after a single IV bolus dose or after stopping the IV infusion. However, this method may be sufficient in clinical practice. As the second blood sample is taken closer to the time for steady state, the accuracy of this method improves. At the 30th hour, for example, the plasma concentration would be 99% of the true steady-state value (corresponding to 30/6 or 5 elimination half-lives), and less error would result in applying Equation 5.8.

When Equation 5.8 was used as in the example above to calculate the drug $t_{1/2}$ of the patient, the second plasma drug concentration was assumed to be the theoretical C_{SS}. As demonstrated below, when $t_{1/2}$ and the corresponding values are substituted,

$$\log\left(\frac{C_{SS}-5.5}{C_{SS}}\right) = -\frac{(0.231)(8)}{2.3}$$

$$\frac{C_{SS}-5.5}{C_{SS}} = 0.157$$

$$C_{SS} = 6.5 \text{ mg/L}$$

(Note that C_{SS} is in fact the same as the concentration at 24 hours in the example above.)

In practice, before starting an IV infusion, an appropriate infusion rate (R) is generally calculated from Equation 5.8 using literature values for C_{SS}, k, and V_D or Cl_T. Two plasma samples are taken and the sampling times recorded. The second sample should be taken near the theoretical time for steady state. Equation 5.8 would then be used to calculate a $t_{1/2}$. If the elimination half-life calculated confirms that the second sample was taken at steady state, the plasma concentration is simply assumed as the steady-state concentration and a new infusion rate may be calculated.

 # EXAMPLE 2

If the desired therapeutic plasma concentration is 8 mg/L for the above patient (Example 1), what is a suitable infusion rate for the patient?

Solution

From Example 1, the trial infusion rate was 15 mg/hr. Assuming the second blood sample is the steady-state level, 6.5 mg/mL, the clearance of the patient is

$$C_{SS} = \frac{R}{Cl}$$

$$Cl = \frac{R}{C_{SS}} = 15/6.5 = 2.31 \text{ L/hr}$$

The new infusion rate should be

$$R = C_{SS} \times Cl = 8 \times 2.31 = 18.48 \text{ mg/hr}$$

In this example, the $t_{1/2}$ of this patient is a little shorter, about 3 hours, compared to 3–6 hours reported for the general population. Therefore, the infusion rate should be a little greater in order to maintain the desired steady-state level of 15 mg/L.

Equation 5.7 or the steady-state clearance method has been applied to the clinical infusion of drugs. The method was regarded as simple and accurate compared with other methods, including the two-point method (Hurley and McNeil, 1988).

LOADING DOSE PLUS IV INFUSION: ONE-COMPARTMENT MODEL

The *loading dose*, D_L, or initial bolus dose of a drug, is used to obtain desired concentrations as rapidly as possible. The concentration of drug in the body for a one-compartment model after an IV bolus dose is described by

$$C_1 = C_0 e^{-kt} = \frac{D_L}{V_D} e^{-kt} \tag{5.9}$$

and concentration by infusion at the rate R is

$$C_2 = \frac{R}{V_D k} = (1 - e^{-kt}) \tag{5.10}$$

Assume that an IV bolus dose D_L of the drug is given and that an IV infusion is started at the same time. The total concentration C_p at t hours after the start of infusion is $C_1 + C_2$, due to the sum contributions of bolus and infusion, or

$$C_p = C_1 + C_2$$

$$C_p = \frac{D_L}{V_D} e^{-kt} + \frac{R}{V_D k}(1 - e^{-kt})$$

$$C_p = \frac{D_L}{V_D} e^{-kt} + \frac{R}{V_D k} - \frac{R}{V_D k} e^{-kt}$$

$$C_p = \frac{R}{V_D k} + \left(\frac{D_L}{V_D} e^{-kt} - \frac{R}{V_D k} e^{-kt} \right) \tag{5.11}$$

Let the loading dose (D_L) equal the amount of drug in the body at steady state:

$$D_L = C_{SS} V_D$$

From Equation 5.4, $C_{SS} V_D = R/k$. Therefore,

$$D_L = \frac{R}{k} \tag{5.12}$$

Substituting $D_L = R/k$ in Equation 5.11 makes the expression in parentheses in Equation 5.11 cancel out. Equation 5.11 reduces to Equation 5.13, which is the same expression for C_{SS} or steady-state plasma concentration:

$$C_p = \frac{R}{V_D k} \tag{5.13}$$

$$C_{SS} = \frac{R}{V_D k} \tag{5.14}$$

Therefore, if an IV loading dose of R/k is given, followed by an IV infusion, steady-state plasma drug concentrations are obtained immediately and maintained (Fig. 5-4). In this situation, steady state is also achieved in a one-compartment model, since rate in = rate out ($R = dD_B/dt$).

The loading dose needed to get immediate steady-state drug levels can also be found by the following approach.

Loading dose equation:

$$C_1 = \frac{D_L}{V_D} e^{-kt}$$

Infusion equation:

$$C_2 = \frac{R}{V_D k} (1 - e^{-kt})$$

Adding up the two equations yields Equation 5.15, an equation describing simultaneous infusion after a loading dose:

$$C_2 = \frac{D_L}{V_D} e^{-kt} + \frac{R}{V_D k} (1 - e^{-kt}) \tag{5.15}$$

By differentiating this equation at steady state, we obtain

$$\frac{dC_p}{dt} = 0 = \frac{-D_L k}{V_D} e^{-kt} + \frac{Rk}{V_D k} e^{-kt} \tag{5.16}$$

$$0 = e^{-kt} \left(\frac{-D_L k}{V_D} + \frac{R}{V_D} \right)$$

Figure 5-4. IV Infusion with loading dose D_L. The loading dose is given by IV bolus injection at the start of the infusion. Plasma drug concentrations decline exponentially after D_L whereas they increase exponentially during the infusion. The resulting plasma drug concentration-versus-time curve is a straight line due to the summation of the two curves.

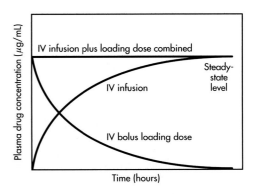

$$\frac{D_L k}{V_D} = \frac{R}{V_D} \tag{5.17}$$

$$D_L = \frac{R}{k} = \text{loading dose}$$

In order to maintain instant steady-state level $[(dC_p/dt) = 0]$, the loading dose should be equal to R/k.

For a one-compartment drug, if the D_L and infusion rate are calculated such that C_0 and C_{SS} are the same and both D_L and infusion are started concurrently, then steady state and C_{SS} will be achieved immediately after the loading dose is administered (Fig. 5-4). Similarly, in Figure 5-5, curve *b* shows the blood level after a single loading dose of R/k plus infusion from which the concentration desired at steady state is obtained. If the D_L is not equal to R/k, then steady state will not occur immediately. If the loading dose given is larger than R/k, the plasma drug concentration takes longer to decline to the concentration desired at steady state (curve *a*). If the loading dose is lower than R/k, the plasma drug concentrations will increase slowly to desired drug levels (curve *c*), but more quickly than without any loading dose.

Another method for the calculation of loading dose D_L is based on knowledge of the desired steady-state drug concentration C_{SS} and the apparent volume of distribution V_D for the drug, as shown in Equation 5.18.

$$D_L = C_{SS} V_D \tag{5.18}$$

For many drugs, the desired C_{SS} is reported in the literature as the effective therapeutic drug concentration. The V_D and the elimination half-life are also available for these drugs.

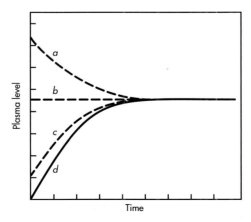

Figure 5-5. Intravenous infusion with loading doses *a*, *b*, and *c*. Curve *d* represents an IV infusion without a loading dose.

PRACTICE PROBLEMS

1. A physician wants to administer an anesthetic agent at a rate of 2 mg/hr by IV infusion. The elimination rate constant is 0.1 hr^{-1}, and the volume of distribution (one compartment) is 10 L. What loading dose should be recommended if the doctor wants the drug level to reach 2 μg/mL immediately?

Solution

$$C_{SS} = \frac{R}{V_D k} = \frac{2000}{(10 \times 10^3)(0.1)} = 2 \ \mu g/mL$$

To reach C_{SS} instantly,

$$D_L = \frac{R}{k} = \frac{2 \ mg/hr}{0.1/hr} \qquad D_L = 20 \ mg$$

2. What is the concentration of a drug 6 hours after administration of a loading dose of 10 mg and simultaneous infusion at 2 mg/hr (the drug has a $t_{1/2}$ of 3 hr and a volume of distribution of 10 L)?

Solution

$$k = \frac{0.693}{3 \ hr}$$

$$C_p = \frac{D_L}{V_D} e^{-kt} - \frac{R}{V_D k}(1 - e^{-kt})$$

$$C_p = \frac{10,000}{10,000} e^{-(0.693/3)(6)} - \frac{2,000}{(10,000)(0.693/3)}(1 - e^{-(0.693/3)(6)})$$

$$C_p = 0.90 \ \mu g/mL$$

3. Calculate the drug concentration in the blood after infusion has been stopped.

Solution

This concentration can be calculated in two parts (see Fig. 5-2, point A). First, calculate the concentration of drug during infusion; and second, calculate the final infusion concentration, C_0. Then use the IV bolus dose equation ($C = C_0 e^{-kt}$) for calculations for any further point in time. For convenience, the two equations can be combined as follows.

$$C_p = \frac{R}{V_D k}(1 - e^{-kb}) e^{-k(t-b)} \qquad\qquad \textbf{(5.19)}$$

where b = length of time of infusion period, t = total time (infusion and postinfusion), and $t - b$ = length of time after infusion has stopped.

4. A patient was infused for 6 hours with a drug ($k = 0.01$ hr^{-1}; $V_D = 10$ L) at a rate of 2 mg/hr. What is the concentration of the drug in the body 2 hours after cessation of the infusion?

Solution

Using Equation 5.19,

$$C_p = \frac{200}{(0.01)(10,000)} (1 - e^{-0.01(6)}) e^{-0.01(8-6)}$$

$$C_p = 1.14 \ \mu g/mL$$

Alternatively, when infusion stops, C_p' is calculated:

$$C_p' = \frac{R}{V_D k} (1 - e^{-kt})$$

$$C_p' = \frac{2,000}{0.01 \times 10,000} (1 - e^{-0.01(6)})$$

$$C = C_p' e^{-0.01(2)}$$

$$C = 1.14 \ \mu g/mL$$

The two approaches should give the same answer.

5. An adult male asthmatic patient (78 kg, 48 years old) with a history of heavy smoking was given an IV infusion of aminophylline at a rate of 0.5 mg/kg per hr. A loading dose of 6 mg/kg was given by IV bolus injection just prior to the start of the infusion. At 2 hours after the start of the IV infusion, the plasma theophylline concentration was measured and found to contain 5.8 $\mu g/mL$ of theophylline. The apparent V_D for theophylline is 0.45 L/kg. Aminophylline is the ethylenediamine salt of theophylline and contains 80% of theophylline base.

Because the patient was responding poorly to the aminophylline therapy, the physician wanted to increase the plasma theophylline concentration in the patient to 10 $\mu g/mL$. What dosage recommendation would you give the physician? Would you recommend another loading dose?

Solution

If no loading dose is given and the IV infusion rate is increased, the time to reach steady-state plasma drug concentrations will be about 4 to 5 $t_{1/2}$ to reach 95% of C_{SS}. Therefore, a second loading dose should be recommended to rapidly increase the plasma theophylline concentration to 10 $\mu g/mL$. The infusion rate must also be increased to maintain this desired C_{SS}.

The calculation of loading dose D_L must consider the present plasma theophylline concentration.

$$D_L = \frac{V_D(C_{p,\text{desired}} - C_{p,\text{present}})}{(S)(F)} \qquad (5.20)$$

where S is the salt form of the drug and F is the fraction of drug bioavailable. For aminophylline, S is equal to 0.80, and for an IV bolus injection, F is equal to 1.

$$D_L = \frac{(0.45 \text{ L/kg})(78 \text{ kg})(10 - 5.8 \text{ mg/L})}{(0.8)(1)}$$

$D_L = 184$ mg aminophylline

The maintenance IV infusion rate may be calculated after estimation of the patient's clearance, Cl_T. Because a loading dose and an IV infusion of 0.5 mg/hr per kilogram was given to the patient, the plasma theophylline concentration of 5.8 mg/L is at steady-state C_{SS}. Total clearance may be estimated by

$$Cl_T = \frac{R}{C_{SS,\text{present}}} = \frac{(0.6 \text{ mg/hr kg})(78 \text{ kg})}{5.8 \text{ mg/L}}$$

$Cl_T = 8.07$ L/hr   or   1.72 mL/min per kg

The usual Cl_T for adult, nonsmoking patients with uncomplicated asthma is approximately 0.65 mL/min per kilogram. Heavy smoking is known to increase Cl_T for theophylline.

The new IV infusion rate, R', is calculated by

$$R' = C_{SS,\text{desired}} \, Cl_T$$

$$R' = \text{mg/L} \times 8.07 \text{ L/hr} = 80.7 \text{ mg/hr} \text{ or } 1.03 \text{ mg/hr per kg}$$

6. An adult male patient (43 years old, 80 kg) is to be given an antibiotic by IV infusion. According to the literature, the antibiotic has an elimination $t_{1/2}$ of 2 hours, a V_D of 1.25 L/kg, and is effective at a plasma drug concentration of 14 mg/L. The drug is supplied in 5-mL ampuls containing 150 mg/mL.

a. Recommend a starting infusion rate in milligrams per hour and liters per hour.

Solution

Assume the effective plasma drug concentration is the target drug concentration or C_{SS}.

$$R = C_{SS} k V_D$$

$$R = (14 \text{ mg/L})(0.693/2 \text{ hr})(1.5 \text{ L/kg})(80 \text{ kg})$$

$$R = 485.1 \text{ mg/hr}$$

Because the drug is supplied at a concentration of 150 mg/mL,

$$(485.1 \text{ mg})(\text{mL}/150 \text{ mg}) = 3.23 \text{ mL}$$

Thus, $R = 3.23$ mL/hr.

b. Blood samples were taken from the patient at 12, 16, and 24 hours after the start of the infusion. Plasma drug concentrations were as shown below:

t (hr)	C_p (mg/L)
12	16.1
16	16.3
24	16.5

From this additional data, calculate the total body clearance Cl_T for the drug in this patient.

Solution

Because the plasma drug concentrations at 12, 16, and 24 hours were similar, steady state has essentially been reached. (Note: The continuous increase in plasma drug concentrations could be caused by drug accumulation due to a second tissue compartment, or could be due to variation in the drug assay.) Assuming a C_{SS} of 16.3 mg/mL, Cl_T is calculated.

$$Cl_T = \frac{R}{C_{SS}} = \frac{485.1 \text{ mg/hr}}{16.3 \text{ mg/L}} = 29.8 \text{ L/hr}$$

c. From the above data, estimate the elimination half-life for the antibiotic in this patient.

Solution

Generally, the apparent volume of distribution (V_D) is less variable than $t_{1/2}$. Assuming that the literature value for V_D is 1.25 L/kg, then $t_{1/2}$ may be estimated from the Cl_T.

$$Cl_T = kV_D$$

$$k = \frac{Cl_T}{V_D} = \frac{29.9 \text{ L/hr}}{(1.25 \text{ L/kg})(80 \text{ kg})} = 0.299 \text{ hr}^{-1}$$

$$t_{1/2} = \frac{0.693}{0.299 \text{ hr}^{-1}} = 2.32 \text{ hr}$$

Thus the $t_{1/2}$ for the antibiotic in this patient is 2.32 hours, which is in good agreement with the literature value of 2 hours.

d. After reviewing pharmacokinetics of the antibiotic in this patient, should the infusion rate for the antibiotic be changed?

Solution

To decide whether the infusion rate should be changed, the clinical pharmacist must consider the pharmacodynamics and toxicity of the drug. Assuming the drug has a wide therapeutic window and shows no sign of adverse drug toxicity, the infusion rate of 485.1 mg/hr, calculated according to pharmacokinetic literature values for the drug, appears to be correct.

$$C_{\mathrm{p}} = \frac{R}{Cl}(1 - e^{-(Cl/V_{\mathrm{D}})t})$$

ESTIMATION OF DRUG CLEARANCE AND V_{D} FROM INFUSION DATA

The plasma concentration of a drug during constant infusion was described in terms of volume of distribution and elimination constant k in Equation 5.2. Alternatively, the equation may be described in terms of clearance by substituting for k into Equation 5.2 with $k = Cl/V_{\mathrm{D}}$:

$$C_{\mathrm{p}} = \frac{R}{Cl}(1 - e^{-(Cl/V_{\mathrm{D}})t}) \tag{5.21}$$

The drug concentration in this physiologic model is described in terms of volume of distribution of V_{D} and total body clearance (Cl). The independent parameters are clearance and volume of distribution; k is viewed as a dependent variable that depends on Cl and V_{D}. In this model, the time to reach steady state and the resulting steady-state concentration will be dependent on both clearance and volume of distribution. When a constant volume of distribution is evident, the time to reach steady state is then inversely related to clearance. Thus, drugs with small clearance will take a long time to reach steady state. Although this newer approach is preferred by some clinical pharmacists, the alternative approach to parameter estimation was known for some time in classical pharmacokinetics. Equation 5.21 has been applied in population pharmacokinetics to estimate both Cl and V_{D} in individual patients with one or more data points. However, clearance in patients may differ greatly from subjects in the population, especially subjects with different renal functions. Unfortunately, the plasma samples taken at time equivalent to less than one half-life after infusion was started may not be very discriminating, due to the small change in the drug concentration. Blood samples taken at 3–4 half-lives later are much more reflective of the difference in clearance.

INTRAVENOUS INFUSION OF TWO-COMPARTMENT MODEL DRUGS

Many drugs given by IV infusion follow two-compartment kinetics. For example, the respective distributions of theophylline and lidocaine in humans are described by the two-compartment open model. With two-compartment model drugs, IV infusion requires a distribution and equilibration of the drug before a stable blood level is reached. During a constant IV infusion, drug in the tissue compartment is in distribution equilibrium with the plasma; thus, constant C_{SS} levels also result in constant drug concentrations in the tissue; ie, no *net* change in the amount of drug in the tissue occurs at steady state. Although some clinicians assume that tissue and plasma concentrations are equal when fully equilibrated, kinetic models predict only that the rates of drug transfer into and out of the compartments are equal at steady state. In other words, drug concentrations in the tissue are also constant, but may differ from plasma concentrations.

The time needed to reach a steady-state blood level depends entirely on the distribution half-life of the drug. The equation describing plasma drug concentration as a function of time is as follows:

$$C_p = \frac{R}{V_p k}\left[1 - \left(\frac{k - b}{a - b}\right)e^{-at} - \left(\frac{a - k}{a - b}\right)e^{-bt}\right] \tag{5.22}$$

where a and b are hybrid rate constants and R is the rate of infusion. At steady state (ie, $t = \infty$), Equation 5.22 reduces to

$$C_{SS} = \frac{R}{V_p k} \tag{5.23}$$

By rearranging this equation, the infusion rate for a desired steady-state plasma drug concentration may be calculated.

$$R = C_{SS}V_p k \tag{5.24}$$

LOADING DOSE PLUS IV INFUSION: TWO-COMPARTMENT MODEL

Drugs with long half-lives require a loading dose to more rapidly attain steady-state plasma drug levels. It is clinically desirable to achieve rapid therapeutic drug levels by using a loading dose. However, for drugs that follow the two-compartment pharmacokinetic model, the drug distributes slowly into extravascular tissues (compartment 2). Thus, drug equilibrium is not immediate. The plasma drug concentration of a drug that follows a two-compartment model after various loading doses is shown in Figure 5-6. If a loading dose is given too rapidly, the drug may initially give

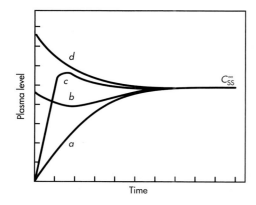

Figure 5-6. *Plasma drug level after various loading doses and rates of infusion for a drug that follows a two-compartment model: a, no loading dose; b, loading dose = R/k (rapid infusion); c, loading dose = R/b (slow infusion); and d, loading dose = R/b (rapid infusion).*

excessively high concentrations in the plasma (central compartment), which then decreases as drug equilibrium is reached (Fig. 5-6). It is not possible to maintain an instantaneous, stable steady-state blood level for a two-compartment model drug with a zero-order rate of infusion. Therefore, a loading dose produces an initial blood level either slightly higher or lower than the steady-state blood level. To overcome this problem, several IV bolus injections given as short intermittent IV infusions may be used as a method for administering a loading dose to the patient (see Chapter 8).

Apparent Volume of Distribution at Steady State, Two-Compartment Model

After administration of any drug that follows two-compartment kinetics, plasma drug levels will decline due to elimination, and some redistribution will occur as drug in tissue diffuses back into the plasma fluid. The volume of distribution at steady state, $(V_D)_{SS}$, is the "hypothetical space" in which the drug is assumed to be distributed. The product of the plasma drug concentration with $(V_D)_{SS}$ will give the total amount of drug in the body at that time period, such that $C_{pSS} \times (V_D)_{SS} =$ amount of drug in the body at steady state. At steady-state conditions, the rate of drug entry into the tissue compartment from the central compartment is equal to the rate of drug exit from the tissue compartment into the central compartment. These rates of drug transfer are described by the following expressions:

$$D_t k_{21} = D_p k_{12} \tag{5.25}$$

$$D_t = \frac{k_{12} D_p}{k_{12}} \tag{5.26}$$

where D_t is the amount of drug in the tissue compartment. Because the amount of drug in the central compartment, D_p, is equal to $V_p C_p$, by substitution in the above equation,

$$D_t = \frac{k_{12} C_p V_p}{k_{21}} \tag{5.27}$$

The total amount of drug in the body at steady state is equal to the sum of the amount of drug in the tissue compartment, D_t, and the amount of drug in the central compartment, D_p. Therefore, the apparent volume of drug at steady state $(V_D)_{SS}$ may be calculated by dividing the total amount of drug in the body by the concentration of drug in the central compartment at steady state:

$$(V_D)_{SS} = \frac{D_p + D_t}{C_p} \tag{5.28}$$

By substitution of Equation 5.27 into Equation 5.28, and by expressing D_p as $V_p C_p$, a more useful equation for the calculation of $(V_D)_{SS}$ is obtained:

$$(V_D)_{SS} = \frac{C_p V_p + k_{12} V_p C_p / k_{21}}{C_p} \tag{5.29}$$

which reduces to

$$(V_D)_{SS} = V_p + \frac{k_{12}}{k_{21}} V_p \tag{5.30}$$

In practice, Equation 5.30 is used to calculate $(V_D)_{SS}$. The $(V_D)_{SS}$ is a function of the transfer constants, k_{12} and k_{21}, which represent the rate constants of drug going into and out of the tissue compartment, respectively. The magnitude of $(V_D)_{SS}$ is dependent on the hemodynamic factors responsible for drug distribution and on the physical properties of the drug, properties which, in turn, determine the relative amount of intra- and extravascular drug.

Another volume term used in two-compartment modeling is $(V_D)_b$ (see Chapter 4). $(V_D)_b$ is often calculated from total body clearance divided by b. Unlike the steady-state volume of distribution, $(V_D)_{SS}$, $(V_D)_b$ is influenced by drug elimination in the beta "b" phase. Reduced drug clearance from the body may increase the area under the curve, AUC, such that $(V_D)_b$ is either reduced or unchanged, depending on the value of b as shown in Equation 4.30 (see Chapter 4):

$$(V_D)_b = (V_D)_{area} = \frac{D_0}{b[AUC]_0^\infty} \tag{4.30}$$

Unlike $(V_D)_b$, $(V_D)_{SS}$ is not affected by changes in drug elimination. $(V_D)_{SS}$ reflects the true distributional volume occupied by the plasma and the tissue pool when steady state is reached. Although this volume is not useful in calculating the amount of drug in the body during pre-steady state, $(V_D)_{SS}$ multiplied by the steady-state plasma drug concentration, C_{SS}, yields the amount of drug in the body. This volume is often used to determine the loading drug dose necessary to upload the body to a desired plasma drug concentration. As shown by Equation 4.30, $(V_D)_{SS}$ is several times greater than V_p, which represents the volume of the plasma compartment, but differs somewhat in value depending on the transfer constants.

PRACTICAL FOCUS

Questions

1. Do you agree with the following statements for a drug that is described by a two-compartment pharmacokinetic model? At steady state, the drug is well equilibrated between the plasma and the tissue compartment, $C_p = C_t$, and the rates of drug diffusion into and from the plasma compartment are equal. The steady-state volume of distribution is much larger than the initial volume, V_i, or the original plasma volume, V_p, of the central compartment. The loading dose is often calculated using the $(V_D)_{SS}$ instead of V_p.

2. Azithromycin may be described by a plasma and a tissue compartment model (refer to Chapter 4).

3. "Rapid distribution of azithromycin into cells causes higher concentration in the tissues than in the plasma. . . ." Does this statement conflict with the steady-state concept?

4. Why is a loading dose used?

Solutions

1. For a drug that follows a multiple-compartment model, the rates of drug diffusion into the tissues from the plasma and from the tissues into the plasma are equal at steady state. However, the tissue drug concentration is generally not equal to the plasma drug concentration.

2. When plasma drug concentration data are used alone to describe the disposition of the drug, no information on tissue drug concentration is known, and no model will predict actual tissue drug concentrations. To account for the mass balance (drug mass/volume = body drug concentration) of drug present in the body (tissue and plasma pool) at any time after dosing, the body drug concentration is assumed to be the plasma drug concentration. In reality, azithromycin tissue concentration is much higher. Therefore, the calculated volume of the tissue compartment is much bigger (31.1 L/kg) than its actual volume.

The product of the steady-state apparent $(V_D)_{SS}$ and the steady-state plasma drug concentration (C_{SS}) estimates the amount of drug present in the body. The amount of drug present in the body may be important information for toxicity considerations, but may be used as a therapeutic end point. In most cases, the therapeutic drug at the site of action accounts for only a small fraction of total drug in the tissue compartment. The pharmacodynamic profile may be described as a separate compartment (see effect compartment in Chapter 19). Based on pharmacokinetic and biopharmaceutic studies, the factors that account for high tissue concentrations include diffusion constant, lipid solubility, and tissue binding to cell components. A ratio measuring the relative drug concentration in tissue and plasma is the partition coefficient, which is helpful in predicting the distribution of a drug into tissues. Ultimately, studies of tissue drug distribution using radiolabeled drug are much more useful.

The real tissue drug level will differ from the plasma drug concentration depending on the partitioning of drug in tissues and plasma. $(V_D)_b$ is a volume of distribution often calculated because it is easier to calculate than $(V_D)_{SS}$. This volume of distribution, $(V_D)_b$, allows the area under the curve to be calculated, an area that has been related to toxicities associated with many cancer chemotherapy agents. Many values for apparent volumes of distribution reported in the clinical literature are obtained using the area equation. Some early pharmacokinetic literature includes only the steady-state volume of distribution, which approximates the $(V_D)_b$ but is substantially smaller in many cases. In general, both volume terms reflect extravascular drug distribution. $(V_D)_b$ appears to be much more affected by the dynamics of drug disposition in the beta phase, whereas $(V_D)_{SS}$ reflects more accurately the inherent distribution of the drug.

3. When drugs are given in a multiple-dose regimen, a loading dose may be given to achieve steady-state drug concentrations more rapidly.

FREQUENTLY ASKED QUESTIONS

1. What is the main reason for giving a drug by slow IV infusion?
2. Why do we use a loading dose to rapidly achieve therapeutic concentration for a drug with a long elimination half-life, instead of increasing the rate of drug infusion or increasing the size of the infusion dose?
3. What are some of the complications involved with IV infusion?

LEARNING QUESTIONS

1. A female patient (35 years old, 65 kg) with normal renal function is to be given a drug by IV infusion. According to the literature, the elimination half-life of this drug is 7 hours and the apparent V_D is 23.1% of body weight. The pharmacokinetics of this drug assumes a first-order process. The desired steady-state plasma level for this antibiotic is 10 μg/mL.

   a. Assuming no loading dose, how long after the start of the IV infusion would it take to reach 95% of the C_{SS}?

   b. What is the proper loading dose for this antibiotic?

   c. What is the proper infusion rate for this drug?

   d. What is the total body clearance?

   e. If the patient suddenly develops partial renal failure, how long would it take for a new steady-state plasma level to be established (assume that 95% of the C_{SS} is a reasonable approximation)?

   f. If the total body clearance declined 50% due to partial renal failure, what new infusion rate would you recommend to maintain the desired steady-state plasma level of 10 μg/mL?

2. An anticonvulsant drug was given as (a) a single IV dose and (b) a constant IV infusion. The serum drug concentrations are as presented in Table 5.2.

   a. What is the steady-state plasma drug level?

   b. What is the time for 95% steady-state plasma drug level?

   c. What is the drug clearance?

   d. What is the plasma concentration of the drug 4 hours after stopping infusion? (Infusion was stopped after 24 hours.)

   e. What is the infusion rate for a patient weighing 75 kg to maintain a steady-state drug level of 10 μg/mL?

   f. What is the plasma drug concentration 4 hours after an IV dose of 1 mg/kg followed by a constant infusion of 0.2 mg/kg per hour?

TABLE 5.2   Serum Drug Concentrations for a Hypothetical Anticonvulsant Drug

	CONCENTRATION IN PLASMA (μg/mL)	
TIME (hr)	Single IV Dose (1 mg/kg)	Constant IV Infusion (0.2 mg/kg per hr)
0	10.0	0
2	6.7	3.3
4	4.5	5.5
6	3.0	7.0
8	2.0	8.0
10	1.35	8.6
12		9.1
18		9.7
24		9.9

3. An antibiotic is to be given by IV infusion. How many milliliters per minute should a sterile drug solution containing 25 mg/mL be given to a 75-kg adult male patient to achieve an infusion rate of 1 mg/kg per hour?

4. An antibiotic drug is to be given to an adult male patient (75 kg, 58 years old) by IV infusion. The drug is supplied in sterile vials containing 30 mL of the antibiotic solution at a concentration of 125 mg/mL. What rate in milliliters per hour would you infuse this patient to obtain a steady-state concentration of 20 μg/mL? What loading dose would you suggest? Assume the drug follows the pharmacokinetics of a one-compartment open model. The apparent volume of distribution of this drug is 0.5 L/kg, and the elimination half-life is 3 hours.

5. According to the manufacturer, a steady-state serum concentration of 17 μg/mL was measured when the antibiotic cephradine (Velosef, Bristol-Meyers, Squibb) was given by IV infusion to 9 adult male volunteers (average weight, 71.7 kg) at a rate of 5.3 mg/kg hr for 4 hours.

   a. Calculate the total body clearance for this drug.

   b. When the IV infusion was discontinued, the cephradine serum concentration decreased exponentially, declining to 1.5 μg/mL at 6.5 hours after the start of the infusion. Calculate the elimination half-life.

   c. From the information above, calculate the apparent volume of distribution.

   d. Cephradine is completely excreted unchanged in the urine, and studies have shown that probenecid given concurrently causes elevation of the serum cephradine concentration. What is the probable mechanism for this interaction of probenecid with cephradine?

6. Calculate the excretion rate at steady state for a drug given by IV infusion at a rate of 30 mg/hr. The C_{SS} is 20 μg/mL. If the rate of infusion were increased to 40 mg/hr, what would be the new steady-state drug concentration, C_{SS}? Would the excretion rate for the drug at the new steady state be the same? Assume first-order elimination kinetics and a one-compartment model.

7. An antibiotic is to be given to an adult male patient (58 years old, 75 kg) by IV infusion. The elimination half-life is 8 hours and the apparent volume of distribution is 1.5 L/kg. The drug is supplied in 60-mL ampules at a drug

concentration of 15 mg/mL. The desired steady-state drug concentration is 20 μg/mL.

a. What infusion rate, in milliliters per hour, would you recommend for this patient?

b. What loading dose would you recommend for this patient? By what route of administration would you give the loading dose? When?

c. Why should a loading dose be recommended?

d. According to the manufacturer, the recommended starting infusion rate is 15 mL/hr. Do you agree with this recommended infusion rate for your patient? Give a reason for your answer.

e. If you were to monitor the patient's serum drug concentration, when would you request a blood sample? Give a reason for your answer.

f. The observed serum drug concentration is higher than anticipated. Give two possible reasons based on sound pharmacokinetic principles that would account for this observation.

8. Which of the following statements **(a–e)** is/are true regarding the time to reach steady state for the three drugs below.

	Drug A	**Drug B**	**Drug C**
Rate of infusion (mg/hr)	10	20	15
k (hr^{-1})	0.5	0.1	0.05
Cl (L/hr)	5	20	5

a. Drug A takes the longest time to reach steady state.

b. Drug B takes the longest time to reach steady state.

c. Drug C takes the longest time to reach steady state.

d. Drug A takes 6.9 hours to reach steady state.

e. None of the above is true.

9. The steady-state drug concentration of a cephalosporin after constant infusion of 250 mg/hr is 45 μg/mL. What is the drug clearance of this cephalosporin?

10. Some clinical pharmacists assumed that, at steady state when equilibration is reached between the plasma and the tissue, the tissue drug concentration would be the same as the plasma. Do you agree?

REFERENCE

Hurley SF, McNeil JJ: A comparison of the accuracy of a least-squares regression, a Bayesian, Chiou's and the steady-state clearance method of individualizing theophylline dosage. *Clin Pharmacokinet* **14:**311–320, 1988

BIBLIOGRAPHY

Gibaldi M: Estimation of the pharmacokinetic parameters of the two-compartment open model from postinfusion plasma concentration data. *J Pharm Sci* **58:**1133–1135, 1969

Koup J, Greenblatt D, Jusko W, et al: Pharmacokinetics of digoxin in normal subjects after intravenous bolus and infusion dose. *J Pharmacokinet Biopharm* **3:**181–191, 1975

Loo J, Riegelman S: Assessment of pharmacokinetic constants from postinfusion blood curves obtained after IV infusion. *J Pharm Sci* **59:**53–54, 1970

Loughnam PM, Sitar DS, Ogilvie RI, Neims AH: The two-compartment open system kinetic model: A review of its clinical implications and applications. *J Pediatr* **88:**869-873, 1976

Mitenko P, Ogilvie R: Rapidly achieved plasma concentration plateaus, with observations on theophylline kinetics. *Clin Pharmacol Ther* **13:**329–335, 1972

Riegelman JS, Loo JC: Assessment of pharmacokinetic constants from postinfusion blood curves obtained after IV infusion. *J Pharm Sci* **59:**53, 1970

Sawchuk RJ, Zaske DE: Pharmacokinetics of dosing regimens which utilize multiple intravenous infusions: Gentamicin in burn patients. *J Pharmacokinet Biopharm* **4:**183–195, 1976

Wagner J: A safe method for rapidly achieving plasma concentration plateaus. *Clin Pharmacol Ther* **16:**691–700, 1974

6

DRUG ELIMINATION AND CLEARANCE

DRUG ELIMINATION

Drugs are removed from the body by various elimination processes. *Drug elimination* refers to the irreversible removal of drug from the body by all routes of elimination. Drug elimination is usually divided into two major components: excretion and biotransformation.

Drug excretion is the removal of the intact drug. Nonvolatile drugs are excreted mainly by renal excretion, a process in which the drug passes through the kidney to the bladder and ultimately into the urine. Other pathways for drug excretion may include the excretion of drug into bile, sweat, saliva, milk (via lactation), or other body fluids. Volatile drugs, such as gaseous anesthetics or drugs with high volatility, are excreted via the lungs into expired air.

Biotransformation or *drug metabolism* is the process by which the drug is chemically converted in the body to a metabolite. Biotransformation is usually an enzymatic process. A few drugs may also be changed chemically by a nonenzymatic process (eg, ester hydrolysis). The enzymes involved in the biotransformation of drugs are located mainly in the liver (Chapter 13). Other tissues such as kidney, lung, small intestine, and skin also contain biotransformation enzymes.

Drug elimination in the body involves many complex rate processes. Although organ systems have specific functions, the tissues within the organs are not structurally homogeneous, and elimination processes may vary in each organ. In Chapter 3, elimination was modeled by an overall first-order elimination rate process. In this chapter, drug elimination is described in terms of clearance from a well-stirred compartment containing uniform drug distribution. The term *clearance* describes the process of drug elimination from the body or from a single organ without identifying the individual processes involved. Clearance may be defined as the volume of fluid cleared of drug from the body per unit of time. The units for clearance are milliliters per minute (mL/min) or liters per hour (L/hr). The volume concept is simple and convenient, because all drugs are dissolved and distributed in the fluids of the body.

The advantage of the clearance approach is that clearance applies to all elimination rate processes, regardless of the mechanism for elimination. In addition, for first–order elimination processes, clearance is a constant, whereas drug elimination rate is not constant. For example, clearance considers that a certain portion or percent of the distribution volume is cleared of drug over a given time period. This basic concept (also see Chapter 3) will be elaborated upon after a review of the anatomy and physiology of the kidney.

THE KIDNEY

The liver (see Chapter 11) and kidney are the two major drug elimination organs in the body, though drug elimination can also occur almost anywhere in the body. The kidney is the main excretory organ for the removal of metabolic waste products and plays a major role in maintaining the normal fluid volume and electrolyte composition in the body. To maintain salt and water balance, the kidney excretes excess electrolytes, water, and waste products while conserving solutes necessary for proper body function. In addition, the kidney has two endocrine functions: (1) secretion of renin, which regulates blood pressure; and (2) secretion of erythropoietin, which stimulates red blood cell production.

Anatomic Considerations

The kidneys are located in the peritoneal cavity. A general view is shown in Figure 6-1 and a longitudinal view in Figure 6-2. The outer zone of the kidney is called the *cortex*, and the inner region is called the *medulla*. The *nephrons* are the basic functional units, collectively responsible for the removal of metabolic waste and the maintenance of water and electrolyte balance. Each kidney contains 1 to 1.5 million nephrons. The *glomerulus* of each nephron starts in the cortex. *Cortical nephrons* have short *loops of Henle* that remain exclusively in the cortex; *juxtamedullary nephrons* have long loops of Henle that extend into the medulla (Fig. 6-3). The longer loops of Henle allow for a greater ability of the nephron to reabsorb water, thereby producing a more concentrated urine.

Figure 6-1.   The general organizational plan of the urinary system.
(From Guyton, 1991, with permission.)

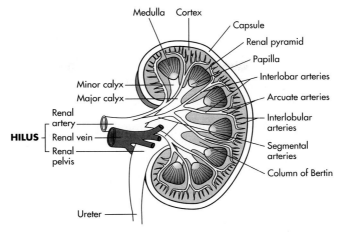

Figure 6-2. Longitudinal section of the kidney, illustrating major anatomical features and blood vessels. (From West, 1985, with permission.)

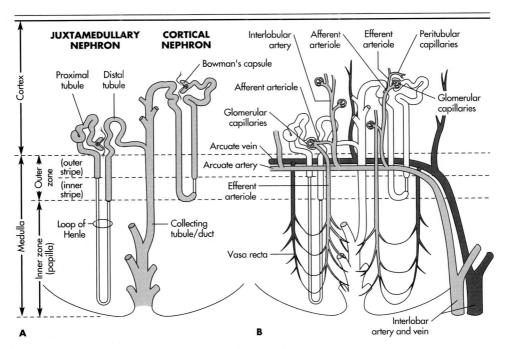

Figure 6-3. Cortical and juxtamedullary nephrons and their vasculature. (From West, 1985, with permission.)

Blood Supply

The kidneys represent about 0.5% of the total body weight and receive approximately 20–25% of the cardiac output. The kidney is supplied by blood via the renal artery, which subdivides into the interlobar arteries penetrating within the kidney and branching farther into the afferent arterioles. Each afferent arteriole carries blood toward a single nephron into the glomerular portion of the nephron (*Bowman's capsule*). The filtration of blood occurs in the glomeruli in Bowman's capsule. From the capillaries (*glomerulus*) within Bowman's capsule, the blood flows out via the efferent arterioles and then into a second capillary network that surrounds the tubules (*peritubule capillaries* and *vasa recti*), including the loop of Henle, where some water is reabsorbed.

The *renal blood flow* (RBF) is the volume of blood flowing through the renal vasculature per unit time. Renal blood flow exceeds 1.2 L/min or 1700 L/day. *Renal plasma flow* (RPF) is the renal blood flow minus the volume of red blood cells present. Renal plasma flow is an important factor in the rate of drug filtration at the glomerulus.

$$RPF = RBF - (RBF \times Hct) \tag{6.1}$$

where Hct is hematocrit.

Hct is the fraction of blood cells in the blood, about 45% of the total blood volume, or 0.45. The relationship of renal blood flow to renal plasma flow is given by a rearrangement of Equation 6.1:

$$RPF = RBF(1 - Hct) \tag{6.2}$$

Assuming a hematocrit of 0.45 and a RBF of 1.2 L/min, using the above equation, RPF = 1.2 − (1.2 × 0.45) = 0.66 L/min or 660 mL/min, approximately 950 L/day. The *glomerular filtration rate* (GFR) is about 125 mL/min in an average adult, or about 20% of the RPF. The ratio GFR/RPF is the *filtration fraction*.

Regulation of Renal Blood Flow

Blood flow to an organ is directly proportional to the arteriovenous pressure difference (*perfusion pressure*) across the vascular bed and indirectly proportional to the vascular resistance. The normal renal arterial pressure (Fig. 6-4) is approximately 100 mmHg

Figure 6-4. Approximate pressures at different points in the vessels and tubules of the functional nephron and in the interstitial fluid. (From Guyton, 1991, with permission.)

Figure 6-5. Schematic representation of the effect of mean arterial pressure on GFR and RPF, illustrating the phenomenon of autoregulation. (From West, 1985, with permission.)

and falls to approximately 45–60 mm Hg in the glomerulus (glomerular capillary hydrostatic pressure). This pressure difference is probably due to the increasing vasculature resistance provided by the small diameters of the capillary network. Thus, the GFR is controlled by changes in the glomerular capillary hydrostatic pressure.

In the normal kidney, RBF and GFR remain relatively constant even with large differences in mean systemic blood pressure (Fig. 6-5). The term *autoregulation* refers to the maintenance of a constant blood flow in the presence of large fluctuations in arterial blood pressure. Because autoregulation maintains a relatively constant blood flow, the filtration fraction (GFR/RPF) also remains fairly constant in this pressure range.

Glomerular Filtration and Urine Formation

A normal adult male subject has a GFR of approximately 125 mL/min. About 180 L of fluid per day are filtered through the kidneys. In spite of this large filtration volume, the average urine volume is 1–1.5 L. Up to 99% of the fluid volume filtered at the glomerulus is reabsorbed. Besides fluid regulation, the kidney also regulates the retention or excretion of various solutes and electrolytes (Table 6.1). With the exception of proteins and protein-bound substances, most small molecules are filtered through the glomerulus from the plasma. The filtrate contains some ions, glucose, and essential nutrients as well as waste products, such as urea, phosphate, sulfate, and other substances. The essential nutrients and water are reabsorbed at

TABLE 6.1 Quantitative Aspects of Urine Formation[a]

SUBSTANCE	PER 24 HOURS				PERCENT REABSORBED
	Filtered	Reabsorbed	Secreted	Excreted	
Sodium ion (mEq)	26,000	25,850		150	99.4
Chloride ion (mEq)	18,000	17,850		150	99.2
Bicarbonate ion (mEq)	4,900	4,900		0	100
Urea (mM)	870	460[b]		410	53
Glucose (mM)	800	800		0	100
Water (mL)	180,000	179,000		1,000	99.4
Hydrogen ion			Variable	Variable[c]	
Potassium ion (mEq)	900	900[d]	100	100	100[d]

[a]Quantity of various plasma constituents filtered, reabsorbed, and excreted by a normal adult on an average diet.
[b]Urea diffuses into, as well as out of, some portions of the nephron.
[c]pH or urine is on the acid side (4.5–6.9) when all bicarbonate is reabsorbed.
[d]Potassium ion is almost completely reabsorbed before it reaches the distal nephron. The potassium ion in the voided urine is actively secreted into the urine in the distal tubule in exchange for sodium ion.

From Levine (1990), with permission.

various sites, including the proximal tubule, loops of Henle, and distal tubules. Both active reabsorption and secretion mechanisms are involved. The urine volume is reduced, and the urine generally contains a high concentration of metabolic wastes and eliminated drug products.

RENAL DRUG EXCRETION

Renal excretion is a major route of elimination for many drugs. Drugs that are non-volatile, water soluble, have a low molecular weight (MW), or are slowly biotrans-formed by the liver are eliminated by renal excretion. The processes by which a drug is excreted via the kidneys may include any combination of the following:

- Glomerular filtration
- Active tubular secretion
- Tubular reabsorption

Glomerular filtration is a unidirectional process that occurs for most small molecules (MW < 500), including undissociated (nonionized) and dissociated (ionized) drugs. Protein-bound drugs behave as large molecules and do not get filtered at the glomerulus. The major driving force for glomerular filtration is the hydrostatic pressure within the glomerular capillaries. The kidneys receive a large blood supply (approximately 25% of the cardiac output) via the renal artery, with very little decrease in the hydrostatic pressure.

Glomerular filtration rate (GFR) is measured by using a drug that is eliminated by filtration only (ie, the drug is neither reabsorbed nor secreted). Examples of such drugs are inulin and creatinine. Therefore, the clearance of inulin is equal to the GFR, which is equal to 125–130 mL/min. The value for the GFR correlates fairly well with body surface area. Glomerular filtration of drugs is directly related to the free or nonprotein-bound drug concentration in the plasma. As the free drug concentration in the plasma increases, the glomerular filtration for the drug increases proportionately, thus increasing renal drug clearance for some drugs.

Active tubular secretion is an active transport process. As such, active renal secretion is a carrier-mediated system that requires energy input, because the drug is transported against a concentration gradient. The carrier system is capacity limited and may be saturated. Drugs with similar structures may compete for the same carrier system. Two active renal secretion systems have been identified, systems for (1) weak acids and (2) weak bases. For example, probenecid competes with penicillin for the same carrier system (*weak acids*). Active tubular secretion rate is dependent on renal plasma flow. Drugs commonly used to measure active tubular secretion include *p*-amino-hippuric acid (PAH) and iodopyracet (Diodrast). These substances are both filtered by the glomeruli and secreted by the tubular cells. Active secretion is extremely rapid for these drugs, and practically all the drug carried to the kidney is eliminated in a single pass. The clearance for these drugs therefore reflects the *effective renal plasma flow* (ERPF), which varies from 425 to 650 mL/min.

For a drug that is excreted solely by glomerular filtration, the elimination half-life may change markedly in accordance with the binding affinity of the drug for plasma proteins. In contrast, drug protein binding has very little effect on the elimination half-life of the drug excreted mostly by active secretion. Because drug protein binding is reversible, drug bound to plasma protein rapidly dissociates as free drug is secreted by the kidneys. For example, some of the penicillins are extensively protein bound, but their elimination half-lives are short due to rapid elimination by active secretion.

Tubular reabsorption occurs after the drug is filtered through the glomerulus and can be an active or a passive process. If a drug is completely reabsorbed (eg, glucose), then the value for the clearance of the drug is approximately zero. For drugs that are partially reabsorbed, clearance values are less than the GFR of 125–130 mL/min.

The reabsorption of drugs that are acids or weak bases is influenced by the pH of the fluid in the renal tubule (ie, urine pH) and the pK_a of the drug. Both of these factors together determine the percentage of dissociated (ionized) and undissociated (nonionized) drug. Generally, the undissociated species is more lipid soluble (less water soluble) and has greater membrane permeability. The undissociated drug is easily reabsorbed from the renal tubule back into the body. This process of drug reabsorption can significantly reduce the amount of drug excreted, depending on the pH of the urinary fluid and the pK_a of the drug. The pK_a of the drug is a constant, but the normal urinary pH may vary from 4.5 to 8.0, depending on diet, pathophysiology, and drug intake. Vegetable and fruit diets or diets rich in carbohydrates result in higher urinary pH, whereas diets rich in protein result in lower urinary pH. Drugs such as ascorbic acid and antacids such as sodium carbonate may decrease (acidify) or increase (alkalinize) the urinary pH, respectively, when administered in large quantities. By far the most important changes in urinary pH are caused by fluids administered intravenously. Intravenous fluids, such as solutions of bicarbonate or ammonium chloride, are used in acid–base therapy. Excretion of these solutions may drastically change urinary pH and alter drug reabsorption and drug excretion by the kidney.

The percentage of ionized weak acid drug corresponding to a given pH can be obtained from the *Henderson–Hesselbalch equation.*

$$pH = pK_a + \log \frac{[\text{ionized}]}{[\text{nonionized}]} \tag{6.3}$$

Rearrangement of this equation yields

$$\frac{[\text{ionized}]}{[\text{nonionized}]} = 10^{pH - pK_a} \tag{6.4}$$

$$\text{Fraction of drug ionized} = \frac{[\text{ionized}]}{[\text{ionized}] + [\text{nonionized}]} \tag{6.5}$$

$$= \frac{10^{pH - pK_a}[\text{nonionized}]}{[\text{ionized}] + [\text{nonionized}]}$$

$$= \frac{10^{pH - pK_a}}{1 + 10^{pH - pK_a}}$$

TABLE 6.2 Effect of Urinary pH and pK$_a$ on the Ionization of Drugs

pH OF URINE	PERCENT OF DRUG IONIZED: pK$_a$=3	PERCENT OF DRUG IONIZED: pK$_a$=5
7.4	100	99.6
5	99	50.0
4	91	9.1
3	50	0.99

The fraction or percent of weak acid drug ionized in any pH environment may be calculated with Equation 6.5. For acidic drugs with pK$_a$ values from 3 to 8, a change in urinary pH affects the extent of dissociation (Table 6.2). The extent of dissociation is more greatly affected by changes in urinary pH for drugs with a pK$_a$ of 5 than with a pK$_a$ of 3. Weak acids with pK$_a$ values of less than 2 are highly ionized at all urinary pH values and are only slightly affected by pH variations.

For a weak base drug, the Henderson–Hasselbalch equation is given as

$$pH = pK_a + \log + \frac{[\text{nonionized}]}{[\text{ionized}]} \tag{6.6}$$

and

$$\text{Percent of drug ionized} = \frac{1 + 10^{pH - pK_a}}{10^{pH - pK_a}} \tag{6.7}$$

The greatest effect of urinary pH on reabsorption occurs with weak base drugs with pK$_a$ values of 7.5–10.5.

From the Henderson–Hesselbalch relationship, a concentration ratio for the distribution of a weak acid or basic drug between urine and plasma may be derived. The urine–plasma (U/P) ratios for these drugs are as follows.

For weak acids,

$$\frac{U}{P} = \frac{1 + 10^{pH_{\text{urine}} - pK_a}}{1 + 10^{pH_{\text{plasma}} - pK_a}} \tag{6.8}$$

For weak bases,

$$\frac{U}{P} = \frac{1 + 10^{pK_a - pH_{\text{urine}}}}{1 + 10^{pK_a - pH_{\text{plasma}}}} \tag{6.9}$$

For example, amphetamine, a weak base, will be reabsorbed if the urine pH is made alkaline and more lipid-soluble nonionized species are formed. In contrast, acidification of the urine will cause the amphetamine to become more ionized (form a salt). The salt form is more water soluble and less likely to be reabsorbed and has a tendency to be excreted into the urine more quickly. In the case of weak acids (such as salicylic acid), acidification of the urine causes greater reabsorption of the drug and alkalinization of the urine causes more rapid excretion of the drug.

PRACTICE PROBLEMS

Let $pK_a = 5$ for an acidic drug. Compare the U/P at urinary pH **(a)** 3, **(b)** 5, and **(c)** 7.

Solution

a. At pH = 3,

$$\frac{U}{P} = \frac{1 + 10^{3-5}}{1 + 10^{7.4-5}} = \frac{1.01}{1 + 10^{2.4}}$$

$$= \frac{1.01}{252} = \frac{1}{252}$$

b. At pH = 5,

$$\frac{U}{P} = \frac{1 + 10^{5-5}}{1 + 10^{7.4-5}} = \frac{2}{1 + 10^{2.4}} = \frac{2}{252}$$

c. At pH = 7,

$$\frac{U}{P} = \frac{1 + 10^{7-5}}{1 + 10^{7.4-5}} = \frac{101}{1 + 10^{2.4}} = \frac{101}{252}$$

In addition to the pH of the urine, the rate of urine flow influences the amount of filtered drug that is reabsorbed. The normal flow of urine is approximately 1–2 mL/min. Nonpolar and nonionized drugs, which are normally well reabsorbed in the renal tubules, are sensitive to changes in the rate of urine flow. Drugs that increase urine flow, such as ethanol, large fluid intake, and methylxanthines (such as caffeine or theophylline), decrease the time for drug reabsorption and promote their excretion. Thus, forced diuresis through the use of diuretics may be a useful adjunct for removing excessive drug in an intoxicated patient, by increasing renal drug excretion.

DRUG CLEARANCE

Drug clearance is a pharmacokinetic term for describing drug elimination from the body without identifying the mechanism of the process. Drug clearance (*body clearance, total body clearance,* or Cl_T) considers the entire body as a single drug-eliminating system from which many unidentified elimination processes may occur. Instead of describing the drug elimination rate in terms of amount of drug removed per time unit (eg, mg/min), drug clearance is described in terms of volume of fluid clear of drug per time unit (eg, mL/min).

There are several definitions of clearance, which are similarly based on volume of drug removed per unit time. The simplest concept of clearance regards the body as a space that contains a definite volume of body fluid (apparent volume of distribution, V_D) in which the drug is dissolved. Drug clearance is defined as the fixed volume of fluid (containing the drug) cleared of drug per unit of time. The units for clearance are volume/time (eg, mL/min, L/hr). For example, if the Cl_T of penicillin is 15 mL/min in a patient and penicillin has a V_D of 12 L, then from the clearance definition, 15 mL of the 12 L will be cleared of drug per minute.

Alternatively, Cl_T may be defined as the rate of drug elimination divided by the plasma drug concentration. This definition expresses drug elimination in terms of the volume of plasma eliminated of drug per unit time. This definition is a practical way to calculate clearance based on plasma drug concentration data.

$$Cl_T = \frac{\text{elimination rate}}{\text{plasma concentration}(C_p)} \tag{6.10}$$

$$Cl_T = \frac{dD_E/dt}{C_p} = \frac{\mu g/\text{min}}{\mu g/\text{mL}} = \text{mL/min} \tag{6.11}$$

where D_E is the amount of drug eliminated and dD_E/dt is the rate of elimination. Rearrangement of Equation 6.11 gives Equation 6.12.

$$\text{Elimination rate} = \frac{dD_E}{dt} = C_p Cl_T \tag{6.12}$$

The two definitions for clearance are similar because dividing the elimination rate by the C_p yields the volume of plasma cleared of drug per minute, as shown in Equation 6.10.

As discussed in previous chapters, a first-order elimination rate, dD_E/dt, is equal to kD_B or kC_pV_D. Based on Equation 6.10, substituting elimination rate for kC_pV_p,

$$Cl_T = \frac{kC_pV_D}{C_p} = kV_D \tag{6.13}$$

Equation 6.13 shows that clearance is the product of V_D and k, both of which are constant. As the plasma drug concentration decreases during elimination, the rate of drug elimination, dD_E/dt, decreases accordingly, but clearance remains constant. Clearance is constant as long as the rate of drug elimination is a first-order process.

EXAMPLE

Penicillin has a Cl_T of 15 mL/min. Calculate the elimination rate for penicillin when the plasma drug concentration, C_p, is 2 μg/mL.

Solution

Elimination rate = $C_p \times Cl_T$ (from Eq. 6.12)

$$\frac{dD_E}{dt} = 2\ \mu g/\text{mL} \times 15\ \text{mL/min} = 30\ \mu g/\text{min}$$

Using the previous penicillin example, assume that the plasma penicillin concentration is 10 μg/mL. From Equation 6.11, the rate of drug elimination is

$$\frac{dD_E}{dt} = 10\ \mu g/\text{mL} \times 15\ \text{mL/min} = 150\ \mu g/\text{min}$$

Thus, 150 μg/min of penicillin is eliminated from the body when the plasma penicillin concentration is 10 μg/mL.

Clearance may be used to estimate the rate of drug elimination at any given concentration. Using the same example, if the elimination rate of penicillin was measured as 150 μg/min when the plasma penicillin concentration was 10 μg/mL, then the clearance of penicillin is calculated from Equation 6.11:

$$Cl_{\text{penicillin}} = \frac{150\ \mu g/\min}{10\ \mu g/mL} = 15\ mL/\min$$

Just as the elimination rate constant (k) represents the sum total of all the rate constants for drug elimination, including excretion and biotransformation, Cl_T is the sum total of all the clearance processes in the body, including clearance through the kidney (renal clearance), lung, and liver (hepatic clearance).

Renal clearance = $k_e V_D$
Lung clearance = $k_l V_D$
Hepatic clearance = $k_m V_D$
Body clearance = $k_e V_D + k_l V_D + k_m V_D = (k_e + k_l + k_n) V_D = kV_D$ **(6.14)**

From Equation 6.14, body clearance Cl_T of a drug is the product of two constants, k and V_D, which reflect all the distribution and elimination processes of the drug in the body. The volume of distribution and elimination rate constant are affected by blood flow, which will be considered below (and in Chapter 10) using a physiologic model.

Clearance values are often normalized on a per-kilogram body–weight basis, such as milliliters per minute kilogram. This approach is similar to the method for expressing V_D, because both pharmacokinetic parameters vary with body weight. The clearance for an individual patient is estimated as the product of the clearance per kilogram multiplied by the body weight (kg) of the patient.

EXAMPLE

Determine the total body clearance for a drug in a 70-kg male patient. The drug follows the kinetics of a one-compartment model and has an elimination half-life of 3 hours with an apparent volume of distribution of 100 mL/kg.

Solution

First determine the elimination rate constant (k) and then substitute properly into Equation 6.13.

$$k = \frac{0.693}{t_{1/2}} = \frac{0.693}{3} = 0.231\ hr^{-1}$$

$Cl_T = 0.231\ hr^{-1} \times 100\ mL/kg = 23.1\ ml/kg\ hr$

For a 70-kg patient,

$Cl_T = 23.1\ mL/kg \times 70\ kg = 1617\ mL/hr$

CLEARANCE MODELS

The calculation of clearance from k and V_D assumes (sometimes incorrectly) a defined model, whereas clearance estimated directly from the plasma drug concentration time curve does not assume any model. Although clearance may be regarded as the product of k and V_D, Equation 6.10 is far more general because the reaction order for the rate of drug elimination, dD_E/dt, is not specified, and the elimination rate may or may not follow first-order kinetics.

Physiologic/Organ Clearance

Clearance may be calculated for any organ involved in the irreversible removal of drug from the body. Many organs in the body have the capacity for drug elimination, including drug excretion and biotransformation. The kidneys and liver are the most common organs involved in excretion and metabolism, respectively. Physiologic pharmacokinetic models are based on drug clearance through individual organs or tissue groups (Fig. 6-6).

For any organ, clearance may be defined as the fraction of blood volume containing drug that flows through the organ and is eliminated of drug per unit time. From this definition, clearance is the product of the blood flow (Q) to the organ, and the extraction ratio (ER). The ER is the fraction of drug extracted by the organ as drug passes through.

$$\text{Clearance} = Q(\text{ER}) \tag{6.15}$$

If the drug concentration in the blood (C_a) entering the organ is greater than the drug concentration of blood (C_v) leaving the organ, then some of the drug has been extracted by the organ (Fig. 6-6). The ER is $C_a - C_v$ divided by the entering drug concentration (C_a), as shown in Equation 6.16.

$$\text{ER} = \frac{C_a - C_v}{C_a} \tag{6.16}$$

ER is a ratio with no units. The value of ER may range from 0 (no drug removed by the organ) to 1 (100% of the drug is removed by the organ). An ER of 0.25 indicates that 25% of the incoming drug concentration is removed by the organ as the drug passes through.

Substituting for ER into Equation 6.15 yields

$$Cl = Q\left(\frac{C_a - C_v}{C_a}\right) \tag{6.17}$$

The physiologic approach to clearance shows that clearance depends on the blood flow rate and the ability of the organ to eliminate drug, whereas the classical

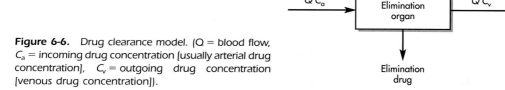

Figure 6-6. Drug clearance model. (Q = blood flow, C_a = incoming drug concentration [usually arterial drug concentration], C_v = outgoing drug concentration [venous drug concentration]).

definitions of clearance is that a constant or static fraction of the volume in which the drug is contained is removed per unit time by the organ. However, clearance measurements using the physiologic approach require invasive techniques to obtain measurements of blood flow and extraction ratio. The physiologic approach has been used to describe hepatic clearance, which is discussed under hepatic elimination (Chap. 11). More classical definitions of clearance have been applied to renal clearance because direct measurements of plasma drug concentration and urinary drug excretion may be obtained. The various approaches for estimating clearance are described in Figure 6-7.

Model-Independent Methods

Clearance is commonly used to describe first-order drug elimination from compartment models such as the one-compartment model, $C(t) = C_p = C_p^0 e^{-kt}$ in which the distribution volume and elimination rate constant are well defined. Clearance estimated directly from the plasma drug concentration–time curve does not assume any model. However, any elimination process other than a first-order rate process becomes complex and difficult to relate clearance to a compartment model.

Model-independent methods are *noncompartment* model approaches used to calculate certain pharmacokinetic parameters such as clearance and bioavailability (F). The major advantage of model-independent methods is that no assumption for a specific compartment model is required to analyze the data. Moreover, the volume of distribution and the elimination rate constant need not be determined

Compartment model

$V_D\,C_p$ k

Static volume and first-order elimination is assumed.
Plasma flow is not considered. $Cl_T = k\,V_D$.

Physiologic model

$Q\,C_a$ $Q\,C_v$

Elimination

Clearance is the product of the plasma flow (Q) and the extraction ratio (ER).
Thus $Cl_T = Q\,\text{ER}$

Model independent

$?V\,C_p$ $?k$

Volume and elimination rate constant not defined. $Cl_T = \text{Dose}/[\text{AUC}]_0^\infty$.

Figure 6-7.   *General approaches to clearance. Volume and elimination rate constant not defined.*

directly from the equation that best fits the plasma drug concentration–time curve.

Clearance can be determined directly from the plasma–time concentration curve by

$$Cl = \int_0^\infty \frac{D_0}{C(t)\ dt} \tag{6.18}$$

where D_0 is the dose and $C(t)$ is an unknown function that describes the declining plasma drug concentrations.

In the compartment model, $C(t) = C_p = C_p^0 e^{-kt}$ can be different mathematical functions that describe the individual pharmacokinetics of the drug. Using the non-compartment approach, the general equation uses area under the curve of the plasma drug concentration curve, $[\text{AUC}]_0^\infty$ for the calculation of clearance.

$$Cl_r = \frac{D_0}{[\text{AUC}]_0^\infty} \tag{6.19}$$

where D_0 is the dose and $[\text{AUC}]_0^\infty = \int_0^\infty C_p\ dt$

Because $[\text{AUC}]_0^\infty$ is calculated from the plasma drug concentration–time curve from 0 to infinity using the trapezoidal rule, no compartmental model is assumed. However, to extrapolate the data to infinity to obtain the residual $[\text{AUC}]_t^\infty$ or (C_{p_t}/k), first-order elimination is usually assumed. This calculation of Cl_T is referred to as a noncompartment or model-independent method. In this case, if the drug follows the kinetics of a one-compartment model, the Cl_T is numerically similar to the product of V_D and k obtained by fitting the data to a one-compartment model.

RENAL CLEARANCE

Renal clearance, Cl_R, is defined as the volume of plasma that is cleared of drug per unit of time through the kidney. Similarly, renal clearance may be defined as a constant fraction of the V_D in which the drug is contained that is excreted by the kidney per unit of time. More simply, renal clearance is defined as the urinary drug excretion rate (dD_u/dt) divided by the plasma drug concentration (C_p).

$$Cl_R = \frac{\text{excretion rate}}{\text{plasma concentration}} = \frac{dD_u/dt}{C_p} \tag{6.20}$$

An alternative approach to obtaining Equation 6.20 is to consider the mass balance of drug cleared by the kidney and ultimately excreted in the urine. For any drug cleared through the kidney, the rate of the drug passing through kidney (via filtration, reabsorption, and/or active secretion) must equal the rate of drug excreted in the urine.

Rate of drug passing through kidney = rate of drug excreted

$$Cl_R \times C_p = Q_u \times C_u \tag{6.21}$$

$$\text{mL/min} \times \text{mg/mL} = \text{mL/min} \times \text{mg/mL}$$

where Cl_R is renal clearance, C_p is plasma drug concentration, Q_u is the rate of urine flow, and C_u is the urine drug concentration. Rearrangement of Equation 6.21 gives

$$Cl_R = \frac{Q_u C_u}{C_p} = \frac{\text{excretion rate}}{C_p} \tag{6.22}$$

because the excretion rate $= Q_u C_u = dD_u/dt$, Equation 6.22 is the equivalent of Equation 6.20.

Comparison of Drug Excretion Methods

Renal clearance may be measured without regard to the physiologic mechanisms involved in this process. From a physiologic viewpoint, however, renal clearance may be considered as the ratio of the sum of the glomerular filtration and active secretion rates less the reabsorption rate divided by the plasma drug concentration:

$$Cl_R = \frac{\text{filtration rate} + \text{secretion rate} - \text{reabsorption rate}}{C_p} \tag{6.23}$$

The actual renal clearance of a drug is not generally obtained by direct measurement. The clearance value for the drug is often compared to that of a standard reference, such as inulin, which is cleared completely through the kidney by glomerular filtration only. The *clearance ratio,* which is the ratio of drug clearance to inulin clearance, may give an indication for the mechanism of renal excretion of the drug (Table 6.3). However, further renal drug excretion studies are necessary to confirm unambiguously the mechanism of excretion.

A method to quantify renal drug excretion is to consider the kinetic nature of the elimination processes. For this consideration, some of the detailed steps in the elimination process may be omitted or simplified. For example, assume that the body fluid volume is the V_D and that the plasma drug concentration, C_p, is changing after an intravenous bolus injection.

TABLE 6.3 Comparison of Clearance of a Sample Drug to Clearance of a Reference Drug, Inulin

CLEARANCE RATIO	PROBABLE MECHANISM OF RENAL EXCRETION
$\dfrac{Cl_{drug}}{Cl_{inulin}} < 1$	Drug is partially reabsorbed
$\dfrac{Cl_{drug}}{Cl_{inulin}} = 1$	Drug is filtered only
$\dfrac{Cl_{drug}}{Cl_{inulin}} > 1$	Drug is actively secreted

TABLE 6.4 Urinary Drug Excretion Rate[a]

TIME (min)	C_p (μg/ml)	EXCRETION RATE (μg/min) (Drug filtered by GFR per min)
0	$(C_p)_0$	$(C_p)_0 \times 125$
1	$(C_p)_1$	$(C_p)_1 \times 125$
2	$(C_p)_2$	$(C_p)_2 \times 125$
t	$(C_p)_t$	$(C_p)_t = 125$

[a]Assumes that the drug is excreted by filtration only and that the GFR is 125 mL/min.

Filtration Only

If glomerular filtration is the sole process for drug excretion and no drug is reabsorbed, then the amount of drug filtered at any time (*t*) will always be $C_p \times$ GFR (Table 6.4). Likewise, if the Cl_R of the drug is by glomerular filtration only, as in the case of inulin, then $Cl_R =$ GFR. Otherwise, Cl_R represents all the processes by which the drug is cleared through the kidney, including any combination of filtration, reabsorption, and active secretion.

Note that the quantity of drug excreted per minute is always the plasma concentration (C_p) multiplied by a constant (eg, 125 mL/min), which in this case is also the renal clearance for the drug. The glomerular filtration rate may be treated as a first-order process relating to C_p. The rate of drug excretion using a compartment approach and physiologic approach are compared in Equations 6.22 and 6.23.

$$\frac{dD_u}{dt} = k_e V_D C_p \text{ (compartment)} \tag{6.24}$$

$$\frac{dD_u}{dt} = Cl_R C_p \text{ (physiologic)} \tag{6.25}$$

Equating 6.24 with 6.25,

$$k_e V_D C_p = Cl_R C_p$$

$$k_e = \frac{Cl_R}{V_D} \tag{6.26}$$

Equation 6.26 shows that, in the absence of other processes of drug elimination, the excretion rate constant is a fractional constant reflecting the volume pumped out per unit time due to GFR relative to the volume of the body compartment (V_D).

In the one-compartment model, a drug is assumed to be uniformly and instantly equilibrated. However, the renal plasma drug concentration entering the kidney (arterial drug concentration) is always higher than the venous plasma drug concentration leaving the kidney. In spite of this inconsistency, the rate of drug elimination is properly adjusted in the estimation of the first-order elimination rate constant (*k*) given in Equation 6.25 if the overall plasma drug concentration profile is adequately described. If the pharmacokinetic parameters are properly calculated to fit the data, the parameters k and V_D reflect the underlying kinetic processes.

Filtration and Reabsorption

For a drug with a *reabsorption fraction* of *fr*, the drug excretion rate is reduced, and Equation 6.25 is restated as Equation 6.27:

$$\frac{dD_u}{dt} = Cl_R(1 - fr)C_p \qquad\qquad (6.27)$$

Equating the right sides of Equations 6.27 and 6.24 indicates that the first-order rate constant (k_e) in the compartment model is equivalent to $Cl_R\,(1 - fr)/V_D$. In this case, the excretion rate constant is affected by the reabsorption fraction (fr) and the GFR. Because these two parameters generally remain constant, the general adoption of a first-order elimination process to describe renal drug excretion is a reasonable approach.

Filtration and Active Secretion

For a drug that is primarily filtered and secreted, with negligible reabsorption, the overall excretion rate will exceed GFR (Table 6.3). At low drug plasma concentrations, active secretion is not saturated, and the drug is excreted by filtration and active secretion. At high concentrations, the percentage of drug excreted by active secretion decreases due to saturation. Clearance decreases because excretion rate decreases (Figure 6-8). Clearance decreases because the total excretion rate of the drug increases to the point where it is approximately equal to the filtration rate (Figure 6-9).

The power of the kinetic approach is that, even lacking any knowledge of GFR, active secretion, or the reabsorption process, modeling the data allows the process of drug elimination to be described quantitatively. If a change to a higher-order elimination rate process occurs, then an additional process besides GFR may be involved. The compartmental analysis aids the ultimate development of a model consistent with physiologic functions of the body.

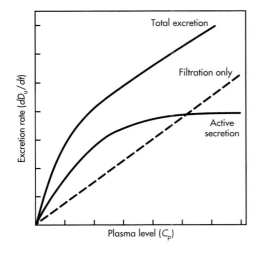

Figure 6-8. Excretion rate-versus-plasma level curves for a drug that demonstrates active tubular secretion and a drug that is secreted by glomerular filtration only.

Figure 6-9.   Graph representing the decline of renal clearance. As the drug plasma level increases to a concentration that saturates the active tubular secretion, glomerular filtration becomes the major component for renal clearance.

 # EXAMPLE

Two drugs, A and B, are entirely eliminated through the kidney by glomerular filtration (125 mL/min), with no reabsorption. Drug A has half the distribution volume of drug B, and the V_D of drug B is 20 L. What are the drug clearances for each drug based on the classical and physiologic approaches?

Solution

Since glomerular filtration of the two drugs is the same, and both drugs are not eliminated by other means, clearance for both drugs depends on renal plasma flow and extraction by the kidney only.

Basing the clearance calculation on the physiologic definition and using Equation 6.17 results in

$$Cl = \frac{Q(C_a - C_v)}{C_a} = 125 \text{ mL/min.}$$

Interestingly, known drug clearance tells little about the dosing differences of the two drugs, although it helps to identify the mechanism of drug elimination. In this example, both drugs have the same clearance.

Basing the calculation on the elimination concept and applying Equation 6.14, k is easily determined, resulting in an obvious difference in $t_{1/2}$ between the two drugs—in spite of similar drug clearance.

$$k_{\text{drug A}} = \frac{Cl}{V_D} = \frac{125 \text{ mL/min}}{10 \times 1000 \text{ mL}} = 0.0125 \text{ min}^{-1}$$

$$k_{\text{drug B}} = \frac{Cl}{V_D} = \frac{125 \text{ mL/min}}{200 \times 1000 \text{ mL}} = 0.00625 \text{ min}^{-1}$$

Here k specifies the fraction of drug eliminated regardless of distributional differences of the drug.

In spite of identical drug clearances, k for drug A is twice that of drug B. Drug A has an elimination half-life of 80 minutes, while that of drug B is 160 minutes—much longer because of the bigger volume of distribution.

DETERMINATION OF RENAL CLEARANCE

Graphical Methods

The clearance is given by the slope of the curve obtained by plotting the rate of drug excretion in urine (dD_u/dt) against C_p (Eq. 6.28). For a drug that is excreted rapidly, dD_u/dt is large, the slope is steeper, and clearance is greater (Fig. 6-10, line A). For a drug that is excreted slowly through the kidney, the slope is smaller (Fig. 6-10, line B).

From Equation 6.20,

$$Cl_R = \frac{dD_u/dt}{C_p}$$

Multiplying both sides by C_p gives

$$Cl_R C_p = \frac{dD_u}{dt} \tag{6.28}$$

By rearranging Equation 6.28 and integrating, one obtains

$$\int_0^{D_u} dD_u = Cl_R \int_0^t C_p \, dt \tag{6.29}$$

$$[D_u]_0^t = Cl_R [\text{AUC}]_0^t \tag{6.30}$$

A graph is then plotted of cumulative drug excreted in the urine versus the area under the concentration–time curve (Fig. 6-11). Renal clearance is obtained from the slope of the curve. The area under the curve can be estimated by the trapezoidal rule or by other measurement methods. The disadvantage of this method is that if a data point is missing, the cumulative amount of drug excreted in the urine is difficult to obtain. However, if the data are complete, then the determination of clearance is more accurate by this method.

Figure 6-10. Rate of drug excretion versus concentration of drug in the plasma. Drug A has a higher clearance than drug B, as shown by the slopes of line A and line B.

Figure 6-11. Cumulative drug excretion versus AUC. The slope is equal to Cl_R.

By plotting cumulative drug excreted in the urine from t_1 to t_2, $[D_u]_{t_1}^{t_2}$ versus $[\text{AUC}]_t^{t_2}$, one obtains an equation similar to that presented previously:

$$\int_{D_u^1}^{D_u^2} dD_u = Cl_R \int_{t_1}^{t_2} C_p \, dt \tag{6.31}$$

$$[D_u]_{t_1}^{t_2} = Cl_R[\text{AUC}]_{t_1}^{t_2} \tag{6.32}$$

The slope is equal to the renal clearance (Fig. 6-12).

Model-Independent Methods

Clearance rates may also be estimated by a single (nongraphical) calculation from knowledge of the $[\text{AUC}]_0^\infty$, the total amount of drug absorbed, FD_0, and the total amount of drug excreted in the urine, D_u^∞. For example, if a single IV bolus drug injection is given to a patient and the $[\text{AUC}]_0^\infty$ is obtained from the plasma drug level–time curve, then total body clearance is estimated by

$$Cl_T = \frac{D_0}{[\text{AUC}]_0^\infty} \tag{6.33}$$

If the total amount of drug excreted in the urine, D_u^∞, has been obtained, then renal clearance is calculated by

$$Cl_R = \frac{D_u^\infty}{[\text{AUC}]_0^\infty} \tag{6.34}$$

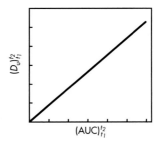

Figure 6-12. Drug excreted versus $(\text{AUC})_{t_1}^{t_2}$. The slope is equal to Cl_R.

The calculations using Equations 6.33 and 6.34 allow for rapid and easily obtainable estimates of drug clearance. However, only a single dose estimate is obtained; therefore, the calculations do not reflect nonlinear changes in the clearance rates, as indicated in Figure 6-8.

Clearance can also be calculated from fitted parameters. If the volume of distribution and elimination constants are known, body clearance (Cl_T), renal clearance (Cl_R), and hepatic clearance (Cl_h) can be calculated according to the following expressions:

$$Cl_T = kV_D \tag{6.35}$$

$$Cl_R = k_e V_D \tag{6.36}$$

$$Cl_h = k_m V_D \tag{6.37}$$

Total body clearance (Cl_T) is equal to the sum of renal clearance and hepatic clearance and is based on the concept that the entire body acts as a drug-eliminating system.

$$Cl_T = Cl_R + Cl_h \tag{6.38}$$

By substitution of Equations 6.35 and 6.36 into Equation 6.38,

$$kV_D = k_e V_D + k_m V_D \tag{6.39}$$

Dividing by V_D on both sides of Equation 6.39,

$$k = k_e + k_m \tag{6.40}$$

PRACTICE PROBLEM

Consider a drug that is eliminated by first-order renal excretion and hepatic metabolism. The drug follows a one-compartment model and is given in a single intravenous or oral dose (Fig. 6-13). Working with the model presented in Figure 6-13, assume that a single dose (100 mg) of this drug is given orally. The drug is 90% systemically available. The total amount of unchanged drug recovered in the urine is 60 mg, and the total amount of metabolite recovered in the urine is 30 mg (expressed as milligram equivalents to the parent drug). According to the literature, the elimination half-life for this drug is 3.3 hours and its apparent volume of distribution is 1000 mL. From the information given, find **(a)** the total body clearance, **(b)** the renal clearance, and **(c)** the nonrenal clearance of the drug.

Solution

a. Total body clearance:

$$Cl_T = kV_D$$

$$Cl_T = \frac{0.693}{3.3(1000)} = 210 \text{ mL/hr}$$

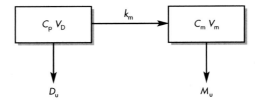

Figure 6-13.   Model of a drug eliminated by first-order renal excretion and hepatic metabolism. (k_e = renal excretion rate constant of parent drug, k_m = metabolism rate constant [conversion of parent drug to metabolite], k_u = renal excretion rate constant of metabolite, D_u = amount of unchanged drug in urine, M_u = amount of metabolite in urine, C_m = plasma concentration of the metabolite, C_p = plasma concentration of the parent drug, V_D = apparent volume of distribution of parent drug, V_m = apparent volume of distribution of metabolite.)

b. Renal clearance. First find k_e:

$$\frac{k_e}{k} = \frac{D_u^\infty}{FD_0} = \frac{D_u^\infty}{M_u^\infty + D_u^\infty} \tag{6.41}$$

$$k_e = \left(\frac{0.693}{3.3}\right)\left(\frac{60}{30 + 60}\right) = 0.14 \text{ hr}^{-1}$$

Then, from Equation 6.36,

$$Cl_R = k_e V_D$$
$$Cl_R = (0.14)(1000) = 140 \text{ mL/hr}$$

c. Nonrenal clearance:

$$Cl_h = Cl_T - Cl_R$$
$$Cl_h = 210 - 140 = 70 \text{ mL/hr}$$

Alternatively,

$$k_m = k - k_e$$
$$k_m = 0.21 - 0.14 = 0.07 \text{ hr}^{-1}$$
$$k_m = k\left[\frac{M_u^\infty}{M_u^\infty + D_u^\infty}\right]$$

$$k_m = 0.21\left(\frac{30}{30 + 60}\right) = 0.07 \text{ hr}^{-1}$$

Applying Equation 6.37,

$$Cl_h = k_m V_D$$
$$Cl_h = (0.07)(1000) = 70 \text{ mL/hr}$$

Calculation of Clearance in Multicompartmental Models

Clearance is a direct measure of elimination from the central compartment, regardless of the number of compartments. The central compartment consists of the plasma and highly perfused tissues in which drug equilibrates rapidly (Chapter 4). The tissues for drug elimination, namely kidney and liver, are considered integral parts of the central compartment.

The first-order elimination rate constant k is a useful measurement for drug elimination in a one-compartment model and can be calculated after IV bolus (Chapter 3), IV infusion (Chapter 5), or even oral (Chapter 7) or multiple doses (Chapter 8) using plasma drug concentrations. The value of k can also be calculated by measuring D_u, drug excreted into the urine (Chapter 3 and below).

In multicompartment models, several methods for the estimation of clearance are possible. The overall elimination rate constant k represents elimination from the central compartment, and total body clearance is the product of k times the volume of the central compartment, V_p.

For the two-compartment model, total body clearance may be estimated according to Equation 6.42 as the product by the elimination rate constant b times $V_{D\beta}$. This latter method gives the same value for clearance. Other methods for calculating total body clearance consider either instantaneous clearance or steady-state clearance, depending on which volume of distribution is chosen. Generally, the various calculations of total body clearance for drugs characterized by multicompartment pharmacokinetics are useful for comparison purposes. For the two-compartment model drug, body clearance can be calculated with the following equation:

$$Cl_T = kV_p \qquad (6.42)$$

or, alternatively,

$$Cl_T = bV_{D_\beta} \qquad (6.43)$$

To obtain renal clearance for drugs demonstrating two-compartment kinetics with metabolism and excretion, the following equation is used:

$$Cl_R = k_e V_p \qquad (6.44)$$

Fraction of Drug Excreted

For many drugs, the total amount of unchanged drug excreted in the urine D_u^∞, may be obtained by direct assay. The ratio of D_u^∞, to the fraction of the dose absorbed, FD_0, is equal to the fraction of drug excreted unchanged in the urine and is also equal to k_e/k.

$$\text{Fraction of drug excreted unchanged in the urine} = f_e = \frac{D_u^\infty}{FD_0} = \frac{k_e}{k} \qquad (6.45)$$

Renal clearance may be determined from the fraction of unchanged drug excreted in the urine and the total body clearance.

$$Cl_R = \frac{D_u^\infty}{FD_0} Cl_T = f_e Cl_T \qquad (6.46)$$

Equation 6.46 can also be expressed as

$$Cl_R = \frac{k_e}{k} Cl_T \qquad (6.47)$$

PRACTICE PROBLEM

An antibiotic is given by IV bolus injection at a dose of 500 mg. The apparent volume of distribution was 21 L and the elimination half-life was 6 hours. Urine was collected for 48 hours, and 400 mg of unchanged drug was recovered. What is the fraction of the dose excreted unchanged in the urine? Calculate k, k_e, Cl_T, Cl_R, and Cl_h.

Solution

Since the elimination half-life, $t_{1/2}$, for this drug is 6 hours, a urine collection for 48 hours represents $8 \times t_{1/2}$, which allows for greater than 99% of the drug to be eliminated from the body. The fraction of drug excreted unchanged in the urine, f_e, is obtained by using Equation 6.47 and recalling that $f = 1$ for drugs given by IV bolus injection.

$$f_e = \frac{400}{500} = 0.8$$

Therefore, 80% of the absorbed dose is excreted in the urine unchanged. Calculations for k, k_e, Cl_T, Cl_R, and Cl_h are given here:

$$k = \frac{0.693}{6} = 0.1155 \text{ hr}^{-1}$$

$$k_e = f_e k = (0.8)(0.1155) = 0.0924 \text{ hr}^{-1}$$
$$Cl_T = (0.1155)(21) = 2.43 \text{ L/hr}$$
$$Cl_R = f_e \, Cl_T = (0.8)(2.43) = 1.94 \text{ L/hr}$$

Alternatively,

$$Cl_R = k_e V_D = (0.0924)(21) = 1.94 \text{ L/hr}$$
$$Cl_h = Cl_T - Cl_R = 2.43 - 1.94 = 0.49 \text{ L/hr}$$

Protein-Bound Drugs

Protein-bound drugs are not eliminated by glomerular filtration. Therefore, Equation 6.18 for the calculation of renal clearance must be modified, because only the free drug is excreted by a linear process. The bound drugs are usually excreted by active secretion, following capacity-limited kinetics. The determination of clearance that separates the two components results in a hybrid clearance. There is no simple way to overcome this problem. Clearance values for a protein-bound drug is therefore calculated with the following equation:

$$Cl_R = \frac{\text{rate of unbound drug excretion}}{\text{concentration of unbound drug in the plasma}} \qquad \textbf{(6.48)}$$

In practice, this equation is not easily applied because the rate of drug excretion is usually determined after collecting urine samples. The drug excreted in the urine is the sum of drug excreted by active tubular secretion and by passive glomerular filtration, minus drug that is reabsorbed. However, it is not possible to distinguish the amount of bound drug actively secreted or reabsorbed from the amount of drug excreted by glomerular filtration. Equation 6.48 can be used for drugs that are protein bound but not actively secreted. Nonlinear drug binding makes clearance less useful due to model complication.

Equation 6.48 is also used in the calculation of free drug concentration in the plasma, where α is the fraction of bound drug and $1 - \alpha$ is the fraction of free drug.

$$(1 - \alpha)\ C_{p,total} = C_{p,free} \qquad \textbf{(6.49)}$$

For most drug studies, the total plasma drug concentration (free plus bound drug) is used in clearance calculations. If renal clearance is corrected for the fraction of drug bound to plasma proteins using Equation 6.48, then the renal clearance for the free drug concentration may have a higher value compared to the uncorrected renal clearance using the total plasma drug concentrations.

Plasma protein binding has very little effect on the renal clearance of actively secreted drugs such as penicillin. For these drugs, the free drug fraction is filtered at the glomerular, whereas the protein-bound drug appears to be stripped from the binding sites and actively secreted into the renal tubules.

RELATIONSHIP OF CLEARANCE TO ELIMINATION HALF-LIFE AND VOLUME OF DISTRIBUTION

The half-life of a drug can be determined if the clearance and V_D are known. From Equation 6.35 we obtain

$$Cl_T = kV_D$$

and

$$k = \frac{0.693}{t_{1/2}}$$

Therefore, by substitution,

$$Cl_T = \frac{0.693\ V_D}{t_{1/2}} \qquad \textbf{(6.50)}$$

TABLE 6.5 Relationships of Clearance, Rate Constant of Elimination, and Elimination Half-Life

	K_e and $t_{1/2}$ IN VARIOUS MEDIA OF DISTRIBUTION		
CLEARANCE[a]	Plasma Water (3,000 mL)	Extracellular Fluid (12,000 mL)	Body Water (41,000 mL)
Partial reabsorption (eg, 30 mL/min)	1.00×10^{-2} (69 min)	2.50×10^{-3} (277 min)	7.32×10^{-4} (947 min)
Glomerular filtration (eg, 130 mL/min)	4.33×10^{-2} (16 min)	1.08×10^{-2} (64 min)	3.17×10^{-3} (219 min)
Tubular secretion (eg, 650 mL/min)	2.17×10^{-1} (3 min)	5.42×10^{-2} (13 min)	1.59×10^{-2} (44 min)

[a]Entries are values for k_e, the rate constant of elimination (in units of min^{-1}); parenthetic entries are corresponding values of the elimination half-life. The clearance given under "partial reabsorption" is arbitrary; any clearance between 0 (complete reabsorption) and 650 mL/min is possible.

From Goldstein et al (1974), with permission.

From Equation 6.50, as Cl_T decreases, which might happen in the case of renal insufficiency, the $t_{1/2}$ for the drug increases. A good relationship of V_D, k, and $t_{1/2}$ is shown in Table 6.5.

Total body clearance, Cl_T, is a more useful index of measurement of drug removal compared to the elimination half-life, $t_{1/2}$. Total body clearance takes into account changes in both the apparent volume of distribution, V_D, and $t_{1/2}$. In overt obesity or edematous conditions, the V_D may change without a marked change in $t_{1/2}$. As will be shown in Chapters 10 and 11, V_D is important in the calculation of the loading dose, whereas Cl_T is important in the calculation of the maintenance dose.

Total body clearance may be calculated by the ratio, $FD_0/[AUC]_0^\infty$, which is considered a model-independent method and assumes no particular pharmacokinetic model for drug elimination.

$$Cl_T = \frac{FD_0}{[AUC]_0^\infty} \tag{6.51}$$

Total Body Clearance of Drugs after Intravenous Infusion

When drugs are administered by intravenous infusion (Chapter 5), the total body clearance is obtained with the following equation:

$$Cl_T = \frac{R}{C_{SS}} \tag{6.52}$$

where C_{SS} is the steady-state plasma drug concentration and R is the rate of infusion. Equation 6.52 is valid for drugs that follow either the one- or the two-compartment open model (see Chapter 4).

PRACTICE PROBLEMS

A new antibiotic is actively secreted by the kidney; V_D is 35 L in the normal adult. The clearance of this drug is 650 mL/min.

1. What is the usual $t_{1/2}$ for this drug?

Solution

$$t_{1/2} = \frac{0.693 \,(35,000 \text{ mL})}{650 \text{ mL/min}}$$

$$t_{1/2} = 37.3 \text{ min}$$

2. What would be the new $t_{1/2}$ for this drug in an adult with partial renal failure whose clearance of the antibiotic was only 75 mL/min?

Solution

$$t_{1/2} = \frac{0.693 \,(35,000 \text{ mL})}{75 \text{ mL/min}}$$

$$t_{1/2} = 323 \text{ min}$$

In patients with renal impairment the $t_{1/2}$ generally changes more drastically than the V_D. The clearance given under partial reabsorption in Table 6.5 is arbitrary; any clearance between 0 (complete reabsorption) and 650 mL/min is possible.

FREQUENTLY ASKED QUESTIONS

1. Is clearance a better parameter to describe drug elimination than half-life? Why is it necessary to use both parameters in the literature?

2. What is an independent parameter in a model? Is clearance an independent parameter of the physiologic model? How is clearance related to parameters in the compartment model?

3. What is the difference between drug clearance and creatinine clearance?

LEARNING QUESTIONS

1. Explain why plasma protein binding will prolong the renal clearance of a drug that is excreted only by glomerular filtration but does not affect the renal clearance of a drug excreted by both glomerular filtration and active tubular secretion.

2. Explain the effect of alkalization or acidification of the urine on the renal clearance of dextroamphetamine sulfate. Dextroamphetamine sulfate is a weak base with a pK_a of 9.4.

3. Theophylline is effective in the treatment of bronchitis at a blood level of 10–20 $\mu g/mL$. At therapeutic range, theophylline follows first-order kinetics. The average $t_{1/2}$ is 3.4 hours, and the range is 1.8 to 6.8 hours. The average volume of distribution is 30 L.

   a. What are the average, upper, and lower clearance limits for theophylline?

   b. The renal clearance of theophylline is 0.36 L/hr. What are the k_m and k_e, assuming all nonrenal clearance (Cl_{NR}) is due to metabolism?

4. A single 250-mg oral dose of an antibiotic is given to a young man (age 32 years, creatinine clearance 122 mL/min, 78 kg). From the literature, the drug is known to have an apparent V_D equal to 21% of body weight and an elimination half-life of 2 hours. The dose is normally 90% bioavailable. Urinary excretion of the unchanged drug is equal to 70% of the absorbed dose.

   a. What is the total body clearance for this drug?

   b. What is the renal clearance for this drug?

   c. What is the probable mechanism for renal clearance of this drug?

5. A drug with an elimination half-life of 1 hour was given to a male patient (80 kg) by intravenous infusion at a rate of 300 mg/hr. At 7 hours after infusion, the plasma drug concentration was 11 $\mu g/mL$.

   a. What is the total body clearance for this drug?

   b. What is the apparent V_D for this drug?

   c. If the drug is not metabolized and is eliminated only by renal excretion, what is the renal clearance of this drug?

   d. What is the probable mechanism for renal clearance of this drug?

6. In order to rapidly estimate the renal clearance of a drug in a patient, a 2-hour postdose urine sample was collected and found to contain 200 mg of drug. A midpoint plasma sample was taken (1 hr postdose) and the drug concentration in plasma was found to be 2.5 mg%. Estimate the renal clearance for this drug in the patient.

7. According to the manufacturer, after the antibiotic cephradine (Velosef), given by IV infusion at rate of 5.3 mg/kg per hour to 9 adult male volunteers (average weight, 71.7 kg), a steady-state serum concentration of 17 $\mu g/mL$ was measured. Calculate the average total body clearance for this drug in adults.

8. Cephradine is completely excreted unchanged in the urine, and studies have shown that probenecid given concurrently causes elevation of the serum cephradine concentration. What is the probable mechanism for the interaction of probenecid with cephradine?

9. Why is clearance used as a measurement of drug elimination, rather than the excretion rate of the drug?

10. What is the advantage of using total body clearance as a measurement of drug elimination compared to using the elimination half-life of the drug?

11. A patient was given 2500 mg of a drug by IV bolus dose, and periodic urinary data was collected. **(a)** Determine the renal clearance of the drug using urinary data. **(b)** Determine total body clearance using the area method. **(c)** Is there any nonrenal clearance of the drug in this patient? What would be the nonrenal clearance, if any? How would you determine clearance using a compartmental approach and compare that with the area method?

Time (hr)	Plasma Urinary Concentration (μg/mL)	Urinary Volume (mL)	Urinary Concentration (μg/mL)
0	250.00	100.00	0.00
1	198.63	125.00	2880.00
2	157.82	140.00	1901.20
3	125.39	100.00	2114.80
4	99.63	80.00	2100.35
5	79.16	250.00	534.01
6	62.89	170.00	623.96
7	49.97	160.00	526.74
8	39.70	90.00	744.03
9	31.55	400.00	133.01
10	25.06	240.00	176.13

REFERENCES

Goldstein A, Aronow L, Kalman SM: *Principles of Drug Action.* New York, Wiley, 1974

Guyton AC: *Textbook of Medical Physiology,* 8th ed. Philadelphia, Saunders, 1991

Levine RR: *Pharmacology: Drug Actions and Reactions,* 4th ed. Boston, Little, Brown, 1990

West JB (ed): *Best and Taylor's Physiological Basis of Medical Practice,* 11th ed. Baltimore, Williams & Wilkins, 1985, p 451

BIBLIOGRAPHY

Cafruny EJ: Renal tubular handling of drugs. *Am J Med* **62**:490–496, 1977

Hewitt WR, Hook JB: The renal excretion of drugs. In Bridges VW, Chasseaud LF (eds.), *Progress in Drug Metabolism,* vol. 7. New York, Wiley, 1983, chap 1

Renkin EM, Robinson RR: Glomerular filtration. *N Engl J Med* **290**:785–792, 1974

Rowland M, Benet LZ, Graham GG: Clearance concepts in pharmacokinetics. *J Pharm Biopharm* **1**:123–136, 1973

Smith H: *The Kidney: Structure and Function in Health and Disease.* New York, Oxford University Press, 1951

Thomson P, Melmon K, Richardson J, et al: Lidocaine pharmacokinetics in advanced heart failure, liver disease and renal failure in humans. *Ann Intern Med* **78**:499–508, 1973

Tucker GT: Measurement of the renal clearance of drugs. *Br J Clin Pharm* **12**:761–770, 1981

Weiner IM, Mudge GH: Renal tubular mechanisms for excretion and organic acids and bases. *Am J Med* **36**:743–762, 1964

Wilkinson GR: Clearance approaches in pharmacology. *Pharmacol Rev* **39**:1–47, 1987

7

PHARMACOKINETICS OF ORAL ABSORPTION

PHARMACOKINETICS OF DRUG ABSORPTION

The pharmacokinetics of drugs following intravenous drug administration are more simple to model compared to extravascular delivery (see Chapters 1–6). Extravascular delivery routes, particularly oral dosing, are important and popular means of drug administration. Unlike intravenous administration, in which the drug is injected directly into the plasma, pharmacokinetic models after extravascular drug administration must consider systemic drug absorption from the site of administration, eg, the lung, the gut, etc., into the plasma. Extravascular drug delivery is further complicated by variables at the absorption site, including possible drug degradation and significant inter- and intrapatient differences in the rate and extent of absorption. Absorption and metabolic variables are characterized using pharmacokinetic methods. The variability in systemic drug absorption can be minimized to some extent by proper biopharmaceutical design of the dosage form to provide predictable and reliable drug therapy (Chapters 14–16). The major advantage of intravenous administration is that the rate and extent of systemic drug input is carefully controlled.

The systemic drug absorption from the gastrointestinal (GI) tract or from any other extravascular site is dependent on (1) the physicochemical properties of the drug, (2) the dosage form used, and (3) the anatomy and physiology of the absorption site. Although this chapter will focus primarily on oral dosing, the concepts discussed here may be easily extrapolated to other extravascular routes. For oral dosing, such factors as surface area of the GI tract, stomach-emptying rate, GI mobility, and blood flow to the absorption site all affect the rate and the extent of drug absorption. In pharmacokinetics, the overall rate of drug absorption may be described as either a first-order or zero-order input process. Most pharmacokinetic models assume first-order absorption unless an assumption of zero-order absorption improves the model significantly or has been verified experimentally.

Figure 7-1. Model of drug absorption and elimination.

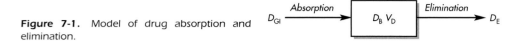

The rate of change in the amount of drug in the body, dD_B/dt, is dependent on the relative rates of drug absorption and elimination (Fig. 7-1). The net rate of drug accumulation in the body at any time is equal to the rate of drug absorption less the rate of drug elimination, regardless of whether absorption is zero-order or first-order.

$$\frac{dD_B}{dt} = \frac{dD_{GI}}{dt} - \frac{dD_E}{dt} \tag{7.1}$$

Where D_{GI} is amount of drug in the gastrointestinal tract and D_E is amount of drug eliminated. A plasma level–time curve showing drug adsorption and elimination rate processes is given in Figure 7-2. During the *absorption phase* of a plasma level–time curve (Fig. 7-2), the rate of drug absorption is greater than the rate of drug elimination. Note that during the absorption phase, elimination occurs *whenever* drug is present in the plasma, even though absorption predominates.

$$\frac{dD_{GI}}{dt} > \frac{dD_E}{dt} \tag{7.2}$$

At the *peak drug concentration* in the plasma (Fig. 7-2) the rate of drug absorption just equals the rate of drug elimination, and there is no net change in the amount of drug in the body.

$$\frac{dD_{GI}}{dt} = \frac{dD_E}{dt} \tag{7.3}$$

Immediately after the time of peak drug absorption, some drug may still be at the absorption site (ie, in the GI tract or other site of administration). However,

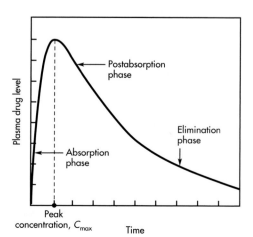

Figure 7-2. Plasma level–time curve for a drug given in a single oral dose. The drug absorption and elimination phases of the curve are shown.

the rate of drug elimination at this time is faster than the rate of absorption, as represented by the *postabsorption phase* in Figure 7-2.

$$\frac{dD_{GI}}{dt} < \frac{dD_E}{dt} \tag{7.4}$$

When the drug at the absorption site becomes depleted, the rate of drug absorption approaches zero, or $dD_{GI}/dt = 0$. The plasma level–time curve (now the *elimination phase*) then represents only the elimination of drug from the body, usually a first-order process. Therefore, during the elimination phase the rate of change in the amount of drug in the body is described as a first-order process,

$$\frac{dD_B}{dt} = -kD_B \tag{7.5}$$

where k is the first-order elimination rate constant.

ZERO-ORDER ABSORPTION MODEL

Zero-order drug absorption from the dosing site into the plasma usually occurs when either the drug is absorbed by a saturable process or a zero-order controlled-release delivery system is used (see Chapter 17). The pharmacokinetic model assuming zero-order absorption is described in Figure 7-3. In this model, drug in the gastrointestinal tract, D_{GI}, is absorbed systemically at a constant rate, k_0. Drug is simultaneously and immediately eliminated from the body by a first-order rate process defined by a first-order rate constant, k. This model is analogous to that of the administration of a drug by intravenous infusion (Chapter 5).

The rate of first-order elimination at any time is equal to $D_B k$. The rate of input is simply k_0. Therefore, the net change per unit time in the body can be expressed as

$$\frac{dD_B}{dt} = k_0 - kD_B \tag{7.6}$$

Integration of this equation with substitution of $V_D C_p$ for D_B produces

$$C_p = \frac{k_0}{V_D k}(1 - e^{-kt}) \tag{7.7}$$

The rate of drug absorption is constant until the amount of drug in the gut, D_{GI}, is depleted. The time for complete drug absorption to occur is equal to D_{GI}/k_0. After this time, the drug is no longer available for absorption from the gut, and Equation 7.7 no longer holds. The drug concentration in the plasma subsequently declines in accordance with a first-order elimination rate process.

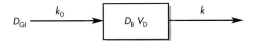

Figure 7-3. One-compartment pharmacokinetic model for zero-order drug absorption and first-order drug elimination.

FIRST-ORDER ABSORPTION MODEL

Although zero-order absorption can occur, absorption is usually assumed to be a first-order process. This model assumes a first-order input across the gut wall and first-order elimination from the body (Fig. 7-4). This model applies mostly to the oral absorption of drugs in solution or rapidly dissolving dosage (immediate release) forms such as tablets, capsules, and suppositories. In addition, drugs given by intramuscular or subcutaneous aqueous injections may also be described using a first-order process.

In the case of a drug given orally, the dosage form first disintegrates if it is given as a solid, then the drug dissolves into the fluids of the GI tract. Only drug in solution is absorbed into the body. The rate of disappearance of drug from the gastrointestinal tract is described by

$$\frac{dD_{GI}}{dt} = -k_a D_{GI} F \tag{7.8}$$

where k_a is the first-order absorption rate constant from the GI tract, F is the fraction absorbed, and D_{GI} is the amount of drug in solution in the GI tract at any time t. Integration of the differential equation (7.8) gives

$$\frac{dD_{GI}}{dt} = D_0 e^{-k_a t} \tag{7.9}$$

where D_0 is the dose of the drug.

The rate of drug elimination is described by a first-order rate process for most drugs and is equal to $-kD_B$. The rate of drug change in the body, dD_B/dt, is therefore the rate of drug in, minus the rate of drug out—as given by the differential equation, Equation 7.10:

$$\frac{dD_B}{dt} = \text{rate in} - \text{rate out}$$

$$\frac{dD_B}{dt} = Fk_a D_{GI} - kD_B \tag{7.10}$$

where F is the fraction of drug absorbed systemically. Since the drug in the gastrointestinal tract also follows a first-order decline (ie, the drug is absorbed across the gastrointestinal wall), the amount of drug in the gastrointestinal tract at any time t is equal to $D_0 e^{-k_a t}$.

$$\frac{dD_B}{dt} = Fk_a D_0 e^{-k_a t} - kD_B$$

The value of F may vary from 1 for a fully absorbed drug to 0 for a drug that is completely unabsorbed. This equation can be integrated to give the general oral

Figure 7-4. One-compartment pharmacokinetic model for first-order drug absorption and first-order elimination.

absorption equation for calculation of the drug concentration (C_p) in the plasma at any time t, as shown below.

$$C_p = \frac{Fk_aD_0}{V_D(k_a - k)}(e^{-kt} - e^{-k_at}) \tag{7.11}$$

A typical plot of the concentration of drug in the body after a single oral dose is presented in Figure 7-5.

The maximum plasma concentration after oral dosing is C_{max}, and the time needed to reach maximum concentration is t_{max}. The t_{max} is independent of dose and is dependent on the rate constants for absorption (k_a) and elimination (k) (Eq. 7.13a). At C_{max}, sometimes called *peak concentration*, the rate of drug absorbed is equal to the rate of drug eliminated. Therefore, the net rate of concentration change is equal to zero. At C_{max}, the rate of concentration change can be obtained by differentiating Equation 7.11, as follows:

$$C_p = \frac{k_aD_0F}{V_D(k_a - k)}(-ke^{-kt} + k_ae^{-k_at}) = 0 \tag{7.12}$$

This can be simplified as follows:

$$-ke^{-kt} + k_ae^{-k_at} = 0 \quad \text{or} \quad ke^{-kt} = k_ae^{-k_at} \tag{7.13}$$

$$\ln k - kt = \ln k_a - k_at$$

$$t_{max} = \frac{\ln k_a - \ln k}{k_a - k} = \frac{\ln(k_a/k)}{k_a - k}$$

$$t_{max} = \frac{2.3 \log(k_a/k)}{k_a - k} \tag{7.13a}$$

As shown in Equation 7.13a, the time for maximum drug concentration, t_{max}, is dependent only on the rate constants k_a and k. In order to calculate C_{max}, the value for t_{max} is determined via Equation 7.13a and then substituted into Equation 7.11, solving for C_{max}. Equation 7.11 shows that C_{max} is directly proportional to the dose

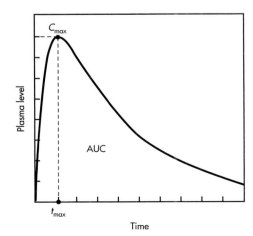

Figure 7-5. Typical plasma level–time curve for a drug given in a single oral close.

of drug given (D_0) and the fraction of drug absorbed (F). Calculation of t_{max} and C_{max} is usually necessary, since direct measurement of the maximum drug concentration may not be possible due to improper timing of the serum samples.

The first-order elimination rate constant may be determined from the elimination phase of the plasma level–time curve (Fig. 7-2). At later time intervals, when drug absorption has been completed, ie, $e^{-k_a t} \approx 0$, Equation 7.11 reduces to

$$C_p = \frac{Fk_a D_0}{V_D(k_a - k)} e^{-kt} \tag{7.14}$$

Taking the natural logarithm of this expression,

$$\ln C_p = \ln \frac{Fk_a D_0}{V_D(k_a - k)} - kt \tag{7.15}$$

Substitution of common logarithms gives

$$\log C_p = \log \frac{Fk_a D_0}{V_D(k_a - k)} - \frac{kt}{2.3} \tag{7.16}$$

With this equation, a graph constructed by plotting $\log C_p$ versus time will yield a straight line with a slope of $-k/2.3$ (Fig. 7-6A).

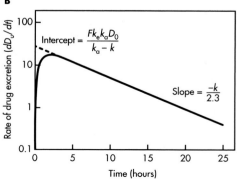

Figure 7-6. **A.** Plasma drug concentration versus time, single oral dose. **B.** Rate of urinary drug excretion versus time, single oral dose.

With a similar approach, urinary drug excretion data may also be used for calculation of the first-order elimination rate constant. The rate of drug excretion after a single oral dose of drug is given by

$$\frac{dD_u}{dt} = \frac{Fk_a k_e D_0}{k_a - k} - (e^{-kt} - e^{-k_a t})$$ (7.17)

where dD_u/dt = rate of urinary drug excretion, k_e = first-order renal excretion constant, and F = fraction of dose absorbed.

A graph constructed by plotting dD_u/dt versus time will yield a curve identical in appearance to the plasma level–time curve for the drug (Fig. 7-7B). After drug absorption is virtually complete, $-e^{-k_a t}$ approaches zero, and Equation 7.17 reduces to

$$\frac{dD_u}{dt} = \frac{Fk_a k_e D_0}{k_a - k} e^{-kt}$$ (7.18)

Taking the natural logarithm of both sides of this expression and substituting for common logarithms, Equation 7.18 becomes

$$\log \frac{dD_u}{dt} = \log \frac{Fk_a k_e D_0}{k_a - k} - \frac{kt}{2.3}$$ (7.19)

A

B

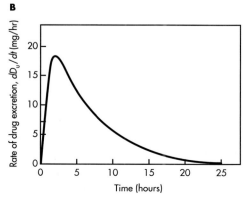

Figure 7-7. A. Plasma drug concentration versus time, single oral dose. **B.** Rate of urinary drug excretion versus time, single oral dose.

Figure 7-8. Cumulative urinary drug excretion versus time, single oral dose. Urine samples are collected at various time periods after the dose. The amount of drug excreted in each sample is added to the amount of drug recovered in the previous urine sample (cumulative addition). The total amount of drug recovered after all the drug is excreted is D_u^∞.

When $\log(dD_u/dt)$ is plotted against time, a graph of a straight line is obtained with a slope of $-k/2.3$ (Fig. 7-6B). Because the rate of urinary drug excretion, dD_u/dt, cannot be determined directly for any given time point, an average rate of urinary drug excretion is obtained (see also Chapter 3), and this value is plotted against the midpoint of the collection period for each urine sample.

To obtain the cumulative drug excretion in the urine, Equation 7.17 must be integrated, as shown below.

$$D_u = \frac{Fk_a k_e D_0}{k_a - k}\left(\frac{e^{-k_a t}}{k_a} - \frac{e^{-kt}}{k}\right) + \frac{Fk_e D_0}{k} \tag{7.20}$$

A plot of D_u versus time will give the urinary drug excretion curve described in Figure 7-8. When all of the drug has been excreted, at $t = \infty$, Equation 7.20 reduces to

$$D_u^\infty = \frac{Fk_e D_0}{k} \tag{7.21}$$

where D_u^∞ is the maximum amount of active or parent drug excreted.

Determination of Absorption Rate Constants from Oral Absorption Data

Method of Residuals

Assuming $k_a \gg k$ in Equation 7.11, the value for the second exponential will become insignificantly small with time (ie, $e^{-k_a t} \approx 0$) and can therefore be omitted. When this is the case, drug absorption is virtually complete. Equation 7.11 then reduces to Equation 7.22.

$$C_p = \frac{Fk_a D_0}{V_D(k_a - k)}e^{-kt} \tag{7.22}$$

From this, one may also obtain the intercept of the y axis (Fig. 7-9).

$$\frac{Fk_a D_0}{V_D(k_a - k)} = A$$

where A is a constant. Thus, Equation 7.22 becomes

$$C_p = Ae^{-kt} \tag{7.23}$$

This equation, which represents first-order drug elimination, will yield a linear plot on semilog paper. The slope is equal to $-k/2.3$. The value for k_a can be obtained

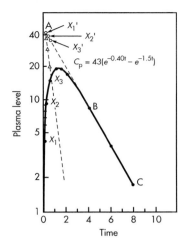

Figure 7-9. Plasma level–time curve for a drug demonstrating first-order absorption and elimination kinetics. The equation of the curve is obtained by the method of residuals.

by using the method of residuals or a feathering technique, as described in Chapter 4. The value of k_a is obtained by the following procedure:

1. Plot the drug concentration versus time on semilog paper with the concentration values on the logarithmic axis (Fig. 7-9).
2. Obtain the slope of the terminal phase (line BC, Fig. 7-9) by extrapolation.
3. Take any points on the upper part of line BC (eg, x_1', x_2', x_3', . . .) and drop vertically to obtain corresponding points on the curve (eg, x_1, x_2, x_3, . . .).
4. Read the concentration values at x_1 and x_1', x_2 and x_2', x_3 and x_3', and so on. Plot the values of the differences at the corresponding time points Δ_1, Δ_2, Δ_3, ... A straight line will be obtained with a slope of $-k_a/2.3$ (Fig. 7-9).

When using the method of residuals, a minimum of three points should be used to define the straight line. Data points occurring shortly after t_{max} may not be accurate, because drug absorption is still continuing at that time. Because this portion of the curve represents the postabsorption phase, only data points from the elimination phase should be used to define the rate of drug absorption as a first-order process.

If drug absorption begins immediately after oral administration, the residual lines obtained by feathering the plasma level–time curve (as shown in Fig. 7-9) will intersect on the y axis at point A. The value of this y intercept, A, represents a hybrid constant composed of k_a, k, V_D, and FD_0. The value of A has no direct physiologic meaning (see Eq. 7.23).

$$A = \frac{Fk_a D_0}{V_D (k_a - k)}$$

The value for A, as well as the values for k and k_a, may be substituted back into Equation 7.11 to obtain a general theoretical equation that will describe the plasma level–time curve.

Lag Time

In some individuals, absorption of drug after a single oral dose does not start immediately, due to such physiologic factors as stomach-emptying time and intestinal

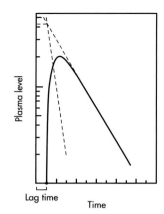

Figure 7-10. The lag time can be determined graphically if the two residual lines obtained by feathering the plasma level–time curve intersect at a point where $t > 0$.

motility. The time delay prior to the commencement of first-order drug absorption is known as *lag time*.

The lag time for a drug may be observed if the two residual lines obtained by feathering the oral absorption plasma level–time curve intersect at a point greater than $t = 0$ on the x axis. The time at the point of intersection on the x axis is the lag time (Fig. 7-10).

The lag time, t_0, represents the beginning of drug absorption and should not be confused with the pharmacologic term *onset time*, which represents latency, eg, the time required for the drug to reach minimum effective concentration.

Two equations can adequately describe the curve in Figure 7-10. In one, the lag time t_0 is subtracted from each time point, as shown in Equation 7.24.

$$C_p = \frac{F k_a D_0}{V_D(k_a - k)} \left(e^{-k(t - t_0)} - e^{-k_a(t - t_0)} \right) \tag{7.24}$$

where $F k_a D_0 / V_D(k_a - k)$ is the y value at the point of intersection of the residual lines in Figure 7-10.

The second expression that describes the curve in Figure 7-10 omits the lag time, as follows:

$$C_p = B e^{-kt} - A e^{-k_a t} \tag{7.25}$$

where A and B represents the intercepts on the y axis after extrapolation of the residual lines for absorption and elimination, respectively.

Flip-Flop of k_a and k

In using the method of residuals to obtain estimates of k_a and k, the terminal phase of an oral absorption curve is usually represented by k whereas the steeper slope is represented by k_a (Fig. 7-11). In a few cases, the elimination rate constant k obtained from oral absorption data does not agree with that obtained after intravenous bolus injection. For example, the k obtained after an intravenous bolus injection of a bronchodilator was 1.72 hr^{-1}, whereas the k calculated after oral administration was 0.7 hr^{-1} (Fig. 7-11). When k_a was obtained by the method of residuals, the rather surprising result was that the k_a was 1.72 hr^{-1}.

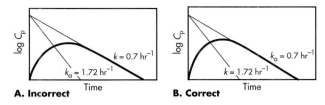

Figure 7-11.   Flip-flop of k_a and k. Because $k > k_a$, the right-hand figure and slopes represent the correct values for k_a and k.

Apparently, the k_a and k obtained by the method of residuals has been interchanged. This phenomenon is called *flip-flop* of the absorption and elimination rate constants. Flip-flop, or the reversal of the rate constants, may occur whenever k_a and k are estimated from oral drug absorption data. Use of computer methods does not ensure against flip-flop of the two constants estimated.

In order to demonstrate unambiguously that the steeper curve represents the elimination rate for a drug given extravascularly, the drug must be given by intravenous injection into the same patient. After intravenous injection, the decline in plasma drug levels over time represents the true elimination rate. The relationship between k_a and k on the shape of the plasma drug concentration–time curve for a constant dose of drug given orally is shown in Figure 7-11.

Most of the drugs observed to have flip-flop characteristics are drugs with fast elimination (ie, $k > k_a$). Drug absorption of most drug solutions or fast-dissolving products are essentially complete or at least half-complete within an hour (ie, absorption half-life of 0.5 or 1 hr, corresponding to a k_a of 1.38 hr^{-1} or 0.69 hr^{-1}). Because most of the drugs used orally have longer elimination half-lives compared to absorption half-lives, the assumption that the smaller slope or smaller rate constant (ie, the terminal phase of the curve in Fig. 7-11) should be used as the elimination constant is generally correct.

For drugs that have a large elimination rate constant ($k > 0.69$ hr^{-1}), the chance for flip-flop of k_a and k is much greater. The drug isoproterenol, for example, has an oral elimination half-life of only a few minutes, and flip-flop of k_a and k has been noted (Portmann, 1970). Similarly, salicyluric acid was flip-flopped when oral data were plotted. The k for salicyluric acid was much larger than its k_a (Levy et al, 1969). Many experimental drugs show flip-flop of k and k_a, whereas few marketed oral drugs do. Drugs with a large k are usually considered to be unsuitable for an oral drug product due to their large elimination rate constant, corresponding to a very short elimination half-life. An extended-release drug product may slow the absorption of a drug, such that the k_a is smaller than the k and producing a flip-flop situation.

Determination of k_a by Plotting Percent of Drug Unabsorbed versus Time (Wagner–Nelson Method)

After a single oral dose of a drug, the total dose should be completely accounted for in the amount present in the body, the amount present in the urine, and the amount present in the GI tract. Therefore, dose (D_0) is expressed as follows:

$$D_0 = D_{GI} + D_B + D_u \tag{7.26}$$

Let $\mathrm{Ab} = D_\mathrm{B} + D_\mathrm{u}$ = amount of drug absorbed and let Ab^∞ = amount of drug absorbed at $t = \infty$. At any given time the fraction of drug absorbed is $\mathrm{Ab}/\mathrm{Ab}^\infty$, and the fraction of drug unabsorbed is $1 - (\mathrm{Ab}/\mathrm{Ab}^\infty)$. The amount of drug excreted at any time t can be calculated as

$$D_\mathrm{u} = kV_\mathrm{D}[\mathrm{AUC}]_0^t \qquad (7.27)$$

The amount of drug in the body (D_B), at any time, $= C_\mathrm{p}V_\mathrm{D}$. At any time t, the amount of drug absorbed (Ab) is

$$\mathrm{Ab} = C_\mathrm{p}V_\mathrm{D} + kV_\mathrm{D}[\mathrm{AUC}]_0^t \qquad (7.28)$$

At $t = \infty$, $C_p^\infty = 0$ (ie, plasma concentration is negligible), and the total amount of drug absorbed is

$$\mathrm{Ab}^\infty = 0 + kV_\mathrm{D}[\mathrm{AUC}]_0^\infty \qquad (7.29)$$

The fraction of drug absorbed at any time is

$$\frac{\mathrm{Ab}}{\mathrm{Ab}^\infty} = \frac{C_\mathrm{p}V_\mathrm{D} + kV_\mathrm{D}[\mathrm{AUC}]_0^t}{kV_\mathrm{D}[\mathrm{AUC}]_0^\infty} \qquad (7.30)$$

$$\frac{\mathrm{Ab}}{\mathrm{Ab}^\infty} = \frac{C_\mathrm{p} + k[\mathrm{AUC}]_0^t}{k[\mathrm{AUC}]_0^\infty} \qquad (7.31)$$

The fraction unabsorbed at any time t is

$$1 - \frac{\mathrm{Ab}}{\mathrm{Ab}^\infty} = 1 - \frac{C_\mathrm{p} + k[\mathrm{AUC}]_0^t}{k[\mathrm{AUC}]_0^\infty} \qquad (7.32)$$

The drug remaining in the GI tract at any time t is

$$D_\mathrm{GI} = D_0 e^{-k_\mathrm{a}t} \qquad (7.33)$$

Therefore, the fraction of drug remaining is

$$\frac{D_\mathrm{GI}}{D_0} = e^{-k_\mathrm{a}t} \qquad \log \frac{D_\mathrm{GI}}{D_0} = \frac{-k_\mathrm{a}t}{2.3} \qquad (7.34)$$

Because D_GI/D_0 is actually the fraction of drug *unabsorbed*—that is, $1 - (\mathrm{Ab}/\mathrm{Ab}^\infty)$—a plot of $1 - (\mathrm{Ab}/\mathrm{Ab}^\infty)$ versus time gives $-k_\mathrm{a}/2.3$ as the slope (Fig. 7-12).

The following steps should be useful in determination of k_a:

1. Plot log concentration of drug versus time.
2. Find k from the terminal part of the slope when the slope $= -k/2.3$.
3. Find $[\mathrm{AUC}]_0^t$ by plotting C_p versus t.
4. Find $k[\mathrm{AUC}]_0^t$ by multiplying each $[\mathrm{AUC}]_0^t$ by k.
5. Find $[\mathrm{AUC}]_0^\infty$ by adding up all the [AUC] pieces, from $t = 0$ to $t = \infty$.
6. Determine the $1 - (\mathrm{Ab}/\mathrm{Ab}^\infty)$ value corresponding to each time point t by using Table 7.1.
7. Plot $1 - (\mathrm{Ab}/\mathrm{Ab}^\infty)$ versus time on semilog paper, with $1 - (\mathrm{Ab}/\mathrm{Ab}^\infty)$ on the logarithmic axis.

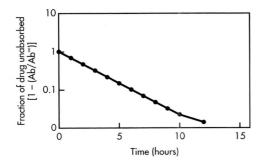

Figure 7-12.   Semilog graph of data in Table 7.2, depicting the fraction of drug unabsorbed versus time using the Wagner–Nelson method.

If the fraction of drug unabsorbed, $1 - Ab/Ab^\infty$, gives a linear regression line on a semilog graph, then the rate of drug absorption, dD_{GI}/dt, is a first-order process. Recall that $1 - Ab/Ab^\infty$ is equal to dD_{GI}/dt (Fig. 7-12).

As the drug approaches 100% absorption, C_p becomes very small and difficult to assay accurately. Consequently, the terminal part of the line described by $1 - Ab/Ab^\infty$ versus time tends to become scattered or nonlinear. This terminal part of the curve is excluded, and only the initial linear segment of the curve is used for the estimate of the slope.

PRACTICE PROBLEM

Drug concentrations in the blood at various times are listed in Table 7.1. Assuming the drug follows a one-compartment model, find the k_a, and compare it with the k_a value obtained by the method of residuals.

Solution

The AUC is approximated by the trapezoidal rule. This method is fairly accurate when there are sufficient data points. The area between each time point is calculated as

$$[\text{AUC}]_{t_{n-1}}^{t_n} = \frac{C_{n-1} + C_n}{2}(t_n - t_{n-1}) \tag{7.35}$$

where C_n and C_{n-1} are concentrations. For example, at $n = 6$, the [AUC] is

$$\frac{6.28 + 6.11}{2}(6 - 5) = 6.20$$

To obtain $[\text{AUC}]_0^\infty$, add all the area portions under the curve from zero to infinity. In this case, 48 hours is long enough to be considered as infinity, because the blood concentration at that point already has fallen to an insignificant drug concentration, $0.1 \ \mu g/mL$. The rest of the needed information is given in Table 7.1. Notice that k is

TABLE 7.1 Blood Concentrations and Associated Data for a Hypothetical Drug

TIME t_n (hr)	CONCENTRATION C_P (μg/mL)	$[AUC]_{t_{n-1}}^{t_n}$	$[AUC]_0^t$	$k[AUC]_0^t$	$C_p + k[AUC]_0^t$	$\dfrac{Ab}{Ab^\infty}$	$\left(1 - \dfrac{Ab}{Ab^\infty}\right)$
0	0.	0.	0.				1.000
1	3.13	1.57	1.57	0.157	3.287	0.328	0.672
2	4.93	4.03	5.60	0.560	5.490	0.548	0.452
3	5.86	5.40	10.99	1.099	6.959	0.695	0.305
4	6.25	6.06	17.05	1.705	7.955	0.794	0.205
5	6.28	6.26	23.31	2.331	8.610	0.856	0.140
6	6.11	6.20	29.51	2.951	9.061	0.905	0.095
7	5.81	5.96	35.47	3.547	9.357	0.934	0.066
8	5.45	5.63	41.10	4.110	9.560	0.955	0.045
9	5.06	5.26	46.35	4.635	9.695	0.968	0.032
10	4.66	4.86	51.21	5.121			
12	3.90	8.56	59.77	5.977			
14	3.24	7.14	66.91	6.691			
16	2.67	5.92	72.83	7.283			
18	2.19	4.86	77.69	7.769			
24	1.20	10.17	87.85	8.785			
28	0.81	4.02	91.87	9.187			
32	0.54	2.70	94.57	9.457			
36	0.36	1.80	96.37	9.637			
48	0.10	2.76	99.13	9.913			

$k = 0.1$ hr^{-1}

obtained from the plot of log C_p versus t; k was found to be 0.1 hr^{-1}. The plot of $1 - (Ab/Ab^\infty)$ versus t on semilog paper is shown in Figure 7-12.

A more complete method of obtaining the is to estimate the residual area from the last observed plasma concentration, C_{p_n} at t_n to time equal to infinity. This equation is

$$[AUC]_t^\infty = \frac{C_{p_n}}{k} \tag{7.36}$$

The total $[AUC]_0^\infty$ is the sum of the areas obtained by the trapezoidal rule, $[AUC]_0^\infty$, and the residual area $[AUC]_t^\infty$, as described in the following expression:

$$[AUC]_0^\infty = [AUC]_0^t + [AUC]_t^\infty \tag{7.37}$$

Estimation of k_a from Urinary Data

The absorption rate constant may also be estimated from urinary excretion data, using a plot of percent of drug unabsorbed versus time. For a one-compartment model:

Ab = total amount of drug absorbed—that is, the amount of drug in the body plus the amount of drug excreted

D_B = amount of drug in the body

D_u = amount of unchanged drug excreted in the urine

C_p = plasma drug concentration

D_E = total amount of drug eliminated (drug and metabolites)

$$Ab = D_B + D_E \tag{7.38}$$

The differential of Equation 7.38 with respect to time gives

$$\frac{d\text{Ab}}{dt} = \frac{dD_B}{dt} + \frac{dD_E}{dt} \tag{7.39}$$

Assuming first-order elimination kinetics with renal elimination constant k_e,

$$\frac{dD_u}{dt} = k_e D_B = k_e V_D C_p \tag{7.40}$$

Assuming a one-compartment model,

$$V_D C_p = D_B$$

Substituting $V_D C_p$ into Equation 7.39,

$$\frac{d\text{Ab}}{dt} = V_D \frac{dC_p}{dt} + \frac{dD_E}{dt} \tag{7.41}$$

And rearranging Equation 7.40,

$$C_p = \frac{1}{k_e V_D}\left(\frac{dD_u}{dt}\right) \tag{7.42}$$

$$\frac{dC_p}{dt} = \frac{d\,(dD_u/dt)}{dt\, k_e V_D} \tag{7.43}$$

Substituting for dC_p/dt into Equation 7.41 and kD_u/k_e for D_E,

$$\frac{d\text{Ab}}{dt} = \frac{d\,(D_u/dt)}{k_e\, dt} + \frac{k}{k_e}\left(\frac{dD_u}{dt}\right) \tag{7.44}$$

When the above expression is integrated from zero to time t,

$$\text{Ab}_t = \frac{1}{k_e}\left(\frac{dD_u}{dt}\right)t + \frac{k}{k_e}(D_u)t \tag{7.45}$$

At $t = \infty$ all the drug that is ultimately absorbed is expressed as Ab^∞ and $dD_u/dt = 0$. The total amount of drug absorbed is

$$\text{Ab}^\infty = \frac{k}{k_e}D_u^\infty$$

where D_u^∞ is the total amount of unchanged drug excreted in the urine.

The fraction of drug absorbed at any time t is equal to the amount of drug absorbed at this time, Ab_t, divided by the total amount of drug absorbed, Ab^∞.

$$\frac{\text{Ab}_t}{\text{Ab}^\infty} = \frac{(dD_u/dt)_t + k(D_u)_t}{kD_u^\infty} \tag{7.46}$$

A plot of the fraction of drug unabsorbed, $1 - \text{Ab}/\text{Ab}^\infty$, versus time gives $-k_a/2.3$ as the slope from which the absorption rate constant is obtained (Fig. 7-12; refer to Eq. 7-34).

When collecting urinary drug samples for the determination of pharmacokinetic parameters, one should obtain a valid urine collection as discussed in Chapter 3. If the drug is rapidly absorbed, it may be difficult to obtain multiple early urine samples to describe the absorption phase accurately. Moreover, drugs with very slow absorption will have low concentrations, which may present analytical problems.

Effect of k_a and k on C_{max}, t_{max}, and AUC

Changes in k_a and k may affect t_{max}, C_{max}, and AUC as shown in Table 7.2. If the values for k_a and k are reversed, then the same t_{max} is obtained, but the C_{max} and AUC are different. If the elimination rate constant is kept at 0.1 hr^{-1} and the k_a changes from 0.2 to 0.6 hr^{-1} (absorption rate increases), then the t_{max} becomes shorter (from 6.93 to 3.58 hr), the C_{max} increases (from 5.00 to 6.99 $\mu g/mL$), but the AUC remains constant (100 μg hr/mL). In contrast, when the absorption rate constant is kept at 0.3 hr^{-1} and k changes from 0.1 to 0.5 hr^{-1} (elimination rate increases), then the t_{max} decreases (from 5.49 to 2.55 hr), the C_{max} decreases (from 5.77 to 2.79 $\mu g/mL$), and the AUC decreases (from 100 to 20 μg hr/mL). Graphical representations for the relationships of k_a and k on the time for peak absorption and the peak drug concentrations are shown in Figures 7-13 and 7-14.

Determination of k_a from Two-Compartment Oral Absorption Data (Loo–Riegelman Method)

Plotting the percent of drug unabsorbed versus time to determine the k_a may be calculated for a drug exhibiting a two-compartment kinetic model. As in the method used previously to obtain an estimate of the k_a, no limitation is placed on the order of the absorption process. However, this method does require that the drug be given intravenously as well as orally to obtain all the necessary kinetic constants.

TABLE 7.2 Effects of the Absorption Rate Constant and Elimination Rate[a]

ABSORPTION RATE CONSTANT k_a (hr^{-1})	ELIMINATION RATE CONSTANT k (hr^{-1})	t_{max} (hr)	C_{max} ($\mu g/mL$)	AUC (μg hr/mL)
0.1	0.2	6.93	2.50	50
0.2	0.1	6.93	5.00	100
0.3	0.1	5.49	5.77	100
0.4	0.1	4.62	6.29	100
0.5	0.1	4.02	6.69	100
0.6	0.1	3.58	6.99	100
0.3	0.1	5.49	5.77	100
0.3	0.2	4.05	4.44	50
0.3	0.3	3.33	3.68	33.3
0.3	0.4	2.88	3.16	25
0.3	0.5	2.55	2.79	20

[a] t_{max} = peak plasma concentration, C_{max} = peak drug concentration, AUC = area under the curve. Values are based on a single oral dose (100 mg) that is 100% bioavailable ($F = 1$) and has an apparent V_D of 10 L. The drug follows a one-compartment open model. t_{max} is calculated by Eq. 7.13 and C_{max} is calculated by Eq. 7.11. The AUC is calculated by the trapezoidal rule from 0 to 24 hours.

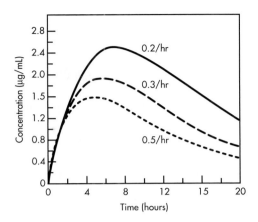

Figure 7-13. Effect of a change in the absorption rate constant, k_a, on the plasma drug concentration-versus-time curve. Dose of drug is 100 mg, V_D is 10 L, and k is 0.1 hr^{-1}.

Figure 7-14. Effect of a change in the elimination rate constant, k, on the plasma drug concentration-versus-time curve. Dose of drug is 100 mg, V_D is 10 L, and k_a is 0.1 hr^{-1}.

After oral administration of a dose of a drug that exhibits two-compartment model kinetics, the amount of drug absorbed is calculated as the sum of the amounts of drug in the central compartment (D_p) and in the tissue compartment (D_t) and the amount of drug eliminated by all routes (D_u) (Fig. 7-15).

$$Ab = D_p + D_t + D_u \tag{7.47}$$

Each of these terms may be expressed in terms of kinetics constants and plasma drug concentrations, as follows:

$$D_p = V_p C_p \tag{7.48}$$

$$D_t = V_t C_t \tag{7.49}$$

$$\frac{dD_u}{dt} = k V_p C_p \tag{7.50}$$

$$D_u = k V_p [\mathrm{AUC}]_0^t$$

Substituting the above expression for D_p and D_u into Equation 7.46,

$$Ab = V_p C_p + D_t + k V_p [\mathrm{AUC}]_0^t \tag{7.51}$$

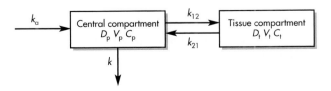

Figure 7-15. Two-compartment pharmacokinetic mode. Drug absorption and elimination occur from the central compartment.

By dividing this equation by V_p to express the equation on drug concentrations, we obtain

$$\frac{Ab}{V_p} = C_p + \frac{D_t}{V_p} + k[AUC]_0^t \tag{7.52}$$

At $t = \infty$ this equation becomes

$$\frac{Ab}{V_p} = k[AUC]_0^\infty \tag{7.53}$$

Equation 7.53 divided by Equation 7.54 gives the fraction of drug absorbed at any time.

$$\frac{Ab}{Ab^\infty} = \frac{C_p + \left(\dfrac{D_t}{V_p}\right) + k[AUC]_0^t}{k[AUC]_0^\infty} \tag{7.54}$$

A plot of the fraction of drug unabsorbed, $1 - Ab/Ab^\infty$, versus time gives $-k_a/2.3$ as the slope from which the value for the absorption rate constant is obtained (refer to Eq. 7-34).

C_p and $k[AUC]_0^t$ are calculated from a plot of C_p versus time. Values for (D_t/V_p) can be approximated by the Loo–Riegelman method, as follows:

$$(C_t)_{t_n} = \frac{k_{12} \Delta C_p \Delta t}{2} + \frac{k_{12}}{k_{21}}(C_p)_{t_{n-1}}(1 - e^{-k_{21}\Delta t}) + (C_t)_{t_{n-1}} e^{-k_{21}\Delta t} \tag{7.55}$$

where C_t is D_t/V_p, or apparent tissue concentration; $t =$ time of sampling for sample n; $t_{n-1} =$ time of sampling for the sampling point preceding sample n; and $(C_p)_{t_{n-1}} =$ concentration of drug at central compartment for sample $n - 1$.

Calculation of C_t values is shown in Table 7.3, using a typical set of oral absorption data. After calculation of C_t values, the percent of drug unabsorbed is calculated with Equation 7.54, as shown in Table 7.4. A plot of percent of drug unabsorbed versus time on semilog graph paper gives a k_a of approximately 0.5 hr^{-1}.

For calculation of the k_a by this method, the drug must be given intravenously to allow evaluation of the distribution and elimination rate constants. For drugs that cannot be given by the IV route, the k_a cannot be calculated by the Loo–Riegelman method. For these drugs, given by the oral route only, the Wagner–Nelson method, which assumes a one-compartment model, may be used to provide an initial estimate of k_a. If the drug is given intravenously, there is no way of knowing whether there is any variation in the values for the elimination rate constant k and the distributive rate constants k_{12} and k_{21}. Such variations alter the rate constants. Therefore, a one-compartment model is frequently used to fit the plasma curves after an oral or intramuscular dose. The plasma level predicted from the k_a obtained by this method does deviate from the actual plasma level. However, in many instances, this deviation is not significant.

Cumulative Relative Fraction Absorbed

The fraction of drug absorbed at any time t (Eq. 7.31) may be summed or cumulated for each time period for which a plasma drug sample was obtained. From

TABLE 7.3 Calculation of C_t Values[a]

$(C_p)_{t_n}$	$(t)_{t_n}$	ΔC_p	Δt	$\dfrac{(k_{12}\Delta C_p \Delta t)}{2}$	$(C_p)_{t_{n-1}}$	$(k_{12}/k_{21}) \times$ $(1 - e^{-k_{21}\Delta t})$	$(C_p)_{t_{n-1}} k_{12}/k_{21} \times$ $(1 - e^{-k_{21}\Delta t})$	$(C_t)_{t_{n-1}} e^{-k_{21}\Delta t}$	$(C_t)_{t_n}$
3.00	0.5	3.0	0.5	0.218	0	0.134	0	0	0.218
5.20	1.0	2.2	0.5	0.160	3.00	0.134	0.402	0.187	0.749
6.50	1.5	1.3	0.5	0.094	5.20	0.134	0.697	0.642	1.433
7.30	2.0	0.8	0.5	0.058	6.50	0.134	0.871	1.228	2.157
7.60	2.5	0.3	0.5	0.022	7.30	0.134	0.978	1.849	2.849
7.75	3.0	0.15	0.5	0.011	7.60	0.134	1.018	2.442	3.471
7.70	3.5	−0.05	0.5	−0.004	7.75	0.134	1.039	2.976	4.019
7.60	4.0	−0.10	0.5	−0.007	7.70	0.134	1.032	3.444	4.469
7.10	5.0	−0.50	1.0	−0.073	7.60	0.250	1.900	3.276	5.103
6.60	6.0	−0.50	1.0	−0.073	7.10	0.250	1.775	3.740	5.442
6.00	7.0	−0.60	1.0	−0.087	6.60	0.250	1.650	3.989	5.552
5.10	9.0	−0.90	2.0	−2.261	6.00	0.432	2.592	2.987	5.318
4.40	11.0	−0.70	2.0	−0.203	5.10	0.432	2.203	2.861	4.861
3.30	15.0	−1.10	4.0	−0.638	4.40	0.720	3.168	1.361	3.891

[a]Calculated with the following rate constants: $k_{12} = 0.29$ hr^{-1}, $k_{21} = 0.31^{-1}$.

Adapted with permission from Loo and Riegelman (1968).

TABLE 7.4 *Calculation of Percentage Unabsorbed*[a]

TIME (hr)	$(C_p)_{t_n}$	$[AUC]_{t_{n-1}}^{t_n}$	$[AUC]_{t_0}^{t_n}$	$k[AUC]_{t_0}^{t_n}$	$(C_t)_{t_n}$	Ab/V_p	$\% Ab/V_p$	$100\% - Ab/V_p\%$
0.5	3.00	0.750	0.750	0.120	0.218	3.338	16.6	83.4
1.0	5.20	2.050	2.800	0.448	0.749	6.397	31.8	68.2
1.5	6.50	2.925	5.725	0.916	1.433	8.849	44.0	56.0
2.0	7.30	3.450	9.175	1.468	2.157	10.925	54.3	45.7
2.5	7.60	3.725	12.900	2.064	2.849	12.513	62.2	37.8
3.0	7.75	3.838	16.738	2.678	3.471	13.889	69.1	30.9
3.5	7.70	3.863	20.601	3.296	4.019	15.015	74.6	25.4
4.0	7.60	3.825	24.426	3.908	4.469	15.977	79.4	20.6
5.0	7.10	7.350	31.726	5.084	5.103	17.287	85.9	14.1
6.0	6.60	6.850	38.626	6.180	5.442	18.222	90.6	9.4
7.0	6.00	6.300	44.926	7.188	5.552	18.740	93.1	6.9
9.0	5.10	11.100	56.026	8.964	5.318	19.382	96.3	3.7
11.0	4.40	9.500	65.526	10.484	4.861	19.745	98.1	1.9
15.0	3.30	15.400	80.926	12.948	3.891	20.139	100.0	0

[a] $Ab/V_p = (C_p) + k[AUC]_0^{t_n} + (C_t)_{t_n}$

$(C_t)_{t_n} = k_{12} \Delta C_p \Delta t / 2 + k_{12}/k_{21} (C_p)_{t_{n-1}} (1 - e^{-k_{21} \Delta t}) + (C_t)_{t_{n-1}} e^{-k_{21} \Delta t}$

$k = 0.16; k_{12} = 0.29; k_{21} = 0.31$

Equation 7.31, the term Ab/Ab^∞ becomes the *cumulative relative fraction absorbed* (CRFA).

$$CRFA = \frac{C_{p_t} + k[AUC]_0^t}{k[AUC]_0^\infty} \tag{7.56}$$

where C_{p_t} is the plasma concentration at time t.

In the Wagner–Nelson equation, Ab/Ab^∞ or CRFA will eventually equal unity, or 100%, even though the drug may not be 100% systemically bioavailable. The percent of drug absorbed is based on the total amount of drug absorbed (Ab^∞) rather than the dose D_0. Because the amount of the drug ultimately absorbed, Ab^∞, is equal to $k[AUC]_0^\infty$, the numerator will always equal the denominator, whether the drug is 10, 20, or 100% bioavailable. The percent of drug absorbed based on Ab/Ab^∞ is therefore different from the real percent of drug absorbed unless $F = 1$. However, for the calculation of k_a, the method is acceptable.

To determine the real percent of drug absorbed, a modification of the Wagner–Nelson equation was suggested by Welling (1986). A reference drug product was administered and plasma drug concentrations were determined over time. CRFA was then estimated by dividing Ab/Ab_{ref}^∞, where Ab is the cumulative amount of drug absorbed from the drug product and Ab_{ref}^∞ is the cumulative final amount of drug absorbed from a reference dosage form. In this case, the denominator of Equation 7.56 is modified as follows:

$$CRFA = \frac{C_p + k[AUC]_0^\infty}{k_{ref}[AUC]_{ref}^\infty} \tag{7.57}$$

Figure 7-16. Fraction of drug absorbed. (Wagner–Nelson method).

Figure 7-17. Mean cumulative relative fractions of tolazamide absorbed as a function of time. (From Welling et al, 1982, with permission.)

where k_{ref} and $[AUC]_{ref}^{\infty}$ are the elimination constant and the area under the curve determined from the reference product. The terms in the numerator of Equation 7.57 refer to the product, as in Equation 7.56.

Each fraction of drug absorbed is cumulated and plotted against the time interval in which the plasma drug sample was obtained (Fig. 7-16). An example of the relationship of CRFA versus time for the absorption of tolazamide from four different drug products is shown in Figure 7-17. The data for Figure 7-18 were obtained from the serum tolazamide levels–time curves in Figure 7-17. The CRFA–time graph provides a visual image of the relative rates of drug absorption from various drug products. If the CRFA–time curve is a straight line, then the drug was absorbed from the drug product at an apparent zero-order absorption rate.

SIGNIFICANCE OF ABSORPTION RATE CONSTANTS

The overall rate of systemic drug absorption from an orally administered solid dosage form encompasses many individual rate processes, including dissolution of the drug, GI motility, blood flow, and transport of the drug across the capillary membranes and into the systemic circulation. The rate of drug absorption represents the net result of all these processes. The selection of a model with either first-order or zero-order absorption is generally empirical.

The actual drug absorption process may be zero-order, first-order, or a combination of rate processes that is not easily quantitated. For many immediate-release

Figure 7-18. Mean serum tolazamide levels as a function of time. (From Welling et al, 1982, with permission.)

dosage forms, the absorption process is first-order due to the physical nature of drug diffusion. For certain controlled-release drug products, the rate of drug absorption may be more appropriately described by a zero-order rate constant.

The calculation of k_a is useful in designing a multiple-dosage regimen. Knowledge of the k_a and k allows for the prediction of peak and trough plasma drug concentrations following multiple dosing. In bioequivalence studies, drug products are given in chemically equivalent (ie, pharmaceutical equivalents) doses, and the respective rates of systemic absorption may not differ markedly. Therefore, for these studies, t_{max}, or time of peak drug concentration, can be very useful in comparing the respective rates of absorption of a drug from chemically equivalent drug products.

FREQUENTLY ASKED QUESTIONS

1. What is the absorption half-life of a drug and how is it determined?
2. When one simulates drug absorption with the oral one-compartment model, would a greater absorption rate constant result in a greater amount of drug absorbed?
3. How do you explain that k_a is often greater than k with most drugs?
4. Drug clearance is dependent on dose and area under the time–drug concentration curve. Would drug clearance be affected by the rate of absorption?
5. In switching a drug from IV to oral dosing, what is the most important consideration?

LEARNING QUESTIONS

1. Plasma samples from a patient were collected after an oral bolus dose of 10 mg of a new benzodiazepine solution as follows:

Time (hr)	Concentration (ng/mL)
0.25	2.85
0.50	5.43
0.75	7.75
1.00	9.84
2.00	16.20
4.00	22.15
6.00	23.01
10.00	19.09
14.00	13.90
20.00	7.97

From the data above:

a. Determine the elimination constant of the drug.

b. Determine k_a by feathering.

c. Determine the equation that describes the plasma drug concentration of the new benzodiazepine.

2. Assuming that the drug in Question 1 is 80% absorbed, find **(a)** the absorption constant, k_a; **(b)** the elimination half-life, $t_{1/2}$; **(c)** the t_{max}, or time of peak drug concentration; and **(d)** the volume of distribution of the patient.

3. Contrast the percent of drug-unabsorbed methods for the determination of rate constant for absorption, k_a, in terms of **(a)** pharmacokinetic model, **(b)** route of drug administration, and **(c)** possible sources of error.

4. What is the error inherent in the measurement of k_a for an orally administered drug that follows a two-compartment model when a one-compartment model is assumed in the calculation?

5. What are the main pharmacokinetic parameters that influence **(a)** time for peak drug concentration and **(b)** peak drug concentration?

6. Name a method of drug administration that will provide a zero-order input.

7. A single oral dose (100 mg) of an antibiotic was given to an adult male patient (43 years, 72 kg). From the literature, the pharmacokinetics of this drug fit a one-compartment open model. The equation that best fits the pharmacokinetics of the drug is

$$C_p = 45(e^{-0.17t} - e^{-1.5t})$$

From the equation above, calculate **(a)** t_{max}, **(b)** C_{max}, and **(c)** $t_{1/2}$ for the drug in this patient. Assume C_p is in $\mu g/mL$ and the first-order rate constants are in hours^{-1}.

8. Two drugs, A and B, have the following pharmacokinetic parameters after a single oral dose of 500 mg:

Drug	k_a (hr^{-1})	k (hr^{-1})	V_D (mL)
A	1.0	0.2	10,000
B	0.2	1.0	20,000

Both drugs follow a one-compartment pharmacokinetic model and are 100% bioavailable.

a. Calculate the t_{max} for each drug.

b. Calculate the C_{max} for each drug.

9. The bioavailability of phenylpropanolamine hydrochloride was studied in 24 adult male subjects. The following data represent the mean blood phenylpropanolamine hydrochloride concentrations (ng/mL) after the oral administration of a single 25-mg dose of phenylpropanolamine hydrochloride solution.

Time (hr)	Concentration (ng/mL)	Time (hr)	Concentration (ng/mL)
0	0	3	62.98
0.25	51.33	4	52.32
0.5	74.05	6	36.08
0.75	82.91	8	24.88
1.0	85.11	12	11.83
1.5	81.76	18	3.88
2	75.51	24	1.27

a. From the data, obtain the rate constant for absorption, k_a, and the rate constant for elimination, k, by the method of residuals.

b. Is it reasonable to assume that $k_a > k$ for a drug in a solution? How would you determine unequivocally which rate constant represents the elimination constant k?

c. From the data, which method, Wagner–Nelson or Loo–Riegelman, would be more appropriate to determine the order of the rate constant for absorption?

d. From your values, calculate the theoretical t_{max}. How does your value relate to the observed t_{max} obtained from the subjects?

e. Would you consider the pharmacokinetics of phenylpropanolamine HCl to follow a one-compartment model? Why?

REFERENCES

Levy G, Amsel LP, Elliot HC: Kinetics of salicyluric acid elimination in man. *J Pharm Sci* **58**:827–829, 1969

Loo JCK, Riegelman S: New method for calculating the intrinsic absorption rate of drugs. *J Pharm Sci* **57**:918–928, 1968

Portmann G: Pharmacokinetics. In Swarbrick J (ed), *Current Concepts in the Pharmaceutical Sciences,* vol 1. Philadelphia, Lea & Febiger, 1970, Chap 1

Welling PG: *Pharmacokinetics: Processes and Mathematics.* ACS monograph 185. Washington, DC, American Chemical Society, 1986, pp 174–175

Welling PG, Patel RB, Patel UR, et al: Bioavailability of tolazamide from tablets: Comparison of in vitro and in vivo results. *J Pharm Sci* **71**:1259, 1982

Wagner JG: Use of computers in pharmacokinetics. *Clin Pharmacol Ther* **8**:201–218, 1967

BIBLIOGRAPHY

Boxenbaum HG, Kaplan SA: Potential source of error in absorption rate calculations. *J Pharmacokinet Biopharm* **3**:257–264, 1975

Boyes R, Adams H, Duce B: Oral absorption and disposition kinetics of lidocaine hydrochloride in dogs. *J Pharmacol Exp Ther* **174**:1–8, 1970

Dvorchik BH, Vesell ES: Significance of error associated with use of the one-compartment formula to calculate clearance of 38 drugs. *Clin Pharmacol Ther* **23**:617–623, 1978

Wagner JG, Nelson E: Kinetic analysis of blood levels and urinary excretion in the absorptive phase after single doses of drug. *J Pharm Sci* **53**:1392, 1964

8

MULTIPLE-DOSAGE REGIMENS

In earlier chapters of this book we have discussed single-dose drug administration. After single-dose drug administration, the plasma drug level rises above and then falls below the *minimum effective concentration* (MEC), resulting in a decline in therapeutic effect. To maintain prolonged therapeutic activity, many drugs are given in a multiple-dosage regimen. The plasma levels of drugs given in multiple doses must be maintained within the narrow limits of the therapeutic window (eg, plasma drug concentrations above the MEC but below the *minimum toxic concentration* or MTC) to achieve optimal clinical effectiveness. Among these drugs are antibacterials, cardiotonics, anticonvulsants, and hormones. Ideally, a dosage regimen is established for each drug to provide the correct plasma level without excessive fluctuation and drug accumulation outside the therapeutic window.

For certain drugs, such as antibiotics, a desirable MEC can be determined. Some drugs that have a narrow therapeutic range (eg, digoxin and phenytoin) require definition of the therapeutic minimum and maximum nontoxic plasma concentrations (MEC and MTC, respectively). In calculating a multiple-dose regimen, the desired or *target* plasma drug concentration must be related to a therapeutic response, and the multiple-dose regimen must be designed to produce plasma concentrations within the therapeutic window.

There are two main parameters that can be adjusted in developing a dosage regimen: (1) the size of the drug dose and (2) τ, the frequency of drug administration (ie, the time interval between doses).

DRUG ACCUMULATION

To calculate a multiple-dose regimen for a patient or patients, pharmacokinetic parameters are first obtained from the plasma level–time curve generated by single-dose drug studies. With these pharmacokinetic parameters and knowledge of the size of the dose and dosage interval (τ), the complete plasma level–time curve or the plasma level may be predicted at any time after the beginning of the dosage regimen.

Figure 8-1. Simulated data showing blood levels after administration of multiple doses and accumulation of blood levels when equal doses are given at equal time intervals.

To calculate multiple-dose regimens, it is necessary to decide whether successive doses of drug will have any effect on the previous dose. The principle of *superposition* assumes that early doses of drug do not affect the pharmacokinetics of subsequent doses. Therefore, the blood levels after the second, third, or nth dose will overlay or superimpose the blood level attained after the $(n-1)$th dose. In addition, the AUC ($\int_0^\infty C_p\, dt$) following the administration of a single dose equals the AUC($\int_{t_1}^{t_2} C_p\, dt$) during a dosing interval at steady state (Fig. 8-1).

The principle of *superposition* allows one to project the plasma drug concentration–time curve of a drug after multiple consecutive doses based on the plasma drug concentration–time curve obtained after a single dose. The basic assumptions are that the drug is eliminated by first-order kinetics and that the pharmacokinetics of the drug after a single dose (first dose) are not altered after taking multiple doses.

The plasma drug concentrations after multiple doses may be predicted from the plasma drug concentrations obtained after a single dose. In Table 8.1, the plasma drug concentrations from 0 to 24 hours are measured after a single dose. A constant dose of drug is given every 4 hours and plasma drug concentrations after each dose are generated using the data after the first dose. Thus, the *predicted* plasma drug concentration in the patient is the total drug concentration obtained by adding the residual drug concentration obtained after each previous dose. The superposition principle may be used to predict drug concentrations after multiple doses of many drugs. Because the superposition principle is an overlay method, it may be used to predict drug concentrations after multiple doses given at either *equal* or *unequal* dosage intervals. For example, the plasma drug concentrations may be predicted after a drug dose is given every 8 hours, or 3 times a day before meals at 8 AM, 12 noon, and 6 PM.

There are situations, however, in which the superposition principle does not apply. In these cases, the pharmacokinetics of the drug change after multiple dosing due to various factors, including changing pathophysiology in the patient, saturation of a drug carrier system, enzyme induction, and enzyme inhibition. Drugs that follow nonlinear pharmacokinetics (Chapter 9) generally do not have predictable plasma drug concentrations after multiple doses using the superposition principle.

If the drug is administered at a fixed dose and a fixed dosage interval, as is the case with multiple-dose regimens, the amount of drug in the body will increase and then plateau to a mean plasma level higher than the peak C_p obtained from the initial dose (Figs. 8-1 and 8-2). When the second dose is given after a time interval

TABLE 8.1 Predicted Plasma Drug Concentrations for Multiple-Dose Regimen Using the Superposition Principle[a]

DOSE NUMBER	TIME (hr)	PLASMA DRUG CONCENTRATION (μg/mL)						TOTAL
		Dose 1	Dose 2	Dose 3	Dose 4	Dose 5	Dose 6	
1	0	0						0
	1	21.0						21.0
	2	22.3						22.3
	3	19.8						19.8
2	4	16.9	0					16.9
	5	14.3	21.0					35.3
	6	12.0	22.3					34.3
	7	10.1	19.8					29.9
3	8	8.50	16.9	0				25.4
	9	7.15	14.3	21.0				42.5
	10	6.01	12.0	22.3				40.3
	11	5.06	10.1	19.8				35.0
4	12	4.25	8.50	16.9	0			29.7
	13	3.58	7.15	14.3	21.0			46.0
	14	3.01	6.01	12.0	22.3			43.3
	15	2.53	5.06	10.1	19.8			37.5
5	16	2.13	4.25	8.50	16.9	0		31.8
	17	1.79	3.58	7.15	14.3	21.0		47.8
	18	1.51	3.01	6.01	12.0	22.3		44.8
	19	1.27	2.53	5.06	10.1	19.8		38.8
6	20	1.07	2.13	4.25	8.50	16.9	0	32.9
	21	0.90	1.79	3.58	7.15	14.3	21.0	48.7
	22	0.75	1.51	3.01	6.01	12.0	22.3	45.6
	23	0.63	1.27	2.53	5.06	10.1	19.8	39.4
	24	0.53	1.07	2.13	4.25	8.50	16.9	33.4

[a]A single oral dose of 350 mg was given and the plasma drug concentrations were measured for 0–24 hr. The same plasma drug concentrations are assumed to occur after doses 2–6. The total plasma drug concentration is the sum of the plasma drug concentrations due to each dose. For this example, $V_D = 10$ L, $t_{1/2} = 4$hr, and $k_a = 1.5$ hr^{-1}. The drug is 100% bioavailable and follows the pharmacokinetics of a one-compartment open model.

shorter than the time required to "completely" eliminate the previous dose, *drug accumulation* will occur in the body. In other words, the plasma concentrations following the second dose will be higher than corresponding plasma concentrations immediately following the first dose. However, if the second dose is given after a time interval longer than the time required to eliminate the previous dose, drug will not accumulate (Table 8.1).

As repetitive equal doses are given at a constant frequency, the plasma level–time curve plateaus and a steady state is obtained. At steady state, the plasma drug levels fluctuate between C_{max}^{∞} and C_{min}^{∞}. Once steady state is obtained, C_{max}^{∞} and C_{min}^{∞} are constant and remain unchanged from dose to dose. The C_{max}^{∞} is important in determining drug safety. The C_{max}^{∞} should always remain below the minimum toxic concentration. The C_{max}^{∞} is also a good indication of drug accumulation. If a drug produces the same C_{max}^{∞} at steady state, compared with the $(C_{n=1})_{max}$ after the first dose, then there is no drug accumulation. If C_{max}^{∞} is much larger than $(C_{n=1})_{max}$, then there is significant accumulation during the multiple-dose regimen.

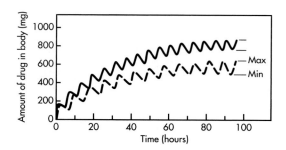

Figure 8-2. Amount of drug in the body as a function of time. Equal doses of drug were given every 6 hours (upper curve) and every 8 hours (lower curve). k_a and k remain constant.

Accumulation is affected by the elimination half-life of the drug and the dosing interval. The index for measuring drug accumulation R is

$$R = \frac{(C^\infty)_{\max}}{(C_{n=1})_{\max}} \qquad (8.1)$$

Substituting for $C_{\max}$ after the first dose and at steady state yields

$$R = \frac{D_0/V_D [1/(1 - e^{-k\tau})]}{D_0/V_D}$$

$$R = \frac{1}{1 - e^{-k\tau}} \qquad (8.2)$$

Equation 8.2 shows that drug accumulation measured with the R index depends on the elimination constant and the dosing interval and is independent of the dose. For a drug given in repetitive oral doses, the time required to reach steady state is dependent on the elimination half-life of the drug and is independent of the size of the dose, the length of the dosing interval, and the number of doses. For example, if the dose or dosage interval of the drug is altered as shown in Figure 8-2, the time required for the drug to reach steady state is the same, but the final steady-state plasma level changes proportionately. Furthermore, if the drug is given at the same dosing rate but as an infusion (eg, 25 mg/hr), the average plasma drug concentrations (C_{av}^∞) will be the same but the fluctuations between $C_{\max}^\infty$ and $C_{\min}^\infty$ will vary (Fig. 8-3). An average steady-state plasma drug concentration is obtained by dividing the area under the curve (AUC) for a dosing period (ie, $\int_{t_1}^{t_2} C_p \, dt$) by the dosing interval τ, at steady state.

An equation for the estimation of the time to reach one-half of the steady-state plasma levels or the accumulation half-life has been described by van Rossum and Tomey (1968).

$$\text{Accumulation } t_{1/2} = t_{1/2}\left(1 + 3.3 \log \frac{k_a}{k_a - k}\right) \qquad (8.3)$$

For IV administration, k_a is very rapid (approaches ∞); k is very small in comparison to k_a and can be omitted in the denominator of Equation 8.3. Thus, Equation 8.3 reduces to

$$\text{Accumulation } t_{1/2} = t_{1/2}\left(1 + 3.3 \log \frac{k_a}{k_a}\right) \qquad (8.4)$$

Figure 8-3. Simulated plasma drug concentration–time curves after IV infusion and oral multiple doses for a drug with an elimination half-life of 4 hours and apparent V_D of 10 L. IV infusion given at a rate of 25 mg/hr, oral multiple doses are 200 mg every 8 hours, 300 mg every 12 hours, and 600 mg every 24 hours.

Because $k_a/k_a = 1$ and $\log 1 = 0$, the accumulation $t_{1/2}$ of a drug administered intravenously is the elimination $t_{1/2}$ of the drug. From this relationship, the time to reach 50% steady-state drug concentrations is dependent on the elimination $t_{1/2}$ and not on the dose or dosage interval.

As shown in Equation 8.4, the accumulation $t_{1/2}$ is directly proportional to the elimination $t_{1/2}$. Table 8.2 gives the accumulation $t_{1/2}$ of drugs with various elimination half-lives given by multiple oral doses (Table 8.2).

From a clinical viewpoint, the time needed to reach 90% of the steady-state plasma concentration is 3.3 times the elimination half-life, whereas the time required to reach 99% of the steady-state plasma concentration is 6.6 times the elimination half-life (Table 8.3). It should be noted from Table 8.3 that at a constant dose size, the shorter the dosage interval, the larger the dosing rate (mg/hr), and the higher the steady-state drug level.

The number of doses for a given drug to reach steady state is dependent on the elimination half-life of the drug and the dosage interval τ (Table 8.3). If the drug is given at a dosage interval equal to the half-life of the drug, then 6.6 doses are required to reach 99% of the theoretical steady-state plasma drug concentration. The number of doses needed to reach steady state is $6.6 t_{1/2}/\tau$, as calculated in the

TABLE 8.2 Effect of Elimination Half-Life and Absorption Rate Constant on Accumulation Half-Life after Oral Administration[a]

ELIMINATION HALF-LIFE (hr)	ELIMINATION RATE CONSTANT (1/hr)	ABSORPTION RATE CONSTANT (1/hr)	ACCUMULATION HALF-LIFE (hr)
4	0.173	1.50	4.70
8	0.0866	1.50	8.67
12	0.0578	1.50	12.8
24	0.0289	1.50	24.7
4	0.173	1.00	5.09
8	0.0866	1.00	8.99
12	0.0578	1.00	13.0
24	0.0289	1.00	25.0

[a]Accumulation half-life is calculated by Equation 8.3, and is the half-time for accumulation of the drug to 90% of the steady-state plasma drug concentration.

far right column of Table 8.3. As discussed in Chapter 5, Table 5.1, it takes 4.32 half-lives to reach 95% of steady state.

REPETITIVE INTRAVENOUS INJECTIONS

The maximum amount of drug in the body following a single rapid IV injection is equal to the dose of the drug. For a one-compartment open model, the drug will be eliminated according to first-order kinetics.

$$D_B = D_0 e^{-kt} \tag{8.5}$$

TABLE 8.3 Interrelation of Elimination Half-Life, Dosage Interval, Maximum Plasma Concentration, and Time to Reach Steady-State Plasma Concentration[a]

ELIMINATION HALF-LIFE (hr)	DOSAGE INTERVAL, τ (hr)	C_{max}^{∞} (μg/mL)	TIME FOR C_{av}^{∞}[b] (hr)	NO. DOSES TO REACH 99% STEADY STATE
0.5	0.5	200	3.3	6.6
0.5	1.0	133	3.3	3.3
1.0	0.5	341	6.6	13.2
1.0	1.0	200	6.6	6.6
1.0	2.0	133	6.6	3.3
1.0	4.0	107	6.6	1.65
1.0	10.0	100[c]	6.6	0.66
2.0	1.0	341	13.2	13.2
2.0	2.0	200	13.2	6.1

[a]A single dose of 1000 mg of three hypothetical drugs with various elimination half-lives but equal volumes of distribution (V_D = 10 L) were given by multiple IV doses at various dosing intervals. All time values are in hours: (C_{max}^{∞}) = maximum steady-state concentration. C_{av}^{∞} = average steady-state plasma concentration. The maximum plasma drug concentration after the first dose of the drug is $(C_{n=1})_{max}$ = 100 μg/mL.
[b]Time to reach 99% of steady-state plasma concentration.
[c]Since the dosage interval, τ, is very large compared to the elimination half-life, no accumulation of drug occurs.

If τ is equal to the dosage interval (ie, the time between the first dose and the next dose), then the amount of drug remaining in the body after several hours can be determined with

$$D_B = D_0 e^{-k\tau} \tag{8.6}$$

The fraction (f) of the dose remaining in the body is related to the elimination constant (k) and the dosage interval (τ) as follows:

$$f = \frac{D_B}{D_0} = e^{-k\tau} \tag{8.7}$$

With any given dose, f depends on k and τ. If τ is large, f will be smaller because D_B (the amount of drug remaining in the body) is smaller.

 # EXAMPLES

1. A patient receives 1000 mg every 6 hours by repetitive IV injection of an antibiotic with an elimination half-life of 3 hours. Assume the drug is distributed according to a one-compartment model and the volume of distribution is 20 L.

   a. Find the maximum and minimum amount of drug in the body.

   b. Determine the maximum and minimum plasma concentration of the drug.

Solution

   a. The fraction of drug remaining in the body is estimated by Equation 8.7. The concentration of the drug declines to one-half after 3 hours ($t_{1/2} = 3$ hr), after which the amount of drug will again decline by one-half at the end of the next 3 hours. Therefore, at the end of 6 hours only one-quarter, or 0.25, of the original dose remains in the body. Thus f is equal to 0.25.

   To use Equation 8.7, we must first find the value of k from the $t_{1/2}$.

   $$k = \frac{0.693}{t_{1/2}} = \frac{0.693}{3} = 0.231 \text{ hr}^{-1}$$

   The time interval τ is equal to 6 hours. From Equation 8.7,

   $$f = e^{-(0.231)(6)}$$
   $$f = 0.25$$

   In this example, 1000 mg of drug is given intravenously, so the amount of drug in the body is immediately increased by 1000 mg. At the end of the dosage interval (ie, before the next dose), the amount of drug remaining in the body is 25% of the amount of drug present just after the previous dose, because $f = 0.25$.

TABLE 8.4 Fraction of the Dose in the Body before and after Intravenous Injections of a 1000-mg Dose[a]

	AMOUNT OF DRUG IN BODY	
NUMBER OF DOSES	Before Dose	After Dose
1	0	1000
2	250	1250
3	312	1312
4	328	1328
5	332	1332
6	333	1333
7	333	1333
∞	333	1333

[a]$f = 0.25$.

Thus, if the value of f is known, a table can be constructed relating the fraction of the dose in the body before and after rapid IV injection (Table 8.4).

From Table 8.4 the maximum amount of drug in the body is 1333 mg and the minimum amount of drug in the body is 333 mg. The difference between the maximum and minimum values, D_0, will always equal the injected dose.

$$D_{max} - D_{min} = D_0 \tag{8.8}$$

In this example,

$$1333 - 333 = 1000 \text{ mg}$$

D_{max}^{∞} can also be calculated directly by the relationship

$$D_{max}^{\infty} = \frac{D_0}{1 - f} \tag{8.9}$$

Substituting known data, we obtain

$$D_{max}^{\infty} = \frac{1000}{1 - 0.25} = 1333 \text{ mg}$$

then, from Equation 13.8,

$$D_{min}^{\infty} = 1333 - 1000 = 333 \text{ mg}$$

The average amount of drug in the body at steady state, D_{av}^{∞}, can be found by Equation 8.10 or Equation 8.11. F is the fraction of dose absorbed. For an IV injection, F is equal to 1.0.

$$D_{av}^{\infty} = \frac{FD_0}{k\tau} \tag{8.10}$$

$$D_{av}^{\infty} = \frac{FD_0 1.44 t_{1/2}}{\tau} \tag{8.11}$$

Equations 8.10 and 8.11 can be used for repetitive dosing at constant time intervals and for any route of administration as long as elimination occurs from the central compartment. Substitution of values from the example into Equation 8.11 gives

$$D_{\text{av}}^{\infty} = \frac{(1)\,(1000)\,(1.44)\,(3)}{6} = 720 \text{ mg}$$

Since the drug in the body declines exponentially (ie, first-order drug elimination), the value D_{av}^{∞} is not the arithmetic mean of D_{max}^{∞} and D_{min}^{∞}. The limitation of using D_{av}^{∞} is that the fluctuations of D_{max}^{∞} and D_{min}^{∞} are not known.

b. To determine the concentration of drug in the body after multiple doses, divide the amount of drug in the body by the volume in which it is dissolved. For a one-compartment model, the maximum, minimum, and steady-state concentrations of drug in the plasma are found by the following equations:

$$C_{\text{max}}^{\infty} = \frac{D_{\text{max}}^{\infty}}{V_{\text{D}}} \tag{8.12}$$

$$C_{\text{min}}^{\infty} = \frac{D_{\text{min}}^{\infty}}{V_{\text{D}}} \tag{8.13}$$

$$C_{\text{av}}^{\infty} = \frac{D_{\text{av}}^{\infty}}{V_{\text{D}}} \tag{8.14}$$

A more direct approach to finding C_{max}^{∞}, C_{min}^{∞}, and C_{av}^{∞} is

$$C_{\text{max}}^{\infty} = \frac{C_{\text{p}}^{0}}{1 - e^{-k\tau}} \tag{8.15}$$

where C_{p}^{0} is equal to D_{0}/V_{D}.

$$C_{\text{min}}^{\infty} = \frac{C_{\text{p}}^{0} e^{-k\tau}}{1 - e^{-k\tau}} \tag{8.16}$$

$$C_{\text{av}}^{\infty} = \frac{FD_{0}}{V_{\text{D}} k\tau} \tag{8.17}$$

For this example, the values for C_{max}^{∞}, C_{min}^{∞}, and C_{av}^{∞} are 66.7, 16.7, and 36.1 μg/mL, respectively.

As mentioned, C_{av}^{∞} is not the arithmetic mean of C_{max}^{∞} and C_{min}^{∞} because plasma drug concentration declines exponentially. The C_{av}^{∞} is equal to the AUC($\int_{t_1}^{t_2} C_{\text{p}}\, dt$) for a dosage interval at steady state divided by the dosage interval τ.

$$C_{\text{av}}^{\infty} = \frac{[\text{AUC}]_{t_1}^{t_2}}{\tau} \tag{8.18}$$

The AUC is related to the amount of drug absorbed divided by total body clearance (Cl), as shown in the following equation.

$$[\text{AUC}]_{t_1}^{t_2} = \frac{FD_0}{Cl_T} = \frac{FD_0}{kV_D} \tag{8.19}$$

Substitution of FD_0/kV_D for AUC in Equation 8.18 gives Equation 8.17. Equation 8.17 or 8.18 can be used to obtain C_{av}^{∞} after a multiple-dose regimen regardless of the route of administration.

It is sometimes desirable to know the plasma drug concentration at any time after the administration of n doses of drug. The general expression for calculating this plasma drug concentration is

$$C_p = \frac{D_0}{V_D}\left(\frac{1 - e^{-nk\tau}}{1 - e^{-k\tau}}\right)e^{-kt} \tag{8.20}$$

where n is the number of doses given and t is the time after the nth dose.

At steady state, $e^{-nk\tau}$ approaches zero and Equation 8.20 reduces to

$$C_p^{\infty} = \frac{D_0}{V_D}\left(\frac{1}{1 - e^{-k\tau}}\right)e^{-kt} \tag{8.21}$$

where C_p^{∞} is the steady-state drug concentration at time t after the dose.

2. The patient in the previous example received 1000 mg of an antibiotic every 6 hours by repetitive IV injection. The drug has an apparent volume of distribution of 20 L and elimination half-life of 3 hours. Calculate (a) the plasma drug concentration C_p at 3 hours after the second dose, (b) the steady-state plasma drug concentration C_p^{∞} at 3 hours after the last dose, (c) C_{max}^{∞}, (d) C_{min}^{∞}, and (e) C_{SS}.

Solution

a. The C_p at 3 hours after the second dose. Use Equation 8.20 and let $n = 2$, $t = 3$ hours, and make other appropriate substitutions.

$$C_p = \frac{1000}{20}\left(\frac{1 - e^{-(2)(0.231)(6)}}{1 - e^{-(0.231)(6)}}\right)e^{-0.231(3)}$$

$$C_p = 31.3 \text{ mg/L}$$

b. The C_p^{∞} at 3 hours after the last dose. Because steady state is reached, use Equation 8.21 and perform the following calculation.

$$C_p^{\infty} = \frac{1000}{20}\left(\frac{1}{1 - e^{-0.231(6)}}\right)e^{-0.231(3)}$$

$$C_p^{\infty} = 33.3 \text{ mg/L}$$

c. The C_{max}^{∞} is calculated from Equation 8.15.

$$C_{max}^{\infty} = \frac{1000/20}{1 - e^{-(0.231)(6)}} = 66.7 \text{ mg/L}$$

d. The $C_{\min}^{\infty}$ may be estimated as the drug concentration after the dosage interval τ, or just before the next dose.

$$C_{\min}^{\infty} = C_{\max}^{\infty}\, e^{-kt} = 66.7 e^{-(0.231)(6)} = 16.7 \text{ mg/L}$$

e. The C_{SS} is estimated by Equation 8.17. Because the drug is given by IV bolus injections, $F = 1$.

$$C_{SS} = \frac{1000}{(0.231)(20)(6)} = 36.1 \text{ mg/L}$$

C_{av}^{∞} is represented as C_{SS} in some references.

Problem of a Missed Dose

Equation 8.22 describes the plasma drug concentration t hours after the nth dose was administered; the doses are administered τ hours apart according to a multiple-dose regimen:

$$C_{p} = \frac{D_{0}}{V_{D}}\left(\frac{1 - e^{-nk\tau}}{1 - e^{-k\tau}}\right)e^{-kt} \tag{8.22}$$

Concentration contributed by the missing dose is

$$C'_{p} = \frac{D_{0}}{V_{D}}e^{-kt_{\text{miss}}} \tag{8.23}$$

in which t_{miss} = time elapsed since the scheduled dose was missed. Subtracting Equation 8.23 from Equation 8.20 corrects for the missing dose as shown in Equation 8.24.

$$C_{p} = \frac{D_{0}}{V_{D}}\left[\left(\frac{1 - e^{-nk\tau}}{1 - e^{-k\tau}}\right)e^{-kt} - e^{-kt_{\text{miss}}}\right] \tag{8.24}$$

Note: If steady state is reached (ie, either n = large or after many doses), the equation simplifies to Equation 8.25. Equation 8.25 is useful when steady state is reached.

$$C_{p} = \frac{D_{0}}{V_{D}}\left(\frac{e^{-kt}}{1 - e^{-kt}}\right) - e^{-kt_{\text{miss}}} \tag{8.25}$$

Generally, if the missing dose is recent, it will affect the present drug level more. If the missing dose is several half-lives later ($>5t_{1/2}$), the missing dose may be omitted because it will be very small. Equation 8.24 accounts for one missing dose, but several missing doses can be subtracted in a similar way if necessary.

EXAMPLE

A cephalosporin ($k = 0.2 \text{ hr}^{-1}$, $V_D = 10$ L) was administered by IV multiple dosing; 100 mg was injected every 6 hours for 6 doses. What was the plasma drug concentration 4 hours after the 6th dose (ie, 40 hours later) if **(a)** the 5th dose was omitted, **(b)** the 6th dose was omitted, **(c)** the 4th dose was omitted?

Solution

Substitute $k = 0.2 \text{ hr}^{-1}$, $V_D = 10$ L, $D = 100$ mg, $n = 6$, $t = 4$ hr, and $\tau = 6$ hr into equation 8.20 and evaluate:

$$C_p = 6.425 \text{ mg/L}$$

If no dose was omitted, then 4 hours after the 6th injection, C_p would be 6.425 mg/L.

(a) Missing the 5th dose, its contribution must be subtracted off, $t_{miss} = 6 + 4 = 10$ hours (the time elapsed since missing the dose):

$$C_p' = \frac{D_0}{V_D} e^{-kt_{miss}} = \frac{100}{10} e^{-(0.2 \times 10)} = 10 \times 0.1353 = 1.353 \text{ mg/L}$$

Drug concentration correcting for the missing dose $= 6.425 - 1.353 = 5.072$ mg/L.

(b) If the 6th dose is missing, $t_{miss} = 4$ hours:

$$C_p' = \frac{D_0}{V_D} e^{-kt_{miss}} = \frac{100}{10} e^{-(0.2 \times 4)} = 4.493 \text{ mg/L}$$

Drug concentration correcting for the missing dose $= 6.425 - 4.493 = 1.932$ mg/L.

(c) If the 4th dose is missing, $t_{miss} = 12 + 4 = 16$ hours:

$$C_p' = \frac{D_0}{V_D} e^{-kt_{miss}} = \frac{100}{10} e^{-(0.2 \times 16)} = 0.408 \text{ mg/L}$$

The drug concentration corrected for the missing dose $= 6.425 - 0.408 = 6.017$ mg/L.

Note: The effect of a missing dose becomes less pronounced at a later time. A strict dose regimen compliance is advised for all drugs. With some drugs, missing a dose can have a serious effect on therapy. For example, compliance is important for the anti-HIV1 drugs such as protease inhibitors.

Early or Late Dose Administration during Multiple Dosing

When one of the drug doses is taken earlier or later than scheduled, the resulting plasma drug concentration can still be calculated based on the principle of superposition. The dose can be treated as missing, with the late or early dose added back to take into account the actual time of dosing, using Equation 8.26.

$$C_p = \frac{D_0}{V_D}\left(\frac{1 - e^{-nkt}}{1 - e^{-kt}}e^{-kt} - e^{-kt_{miss}} + e^{-kt_{actual}}\right) \tag{8.26}$$

in which t_{miss} = time elapsed since the dose (late or early) is scheduled, and t_{actual} = time elapsed since the dose (late or early) is actually taken. Using a similar approach, a second missed dose can be subtracted from Equation 8.20. Similarly, a second late/early dose may be corrected by subtracting the scheduled dose followed by adding the actual dose. Similarly, if a different dose is given, the regular dose may be subtracted and the new dose added back.

EXAMPLE

Assume the same drug as above (ie, $k = 0.2$ hr^{-1}, $V_D = 10$ L) was given by multiple IV bolus injections and that at a dose of 100 mg every 6 hours for 6 doses. What is the plasma drug concentration 4 hours after the 6th dose, if the 5th dose were given an hour late?

Substitute into Equation 8.26 for all unknowns: $k = 0.2$ hr^{-1}, $V_D = 10$ L, $D = 100$ mg, $n = 6$, $\tau = 4$ hr, $\tau = 6$ hr, t-miss $= 6 + 4 = 10$ hr, $t_{actual} = 9$ hr (taken 1 hour late, ie, 5 hours before the 6th dose).

$$C_p = \frac{D_0}{V_D}\left(\frac{1 - e^{-nk\tau}}{1 - e^{-k\tau}}e^{-k\tau} - e^{kt_{miss}} + e^{-kt_{actual}}\right)$$

$$C_p = 6.425 - 1.353 + 1.653 = 6.725 \text{ mg/L}$$

Note: 1.353 mg/L was subtracted and 1.653 mg/mL was added because the 5th dose was not given as planned, but was given 1 hour later.

INTERMITTENT INTRAVENOUS INFUSION

Intermittent IV infusion is a method of successive short IV drug infusions in which the drug is given by IV infusion for a short period of time followed by a drug elimination period, then followed by another short IV infusion (Fig. 8-4). In drug regimens involving short IV infusion, the drug may not reach steady state. The rational for intermittent IV infusion is to prevent transient high drug concentrations and accompanying side effects. Many drugs are better tolerated when infused slowly over time compared to IV bolus dosing.

Administering One or More Doses by Constant Infusion: Superposition of Several IV Infusion Doses

For a continuous IV infusion (see Chapter 6):

$$C_p = \frac{R}{Cl}(1 - e^{-kt}) = \frac{R}{kV_D}(1 - e^{-kt}) \qquad (8.27)$$

Equation 8.27 may be modified to determine drug concentration after one or more short IV infusions for a specified time period (Eq. 8.28).

$$C_p = \frac{D}{t_{inf}V_D k}(1 - e^{-kt}) \qquad (8.28)$$

where R = rate of infusion = D/t_{inf}, D = size of infusion dose, and t_{inf} = infusion period.

After the infusion is stopped, the drug concentration post-IV infusion is obtained using the first-order equation for drug elimination:

$$C_p = C_{stop}e^{-kt} \qquad (8.29)$$

where C_{stop} = concentration when infusion stops, t = time elapsed since infusion stopped.

EXAMPLE

An antibiotic was infused with a 40-mg IV dose over 2 hours. Ten hours later, a second dose of 40 mg was infused, again over 2 hours. **(a)** What is the plasma drug concentration 2 hours after the start of the first infusion? **(b)** What is the plasma drug concentration 5 hours after the second dose infusion was started? Assume $k = 0.2$ hr^{-1}, $V_D = 10$ L for the antibiotic.

Solution

The predicted plasma drug concentrations after the first and second IV infusions are shown in Table 8.5. Using the principle of superposition, the total plasma drug concentration is the sum of the residual drug concentrations due to the first IV infusion (column 3) and the drug concentrations due to the second IV infusion (column 4). A graphical representation of these data is shown in Figure 8-4.

   a. The plasma drug concentration at 2 hours after the first IV infusion starts is calculated from Equation 8.28.

$$C_p = \frac{40/2}{10 \times 0.2}(1 - e^{-0.2(2)}) = 3.30 \text{ mg/L}$$

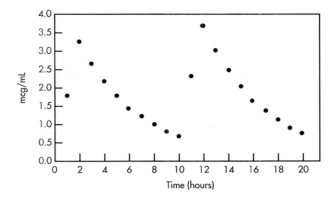

Figure 8-41.   Plasma drug concentration after two doses by IV infusion. Data from Table 8.5.

b. From Table 8.5, the plasma drug concentration at 15 hours (ie, 5 hours after the start of the second IV infusion) is 2.06 μg/mL. At 5 hours after the second IV infusion starts, the plasma drug concentration is the sum of the residual plasma drug concentrations from the first 2-hour infusion according to first-order elimination and the residual plasma drug concentrations from the second 2-hour IV infusion as shown in the following scheme:

The plasma drug concentration is calculated using the first-order elimination equation, where C_{stop} is the plasma drug concentration at the stop of the 2-hour IV infusion.

The plasma drug concentration after the completion of the first IV infusion, when $t = 13$ hours is

$$C_p = C_{stop}\ e^{-kt} = 3.30e^{-0.2\times13} = 0.25 \text{ mg/L}$$

The plasma drug concentration 5 hours after the second IV infusion is

$$C_p = C_{stop}e^{-kt} = 3.30e^{-0.2\times3} = 1.81\ \mu\text{g/mL}$$

The total plasma drug concentration 5 hours after the start of the second IV infusion is

$$0.25 \text{ mg/L} + 1.81 \text{ mg/L} = 2.06 \text{ mg/L.}$$

TABLE 8.5   Drug Concentration after Two Intravenous Infusions[a]

	TIME (hr)	PLASMA DRUG CONCENTRATION AFTER INFUSION 1	PLASMA DRUG CONCENTRATION AFTER INFUSION 2	TOTAL PLASMA DRUG CONCENTRATION
Infusion 1 begins	0	0		0
	1	1.81		1.81
Infusion 1 stopped	2	3.30		3.30
	3	2.70		2.70
	4	2.21		2.21
	5	1.81		1.81
	6	1.48		1.48
	7	1.21		1.21
	8	0.99		0.99
	9	0.81		0.81
Infusion 2 begins	10	0.67	0	0.67
	11	0.55	1.81	2.36
Infusion 2 stopped	12	0.45	3.30	3.74
	13	0.37	2.70	3.07
	14	0.30	2.21	2.51
	15	0.25	1.81	2.06

[a]Drug is given by a 2-hour infusion separated by a 10-hour drug elimination interval. All drug concentrations are in $\mu g/mL$. The declining drug concentration after the first infusion dose and the drug concentration after the second infusion dose gives the total plasma drug concentration.

CLINICAL EXAMPLE

Gentamicin sulfate was given to an adult male patient (57 years old, 70 kg) by intermittent IV infusions. One-hour IV infusions of 90 mg of gentamicin were given at 8-hour intervals. Gentamicin clearance is similar to creatinine clearance and was estimated as 7.2 L/hr with an elimination half-life of 3 hours.

a. What is the plasma drug concentration after the first IV infusion?

b. What is the peak plasma drug concentration, C_{pk}, and the trough plasma drug concentration, C_{min}, at steady state?

Solution

a. The plasma drug concentration directly after the first infusion is calculated from Equation 8.27, where $R = 90$ mg/hr, $Cl = 7.2$ L/hr, and $k = 0.231$ hr^{-1}. The time for infusion, t_{int}, is 1 hour.

$$C_{p} = \frac{90}{7.2} \left(1 - e^{-(0.231)(1)}\right) = 2.58 \text{ mg/L}$$

b. The C_{pk} at steady state may be obtained from Equation 8.30.

$$C_{pk} = \frac{R(1 - e^{-kt_{inf}})}{Cl} \frac{1}{(1 - e^{-k\tau})} \tag{8.30}$$

where C_{pk} is the peak drug concentration following the nth infusion, at steady state, t_{inf} is the time for infusion, and τ is the dosage interval. The term $1/(1 - e^{-kt})$ is the accumulation factor for repeated drug administration.

Substitution in Equation 8.30 gives

$$C_{pk} = \frac{90\,(1 - e^{-(0.231)(1)})}{7.2} \times \frac{1}{(1 - e^{-(0.231)(8)})} = 3.06 \text{ mg/L}$$

The plasma drug concentration at any time after the last infusion at steady state is obtained by Equation 8.31 and assumes that plasma drug concentrations decline according to first-order elimination kinetics.

$$C_{pk} = \frac{R\,(1 - e^{-kt_{inf}})}{Cl} \times \frac{1}{(1 - e^{-k\tau})} \times e^{-kt_{inf}} \tag{8.31}$$

where t_{inf} is the time for infusion and t is the time after the start of the infusion.

The trough plasma drug concentration, C_{min}, at steady state is the drug concentration just before the start of the next IV infusion or after a dosage interval equal to 8 hours after the infusion stopped. Equation 8.31 can be used to determine the plasma drug concentration at any time after the last infusion is stopped (after steady state has been reached).

$$C_{min} = \frac{90\,(1 - e^{-(0.231)(1)})}{7.2} \times \frac{e^{-(0.231)(9-1)}}{(1 - e^{-(0.231)(8)})} = 0.48 \text{ mg/L}$$

ESTIMATION OF k AND V_D OF AMINOGLYCOSIDES IN CLINICAL SITUATIONS

As illustrated above, antibiotics are often infused intravenously by multiple doses, so it is desirable to adjust the recommended starting dose based on the patient's individual k and V_D values. According to Sawchuk and Zaske (1976), individual parameters for aminoglycoside pharmacokinetics may be determined in a patient by using a limited number of plasma drug samples taken at appropriate time intervals. The equation was simplified by replacing an elaborate model with the one-compartment model to describe drug elimination and appropriately avoiding the distributive phase. The plasma sample should be collected 15 to 30 minutes postinfusion (with infusion lasting about 60 minutes) and, in patients with poor renal function, 1 to 2 hours postinfusion, to allow adequate tissue distribution. The second and third blood samples should be collected about 2 to 3 half-lives later, in order to get a good estimation of the slope. The data may be determined graphically or by regression analysis using a scientific calculator or computer program.

$$V_D = \frac{R(1 - e^{-kt_{inf}})}{[C_{SS,max} - C_{SS,min}e^{-kt_{inf}}]} \tag{8.32}$$

The dose of aminoglycoside is generally fixed by the desirable peak, $C_{SS,max}$, and trough plasma concentration, $C_{SS,min}$. For example, $C_{SS,min}$ for gentamicin may be set at 6–10 μg/mL with the steady-state trough level, $C_{SS,min}$, generally about 0.5–2 μg/mL, depending on the severity of the infection and renal considerations. The upper range is used only for life-threatening infections. The infusion rate for any desired peak drug concentration may be calculated using Equation 8.33.

$$R = \frac{V_D k C_{SS,max}(1 - e^{-k\tau})}{(1 - e^{-kt_{inf}})} \tag{8.33}$$

The dosing interval τ between infusions may be adjusted to obtain a desired concentration.

MULTIPLE-ORAL-DOSE REGIMEN

Figures 8-1 and 8-2 present typical cumulation curves for the concentration of drug in the body after multiple oral doses given at a constant dosage interval. The plasma concentration at any time during an oral or extravascular multiple-dose regimen, assuming a one-compartment model and constant doses and dose interval, can be determined as follows:

$$C_p = \frac{Fk_a D_0}{V_D(k - k_a)}\left[\left(\frac{1 - e^{-nk_a\tau}}{1 - e^{-k_a\tau}}\right)e^{-k_a t} - \left(\frac{1 - e^{-nk\tau}}{1 - e^{-k\tau}}\right)e^{-kt}\right] \tag{8.34}$$

where n = number of doses, τ = dosage interval, F = fraction of dose absorbed, and t = time after administration of n doses.

The mean plasma level at steady state, C_{av}^{∞}, is determined by a similar method to that employed for repeat IV injections. Equation 8.17 can be used for finding C_{av}^{∞} for any route of administration.

$$C_{av}^{\infty} = \frac{FD_0}{V_D k\tau} \tag{8.17}$$

Because proper evaluation of F and V_D requires IV data, the AUC of a dosing interval at steady state may be substituted in Equation 8.17 to obtain

$$C_{av}^{\infty} = \frac{\int_0^{\infty} C_p\, dt}{\tau} = \frac{[AUC]_0^{\infty}}{\tau} \tag{8.35}$$

One can see from Equation 8.17 that the magnitude of C_{av}^{∞} is directly proportional to the size of the dose and the extent of drug absorbed. Furthermore, if the dosage interval (τ) is shortened, then the value for C_{av}^{∞} will increase. The C_{av}^{∞} will be predictably higher for drugs distributed in a small V_D (eg, plasma water) or that have long elimination half-lives than for drugs distributed in a large V_D (eg, total body water) or that have very short elimination half-lives. Because body clearance (Cl_T) is equal to kV_D, substitution into Equation 8.17 yields

$$C_{av}^{\infty} = \frac{FD_0}{Cl_T \tau} \tag{8.36}$$

Thus, if Cl_T decreases, C_{av}^{∞} will increase.

The C_{av}^{∞} does not give information concerning the fluctuations in plasma concentration (C_{max}^{∞} and C_{min}^{∞}). In multiple-dose regimens, C_p at any time can be obtained using Equation 8.34, where $n = n$th dose. At steady state, the drug concentration can be determined by letting n equal infinity. Therefore, $e^{-nk\tau}$ becomes approximately equal to zero and Equation 8.22 becomes

$$C_p^{\infty} = \frac{k_a FD_0}{V_D(k_a - k)} \left[\left(\frac{1}{1 - e^{-k\tau}} \right) e^{-kt} - \left(\frac{1}{1 - e^{k_a\tau}} \right) e^{-k_a t} \right] \tag{8.37}$$

The maximum and minimum drug concentrations (C_{max}^{∞} and C_{min}^{∞}) can be obtained with the following equations:

$$C_{max}^{\infty} = \frac{FD_0}{V_D} \left(\frac{1}{1 - e^{-k\tau}} \right) e^{-kt_p} \tag{8.38}$$

$$C_{min}^{\infty} = \frac{k_a FD_0}{V_D(k_a - k)} \left(\frac{1}{1 - e^{-k\tau}} \right) e^{-k\tau} \tag{8.39}$$

The time at which maximum (peak) plasma concentration (or t_{max}) occurs following a single oral dose is

$$t_{max} = \frac{2.3}{k_a - k} \log \frac{k_a}{k} \tag{8.40}$$

whereas the peak plasma concentration, t_p, following multiple doses is given by Equation 8.37.

Large fluctuations between C_{max}^{∞} and C_{min}^{∞} can be hazardous, particularly with drugs that have a narrow therapeutic index. The larger the number of divided doses, the smaller the fluctuations in the plasma drug concentrations. For example, a 500-mg dose of drug given every 6 hours will produce the same C_{av}^{∞} value as a 250-mg dose of the same drug given every 3 hours, while the C_{max}^{∞} and C_{min}^{∞} fluctuations for the latter dose will be decreased by one-half (see Figure 8.3). With drugs that have a narrow therapeutic index, the dosage interval should not be longer than the elimination half-life.

EXAMPLE

An adult male patient (46 years old, 81 kg) was given orally 250 mg of tetracycline hydrochloride every 8 hours for 2 weeks. From the literature, tetracycline hydrochloride is about 75% bioavailable and has an apparent volume of distribution of 1.5 L/kg. The elimination half-life is about 10 hours. The absorption rate constant is 0.9 hr^{-1}. From this information, calculate (a) C_{max} after the first dose, (b) C_{min} after the first dose, (c) plasma drug concentration C_p at 4 hours after the 7th dose, (d) maximum plasma drug concentration at steady-state C_{max}^∞, (e) minimum plasma drug concentration at steady-state C_{min}^∞, and (f) average plasma drug concentration at steady-state C_{av}^∞.

Solution

a. C_{max} after the first dose occurs at t_{max}. Therefore, using Equation 8.40,

$$t_{max} = \frac{2.3}{0.9 - 0.07} \log\left(\frac{0.9}{0.07}\right)$$

$$t_{max} = 3.07$$

Then substitute t_{max} into the following equation for a single oral dose (one-compartment model) to obtain C_{max}.

$$C_{max} = \frac{FD_0 k_a}{V_D(k_a - k)} \left(e^{-kt_{max}} - e^{-k_a t_{max}}\right)$$

$$C_{max} = \frac{(0.75)(250)(0.9)}{(121.5)(0.9 - 0.07)} \left(e^{-0.07(3.07)} - e^{-0.9(3.07)}\right)$$

$$C_{max} = 1.28 \text{ mg/L}$$

b. C_{min} after the first dose occurs just before the administration of the next dose of drug. Therefore, set $t = 8$ hours and solve for C_{min}.

$$C_{min} = \frac{(0.75)(250)(0.9)}{(121.5)(0.9 - 0.07)} \left(e^{-0.07(8)} - e^{-0.9(8)}\right)$$

$$C_{min} = 0.95 \text{ mg/L}$$

c. C_p at 4 hours after the 7th dose may be calculated using Equation 8.34, letting $n = 7$, $t = 4$, $\tau = 8$, and making the appropriate substitutions.

$$C_p = \frac{(0.75)(250)(0.9)}{(121.5)(0.07 - 0.9)} \times \left[\left(\frac{1 - e^{-(7)(0.9)(8)}}{1 - e^{-0.9(8)}}\right)e^{-0.9(4)} - \left(\frac{1 - e^{-(7)(0.07)(8)}}{1 - e^{-(0.07)(8)}}\right)e^{-0.07(4)}\right]$$

$$C_p = 2.86 \text{ mg/L}$$

d. $C_{\mathrm{max}}^{\infty}$ at steady state: t_{p} at steady state is obtained from Equation 8.37.

$$t_{\mathrm{p}} = \frac{1}{k_{\mathrm{a}} - k} \ln\left[\frac{k_{\mathrm{a}}(1 - e^{-k\tau})}{k(1 - e^{-k_{\mathrm{a}}\tau})}\right] \tag{8.41}$$

$$t_{\mathrm{p}} = \frac{1}{0.9 - 0.07} \ln\left[\frac{0.9(1 - e^{-(0.07)(8)})}{0.07(1 - e^{-(0.9)(8)})}\right]$$

$$t_{\mathrm{p}} = 2.05 \text{ hr}$$

Then $C_{\mathrm{max}}^{\infty}$ is obtained using Equation 8.38.

$$C_{\mathrm{max}}^{\infty} = \frac{0.75(250)}{121.5}\left(\frac{1}{1 - e^{-0.07(8)}}\right)e^{-0.07(2.05)}$$

$$C_{\mathrm{max}}^{\infty} = 3.12 \text{ mg/L}$$

e. $C_{\mathrm{min}}^{\infty}$ at steady state is calculated from Equation 8.39.

$$C_{\mathrm{min}}^{\infty} = \frac{(0.9)(0.75)(250)}{(121.5)(0.9 - 0.07)}\left(\frac{1}{1 - e^{-0.07(8)}}\right)e^{-(0.7)(8)}$$

$$C_{\mathrm{min}}^{\infty} = 2.23 \text{ mg/L}$$

f. $C_{\mathrm{min}}^{\infty}$ at steady state is calculated from Equation 8.17.

$$C_{\mathrm{av}}^{\infty} = \frac{(0.75)(250)}{(121.5)(0.07)(8)}$$

$$C_{\mathrm{av}}^{\infty} = 2.76 \text{ mg/L}$$

LOADING DOSE

Since extravascular doses require time for absorption into the plasma to occur, therapeutic effects are delayed until sufficient plasma concentrations are achieved. To reduce the onset time of the drug—that is, the time it takes to achieve the minimum effective concentration (assumed to be equivalent to the C_{av}^{∞})—a loading (priming) or initial dose of drug is given. The main objective of the loading dose is to achieve desired plasma concentrations, C_{av}^{∞}, as quickly as possible. If the drug follows one-compartment pharmacokinetics, then in theory, steady state is also achieved immediately following the loading dose. Thereafter, a maintenance dose is given to maintain C_{av}^{∞} and steady state so that the therapeutic effect is also maintained. In practice, a loading dose may be given as a bolus dose or a short-term loading IV infusion.

As discussed earlier, the time required for the drug to accumulate to a steady-state plasma level is dependent mainly on its elimination half-life. The time needed to reach 90% of C_{av}^{∞} is approximately 3.3 half-lives, and the time required to reach 99% of C_{av}^{∞} is equal to approximately 6.6 half-lives. For a drug with a half-life of 4 hours, it will take approximately 13 and 26 hours to reach 90% and 99% of C_{av}^{∞}, respectively.

For drugs absorbed rapidly in relation to elimination ($k_a \gg k$) and are distributed rapidly, the loading dose D_L can be calculated as follows:

$$\frac{D_L}{D_0} = \frac{1}{(1 - e^{-k_a \tau})(1 - e^{-k\tau})} \tag{8.42}$$

For extremely rapid absorption, as when the product of $k_a \tau$ is large or in the case of IV infusion, $e^{-k_a \tau}$ becomes approximately zero and Equation 8.42 reduces to

$$\frac{D_L}{D_0} = \frac{1}{1 - e^{-k\tau}} \tag{8.43}$$

The loading dose should approximate the amount of drug contained in the body at steady state. The dose ratio is equal to the loading dose divided by the maintenance dose.

$$\text{Dose ratio} = \frac{D_L}{D_0} \tag{8.44}$$

As a general rule, the dose ratio should be equal to 2.0 if the selected dosage interval is equal to the elimination half-life. Figure 8-5 shows the plasma level–time curve for dosage regimens with equal maintenance doses but different loading doses. A rapid approximation of loading dose, D_L, may be estimated from

$$D_L = \frac{V_D C_{av}^{\infty}}{(S)(F)} \tag{8.45}$$

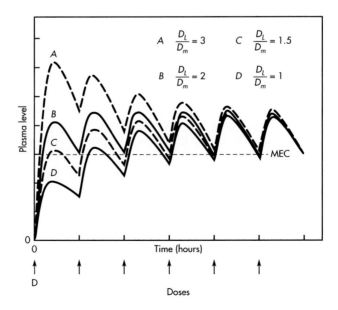

Figure 8-5.   Concentration curves for dosage regimens with equal maintenance doses (D) and dosage intervals (τ) and different dose ratios.
(From Kruger-Thiemer 1968, with permission.)

where C_{av}^∞ is the desired plasma drug concentration, S is the salt form of the drug, and F is the fraction of drug bioavailability.

Equation 8.45 assumes very rapid drug absorption from an immediate-release dosage form. The D_L calculated by this method has been used in clinical situations for which only an approximation of the D_L is needed.

These calculations for loading doses are not applicable to drugs that demonstrate multicompartment kinetics. Such drugs distribute slowly into extravascular tissues, and drug equilibration and steady state may not occur until after the apparent plateau is reached in the vascular (central) compartment.

DETERMINATION OF BIOAVAILABILITY AND BIOEQUIVALENCE IN A MULTIPLE-DOSE REGIMEN

In evaluating drug bioavailability information, one must consider the experimental design used to obtain the data. Otherwise, differences due to an artifact might be mistaken for real differences in bioavailability. Estimation of the absorption rate constant during multiple dosing is difficult, because the residual drug from the previous dose superimposes on the dose that follows. However, the data obtained in multiple doses are useful in calculating a steady-state plasma level.

Bioavailability may be determined during a multiple-dose regimen only after a steady-state plasma drug level has been reached. As discussed, the time needed to reach the steady-state plasma level is related to the elimination half-life, $t_{1/2}$, of the drug. As observed in Table 8.3, it takes approximately 6.6 half-lives to reach 99% of the C_{av}^∞.

The parameters for bioavailability of a drug using plasma-level data from a multiple-dose regimen are similar to those obtained with a single-dose regimen. In the former case, the first plasma samples are taken just before the second dose of the drug. Thereafter, plasma samples are taken periodically after the dose is administered, in order to describe the entire plasma level–time curve adequately (Fig. 8-1). Parameters including AUC, time for peak drug concentration, and peak drug concentration are then used to describe the bioavailability of the drug.

The extent of bioavailability, measured by assuming the $[AUC]_0^\infty$, is dependent on clearance:

$$[AUC]_0^\infty = \frac{FD_0}{Cl_T} \tag{8.46}$$

Determination of bioavailability using multiple doses reveals changes that are normally not detected in a single-dose study. For example, nonlinear pharmacokinetics may occur after multiple drug doses, due to the higher plasma drug concentrations saturating an enzyme system involved in absorption or elimination of the drug. With some drugs, a drug-induced malabsorption syndrome can also alter the percentage of drug absorbed. In this case, drug bioavailability may decrease after repeated doses if the fraction of the dose absorbed (F) decreases or if the total body clearance (kV_D) increases.

BIOEQUIVALENCE STUDIES

A bioequivalence study may be performed using a multiple-dose study design. Multiple doses of the same drug are given consecutively to reach steady-state plasma drug levels. The multiple-dose study is designed as a steady-state, randomized, two-treatment, two-way, crossover study comparing equal doses of the test and reference products in adult, healthy subjects. Each subject receives either the test or reference product separated by a "washout" period, which is the time needed for the drug to be completely eliminated from the body.

To ascertain that the subjects are at steady state, three consecutive trough concentrations (C_{min}) are determined. The last morning dose is given to the subject after an overnight fast, with continual fasting for at least 2 hours following dose administration. Blood sampling is then performed similar to the single-dose study (see also Chapter 15).

Pharmacokinetic analysis includes calculation for each subject of the steady-state area under the curve (AUC_{0-t}), t_{max}, C_{min}, C_{max}, and the percent fluctuation $[100(C_{max} - C_{min})/C_{min}]$. The data are analyzed statistically using analysis of variance (ANOVA) on the log-transformed AUC and C_{max}. To establish bioequivalence, the AUC and C_{max} parameters for the test (generic) product should be within 80–125% of the reference product using a 90% confidence interval.

For some situations, such as hormone replacement therapy, a bioequivalence study may be performed in patients already maintained on the drug. In this case, a washout period would place the patient at substantial risk by being without drug therapy. Therefore, the patient continues on his or her own medication, and blood sampling is performed during a dosage interval (Fig. 8-6, drug product A). Once this is accomplished, the patient begins to take equal oral doses of an alternate drug product. Again, time must be allowed for the theoretical attainment of C_{av}^{∞} with the second drug product. When steady state is reached, the plasma level–time curve for a dosage interval with the second drug product is described (Fig. 8-6, drug product B). Using the same plasma parameters as before, the bioequivalence or lack of bioequivalence may be determined.

Figure 8-6.   Multiple-dose bioequivalency study comparing the bioavailability of drug product B to the bioavailability of drug product A. Blood levels for such studies must be taken after C_{av}^{∞} is reached. The arrow represents the start of therapy with drug product B.

There are a number of advantages to using this method for the determination of bioequivalence: (1) the patient acts as his or her own control; (2) the patient maintains a minimum plasma drug concentration; and (3) the plasma samples after multiple doses contain more drug that can be assayed more accurately. The disadvantages of using this method include the following: (1) the study takes more time to perform, because steady-state conditions must be reached; and (2) sometimes more plasma samples must be obtained from the patient to ascertain that steady state has been reached and to describe the plasma level–time curve accurately.

Because C_{av}^{∞} depends primarily on the dose of the drug and the time interval between doses, the extent of drug systemically available is more important than the rate of drug availability. Small differences in the rate of drug absorption may not be observed with steady-state study comparisons. If there is wide variation in the rate of a drug's availability, then it is possible that initial high blood levels may lead to toxicity.

If the blood level–time curve of the second drug product is comparable to that of the reference drug product, the second product is considered to be bioequivalent. If the second drug has less bioavailability (assuming that only the extent of drug absorption is less than that of the reference drug), the resulting C_{av}^{∞} will be smaller than that obtained with the first drug. Usually the drug manufacturer will perform dissolution and content uniformity tests before performing a bioequivalence study. These *in-vitro* dissolution tests will help to ensure that the C_{av}^{∞} obtained from each drug product *in vivo* will not be largely different from each other. In contrast, if the extent of drug availability is greater in the second drug product, the C_{av}^{∞} will be higher.

 # CLINICAL EXAMPLE

The bioequivalence of two synthetic levothyroxine sodium preparations, Levothroid and Synthroid, were evaluated in 20 hypothyroid patients (Sista and Albert, 1994). The investigation was designed as a two-way crossover study in which the patients who had been diagnosed as hypothyroid by their primary-care physician were given a single 100-μg daily dose of either Levothroid or Synthroid brand levothyroxine sodium tablets for 50 days and then switched over immediately to other treatment for 50 days. Predose blood samples were taken on days 1, 25, 48, 49, and 50 of each phase, and, on day 50, a complete blood sampling was performed. The serum from each blood sample was analyzed for total and free thyroxine (T_4), total and free triiodothyronine (T_3), the major metabolite of T_4, and thyrotropin (TSH).

a. Why were hypothyroid patients used in this study?

b. Why were the subjects dosed for 50 days with each thyroid product?

c. Why were blood samples obtained on days 48, 49, and 50?

d. Why was T_3 measured?

e. Why was TSH measured?

Solution

a. Normal healthy euthyroid subjects would be at risk if they were to take levothyroxine sodium for an extended period of time.

b. The long (50-day) daily dosing for each product was required to obtain steady-state drug levels because of the long elimination half-life of levothyroxine.

c. Serum from blood samples were taken on days 48, 49, and 50 to obtain three consecutive C_{min} drug levels.

d. T_3 is the active metabolite of T_4.

e. The serum TSH concentration is inversely proportional to the free serum T_4 concentrations and gives an indication of the pharmacodynamic activity of the active drug.

DOSAGE REGIMEN SCHEDULES

Predictions of steady-state plasma drug concentrations usually assume the drug is given at a constant dosage interval throughout a 24-hour day. Very often, however, the drug is given only during the waking hours. Niebergall and associates (1974) discussed the problem of scheduling dosage regimens and particularly warned against improper timing of the drug dosage. For example, Figure 8-7 shows the plasma levels of theophylline given three times a day. Notice the large fluctuation between the maximum and minimum plasma levels. In comparison, procainamide was given on a 0.5-g, four-times-a-day maintenance dosage with a 1.0-g loading dose on the first day (Fig. 8-8). However, on the second and third days, plasma levels did not reach the therapeutic range until after the second dose of drug.

Ideally, drug doses should be given at evenly spaced intervals. However, to improve patient compliance, dosage regimens may be designed to fit with the lifestyle of the patient. For example, the patient is directed to take a drug such as amoxicillin four times a day (QID), before meals and at bedtime, for a systemic infection. This dosage regimen will produce unequal dosage intervals during the day, because the patient takes the drug before breakfast, at 0800 hours (8 AM), before lunch, at 1200 hours (12 noon), before dinner, at 1800 hours (6 PM), and before bedtime, at 2300 hours (11 PM). For these drugs, evenly spaced dosage intervals are not that critical to the effectiveness of the antibiotic as long as the plasma drug concentrations are maintained above the *minimum inhibitory concentration* (MIC) for the microorganism.

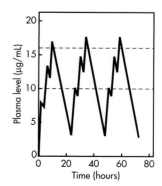

Figure 8-7. *Plasma level–time curve for theophylline given in doses of 160 mg 3 times a day. Dashed lines indicate the therapeutic range.*
(From Niebergall et al 1974, with permission.)

Figure 8-8. *Plasma level–time curve for procainamide given in an initial dose of 1.0 g followed by doses of 0.5 g 4 times a day. Dashed lines indicate the therapeutic range.*
(From Niebergall et at 1974, with permission.)

Patient compliance to multiple dose regimens may be a problem for the patient in following the prescribed dosage regimen. Occasionally, a patient may miss taking the drug dose at the prescribed dosage interval. For drugs with long elimination half-lives (eg, levothyroxine sodium or oral contraceptives), the consequences of one missed dose are minimal, since only a small fraction of drug is lost between daily dosing intervals. The patient should either take the next drug dose as soon as the patient remembers or continue the dosing schedule starting at the next prescribed dosing period. If it is almost time for the next dose, then the skipped dose should not be taken and the regular dosing schedule should be maintained. Generally, the patient should not double the dose of the medication. For specific drug information on missed doses, USP DI II, *Advice for the Patient,* published annually by the United States Pharmacopeia, is a good source of information.

The problems of widely fluctuating plasma drug concentrations may be prevented by using a controlled-release formulation of the drug, or a drug in the same therapeutic class that has a long elimination half-life. The use of extended-release dosage forms allows for less frequent dosing and prevents undermedication between the last evening dose and the first morning dose. Extended-release drug products may improve patient compliance by decreasing the number of doses within a 24-hour period that the patient needs to take. Patients generally show better compliance with a twice-a-day (BID) dosage regimen compared to a three-times-a-day (BID) dosage schedule.

PRACTICE PROBLEMS

1. Patient C.S. is a 35-year-old male weighing 76.6 kg. The patient is to be given multiple IV bolus injections of an antibiotic every 6 hours. The effective concentration of this drug is 15 μg/mL. After the patient is given a single IV dose, the elimination half-life for the drug is determined to be 3.0 hr and the apparent V_D is 196 mL/kg. Determine a multiple IV dose regimen for this drug (assume drug is given every 6 hours).

Solution

$$C_{av}^{\infty} = \frac{FD_0}{V_D k \tau}$$

For IV dose, $F = 1$,

$$D_0 = (15\ \mu g/mL)\left(\frac{0.693}{3\,hr}\right)(196\ mL/kg)\ (6\ hr)$$

$$D_0 = 4.07\ mg/kg\ \text{every 6 hr}$$

Since patient C.S. weighs 76.6 kg, the dose should be as shown:

$$D_0 = (4.07\ mg/kg)(76.6\ kg)$$

$$D_0 = 312\ mg\ \text{every 6 hr}$$

After the condition of this patient has stabilized, the patient is to be given the drug orally for convenience of drug administration. The objective is to design an oral dosage regimen that will produce the same steady-state blood level as the multiple IV doses. The drug dose will depend on the bioavailability of the drug from the drug product, the desired therapeutic drug level, and the dosage interval chosen. Assume that the antibiotic is 90% bioavailable and that the physician would like to continue oral medication every 6 hours.

The average or steady-state plasma drug level is given by

$$C_{av}^{\infty} = \frac{FD_0}{V_D k \tau}$$

Because $k = 0.693/t_{1/2}$,

$$C_{av}^{\infty} = \frac{FD_0 1.44 t_{1/2}}{V_D \tau}$$

Because the literature may give the total body clearance Cl_T for the drug, the above equation is equivalent to

$$C_{av}^{\infty} = \frac{FD_0}{\tau Cl_T}$$

where $Cl_T = kV_D$ for a one-compartment model, or $Cl_T = bV_p$ for a two-compartment model.

$$D_0 = \frac{(15\ \mu g/mL)\,(196\ mL/kg)\,(6\ hr)}{(0.9)\,(1.44)\,(3\ hr)}$$

$$D_0 = 454\ mg/kg$$

Because patient C.S. weighs 76.6 kg, he should be given the following dose:

$$D_0 = (4.54\ mg/kg)(76.6\ kg)$$

$$D_0 = 348\ mg\ \text{every 6 hr}$$

For drugs with equal absorption but slower absorption rates (F is the same but k_a is smaller), the initial dosing period may show a lower blood level; however, the steady-state blood level will be unchanged.

2. In practice, drug products are usually commercially available in certain specified strengths. Using the information provided in the preceding problem, assume that the antibiotic is available in 125-, 250-, and 500-mg tablets. Therefore, the pharmacist or prescriber must now decide which tablets are to be given to the patient. In this case, it may be possible to give the patient 375 mg (eg, one 125-mg tablet and one 250-mg tablet) every 6 hours. However, the C_{av}^{∞} should be calculated to determine if the plasma level is approaching a toxic value. Alternatively, a new dosage interval might be appropriate for the patient. It is very important to design the dosage interval and the dose to be as simple as possible, so that the patient will not be confused and will be able to comply with the medication program properly.

a. What is the new C_{av}^{∞} if the patient is given 375 mg every 6 hours?

Solution

$$C_{av}^{\infty} = \frac{(0.9)\,(375{,}000)\,(1.44)\,(3)}{(196)\,(76.6)\,(6)}$$

$$C_{av}^{\infty} = 16.2\ \mu g/mL$$

Because the therapeutic objective was to achieve a minimum effective concentration (MEC) of 15 $\mu g/mL$, a value of 16.2 $\mu g/mL$ is reasonable.

b. The patient has difficulty in distinguishing tablets of different strengths. Can the patient take a 500-mg dose (eg, two 250-mg tablets)?

Solution

The dosage interval (τ) for the 500-mg tablet would have to be calculated as follows:

$$\tau = \frac{(0.9)\,(500{,}000)\,(1.44)\,(3)}{(196)\,(76.6)\,(15)}$$

$$\tau = 8.63\ hr$$

c. A dosage interval of 8.63 hr is difficult to remember. Is a dosage regimen of 500 mg every 8 hours reasonable?

Solution

$$C_{av}^{\infty} = \frac{(0.9)\,(500{,}000)\,(1.44)\,(3)}{(196)\,(76.6)\,(8)}$$

$$C_{av}^{\infty} = 16.2\ \mu g/mL$$

Notice that a larger dose is necessary if the drug is given at longer intervals.

In designing a dosage regimen, one should consider a regimen that is practical and convenient for the patient. For example, for good compliance, the dosage interval should be spaced conveniently for the patient. In addition, one should consider the commercially available dosage strengths of the prescribed drug product.

The use of Equation 8.17 to estimate a dosage regimen initially has wide utility. The C_{av}^{∞} is equal to the dosing rate divided by the total body clearance of the drug in the patient:

$$C_{av}^{\infty} = \frac{FD_0}{\tau} \frac{1}{Cl_T} \tag{8.47}$$

where FD_0/τ is equal to the dosing rate R, and $1/Cl_T$ is equal to $1/kV_D$.

In designing dosage regimens, the dosing rate D_0/τ is adjusted for the patient's drug clearance to obtain the desired C_{av}^{∞}. For an IV infusion, the zero-order rate of infusion (R) is used to obtain the desired steady-state plasma drug concentration C_{SS}. If R is substituted for FD_0/τ in Equation 8.47, then the following equation for estimating C_{SS} after an IV infusion is obtained:

$$C_{SS} = \frac{R}{Cl_T} \tag{8.48}$$

From Equations 8.47 and 8.48, all dosage schedules having the same dosing rate D_0/τ, or R, will have the same C_{av}^{∞} or C_{SS}, whether the drug is given by multiple doses or by IV infusion. For example, dosage schedules of 100 mg every 4 hours, 200 mg every 8 hours, 300 mg every 12 hours, and 600 mg every 24 hours will yield the same C_{av}^{∞} in the patient. An IV infusion rate of 25 mg/hr in the same patient will give a C_{SS} equal to the C_{av}^{∞} obtained with the multiple-dose schedule (Fig. 8-3; Table 8.6).

TABLE 8.6   Effect of Dosing Schedule on Predicted Steady-State Plasma Drug Concentrations[a]

DOSING SCHEDULE			STEADY-STATE DRUG CONCENTRATION (μg/mL)		
Dose (mg)	1 (hr)	Dosing Rate, D_0/τ (mg/hr)	C_{max}^{∞}	C_{av}^{∞}	C_{min}^{∞}
—	—	25[b]	14.5	14.5	14.5
100	4	25	16.2	14.5	11.6
200	8	25	20.2	14.5	7.81
300	12	25	25.3	14.5	5.03
600	24	25	44.1	14.5	1.12
400	8	50	40.4	28.9	15.6
600	8	75	60.6	43.4	23.4

[a] Drug has an elimination half-life of 4 hours and an apparent V_D of 10 L.
[b] Drug given by IV infusion. The first-order absorption rate constant k_a is 1.2 hr^{-1} and the drug follows a one-compartment open model.

FREQUENTLY ASKED QUESTIONS

1. What are the advantages/disadvantages for giving a drug by a constant IV infusion, intermittent IV infusion, or multiple IV bolus injections? What drugs would most likely be given by each route of administration? Why?

2. Is a loading dose always necessary when placing a patient on a multiple-dose regimen? What are the determining factors?

3. Is the drug accumulation index (R) applicable to any drug given by multiple dose or only to drugs that are eliminated slowly from the body?

4. Does a loading dose significantly affect the steady-state concentration of a drug given by a constant multiple-dose regimen?

5. Give two examples of a drug that requires a loading dose because of its long $t_{1/2}$.

6. Why is the steady-state peak plasma drug concentration often measured sometime after an IV dose is given in a clinical situation?

LEARNING QUESTIONS

1. Gentamicin has an average elimination half-life of approximately 2 hours and an apparent volume of distribution of 20% of body weight. It is necessary to give gentamicin, 1 mg/kg every 8 hours by multiple IV injections, to a 50-kg woman with normal renal function. Calculate **(a)** C_{max}, **(b)** C_{min}, and **(c)** C_{av}^{∞}.

2. A physician wants to give theophylline to a young male asthmatic patient (age 29, 80 kg). According to the literature, the elimination half-life for theophylline is 5 hours and the apparent V_D is equal to 50% of body weight. The plasma level of theophylline required to provide adequate airway ventilation is approximately 10 μg/mL.

    a. The physician wants the patient to take medication every 6 hours around the clock. What dose of theophylline would you recommend (assume theophylline is 100% bioavailable)?

    b. If you were to find that theophylline is available to you only in 225-mg capsules, what dosage regimen would you recommend?

3. What pharmacokinetic parameter is most important in determining the time at which the steady-state plasma drug level (C_{av}^{∞}) is reached?

4. Name two ways in which the fluctuations of plasma concentrations (between C_{max}^{∞} and C_{min}^{∞}) can be minimized for a person on a multiple-dose drug regimen without altering the C_{av}^{∞}.

5. What is the purpose of giving a loading dose?

6. What is the loading dose for an antibiotic ($k = 0.23$ hr^{-1}) with a maintenance dose of 200 mg every 3 hours?

7. What is the main advantage of giving a potent drug by IV infusion as opposed to multiple IV injections?

8. A drug has an elimination half-life of 2 hours and a volume of distribution of 40 L. The drug is given at a dose of 200 mg every 4 hours by multiple IV bolus injections. Predict the plasma drug concentration at 1 hour after the third dose.

9. The elimination half-life of an antibiotic is 3 hours and the apparent volume of distribution is 20% of body weight. The therapeutic window for this drug is from 2 to 10 μg/mL. Adverse toxicity is often observed at drug concentrations above 15 μg/mL. The drug will be given by multiple IV bolus injections.

   a. Calculate the dose for an adult male patient (68 years old, 82 kg) with normal renal function to be given every 8 hours.

   b. Calculate the anticipated C_{max}^{∞} and C_{min}^{∞} values.

   c. Calculate the C_{av}^{∞} value.

   d. Comment on the adequacy of your dosage regimen.

10. Tetracycline hydrochloride (Achromycin V, Lederle) is prescribed for a young adult male patient (28 years old, 78 kg) suffering from gonorrhea. According to the literature, tetracycline HCl is 77% orally absorbed, is 65% bound to plasma proteins, has an apparent volume of distribution of 0.5 L/kg, has an elimination half-life of 10.6 hr, and is 58% excreted unchanged in the urine. The minimum inhibitory drug concentration (MIC) for gonorrhea is 25–30 μg/mL.

    a. Calculate an *exact* maintenance dose for this patient to be given every 6 hours around the clock.

    b. Achromycin V is available in 250-mg and 500-mg capsules. How many capsules (state dose) should the patient take every 6 hours?

    c. What loading dose using the above capsules would you recommend for this patient?

11. The body clearance of sumatriptan (Imitrex) is 250 mL/min. The drug is about 14% bioavailable. What would be the average plasma drug concentration after 5 doses of 100 mg PO every 8 hours in a patient? (Assume steady state was reached.)

12. Cefotaxime has a volume of distribution of 0.17 L/kg and an elimination half-life of 1.5 hr. What is the peak plasma drug concentration in a patient weighing 75 kg after receiving 1 g IV of the drug 3 times daily for 3 days?

REFERENCES

Kruger-Thiemer E: Pharmacokinetics and dose-concentration relationships. In Ariens EJ (ed.), *Physico-Chemical Aspects of Drug Action*. New York, Pergamon, 1968, p 97

Niebergall PJ, Sugita ET, Schnaare RC: Potential dangers of common drug dosing regimens. *Am J Hosp Pharm* **31:**53–59, 1974

Sawchuk RJ, Zaske DE: Pharmacokinetics of dosing regimens which utilize multiple intravenous infusions: Gentamycin in burn patients. *J Pharmacokin Biopharm* **4**(2): 183–195, 1976

Sista S, Albert KS: A two-way crossover, multiple dose bioavailability study of levothyroxine sodium tablets in hypothyroid patients. *Pharm Res,* Oct 1994 (abstract)

Van Rossum JM, Tomey AHM: Rate of accumulation and plateau concentration of drugs after chronic medication. *J Pharm Pharmacol* **30:**390–392, 1968

BIBLIOGRAPHY

Gibaldi M, Perrier D: *Pharmacokinetics,* 2nd ed. New York, Marcel Dekker, 1962, pp 451–457

Levy G: Kinetics of pharmacologic effect. *Clin Pharmacol Ther* **7:**362, 1966

van Rossum JM: Pharmacokinetics of accumulation. *J Pharm Sci* **75:**2162–2164, 1968

Wagner JG: Kinetics of pharmacological response, I: Proposed relationship between response and drug concentration in the intact animal and man. *J Theor Biol* **20:**173, 1968

Wagner JG: Relations between drug concentrations and response. *J Mond Pharm* **14:**279–310, 1971

9

NONLINEAR PHARMACOKINETICS

In previous chapters, linear pharmacokinetic models using simple first-order kinetics were introduced to describe the course of drug disposition and action. These linear models assumed that the pharmacokinetic parameters for a drug would not change when different doses or multiple doses of a drug were given. With some drugs, increased doses or chronic medication can cause deviations from the linear pharmacokinetic profile previously observed with single low doses of the same drug. This *nonlinear* pharmacokinetic behavior is also termed *dose-dependent pharmacokinetics.*

Many of the processes of drug absorption, distribution, biotransformation, and excretion involve enzymes or carrier-mediated systems. For some drugs given at therapeutic levels, one of these specialized processes may become saturated. As shown in Table 9.1, various causes of nonlinear pharmacokinetic behavior are theoretically possible. Besides saturation of plasma protein-binding or carrier-mediated systems, drugs may demonstrate nonlinear pharmacokinetics due to a pathologic alteration in drug absorption, distribution, and elimination. For example, aminoglycosides may cause renal nephrotoxicity, thereby altering renal drug excretion. In addition, gallstone obstruction of the bile duct will alter biliary drug excretion. In most cases, the main pharmacokinetic outcome is a change in the apparent elimination rate constant.

A number of drugs demonstrate *saturation* or *capacity-limited metabolism* in humans. Examples of these saturable metabolic processes include glycine conjugation of salicylate, sulfate conjugation of salicylamide, acetylation of *p*-aminobenzoic acid, and the elimination of phenytoin (Tozer et al, 1981). Drugs that demonstrate saturation kinetics usually show the following characteristics.

1. Elimination of drug does not follow simple first-order kinetics—that is, elimination kinetics are nonlinear.
2. The elimination half-life changes as dose is increased. Usually, the elimination half-life increases with increased dose due to saturation of an enzyme system. However, the elimination half-life might decrease due to "self"-induction of liver biotransformation enzymes, as is observed for carbamazepine.

TABLE 9.1   Examples of Drugs Showing Nonlinear Kinetics

CAUSE[a]	DRUG
GI Absorption	
Saturable transport in gut wall	Riboflavin, gebapentin, L-dopa, baclofen, ceftibuten
Intestinal metabolism	Salicylamide, propranolol
Drugs with low solubility in GI but relatively high dose	Chorothiazide, griseofulvin, danazol
Saturable gastric or GI decomposition	Penicillin G, omeprazole, saquinavir
Distribution	
Saturable plasma protein binding	Phenylbutazone, lidocaine, salicylic acid, ceftriaxone, diazoxide, phenytoin, warfarin, disopyramide
Cellular uptake	Methicillin (rabbit)
Tissue binding	Imiprimine (rat)
CSF transport	Benzylpenicillins
Saturable transport into or out of tissues	Methotrexate
Renal Elimination	
Active secretion	Mezlocillin, para-aminohippuric acid
Tubular reabsorption	Riboflavin, ascorbic acid, cephapirin
Change in urine pH	Salicylic acid, dextroamphetamine
Metabolism	
Saturable metabolism	Phenytoin, salicyclic acid, theophylline, valproic acid[b]
Cofactor or enzyme limitation	Acetaminophen, alcohol
Enzyme induction	Carbamazepine
Altered hepatic blood flow	Propranolol, verapamil
Metabolite inhibition	Diazepam
Biliary Excretion	
Biliary secretion	Iodipamide, sulfobromophthalein sodium
Enterohepatic recycling	Cimetidine, isotretinoin

[a]Hypothermia, metabolic acidosis, altered cardiovascular function, and coma are additional causes of dose and time dependencies in drug overdose.
[b]In guinea pig and probably in some younger subjects.

Compiled by author and from Evans et al (1992), with permission.

3. The area under the curve (AUC) is not proportional to the amount of bioavailable drug.
4. The saturation of capacity-limited processes may be affected by other drugs that require the same enzyme or carrier-mediated system (ie, competition effects).
5. The composition and/or ratio of the metabolites of a drug may be affected by a change in the dose.

Because these drugs have a changing apparent elimination constant with larger doses, prediction of drug concentration in the blood based on a single small dose is difficult. Drug concentrations in the blood can increase rapidly once an elimination process is saturated. In general, metabolism (biotransformation) and active tubular secretion of drugs by the kidney are the processes most usually saturated. Figure 9-1 shows plasma level–time curves for a drug that exhibits *saturable* kinetics. When a large dose is given, a curve is obtained with an initial slow elimination phase followed by a much more rapid elimination at lower blood concentrations

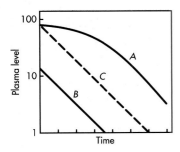

Figure 9-1. Plasma level–time curves for a drug that exhibits a saturable elimination process. Curves *A* and *B* represent high and low doses of durg, respectively, given in a single IV bolus. The terminal slopes of curves *A* and *B* are the same. Curve *C* represents the normal first-order elimination of a different drug.

(curve *A*). With a small dose of the drug, apparent first-order kinetics are observed, because no saturation kinetics occur (curve *B*). If the pharmacokinetic data were estimated only from the blood levels described by curve *B*, then a twofold increase in the dose would give the blood profile presented in curve *C*, which considerably underestimates the drug concentration as well as the duration of action.

In order to determine whether a drug is following dose-dependent kinetics, the drug is given at various dosage levels and a plasma level–time curve is obtained for each dose. The curves should exhibit parallel slopes if the drug follows dose-independent kinetics. Alternatively, a plot of the areas under the plasma level–time curves at various doses should be linear (Figure 9-2).

SATURABLE ENZYMATIC ELIMINATION PROCESSES

The elimination of drug by a saturable enzymatic process is described by *Michaelis–Menten kinetics*. If C_p is the concentration of drug in the plasma, then

$$\text{Elimination rate} = \frac{dC_p}{dt} = \frac{V_{max} C_p}{K_M + C_p} \tag{9.1}$$

where V_{max} is the maximum elimination rate and K_M is the Michaelis constant that reflects the *capacity* of the enzyme system. It is important to note that K_M is not an elimination constant, but is actually a hybrid rate constant in enzyme kinetics, representing both the forward and backward reaction rates and equal to the drug concentration or amount of drug in the body at $0.5 V_{max}$. The values for K_M and V_{max} are dependent on the nature of the drug and the enzymatic process involved.

The elimination rate of a hypothetical drug with a K_M of 0.1 μg/mL and a V_{max} of 0.5 μg/mL per hour is calculated in Table 9.2 by means of Equation 9.1. Because

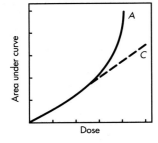

Figure 9-2. Area under the plasma level–time curve versus dose for a drug that exhibits a saturable elimination process. Curve *A* represents dose-dependent or saturable elimination kinetics. Curve *C* represents dose-independent kinetics.

TABLE 9.2   Effect of Drug Concentration on the Elimination Rate and Rate Constant[a]

DRUG CONCENTRATION (μg/mL)	ELIMINATION RATE (μg/mL per hr)	ELIMINATION RATE/ CONCENTRATION[b] (hr^{-1})
0.4	0.400	1.000
0.8	0.444	0.556
1.2	0.462	0.385
1.6	0.472	0.294
2.0	0.476	0.238
2.4	0.480	0.200
2.8	0.483	0.172
3.2	0.485	0.152
10.0	0.495	0.0495
10.4	0.495	0.0476
10.8	0.495	0.0459
11.2	0.496	0.0442
11.6	0.496	0.0427

[a]$K_M = 0.1$ μg/mL, $V_{max} = 0.5$ μg/mL per hour.
[b]The ratio of the elimination rate to the concentration is equal to the rate constant.

the ratio of the elimination rate to drug concentration changes as the drug concentration changes (ie, dC_p/dt is not constant, Eq. 9.1), the rate of drug elimination also changes and is not a first-order or linear process. In contrast, a first-order elimination process would yield the same elimination rate constant at all plasma drug concentrations. At drug concentrations of 0.4–10 μg/mL, the enzyme system is not saturated and the rate of elimination is a mixed or nonlinear process (Table 9.2). At higher drug concentrations, 11.2 μg/mL and above, the elimination rate approaches the maximum velocity (V_{max}) of approximately 0.5 μg/mL per hour. At V_{max}, the elimination rate is a constant and is considered a zero-order process.

Equation 9.1 describes a nonlinear enzyme process that encompasses a broad range of drug concentrations. When the drug concentration C_p is large in relation to K_M ($C_p \gg K_m$), saturation of the enzymes occurs and the value for K_M is negligible. The rate of elimination proceeds at a fixed or constant rate equal to V_{max}. Thus, elimination of drug becomes a zero-order process and Equation 9.1 becomes:

$$-\frac{dC_p}{dt} = \frac{V_{max}C_p}{C_p} = V_{max} \tag{9.2}$$

PRACTICE PROBLEM

Using the hypothetical drug considered in Table 9.2 ($V_{max} = 0.5$ μg/mL per hour, $K_M = 0.1$ μg/mL), how long would it take for the plasma drug concentration to decrease from 20 to 12 μg/mL?

Solution

Because 12 μg/mL is above the saturable level, as indicated in Table 9.2, elimination occurs at a zero-order rate of approximately 0.5 μg/mL per hour.

$$\text{Time needed for the drug to decrease to } 12 \ \mu\text{g/mL} = \frac{20 - 12 \ \mu\text{g}}{0.5 \ \mu\text{g/hr}} = 16 \ \text{hr}$$

A saturable process can also exhibit linear elimination when drug concentrations are much less than enzyme concentrations. When the drug concentration C_p is small in relation to the K_M, the rate of drug elimination becomes a first-order process. The data generated from Equation 9.2 ($C_p \leq 0.05$ μg/mL, Table 9.3) using $K_M = 0.8$ μg/mL and $V_{max} = 0.9$ μg/mL per hour shows that enzymatic drug elimination can change from a nonlinear to a linear process over a restricted concentration range. This is evident because the rate constant (or elimination rate/drug concentration) values are constant. At drug concentrations below 0.05 μg/mL, the ratio of elimination rate to drug concentration has a constant value of 1.1 hr^{-1}. Mathematically, when C_p is much smaller than K_M, C_p in the denominator is negligible and the elimination rate becomes first order.

$$-\frac{dC_p}{dt} = \frac{V_{max} C_p}{C_p + K_M} = \frac{V_{max}}{K_M} C_p$$

$$-\frac{dC_p}{dt} = k' C_p$$

$$(9.3)$$

The first-order rate constant for a saturable process, k', can be calculated from Equation 9.3:

$$k' = \frac{V_{max}}{K_M} = \frac{0.9}{0.8} = {\sim}1.1 \ \text{hr}^{-1}$$

TABLE 9.3   Effect of Drug Concentration on the Elimination Rate and Rate Constant[a]

DRUG CONCENTRATION (C_p) (μg/mL)	ELIMINATION RATE (μg/mL per hr)	ELIMINATION RATE / Concentration (hr^{-1})[b]
0.01	0.011	1.1
0.02	0.022	1.1
0.03	0.033	1.1
0.04	0.043	1.1
0.05	0.053	1.1
0.06	0.063	1.0
0.07	0.072	1.0
0.08	0.082	1.0
0.09	0.091	1.0

[a]$K_M = 0.8$ μg/mL, $V_{max} = 0.9$ μg/mL per hour.
[b]The ratio of the elimination rate to the concentration is equal to the rate constant.

This calculation confirms the data in Table 9.3, because enzymatic drug elimination at drug concentrations below 0.05 μg/mL is a first-order rate process with a rate constant of 1.1 hr^{-1}. Therefore, the $t_{1/2}$ due to enzymatic elimination can be calculated:

$$t_{1/2} = \frac{0.693}{1.1} = 0.63 \text{ hr}$$

 # PRACTICE PROBLEM

How long would it take for the plasma concentration of the drug in Table 9.3 to decline from 0.05 to 0.005 μg/mL?

Solution

Because drug elimination is a first-order process for the specified concentrations,

$$C_p = C_p^0 e^{-kt}$$

$$\log C_p = C_p^0 - \frac{kt}{2.3}$$

$$t = \frac{\log C - \log C_p^0}{k}$$

Because $C_p^0 = 0.05$ μg/mL, $k = 1.1$ hr^{-1}, and $C_p = 0.005$ μg/mL,

$$t = \frac{2.3(\log 0.05 - \log 0.005)}{1.1} = \frac{2.3(-1.30 + 2.3)}{1.1} = \frac{2.3}{1.1} = 2.09 \text{ hr}$$

When given in therapeutic doses, most drugs produce plasma drug concentrations well below K_M for all carrier-mediated enzyme systems affecting the pharmacokinetics of the drug. Therefore, most drugs at normal therapeutic concentrations follow first-order rate processes. Only a few drugs, such as salicylate and phenytoin, tend to saturate the hepatic mixed-function oxidases at higher therapeutic doses. With these drugs, elimination kinetics are first-order with very small doses, mixed order at higher doses, and may approach zero-order with very high therapeutic doses.

DRUG ELIMINATION BY CAPACITY-LIMITED PHARMACOKINETICS: ONE-COMPARTMENT MODEL, IV BOLUS INJECTION

The rate of elimination of a drug that follows capacity-limited pharmacokinetics is governed by the V_{max} and K_M of the drug. Equation 9.1 describes the elimination of a drug that distributes in the body as a single compartment and is eliminated by Michaelis–Menten or capacity-limited pharmacokinetics. If a single IV bolus injection of drug (D_0) is given at $t = 0$, the drug concentration (C_p) in the plasma at any time t may be calculated by an integrated form of Equation 9.1 described by

$$\frac{C_0 - C_p}{t} = V_{max} - \frac{K_M}{t} \ln \frac{C_0}{C_p} \tag{9.4}$$

Alternatively, the amount of drug in the body after an IV bolus injection may be calculated by the following relationship. Equation 9.5 may be used to simulate the decline of drug in the body after various size doses are given, provided the K_M and V_{max} of drug are known.

$$\frac{D_0 - D_t}{t} = V_{max} - \frac{K_M}{t} \ln \frac{D_0}{D_t} \tag{9.5}$$

where D_0 is the amount of drug in the body at $t = 0$. In order to calculate the time for the dose of the drug to decline to a certain amount of drug in the body, Equation 9.5 must be rearranged and solved for time t:

$$t = \frac{1}{V_{max}} \left(D_0 - D_t + K_M \ln \frac{D_0}{D_t} \right) \tag{9.6}$$

The relationship of K_M and V_{max} to the time for an IV bolus injection of drug to decline to a given amount of drug in the body is illustrated in Figures 9-3 and 9-4. Using Equation 9.6, the time for a single 400-mg dose given by IV bolus injection to decline to 20 mg was calculated for a drug with a K_M of 38 mg/L and a V_{max} that varied from 200 to 100 mg/hr (Table 9.4). With a V_{max} of 200 mg/hr, the time for the 400-mg dose to decline to 20 mg in the body is 2.46 hours, whereas when the V_{max} is decreased to 100 mg/hr, the time for the 400-mg dose to decrease to 20 mg is increased to 4.93 hours (Figure 9.3). Thus, there is an inverse relationship between the time for the dose to decline to a certain amount of drug in the body and the V_{max} as shown in Equation 9.6.

Using a similar example, the effect of K_M on the time for a single 400-mg dose given by IV bolus injection to decline to 20 mg in the body is described in

Figure 9-3. Amount of drug in the body versus time for a capacity-limited drug following an IV dose. Data generated using V_{max} of 100 (O) and 200 mg/hr (□). K_M is kept constant.

TABLE 9.4   Capacity-Limited Pharmacokinetics: Effect of V_{max} on the Elimination of Drug[a]

AMOUNT OF DRUG IN BODY (mg)	TIME FOR DRUG ELIMINATION (hr)	
	V_{max} = 200 mg/hr	V_{max} = 100 mg/hr
400	0	0
380	0.109	0.219
360	0.220	0.440
340	0.330	0.661
320	0.442	0.884
300	0.554	1.10
280	0.667	1.33
260	0.781	1.56
240	0.897	1.79
220	1.01	2.02
200	1.13	2.26
180	1.25	2.50
160	1.37	2.74
140	1.49	2.99
120	1.62	3.25
100	1.76	3.52
80	1.90	3.81
60	2.06	4.12
40	2.23	4.47
20	2.46	4.93

[a]A single 400-mg dose is given by IV bolus injection. The drug is distributed into a single compartment and is eliminated by capacity-limited pharmacokinetics. K_M is 38 mg/L. The time for drug to decline from 400 to 20 mg is calculated from Equation 9.6 assuming the drug has V_{max} = 200 mg/hr or V_{max} = 100 mg/hr.

Table 9.5 and Figure 9-4. Assuming V_{max} is constant at 200 mg/hr, the time for the drug to decline from 400 to 20 mg is 2.46 hours when K_M is 38 mg/L; whereas when K_M is 76 mg/L, the time for the drug dose to decline to 20 mg is 3.03 hours. Thus, an increase in K_M (with no change in V_{max}) will increase the time for the drug to be eliminated from the body.

The one-compartment open model with capacity-limited elimination pharmacokinetics adequately describes the plasma drug concentration–time profiles for some drugs. The mathematics needed to describe nonlinear pharmacokinetic

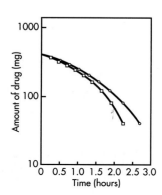

Figure 9-4.   Amount of drug in the body versus time for a capacity-limited drug following an IV dose. Data generated using K_M of 38 mg/L (□) and 76 mg/L (O). V_{max} is kept constant.

TABLE 9.5 Capacity-Limited Pharmacokinetics: Effects of K_M on the Elimination of Drug[a]

AMOUNT OF DRUG IN BODY (mg)	TIME FOR DRUG ELIMINATION (hr)	
	$K_M = 38$ mg/L	$K_M = 76$ mg/L
400	0	0
380	0.109	0.119
360	0.220	0.240
340	0.330	0.361
320	0.442	0.484
300	0.554	0.609
280	0.667	0.735
260	0.781	0.863
240	0.897	0.994
220	1.01	1.12
200	1.13	1.26
180	1.25	1.40
160	1.37	1.54
140	1.49	1.69
120	1.62	1.85
100	1.76	2.02
80	1.90	2.21
60	2.06	2.42
40	2.23	2.67
20	2.46	3.03

[a]A single 400-mg dose is given by IV bolus injection. The drug is distributed into a single compartment and is eliminated by capacity-limited pharmacokinetics. V_{max} is 200 mg/hr. The time for drug to decline from 400 to 20 mg is calculated from Equation 9.6 assuming the drug has $K_M = 38$ mg/L or $K_M = 76$ mg/L.

behavior of drugs that follow two-compartment models and/or have both combined capacity-limited and first-order kinetic profiles are very complex and have little practical application for dosage calculations and therapeutic drug monitoring.

PRACTICE PROBLEMS

1. A drug eliminated from the body by capacity-limited pharmacokinetics has a K_M of 100 mg/L and a V_{max} of 50 mg/hr. If 400 mg of the drug is given to a patient by IV bolus injection, calculate the time for the drug to be 50% eliminated. If 320 mg of the drug is to be given by IV bolus injection, calculate the time for 50% of the dose to be eliminated. Explain why there is a difference in the time for 50% elimination of a 400-mg dose compared to a 320-mg dose.

Solution

Use Equation 9.6 to calculate the time for the dose to decline to a given amount of drug in the body. For this problem, D_t is equal to 50% of the dose D_0.

If the dose is 400 mg,

$$t = \frac{1}{50}\left(400 - 200 + 100 \ \ln \frac{400}{200}\right) = 5.39 \ \text{hr}$$

If the dose is 320 mg,

$$t = \frac{1}{50}\left(320 - 160 + 100 \ \ln \frac{320}{160}\right) = 4.59 \ \text{hr}$$

For capacity-limited elimination, the elimination half-life is dose-dependent, because the drug elimination process is partially saturated. Therefore, small changes in the dose will produce large differences in the time for 50% drug elimination. The parameters K_M and V_{max} determine when the dose is saturated.

2. Using the same drug as in Problem 1, calculate the time for 50% elimination of the dose when the doses are 10 and 5 mg. Explain why the times for 50% drug elimination are similar even though the dose is reduced by one-half.

Solution

As in Practice Problem 1, use Equation 9.6 to calculate the time for the amount of drug in the body at zero time (D0) to decline 50%.
If the dose is 10 mg,

$$t = \frac{1}{50}\left(10 - 5 + 100 \ \ln \frac{10}{5}\right) = 1.49 \ \text{hr}$$

If the dose is 5 mg,

$$t = \frac{1}{50}\left(5 - 2.5 + 100 \ \ln \frac{5}{2.5}\right) = 1.44 \ \text{hr}$$

Whether the patient is given a 10- or a 5-mg dose by IV bolus injection, the times for the amount of drug to decline 50% are approximately the same. For 10- and 5-mg doses the amount of drug in the body is much less than the K_M of 100 mg. Therefore, the amount of drug in the body is well below saturation of the elimination process and the drug declines at a first-order rate.

Determination of K_M and V_{max}

Equation 9.1 relates the rate of drug biotransformation to the concentration of the drug in the body. The same equation may be applied to determine the rate of enzymatic reaction of a drug *in vitro* (Eq. 9.7). When an experiment is performed with solutions of various concentration of drug C, a series of reaction rates (v) may be measured for each concentration. Special plots may then be used to determine K_M and V_{max} (see also Chapter 11).

TABLE 9.6   Information Necessary for Graphic Determination of V_{max} and K_M

OBSERVATION NUMBER	C (μM/mL)	V (μM/mL per min)	1/V (mL per min/μM)	1/C (mL/μM)
1	1	0.500	2.000	1.000
2	6	1.636	0.611	0.166
3	11	2.062	0.484	0.090
4	16	2.285	0.437	0.062
5	21	2.423	0.412	0.047
6	26	2.516	0.397	0.038
7	31	2.583	0.337	0.032
8	36	2.504	0.379	0.027
9	41	2.673	0.373	0.024
10	46	2.705	0.369	0.021

Equation 9.7 may be rearranged into Equation 9.8.

$$v = \frac{V_{max} C}{K_M + C} \tag{9.7}$$

$$\frac{1}{v} = \frac{K_M}{V_{max}} \frac{1}{C} + \frac{1}{V_{max}} \tag{9.8}$$

Equation 9.8 is a linear equation when $1/v$ is plotted against $1/C$. The y-intercept for the line is $1/V_{max}$, and the slope is K_M/V_{max}. An example of a drug reacting enzymatically with rate (v) at various concentrations C is shown in Table 9.6 and Figure 9-5. A plot of $1/v$ versus $1/C$ is shown in Figure 9-6. A plot of $1/v$ versus $1/C$ is linear with an intercept of 0.33 mmol. Therefore,

$$\frac{1}{V_{max}} = 0.33 \text{ min mL}/\mu\text{mol}$$

$$V_{max} = 3 \ \mu\text{mol/mL min}$$

because   the   slope $= 1.65 = K_M/V_{max} = K_M/3$ or $K_M = 3 \times 1.65$ μmol/mL $=$ 5 μmol/mL. Alternatively, K_M may be found from the x intercept, where $-1/K_M$ is equal to the x intercept. (This may be seen by extending the graph to intercept the x axis in the negative region.)

Figure 9-5.   Plot of rate of drug metabolism at various drug concentrations. ($K_M = 0.5 \ \mu$mol/mL, $V_{max} = 3 \ \mu$mol/mL per minute.)

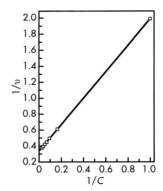

Figure 9-6.   Plot of 1/v versus 1/C for determining K_M and V_{max}.

With this plot (Fig. 9-6), the points are clustered. Other methods are available that may spread the points more evenly. These methods are derived from rearranging Equation 9.8 into Equations 9.9 and 9.10.

$$\frac{C}{v} = \frac{1}{V_{max}}C + \frac{K_M}{V_{max}} \qquad (9.9)$$

$$v = -K_M \frac{v}{C} + V_{max} \qquad (9.10)$$

A plot of C/v versus C would yield a straight line with $1/V_{max}$ as slope and K_M/V_{max} as intercept (Eq. 9.9). A plot of v versus v/C would yield a slope of $-K_M$ and an intercept of V_{max} (Eq. 9.10).

The necessary calculations for making the above plots are shown in Table 9.7. The plots are shown in Figures 9-7 and 9-8. It should be noted that the data are spread out better by the two latter plots. Calculations from the slope show that the same K_M and V_{max} are obtained as in Figure 9-6. When the data are more scattered, one method may be more accurate than the other. A simple approach is to graph the data and examine the linearity of the graphs. The same basic type of plot is used in the clinical literature to determine K_M and V_{max} for individual patients for drugs that undergo capacity-limited kinetics.

TABLE 9.7   Calculations Necessary for Graphic Determination of K_M and V_{max}

C (μM/mL)	v (μM/mL per min)	C/v (min)	v/C (1/min)
1	0.500	2.000	0.500
6	1.636	3.666	0.272
11	2.062	5.333	0.187
16	2.285	7.000	0.142
21	2.423	8.666	0.115
26	2.516	10.333	0.096
31	2.583	12.000	0.083
36	2.634	13.666	0.073
41	2.673	15.333	0.065
46	2.705	17.000	0.058

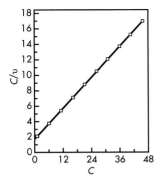

Figure 9-7. Plot of C/v versus C for determining K_M and V_{max}.

Determination of K_M and V_{max} in Patients

Equation 9.7 shows that the rate of drug metabolism (v) is dependent on the concentration of the drug (C). This same basic concept may be applied to the rate of drug metabolism of a capacity-limited drug in the body (Chapter 11). The body may be regarded as a single compartment in which the drug is dissolved. The rate of drug metabolism will vary depending on the concentration of drug C_p as well as on the metabolic rate constants K_M and V_{max} of the drug in each individual.

An example for the determination of K_M and V_{max} is given for the drug phenytoin. Phenytoin undergoes capacity-limited kinetics at therapeutic drug concentrations in the body. To determine K_M and V_{max}, two different dose regimens are given at different times, until steady state is reached. The steady-state drug concentrations are then measured by assay. At steady state, the rate of drug metabolism (v) is assumed to be the same as the rate of drug input R (dose/day). Therefore Equation 9.11 may be written for drug metabolism in the body similar to the way drugs are metabolized *in vitro* (Eq. 9.7). However, steady state will not be reached if the drug input rate, R, is greater than the V_{max}; instead, drug accumulation will continue to occur without reaching a steady-state plateau.

$$R = \frac{V_{max} C_{SS}}{K_M + C_{SS}} \qquad\qquad (9.11)$$

where R = dose/day or dosing rate; C_{SS} = steady-state plasma drug concentration, V_{max} = maximum metabolic rate constant in the body, and K_M = Michaelis–Menten constant of the drug in the body.

Figure 9-8. Plot of v versus v/C for determining K_M and V_{max}.

EXAMPLE

Phenytoin was administered to a patient at dosing rates of 150 and 300 mg/day, respectively. The steady-state plasma drug concentrations were 8.6 and 25.1 mg/L, respectively. Find the K_M and V_{max} of this patient. What dose is needed to achieve a steady-state concentration of 11.3 mg/L?

Solution

There are three methods for solving this problem, all based on the same basic equation (Eq. 9.11).

Method A

Inverting Equation 9.11 on both sides yields

$$\frac{1}{R} = \frac{K_M}{V_{max}} \frac{1}{C_{SS}} + \frac{1}{V_{max}} \tag{9.12}$$

Multiply both sides by $C_{SS} V_{max}$.

$$\frac{V_{max} C_{SS}}{R} = K_M + C_{SS}$$

Rearrange.

$$C_{SS} = \frac{V_{max} C_{SS}}{R} - K_M \tag{9.13}$$

A plot of C_{SS} versus C_{SS}/R is shown in Figure 9-9. V_{max} is equal to the slope, 630 mg/day, and K_M is found from the y intercept, 27.6 mg/L (note the negative intercept).

Method B

From Equation 9.11,

$$RK_M + RC_{SS} = V_{max} C_{SS}$$

Dividing both sides by C_{SS} yields

$$R = V_{max} - \frac{K_M R}{C_{SS}} \tag{9.14}$$

A plot of R versus R/C_{SS} is shown in Figure 9-10. The K_M and V_{max} found are similar to those by the previous method (Fig. 9-9).

Method C

A plot of R versus C_{SS} is shown in Figure 9-11. To determine K_M and V_{max}:

1. Mark points for R of 300 mg/day and C_{SS} of 25.1 mg/L as shown. Connect with a straight line.

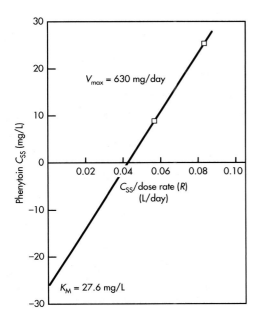

Figure 9-9. Plot of C_{SS} versus C_{SS}/R (method A). (From Witmer and Ritschel, 1984, with permission.)

2. Mark points for R of 150 mg/day and C_{SS} of 8.6 mg/L as shown. Connect with a straight line.

3. Where lines from the first two steps cross is called point A.

4. From point A, read V_{max} on the y axis and K_M on the x axis. (Again, V_{max} of 630 mg/day and K_M of 27 mg/L are found.)

This V_{max} and K_M can be used in Equation 9.11 to find an R to produce the desired C_{SS} of 11.3 mg/L. Alternatively, join point A on the graph to meet 11.3 mg/L on the x axis; R can be read where this line meets the y axis (190 mg/day).

To calculate the dose needed to keep steady-state phenytoin concentration of 11.3 mg/L in this patient, use Equation 9.7.

$$R = \frac{(630 \text{ mg/day})(11.3 \text{ mg/L})}{27 \text{ mg/L} + 11.3 \text{ mg/L}} = \frac{7119}{38.3} = 186 \text{ mg/day}$$

Figure 9-10. Plot of R versus R/C_{SS} or clearance (method B). (From Witmer and Ritschel, 1984, with permission.)

Figure 9-11.   Plot of R versus C_{SS} (method C).
(From Witmer and Ritschel, 1984, with permission.)

This answer compares very closely with the value obtained by the graphic method. All three methods have been used clinically. Vozeh et al (1981) introduced a method that allows for an estimation of phenytoin dose based on steady-state concentration resulting from one dose. This method is based on a statistically compiled nomogram that makes it possible to project a most likely dose for the patient.

Determination of K_M and V_{max} by Direct Method

When steady-state concentrations of phenytoin are known at only two dose levels, there is no advantage in using the graphic method. K_M and V_{max} may be calculated by solving two simultaneous equations formed by substituting C_{ss} and R (Eq. 9.11) with C_1, R_1, C_2, and R_2. The equations contain two unknowns, K_M and V_{max}, and may be solved easily.

$$R_1 = \frac{V_{max} C_1}{K_M + C_1}$$

$$R_2 = \frac{V_{max} C_2}{K_M + C_2}$$

Combining the two equations yields Equation 9.15.

$$K_M = \frac{R_2 - R_1}{(R_1 / C_1) - (R_2 / C_2)} \tag{9.15}$$

where C_1 is steady-state plasma drug concentration after dose 1, C_2 is steady-state plasma drug concentration after dose 2, R_1 is the first dosing rate, and R_2 is the second dosing rate. To calculate K_M and V_{max}, use Equation 9.15 with the values $C_1 = 8.6$ mg/L, $C_2 = 25.1$ mg/L, $R_1 = 150$ mg/day, and $R_2 = 300$ mg/day. The results are

$$K_M = \frac{300 - 150}{(150/8.6) - (300/25.1)} = 27.3 \text{ mg/L}$$

Substitute K_M into either of the two simultaneous equations to solve for V_{max}.

$$150 = \frac{V_{max}(8.6)}{27.3 + 8.6}$$

$$V_{max} = 626 \text{ mg/day}$$

Interpretation of K_M and V_{max}

An understanding of Michaelis–Menten kinetics provides insight into the nonlinear kinetics and helps to avoid dosing a drug at a concentration near enzyme saturation. For example, in the above phenytoin dosing example, since K_M occurs at $0.5 V_{max}$, $K_M = 27.3$ mg/L, the implication is that at a plasma concentration of 27.3 mg/L, enzymes responsible for phenytoin metabolism are eliminating the drug at 50% V_{max}, ie, 0.5×626 mg/day or 313 mg/day. When the subject is receiving 300 mg of phenytoin per day, the plasma drug concentration of phenytoin is 8.6 mg/L, which is considerably below the K_M of 27.3 mg/L. In practice, the K_M in patients can range from 1 to 15 mg/L, V_{max} can range from 100 to 1000 mg/day. Patients with a low K_M tend to have greater changes in plasma concentrations during dosing adjustments. Patients with a smaller K_M (same V_{max}) will show a greater change in the rate of elimination when plasma drug concentration changes compared to subjects with a higher K_M. A subject with the same V_{max}, but different K_M, is shown in Figure 9-12. (For another example, see the slopes of the two curves generated in Figure 9-4).

Dependence of Elimination Half-Life on Dose

For drugs that follow linear kinetics, the elimination half-life is constant and does not change with dose or drug concentration. For a drug that follows nonlinear kinetics, the elimination half-life and drug clearance both change with dose or drug concentration. Generally, the elimination half-life becomes longer, clearance becomes smaller, and the area under the curve becomes disproportionately larger with increasing dose. The relationship between elimination half-life and drug concentration is shown in Equation 9.16. The elimination half-life is dependent on the Michaelis–Menten parameters and concentration.

$$t_{1/2} = \frac{0.693}{V_{max}} (K_M + C_p) \tag{9.16}$$

Some pharmacokineticists prefer not to calculate the elimination half-life of a nonlinear drug because the elimination half-life is not constant. Clinically, if the half-life is increasing as plasma concentration increases, and there is no apparent change in metabolic or renal function, then there is a good possibility that the drug may be metabolized by nonlinear kinetics.

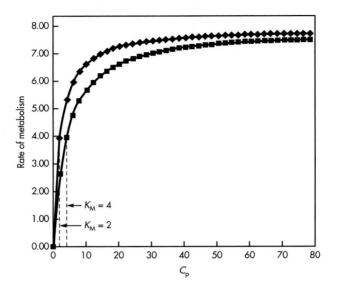

Figure 9-12. Diagram showing the rate of metabolism when V_{max} is constant (8 μg/mL/hr) and K_M is changed ($K_M = 2$ μg/mL for top curve and $K_M = 4$ μg/mL for bottom curve). Note the rate of metabolism is faster for the lower K_M, but saturation starts at lower concentration.

Dependence of Clearance on Dose

The total body clearance of a drug given by IV bolus injection that follows a one-compartment model with Michaelis–Menten elimination kinetics changes with respect to time and plasma drug concentration. Within a certain drug concentration range, an average or mean clearance (Cl_{av}) may be determined. Because the drug follows Michaelis–Menten kinetics, Cl_{av} is dose-dependent. Cl_{av} may be estimated from the area under the curve and the dose given (Wagner et al, 1985).

According to the Michaelis–Menten equation,

$$\frac{dC_p}{dt} = \frac{V_{max} C_p}{K_M + C_p} \tag{9.17}$$

Inverting Equation 9.17 and rearranging yields

$$C_p \, dt = \frac{K_M}{V'_{max}} dC_p - \frac{C_p}{V'_{max}} dC_p \tag{9.18}$$

The area under the curve, $[\text{AUC}]_0^\infty$, is obtained by integration of Equation 9.18 (ie, $[\text{AUC}]_0^\infty = \int_0^\infty C_p \, dt$).

$$\int_0^\infty C_p \, dt = \int_{C_p^0}^\infty \frac{K_M}{V'_{max}} dC_p + \int_{C_p^0}^\infty \frac{C_p}{V'_{max}} dC_p \tag{9.19}$$

where V'_{max} is the maximum velocity for metabolism. Units for V'_{max} are mass/compartment volume per unit time. $V'_{\text{max}} = V_{\text{max}}/V_{\text{D}}$; Wagner et al (1985) used V_{max} in Equation 9.20 as mass/time to be consistent with biochemistry literature, which considers the initial mass of the substrate reacting with the enzyme.

Integration of Equation 9.18 from time 0 to infinity gives Equation 9.20.

$$[\text{AUC}]_0^\infty = \frac{C_{\text{p}}^0}{V_{\text{max}}/V_{\text{D}}}\left(\frac{C_{\text{p}}^0}{2} + K_{\text{M}}\right) \tag{9.20}$$

where V_{D} is the apparent volume of distribution.

Because the dose $D_0 = C_{\text{p}}^0 V_{\text{D}}$, Equation 9.20 may be expressed as

$$[\text{AUC}]_0^\infty = \frac{D_0}{V_{\text{max}}}\left(\frac{C_{\text{p}}^0}{2} + K_{\text{M}}\right) \tag{9.21}$$

To obtain mean body clearance, Cl_{av} is then calculated from the dose and the AUC.

$$Cl_{\text{av}} = \frac{D_0}{[\text{AUC}]_0^\infty} = \frac{V_{\text{max}}}{(C_{\text{p}}^0/2) + K_{\text{M}}} \tag{9.22}$$

$$Cl_{\text{av}} = \frac{V_{\text{max}}}{(D_0/2V_{\text{D}}) + K_{\text{M}}} \tag{9.23}$$

Alternatively, dividing Equation 9.17 by C_{p} gives Equation 9.24, which shows that the clearance of a drug that follows nonlinear pharmacokinetics is dependent on the plasma drug concentration C_{p}, K_{M}, and V_{max}.

$$Cl = \frac{V_{\text{D}}(dC_{\text{p}}/dt)}{C_{\text{p}}} = \frac{V_{\text{max}}}{K_{\text{M}} + C_{\text{p}}} \tag{9.24}$$

Equation 9.22 or 9.23 calculates the average clearance Cl_{av} for the drug after a single IV bolus dose over the entire time course of the drug in the body. For any time period, clearance may be calculated according to Chapter 12 (Eq. 12.10) as

$$Cl_{\text{T}} = \frac{dD_{\text{E}}/dt}{C_{\text{p}}} \tag{9.25}$$

In Chapter 11, the physiologic model based on blood flow and intrinsic clearance is used to describe drug metabolism. The extraction ratios of many drugs are listed in the literature. Actually, extraction ratios are dependent on dose, enzymatic system, blood flow, and for practical purposes, they are often assumed to be constant at normal doses.

Except for phenytoin, there is a paucity of K_{M} and V_{max} data defining the nature of nonlinear drug elimination in patients. However, abundant information is available supporting variable metabolism due to genetic polymorphism (Chapter 11). The clearance (apparent) of many of these drugs in patients who

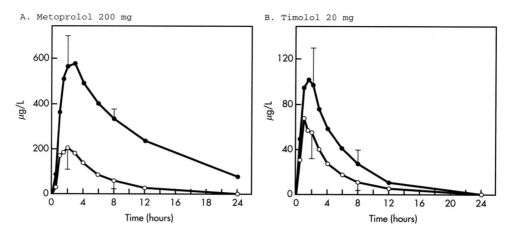

Figure 9-13.   Mean plasma drug concentration versus time profiles following administration of single oral doses of **(A)** metoprolol tartrate 200 mg to 6 extensive metabolizers (EMs) and 6 poor metabolizers (PMs). **(B)** timolol maleate 20 mg to 6 EMs (O) and 4 PMs (●).
(From Lennard et al, 1986, with permission.)

are slow metabolizers changes with dose, although these drugs may exhibit linear kinetics in subjects with the "normal" phenotype. Metoprolol and many β-adrenergic antagonists are extensively metabolized. The plasma levels of metoprolol in slow metabolizers (Lennard et al, 1986) were much greater than other patients, and the AUC, after equal doses, is several times greater among slow metabolizers of metoprolol (Fig. 9-13). A similar picture is observed with another β-adrenergic antagonist, timolol. These drugs have smaller clearance than normal.

EXAMPLE

The dose-dependent pharmacokinetic of sodium valproate (VPA) was studied in guinea pigs at 20, 200, and 600 mg/kg by rapid intravenous infusion. The area under the plasma concentration–time curve increased out of proportion at the 600-mg/kg dose level in all groups (Yu et al, 1987). The total clearance (Cl_T) was significantly decreased and the beta elimination half-life ($t_{1/2}$) was significantly increased at the 600-mg/kg dose level. The dose-dependent kinetics of VPA were due to saturation of metabolism. Metabolic capacity was greatly reduced in young guinea pigs.

Clinically, it is not uncommon to observe similar enzymatic saturation in infants and in special patient populations, whereas drug metabolism may be linear with dose in normal subjects. These patients have lower V_{max} and longer elimination half-life. Variability in drug metabolism is described in Chapters 11 and 12.

EQUATIONS FOR DRUGS DISTRIBUTED AS ONE-COMPARTMENT MODEL AND ELIMINATED BY NONLINEAR PHARMACOKINETICS

The equations presented thus far in this chapter have been for drugs given by IV bolus, distributed as a one-compartment model, and eliminated only by nonlinear pharmacokinetics. The following are useful equations describing other possible routes of drug administration and including mixed drug elimination, by which the drug may be eliminated by both nonlinear (Michaelis–Menten) and linear (first-order) processes.

Mixed Drug Elimination

Drugs may be metabolized to several different metabolites by parallel pathways. At low drug doses corresponding to low drug concentrations at the site of the biotransformation enzymes, the rates of formation of metabolites are first order. However, with higher doses of drug, more drug is absorbed and higher drug concentrations are presented to the biotransformation enzymes. At higher drug concentrations, the enzyme involved in metabolite formation may become saturated, and the rate of metabolite formation becomes nonlinear and approaches zero order. For example, sodium salicylate is metabolized to both a glucuronide and a glycine conjugate (hippurate). The rate of formation of the glycine conjugate is limited by the amount of glycine available. Thus, the rate of formation of the glucuronide continues as a first-order process; whereas the rate of conjugation with glycine is capacity limited.

The equation that describes a drug that is eliminated by both first-order and Michaelis–Menten kinetics after IV bolus injection is given by

$$-\frac{dC_p}{dt} = kC_p + \frac{V'_{max}C_p}{K_M + C_p} \tag{9.26}$$

where k is the first-order rate constant representing the sum of all first-order elimination processes, while the second term of Equation 9.26 represents the saturable process. V'_{max} is simply V_{max} expressed as concentration by dividing by V_D.

Zero-Order Input and Nonlinear Elimination

The usual example of zero-order input is constant IV infusion. If the drug is given by constant IV infusion and is eliminated only by nonlinear pharmacokinetics, then the following equation describes the rate of change of the plasma drug concentration:

$$\frac{dC_p}{dt} = \frac{k_0}{V_D} - \frac{V'_{max}C_p}{K_M + C_p} \tag{9.27}$$

where k_0 is the infusion rate and V_D is the apparent volume of distribution.

First-Order Absorption and Nonlinear Elimination

The relationship that describes the rate of change in the plasma drug concentration for a drug that is given extravascularly (eg, orally), absorbed by first-order absorption, and eliminated only by nonlinear pharmacokinetics, is given by the following equation. C_{GI} is concentration in the GI tract.

$$\frac{dC_p}{dt} = k_a C_{GI} e^{-k_a t} - \frac{V'_{max} C_p}{K_M + C_p} \tag{9.28}$$

where k_a is the first-order absorption rate constant.

If the drug is eliminated by parallel pathways consisting of both linear and nonlinear pharmacokinetics, Equation 9.28 may be extended to Equation 9.29.

$$\frac{dC_p}{dt} = k_a C_{GI} e^{-k_a t} - \frac{V'_{max} C_p}{K_M + C_p} - k C_p \tag{9.29}$$

where k is the first-order elimination rate constant.

CHRONOPHARMACOKINETICS AND TIME-DEPENDENT PHARMACOKINETICS

Chronopharmacokinetics broadly refers to a temporal change in the rate process (such as absorption or elimination) of a drug. The temporal changes in drug absorption or elimination can be cyclical over a constant period (e.g., 24-hour interval), or they may be noncyclical, in which drug absorption or elimination changes over a longer period of time. Chronopharmacokinetics is an important consideration during drug therapy.

Time-dependent pharmacokinetics generally refers to a noncyclical change in the drug absorption or drug elimination rate process over a period of time. Time-dependent pharmacokinetics leads to nonlinear pharmacokinetics. Unlike dose-dependent pharmacokinetics, which involves a change in the rate process when the dose is changed, time-dependent pharmacokinetics may be the result of alteration in the physiology or biochemistry in an organ or a region in the body that influences drug disposition (Levy, 1983).

Time-dependent pharmacokinetics may be due to auto-induction or auto-inhibition of biotransformation enzymes. For example, Pitlick and Levy (1977) have shown that repeated doses of carbamazepine induce the enzymes responsible for its elimination (ie, auto-induction), thereby increasing the clearance of the drug. Auto-inhibition may occur during the course of metabolism of certain drugs (Perrier et al, 1973). In this case, the metabolites formed increase in concentration and further inhibit metabolism of the parent drug. In biochemistry, this phenomenon is known as *product inhibition*. Drugs undergoing time-dependent pharmacokinetic have variable clearance and elimination half-lives. The steady-state concentration of a drug that causes auto-induction may be due to increased clearance over time. Some anticancer drugs are better tolerated at certain times of the day; for example, the antimetabolite drug, fluorouracil (FU) was least toxic when given in the morning to rodents (Von Roemeling, 1991). A list of drugs that demonstrate time dependence is shown in Table 9.8. In pharmacokinetics, it is important to recognize that many isozymes (CYPs) are involved in drug metabolisms. A drug may competitively influence the metabolism of another drug within the same CYP

TABLE 9.8 Drugs Showing Circadian or Time-Dependent Disposition

Cefodizime	Fluorouracil	Ketoprofen	Theophylline
Cisplatin	Heparin	Mequitazine	

From Reinberg (1991).

subfamily. Sometimes, an unrecognized effect from the presence of another drug may be misjudged as a time-dependent pharmacokinetic. Drug metabolism and pharmacogenetics are discussed more extensively in Chapter 12.

Circadian Rhythms and Influence on Drug Response

Circadian rhythms are rhythmic or cyclical changes in plasma drug concentrations that may occur daily, due to normal changes in body functions. Some rhythmic changes that influence body functions and drug response are controlled by genes and subject to modification by environmental factors. The mammalian circadian clock is a self-sustaining oscillator, usually within a period of ~24 hours, that cyclically controls many physiological and behavioral systems. The biological clock attempts to synchronize and respond to changes in length of the daylight cycle and optimize body functions.

Circadian rhythms are regulated through periodic activation of transcription by a set of clock genes. For example, melatonin onset is associated with onset of the quiescent period of cortisol secretion that regulates many functions. Some well-known circadian physiologic parameters are core body temperature (CBT), heart rate (HR), and other cardiovascular parameters. These fundamental physiologic factors can affect disease states, as well as toxicity and therapeutic response to drug therapy. The toxic dose of a drug may vary as much as several-fold, depending on the time of drug administration—during either sleep or wake cycle.

For example, the effects of aminoglycoside administration timing on serum aminoglycoside levels and the incidence of nephrotoxicity were studied in 221 patients (Prins et al, 1997). Each patient received an IV injection of 2–4 mg/kg gentamicin or tobramycin once daily at: (1) between midnight and 7:30 AM, (2) between 8 AM and 3:30 PM, or (3) between 4 PM and 11:30 PM. In this study, no statistically significant differences in drug trough levels (0–4.2 mg/L) or peak drug levels (3.6–26.8 mg/L) were found for the three time periods of drug administration. However, nephrotoxicity occurred significantly more frequently when the aminoglycosides were given during the rest period (midnight to 7:30 AM). Many factors contribute to nephrotoxicity were discussed; the time of administration was considered to be an independent risk factor in the multivariate statistical analysis. Time-dependent pharmacokinetics/pharmacodynamics are important, although it is not always possible to detect the difference in drug concentration clinically because of multivariates.

Another example of circadian changes on drug response involves observations with chronic obstructive pulmonary disease (COPD) patients. Symptoms of hypoxemia may be aggravated in some COPD patients due to changes in respiration during the sleep cycle. Prominent circadian variations have been reported involving the incidence of acute myocardial infarction, sudden cardiac death, and stroke, the leading causes of death in the United States. Platelet aggregation favoring co-agulation is increased after arising in the early morning hours, coincident with the peak incidence of these cardiovascular events, although much remains to be elucidated.

Time-dependent pharmacokinetic and physiologic functions are important considerations in the treatment of certain hypertensive subjects, in whom early-morning rise in blood pressure may increase the risk of stroke or hypertensive crisis. Verapamil is a commonly used antihypertensive. The diurnal pattern of fore-arm vascular resistance (FVR) between hypertensive and normotensive volunteers was studied at 9 PM on 24-hour ambulatory blood pressure monitoring, and the early-morning blood pressure rise was studied in 23 untreated hypertensives and 10 matched, normotensive controls. The diurnal pattern of FVR differed between hypertensives and normotensives, with normotensives exhibiting an FVR decline between 2 PM and 9 PM, while FVR rose at 9 PM in hypertensives. Verapamil appeared to minimize the diurnal variation in FVR in hypertensives, although there were no significant differences at any single time point. Verapamil effectively reduced ambulatory blood pressure throughout the 24-hour period, but it did not blunt the early-morning rate of blood pressure rise despite peak S-verapamil concentrations in the early morning (Nguyen et al, 2000).

Another example of time-dependent pharmacokinetics involves ciprofloxacin. Circadian variation in the urinary excretion of ciprofloxacin was investigated in a crossover study in 12 healthy male volunteers, ages 19–32 years. A significant decrease in the rate and extent of the urinary excretion of ciprofloxacin was observed following administrations at 22:00 versus 10:00 hour, indicating that the rate of excretion during the night time was slower (Sarveshwer Rao et al., 1997).

Clinical and Adverse Toxicity due to Nonlinear Pharmacokinetics

The presence of nonlinear or dose-dependent pharmacokinetics, whether due to saturation of a process involving absorption, first-pass metabolism, binding, or renal excretion, can have significant clinical consequences. However, nonlinear pharmacokinetics may not be noticed in drug studies that use a narrow dose range in patients. In this case, dose estimation may result in disproportionate increases in adverse reactions, but insufficient therapeutic benefits. Nonlinear pharmacokinetics can occur anywhere above, within, or below the therapeutic window.

The problem of nonlinear dose relationship in population pharmacokinetics analysis has been investigated using simulations (Hashimoto et al, 1994, 1995; Jonsson et al, 2000). For example, nonlinear fluvoxamine pharmacokinetics were reported (Jonsson et al, 2000) to be present even at subtherapeutic doses. By using simulated data and applying nonlinear mixed-effects models using NONMEM, the authors also demonstrated that use of nonlinear mixed-effect models in population pharmacokinetics has an important application in the detection and characterization of nonlinear processes (pharmacokinetic and pharmacodynamic). Both first-order (FO) and FO conditional estimation (FOCE) algorithms were used for the population analyses. Population pharmacokinetics are discussed further in Chapter 22.

BIOAVAILABILITY OF DRUGS THAT FOLLOW NONLINEAR PHARMACOKINETICS

The bioavailability of drugs that follow nonlinear pharmacokinetics is difficult to estimate accurately. As shown in Table 9.1, each process of drug absorption, distribution, and elimination is potentially saturable. Drugs that follow linear pharmacokinetics follow the principle of superposition (Chapter 8). The assumption in applying the rule of superposition is that each dose of drug superimposes on the previous dose. Consequently, the bioavailability of subsequent doses is predictable and not affected by the previous dose. In the presence of a saturable pathway for drug absorption, distribution, or elimination, drug bioavailability will change within a single dose or with subsequent (multiple) doses. An example of a drug with dose-dependent absorption is chlorothiazide (Hsu et al, 1987).

The extent of bioavailability is generally estimated using $[AUC]_0^\infty$. If drug absorption is saturation limited in the gastrointestinal tract, then a smaller fraction of drug is absorbed systemically when the gastrointestinal drug concentration is high. A drug with a saturable elimination pathway may also have a concentration-dependent AUC affected by the magnitude of K_M and V_{max} of the enzymes involved in drug elimination (Eq. 9.21). At low C_p, the rate of elimination is first order, even at the beginning of drug absorption from the gastrointestinal tract. As more drug is absorbed, either from a single dose or after multiple doses, systemic drug concentrations increase to levels that saturate the enzymes involved in drug elimination. The body drug clearance changes and the AUC increases disproportionately to the increase in dose (Fig. 9-2).

NONLINEAR PHARMACOKINETICS DUE TO DRUG–PROTEIN BINDING

Protein binding may prolong the elimination half-life of a drug. Drugs that are protein bound must first dissociate into the free or nonbound form to be eliminated by glomerular filtration. The nature and extent of drug–protein binding affects the magnitude of the deviation from normal linear or first-order elimination rate process.

For example, consider the plasma level–time curves of two hypothetical drugs given intravenously in equal doses (Fig. 9-14). One drug is 90% protein bound, whereas the other drug does not bind plasma protein. Both drugs are eliminated solely by glomerular filtration through the kidney.

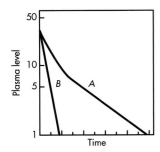

Figure 9-14. Plasma curve comparing the elimination of two drugs given in equal IV doses. Curve *A* represents a drug 90% bound to plasma protein. Curve *B* represents a drug not bound to plasma protein.

The plasma curves in Figure 9-14 demonstrate that the protein-bound drug is more concentrated in the plasma than a drug that is not protein bound, and the protein-bound drug is eliminated at a slower, nonlinear rate. Because the two drugs are eliminated by identical mechanisms, the characteristically slower elimination rate for the protein-bound drug is due to the fact that less free drug is available for glomerular filtration in the course of renal excretion.

The concentration of free drug, C_f, can be calculated at any time, as follows.

$$C_f = C_p (1 - \text{fraction bound}) \tag{9.30}$$

For any protein-bound drug, the free drug concentration (C_f) will always be less than the total drug concentration (C_p).

A careful examination of Figure 9-14 shows that the slope of the bound drug decreases gradually as the drug concentration decreases. This indicates that the percent of drug bound is not constant. *In vivo,* the percent of drug bound usually increases as the plasma drug concentration decreases (see Chapter 10). Since protein binding of drug can cause nonlinear elimination rates, pharmacokinetic fitting of protein-bound drug data to a simple one-compartment model without accounting for binding results in erroneous estimates of the volume of distribution and elimination half-life. Sometimes plasma drug data for drugs that are highly protein bound have been inappropriately fitted to two-compartment models.

Valproic acid (Depakene) shows nonlinear pharmacokinetics that may be due partially to nonlinear protein binding. The free fraction of valproic acid is 10% at a plasma drug concentration of 40 μg/mL and is 18.5% at a plasma drug level of 130 μg/mL. In addition, higher than expected plasma drug concentrations occur in the elderly, hyperlidemic patients, and in patients with hepatic or renal disease.

One-Compartment Model Drug with Protein Binding

The process of elimination of a drug distributed in a single compartment with protein binding is illustrated in Figure 9-15. The one compartment contains both free drug and bound drug, which are dynamically interconverted with rate constants k_1 and k_2. Elimination of drug occurs only with the free drug, at a first-order rate. The bound drug is not eliminated. Assuming a saturable and instantly reversible drug-binding process, where P = protein concentration in plasma, C_f = plasma concentration of free drug, $k_d = k_2/k_1$ = dissociation constant of the protein drug complex, C_p = total plasma drug concentration, and C_b = plasma concentration of bound drug,

$$\frac{C_b}{P} = \frac{(1/k_d)C_f}{1 + (1/k_d)C_f} \tag{9.31}$$

Figure 9-15. One-compartment model with drug–protein binding.

This equation can be rearranged as follows:

$$C_b = \frac{PC_f}{k_d + C_f} = C_p - C_f \tag{9.32}$$

Solving for C_f,

$$C_f = \frac{1}{2}\left[-(P + k_d - C_p) + \sqrt{(P + k_d - C_p)^2 + 4k_d C_p} \right] \tag{9.33}$$

Because the rate of drug elimination is dC_p/dt,

$$\frac{dC_p}{dt} = -kC_f$$

$$\frac{dC_p}{dt} = \frac{-k}{2}\left[-(P + k_d - C_p) + \sqrt{(P + k_d - C_p)^2 + 4k_d C_p} \right] \tag{9.34}$$

This differential equation describes the relationship of changing plasma drug concentrations during elimination. The equation is not easily integrated but can be solved using a numerical method. Figure 9-16 shows the plasma drug concentration curves for a one-compartment protein-bound drug having a volume of distribution of 50 mL/kg and an elimination half-life of 30 minutes. The protein concentration is 4.4% and the molecular weight of the protein is 67,000 Da. At various doses, the pharmacokinetics of elimination of the drug, as shown by the plasma curves, range from linear to nonlinear, depending on the total plasma drug concentration.

Nonlinear drug elimination pharmacokinetics occur at higher doses. Because more free drug is available at higher doses, initial drug elimination occurs more rapidly. For drugs demonstrating nonlinear pharmacokinetics, the free drug concentration may increase slowly at first, but when the dose of drug is raised beyond the protein-bound saturation point, free plasma drug concentrations may rise abruptly. Therefore, the concentration of free drug should always be calculated to make sure the patient receives a proper dose.

Figure 9-16. Plasma drug concentrations for various doses of a one-compartment model durg with protein binding.
(Adapted from Coffey et al, 1971, with permission.)

FREQUENTLY ASKED QUESTIONS

1. Most drugs follow linear pharmacokinetics at therapeutic doses. Why is it important to monitor drug level carefully for dose dependency?

2. What are the main differences in pharmacokinetic parameters between a drug that follows linear and a drug that follows nonlinear pharmacokinetic?

3. What are the main differences between a model based on Michaelis–Menten kinetic (V_{max} and K_M) and the physiologic model that describes hepatic metabolism based on clearance?

4. What is the cause of nonlinear pharmacokinetics that is not dose related?

LEARNING QUESTIONS

1. Define *nonlinear pharmacokinetics*. How do drugs that follow nonlinear pharmacokinetics differ from drugs that follow linear pharmacokinetics?

    a. What is the rate of change in the plasma drug concentration with respect to time, dC_p/dt, when $C_p \ll K_M$?

    b. What is the rate of change in the plasma drug concentration with respect to time, dC_p/dt, when $C_p \gg K_M$?

2. What processes of drug absorption, distribution, and elimination may be considered "capacity limited," "saturated," or "dose dependent?"

3. Drugs, such as phenytoin and salicylates, have been reported to follow dose-dependent elimination kinetics. What changes in pharmacokinetic parameters, including $t_{1/2}$, V_D, AUC, and C_p, could be predicted if the amounts of these drugs administered were increased from low pharmacologic doses to high therapeutic doses?

4. A given drug is metabolized by capacity-limited pharmacokinetics. Assume K_M is 50 μg/mL, V_{max} is 20 μg/mL per hour, and the apparent V_D is 20 L/kg.

    a. What is the reaction order for the metabolism of this drug when given in a single intravenous dose of 10 mg/kg?

    b. How much time is necessary for the drug to be 50% metabolized?

5. How would induction or inhibition of the hepatic enzymes involved in drug biotransformation theoretically affect the pharmacokinetics of a drug that demonstrates nonlinear pharmacokinetics due to saturation of its hepatic elimination pathway?

6. Assume that both the active parent drug and its inactive metabolites are excreted by active tubular secretion. What might be the consequences of increasing the dosage of the drug on its elimination half-life?

7. The drug isoniazid was reported to interfere with the metabolism of phenytoin. Patients taking both drugs together show higher phenytoin levels in the body. Using the basic principles in this chapter, do you expect K_M to increase or decrease in patients taking both drugs? (*Hint:* see Fig. 9-4.)

8. Explain why K_M is often seen to have units of mM/mL and sometimes mg/L.

9. The V_{max} for metabolizing a drug is 10 mmol/hr. The rate of metabolism (v) is 5 μmol/hr when drug concentration is 4 μmol. Which of the following statements is/are true?

   a. K_M is 5 μmol for this drug.

   b. K_M cannot be determined from the information given.

   c. K_M is 4 μmol for this drug.

10. Which of the following statements is/are true regarding the pharmacokinetics of diazepam (98% protein bound) and propranolol (87% protein bound)?

    a. Diazepam has a long elimination half-life because it is difficult to be metabolized due to extensive plasma–protein binding.

    b. Propranolol is an example of a drug with high protein binding but unrestricted (unaffected) metabolic clearance.

    c. Diazepam is an example of a drug with low hepatic extraction.

    d. All of the above.

    e. a and c.

    f. b and c.

11. Which of the following statements describe(s) correctly the properties of a drug that follows nonlinear or capacity-limited pharmacokinetics?

    a. The elimination half-life will remain constant when the dose changes.

    b. The area under the plasma curve (AUC) will increase proportionally as dose increases.

    c. The rate of drug elimination = $C_p \times K_M$.

    d. All of the above.

    e. a and b.

    f. None of the above.

12. The hepatic intrinsic clearances of two drugs are

    Drug A: 1300 mL/min

    Drug B: 26 mL/min

    Which drug is likely to show the greatest increase in hepatic clearance when hepatic blood flow is increased from 1 L/min to 1.5 L/min?

    a. Drug A

    b. Drug B

    c. No change for both drugs

REFERENCES

Coffey J, Bullock FJ, Schoenemann PT: Numerical solution of nonlinear pharmacokinetic equations: Effect of plasma protein binding on drug distribution and elimination. *J Pharm Sci* **60:**1623, 1971

Evans WE, Schentag JJ, Jusko WJ: *Applied Pharmacokinetics—Principles of Therapeutic Drug Monitoring,* 3rd ed. Applied Therapeutics, 1992, pp 2–33

Gibaldi M: Pharmacokinetic aspects of drug metabolism. *Ann NY State Acad Sci* **179:**19, 1971

Hashimoto Y, Odani A, Tanigawara Y, Yasuhara M, Okuno T, Hori R: Population analysis of the dose-dependent pharmacokinetics of zonisamide in epileptic patients. *Biol Pharm Bull* **17:**323–326, 1994

Hashimoto Y, Koue T, Otsuki Y, Yasuhara M, Hori R, Inui K: Simulation for population analysis of Michaelis–Menton kinetics. *J Pharmacokinet Biopharmacol* **23:**205–216, 1995

Hsu F, Prueksaritanont T, Lee MG, Chiou WL: The phenomenon and cause of the dose-dependent oral absorption of chlorothiazide in rats: Extrapolation to human data based on the body surface area concept. *J Pharmacokinet Biopharmacol* **15:**369–386, 1987

Jonsson EN, Wade JR, Karlsson MO: Nonlinearity detection: Advantages of nonlinear mixed-effects modeling. *AAPS Pharmsci* **2**(3), article 32, 2000

Lennard MS, Tucker GT, Woods HF: The polymorphic oxidation of beta-adrenoceptor antagonists— Clinical pharmacokinetic considerations. *Clin Pharmacol* **11:**1–17, 1986

Levy RH: Time-dependent pharmacokinetics. *Pharmacol Ther* **17:**383–392, 1983

Nguyen BN, Parker RB, Noujedehi M, Sullivan JM, Johnson JA: Effects of coerverapamil on circadian pattern of forearm vascular resistance and blood pressure. *J Clin Pharmacol* **40** (suppl):1480–1487, 2000

Perrier D, Ashley JJ, Levy G: Effect of product inhibition in kinetics of drug elimination. *J Pharmacokinet Biopharmacol* **1:**231, 1973

Pitlick WH, Levy RH: Time-dependent kinetics, I. Exponential autoinduction of carbamazepine in monkeys. *J Pharm Sci* **66:**647, 1977

Reinberg AE: Concepts of circadian chronopharmacology. In Hrushesky WJM, Langer R, Theeuwes F (eds), *Temporal Control of Drug Delivery.* New York, Annals of the Academy of Science, 1991, vol 618, p 102

Sarveshwer Rao VV, Rambhau D, Ramesh Rao B, Srinivasu P: Circadian variation in urinary excretion of ciprofloxacin after a single dose oral administration at 1000 and 2200 hours in human subjects. *India Antimicrob Agents Chemother (USA)* **41:**1802–1804, 1997, Kakatiya Univ., Warangal-506 009

Prins JM, Weverling GJ, Van Ketel RJ, Speelman P: Circadian variations in serum levels and the renal toxicity of aminoglycosides in patients. *Clin Pharmacol Therapeut* **62:**106–111, 1997

Tozer TN, et al: In Breimer DD, Speiser P (eds), *Topics in Pharmaceutical Sciences.* New York, Elsevier, 1981, p 4

Von Roemeling R: The therapeutic index of cytotoxic chemotherapy depends upon circadian drug timing. In Hrushesky WJM, Langer R, Theeuwes F (eds), *Temporal Control of Drug Delivery.* New York, Annals of the Academy of Science, 1991, vol 618, pp 292–311

Vozeh S, Muir KT, Sheiner LB: Predicting phenytoin dosage. *J Pharm Biopharm* **9:**131–146, 1981

Wagner JG, Szpunar GJ, Ferry JJ: Michaelis–Menten elimination kinetics: Areas under curves, steady-state concentrations, and clearances for compartment models with different types of input. *Biopharm Drug Disp* **6:**177–200, 1985

Witmer DR, Ritschel WA: Phenytoin isoniazid interaction: A kinetic approach to management. *Drug Intell Clin Pharm* **18:**483–486, 1984

Yu HY, Shen YZ, Sugiyama Y, Hanano M: Dose-dependent pharmacokinetics of valproate in guinea pigs of different ages. *Epilepsia* **28**(6):680–687, 1987

BIBLIOGRAPHY

Amsel LP, Levy G: Drug biotransformation interactions in man, II. A pharmacokinetic study of the simultaneous conjugation of benzoic and salicylic acids with glycine. *J Pharm Sci* **58:**321–326, 1969

Dutta S, Matsumoto Y, Ebling WF: Is it possible to estimate the parameters of the sigmoid E_{max} model with truncated data typical of clinical studies? *J Pharm Sci* **85:**232–239, 1996

Kruger-Theimer E: Nonlinear dose concentration relationships. *Il Farmaco* **23:**718–756, 1968

Levy G: Pharmacokinetics of salicylate in man. *Drug Metab Rev* **9:**3–19, 1979

Levy G, Tsuchiya T: Salicylate accumulation kinetics in man. *N Engl J Med* **287:**430–432, 1972

Ludden TM: Nonlinear pharmacokinetics. Clinical applications. *Clin Pharmacokinet* **20:**429–446, 1991

Ludden TM, Hawkins DW, Allen JP, Hoffman SF: Optimum phenytoin dosage regimen. *Lancet* **1:**307–308, 1979

Mullen PW: Optimal phenytoin therapy: A new technique for individualizing dosage. *Clin Pharm Ther* **23:**228–232, 1978

Mullen PW, Foster RW: Comparative evaluation of six techniques for determining the Michaelis–Menten parameters relating phenytoin dose and steady state serum concentrations. *J Pharm Pharmacol* **31:**100–104, 1979

Tozer TN, Rubin GM: Saturable kinetics and bioavailability determination. In Welling PG, Tse FLS (eds), *Pharmacokinetics: Regulatory, Industrial, Academic Perspectives.* New York, Marcel Dekker, 1988

Van Rossum JM, van Lingen G, Burgers JPT: Dose-dependent pharmacokinetics. *Pharmacol Ther* **21:**77–99, 1983

Wagner J: Properties of the Michaelis–Menten equation and its integrated form which are useful in pharmacokinetics. *J Pharm Biopharm* **1:**103, 1973

PHYSIOLOGIC DRUG DISTRIBUTION AND PROTEIN BINDING

PHYSIOLOGIC FACTORS OF DISTRIBUTION

After a drug is absorbed into plasma, the drug molecules are distributed throughout the body by the systemic circulation. The drug molecules are carried by the blood to the target site (receptor) for drug action and to other (nonreceptor) tissues as well, where side effects or adverse reactions may occur. Drug molecules are distributed to eliminating organs, such as the liver and kidney, and to noneliminating tissues, such as the brain, skin, and muscle. In pregnancy, drugs cross the placenta and may affect the developing fetus. Drugs can also be secreted in milk via the mammillary glands. A substantial portion of the drug may be bound to proteins in the plasma and/or tissues. Lipophilic drugs deposit in fat, from which the drug may be slowly released.

The circulatory system consists of a series of blood vessels; these include the arteries that carry blood to tissues, and the veins that return the blood back to the heart. An average subject (70 kg) has about 5 L of blood, which is equivalent to 3 L of plasma (Fig. 10-1). About 50% of the blood is in the large veins or venous sinuses. The volume of blood pumped by the heart per minute—the cardiac output—is the product of the stroke volume of the heart and the number of heartbeats per minute. An average cardiac output is 0.08 L/left ventricle contraction × 69 contractions (heart beats)/min, or about 5.5 L/min in subjects at rest. The cardiac output may be five to six times higher during exercise. Left ventricular contraction may produce a systolic blood pressure of 120 mm Hg, and moves blood at a linear speed of 300 mm/sec through the aorta. Mixing of a drug solution in the blood occurs rapidly at this flow rate. Drug molecules rapidly diffuse through a network of fine capillaries to the tissue spaces filled with interstitial fluid (Fig. 10-2). The interstitial fluid plus the plasma water is termed *extracellular water*, because these fluids reside outside the cells. Drug molecules may further diffuse from the interstitial fluid across the cell membrane into the cell cytoplasm.

Figure 10-1. Major water volumes (L) in average 70–kg human.

Drug distribution is generally rapid, and most small drug molecules permeate capillary membranes easily. The passage of drug molecules across a cell membrane depends on the physicochemical nature of both the drug and the cell membrane. Cell membranes are composed of protein and a bilayer of phospholipid, which act as a lipid barrier to drug uptake. Thus, lipid-soluble drugs generally diffuse across cell membranes more easily than highly polar or water-soluble drugs. Small drug molecules generally diffuse more rapidly across cell membranes than large drug molecules. If the drug is bound to a plasma protein such as albumin, the drug–protein complex becomes too large for easy diffusion across the cell or even capillary membranes. A comparison of diffusion rates for water-soluble molecules is given in Table 10.1.

Diffusion and Hydrostatic Pressure

The processes by which drugs transverse capillary membranes include passive diffusion and hydrostatic pressure. Passive diffusion is the main process by which most drugs cross cell membranes. *Passive diffusion* (Chapter 13) is the process by which drug molecules move from an area of high concentration to an area of low concentration. Passive diffusion is described by *Fick's law of diffusion:*

$$\text{Rate of drug diffusion} = \frac{dQ}{dt} = \frac{-DKA(C_p - C_t)}{h} \qquad (10.1)$$

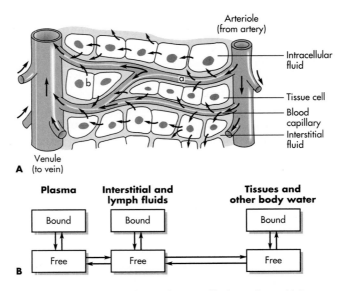

Figure 10-2. Diffusion of drug from capillaries to interstitial spaces.

TABLE 10.1   Permeability of Molecules of Various Sizes to Capillaries

	MOLECULAR WEIGHT	RADIUS OF EQUIVALENT SPHERE A (0.1 mm)	DIFFUSION COEFFICIENT	
			In Water (cm²/sec) × 10⁵	Across Capillary (cm²/sec × 100 g)
Water	18		3.20	3.7
Urea	60	1.6	1.95	1.83
Glucose	180	3.6	0.91	0.64
Sucrose	342	4.4	0.74	0.35
Raffinose	594	5.6	0.56	0.24
Inulin	5,500	15.2	0.21	0.036
Myoglobin	17,000	19	0.15	0.005
Hemoglobin	68,000	31	0.094	0.001
Serum albumin	69,000		0.085	<0.001

From Goldstein et al (1974).

where $C_p - C_t$ is the difference between the drug concentration in the plasma (C_p) and in the tissue (C_t), respectively; A is the surface area of the membrane; h is the thickness of the membrane; K is the lipid–water partition coefficient; and D is the diffusion constant. The negative sign denotes net transfer of drug from inside the capillary lumen into the tissue and extracellular spaces. Diffusion is spontaneous and temperature dependent. Diffusion is distinguished from blood flow-initiated mixing, which involves hydrostatic pressure.

Hydrostatic pressure represents the pressure gradient between the arterial end of the capillaries entering the tissue and the venous capillaries leaving the tissue. Hydrostatic pressure is responsible for penetration of water-soluble drugs into spaces between endothelial cells and possibly into lymph. In the kidneys, high arterial pressure creates a filtration pressure that allows small drug molecules to be filtered in the glomerulus of the renal nephron (see Chapter 6).

Blood flow-induced drug distribution is rapid and efficient, but requires pressure. As blood pressure gradually decreases when arteries branch into the small arterioles, the speed of flow slows and diffusion into the interstitial space becomes diffusion or concentration driven and facilitated by the large surface area of the capillary network. The average pressure of the blood capillary is higher (+18 mm Hg) than the mean tissue pressure (–6 mm Hg), resulting in a net total pressure of 24 mm Hg higher in the capillary over the tissue. This pressure difference is offset by an average osmotic pressure in the blood of 24 mm Hg, pulling the plasma fluid back into the capillary. Thus, on average, the pressures in the tissue and most parts of the capillary are equal, with no net flow of water.

At the arterial end, as the blood newly enters the capillary (Fig. 10-2A), however, the pressure of the capillary blood is slightly higher (about 8 mm Hg) than that of the tissue, causing fluid to leave the capillary and enter the tissues. This pressure is called *hydrostatic* or *filtration pressure*. This filtered fluid (filtrate) is later returned to the venous capillary (Fig. 10-2B) due to a lower venous pressure of about the same magnitude. The lower pressure of the venous blood compared with the tissue fluid is termed *absorptive pressure*. A small amount of fluid returns to the circulation through the lymphatic system.

Distribution Half-Life, Blood Flow, and Drug Uptake by Organs

Because the process of drug transfer from the capillary into the tissue fluid is mainly diffusional, the membrane thickness, diffusion coefficient of the drug, and concentration gradient across the capillary membrane are important factors in determining the rate of drug diffusion. Kinetically, if a drug diffuses rapidly across the membrane in such a way that blood flow is the rate-limiting step in the distribution of drug, then the process is *perfusion* or *flow limited*. A person with congestive heart failure has decreased cardiac output, resulting in impaired blood flow, which may reduce renal clearance through reduced filtration pressure and blood flow. In contrast, if drug distribution is limited by the slow diffusion of drug across the membrane in the tissue, then the process is termed *diffusion* or *permeability limited* (Fig. 10-3). Drugs that are permeability limited may have an increased distribution volume in disease conditions that cause inflammation and increased capillary membrane permeability. The delicate osmotic pressure balance may be altered due to albumin and/or blood loss or due to changes in electrolyte levels in renal and hepatic disease, resulting in net flow of plasma water into the interstitial space (edema). This change in fluid distribution may partially explain the increased extravascular drug distribution during some disease states.

Blood flow, tissue size, and tissue storage are also important in determining the time it takes the drug to become fully distributed. Table 10.2 lists the blood flow and tissue mass for many tissues in the human body. *Drug affinity* for a tissue or organ refers to the partitioning and accumulation of the drug in the tissue. The time for drug distribution is generally measured by the *distribution half-life* or the time for 50% distribution. The factors that determine the distribution constant of a drug into an organ are related to the blood flow to the organ, the volume of the organ, and the partitioning of the drug into the organ tissue, as shown in Equation 10.2.

$$k_d = \frac{Q}{VR} \tag{10.2}$$

where k_d = first-order distribution constant, Q = blood flow to the organ, V = volume of the organ, R = ratio of drug concentration in the organ tissue to drug

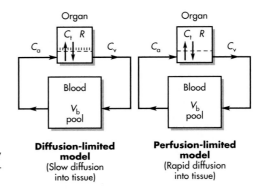

Figure 10-3. Drug distribution to body organs by blood flow (perfusion). **Right.** Tissue with rapid permeability; **Left.** Tissue with slow permeability.

TABLE 10.2   Blood Flow to Human Tissues

TISSUE	PERCENT BODY WEIGHT	PERCENT CARDIAC OUTPUT	BLOOD FLOW (mL/100 g tissue/min)
Adrenals	0.02	1	550
Kidneys	0.4	24	450
Thyroid	0.04	2	400
Liver			
Hepatic	2.0	5	20
Portal		20	75
Portal-drained viscera	2.0	20	75
Heart (basal)	0.4	4	70
Brain	2.0	15	55
Skin	7.0	5	5
Muscle (basal)	40.0	15	3
Connective tissue	7.0	1	1
Fat	15.0	2	1

Adapted with permission from Butler (1972).

concentration in the blood (venous). The *distribution half-life* of the drug to the tissue, $t_{d1/2}$ may easily be determined from the distribution constant, $t_{d1/2} = 0.693/k_d$.

The ratio R must be determined experimentally from tissue samples. With many drugs, however, only animal tissue data are available. Pharmacokineticists have estimated the ratio R based on knowledge of the partition coefficient of the drug. The partition coefficient is a physical property that measures the ratio of the solubility of the drug in the oil phase and in aqueous phase. The partition coefficient ($P_{o/w}$) is defined as a ratio of the drug concentration in the oil phase (usually represented by octanol) divided by the drug concentration in the aqueous phase measured at equilibrium under specified temperature *in vitro* in an oil/water two-layer system (Fig. 10-4). The partition coefficient is one of the most important factors that determine the tissue distribution of a drug.

If each tissue has the same ability to store the drug, then the distribution half-life is governed by the blood flow, Q, and volume (size), V, of the organ. A large blood flow, Q, to the organ decreases the distribution time, whereas a large organ size or volume, V, increases the distribution time because a longer time is needed to fill a large organ volume with drug. Figure 10-5 illustrates the distribution time (for 0, 50, 90, and 95% distribution) for the adrenal gland, kidney, muscle (basal),

Diffusion into oil = $k_{12} C_{water}$

Diffusion into water = $k_{21} C_{oil}$

At steady state, $k_{12} C_{water} = k_{21} C_{oil}$

Figure 10-4.   Diagram showing equilibration of drug between oil and water layer *in vitro*.

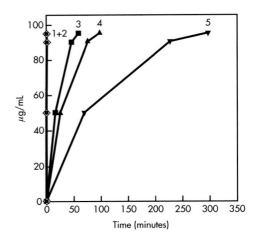

Figure 10-5. Drug distribution in five groups of tissues at various rate of equilibration. (1 = adrenal, 2 = kidney, 3 = skin, 4 = muscle [basal], 5 = fat.)

skin, and fat tissue in an average human subject (ideal body weight, IBW = 70 kg). In this illustration, the blood drug concentration is equally maintained at 100 μg/mL, and the drug is assumed to have equal distribution between all the tissues and blood, ie, when fully equilibrated, the partition or drug concentration ratio (R) between the tissue and the plasma will equal 1. Vascular tissues such as the kidneys and adrenal glands achieve 95% distribution in less than 2 minutes. In contrast, drug distribution time in fat tissues takes 4 hours, while less vascular tissues, such as the skin and muscles, take between 2 and 4 hours (Fig. 10-5). When drug partition of the tissues is the same, the distribution time is dependent only on the tissue volume and its blood flow.

Blood flow is an important consideration in determining how rapid and how much drug reaches the receptor site. Under normal conditions, limited blood flow reaches the muscles. During exercise, the increase in blood flow may change the fraction of drug reaching the muscle tissues. Diabetic patients receiving intramuscular injection of insulin may experience the effects of changing onset of drug action during exercise. Normally, the blood reserve of the body stays mostly in the large veins and sinuses in the abdomen. During injury or when blood is lost, constriction of the large veins redirect more blood to needed areas and, therefore, affect drug distribution. Accumulation of carbon dioxide may lower the pH of certain tissues and may affect the level of drugs reaching those tissues.

Figure 10-6 illustrates the distribution of a drug to three different tissues when the partition of the drug for each tissue varies. For example, the adrenal glands have five times the concentration of the plasma ($R = 5$), while for drug partition for the kidney, $R = 3$, and for basal muscle, $R = 1$. In this illustration, the adrenal gland and kidney take 5 and 3 times as long to be equilibrated with drug. Thus, it can be seen that, even for vascular tissues, high drug partition can take much more time for the tissue to become fully equilibrated. In the example in Figure 10-6, drug administration is continuous (as in IV infusion), since tissue drug levels remain constant after equilibrium.

Some tissues have great ability to store and accumulate drug, as shown by large R values. For example, the antiandrogen drug flutamide and its active metabolite are highly concentrated in the prostate. The prostate drug concentration is 20 times

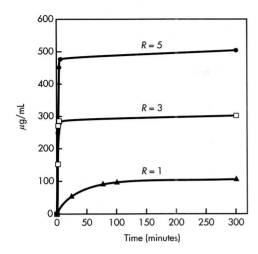

Figure 10-6. Drug distribution in three groups of tissues with various ability to store drug (R) (**top** = adrenal; **middle** = kidney; **bottom** = muscle).

that of the plasma drug concentration; thus, the antiandrogen effect of the drug is not fully achieved until distribution to this receptor site is complete. Digoxin is highly bound to myocardial membranes. Digoxin has a high tissue/plasma concentration ratio ($R = 60-130$) in the myocardium. This high R ratio for digoxin leads to a long distributional phase (see Chapter 4) despite abundant blood flow to the heart. It is important to note that if a tissue has a long distribution half-life, a long time is needed for the drug to leave the tissue when blood level decreases. Understanding drug distribution is important because the activities of many drugs are not well correlated with plasma drug level. Kinetically, both protein binding or favorable solubility in the tissue site lead to longer distribution times.

Chemical knowledge in molecular structure often helps to estimate the lipid solubility of a drug, and a drug with large oil/water partition coefficient tends to have high R values *in vivo*. A reduction in the partition coefficient of a drug often reduces the rate of drug uptake into the brain. This may decrease drug distribution to the central nervous system and decrease undesirable central nervous system side effects. Extensive tissue distribution is kinetically evidenced by an increase in the volume of distribution, while a secondary effect is a prolonged elimination half-life of the drug distributed over a larger volume (thus, more diluted) and, therefore, less efficiently removed by the kidney or the liver. For example, etretinate (a retinoate derivative) for acne treatment has an unusually long elimination half-life of about 100 days (Chien et al, 1992), due to its extensive distribution to body fats. Newly synthesized agents have been designed to reduce lipophilicity and distribution. These new agents have less accumulation and less potential for teratogenicity.

Drug Accumulation

The deposition or uptake of the drug into the tissue is generally controlled by the diffusional barrier of the capillary membrane and other cell membranes. For example, the brain is well perfused with blood, but many drugs with good aqueous solubility have high kidney, liver, and lung concentrations and yet little or negligible brain drug concentration. The brain capillaries are surrounded by a layer of tightly joined *glial* cells that act as a lipid barrier to impede the diffusion of polar or highly ionized drugs. A diffusion-limited model may be necessary to describe the pharmacokinetics of these drugs that are not adequately described by perfusion models.

Tissues receiving high blood flow equilibrate quickly with the drug in the plasma. However, at steady state, the drug may or may not accumulate (concentrate) within the tissue. The accumulation of drug into tissues is dependent on both the blood flow and the affinity of the drug for the tissue. Drug uptake into a tissue is generally reversible. The drug concentration in a tissue with low capacity equilibrates rapidly with the plasma drug concentration and then declines rapidly as the drug is eliminated from the body.

In contrast, drugs with high tissue affinity tend to accumulate or concentrate in the tissue. Drugs with a high lipid/water partition coefficient are very fat soluble and tend to accumulate in lipid or adipose (fat) tissue. In this case, the lipid-soluble drug partitions from the aqueous environment of the plasma into the fat. This process is reversible, but the extraction of drug out of the tissue is so slow that the drug may remain for days or even longer in adipose tissues, long after the drug is depleted from the blood. Because the adipose tissue is poorly perfused with blood, drug accumulation is slow. However, once the drug is concentrated in fat tissue, drug removal from fat may also be slow. For example, the chlorinated hydrocarbon DDT (dichlorodiphenyltrichloroethane) is highly lipid soluble and remains in fat tissue for years.

Drugs may accumulate in tissues by other processes. For example, drugs may accumulate by binding to proteins or other macromolecules in a tissue. Digoxin is highly bound to proteins in cardiac tissue, leading in a large volume of distribution (440 L/70 kg) and long elimination $t_{1/2}$ (approximately 40 hours). Some drugs may complex with melanin in the skin and eye, as observed after long-term administration of high doses of phenothiazine to chronic schizophrenic patients. The antibiotic tetracycline forms an insoluble chelate with calcium. In growing teeth and bones, tetracycline will complex with the calcium and remain in these tissues.

Some tissues have enzyme systems that actively transport natural biochemical substances into the tissues. For example, various adrenergic tissues have a specific uptake system for catecholamines, such as norepinephrine. Thus, amphetamine, which has a phenylethylamine structure similar to norepinephrine, is actively transported into adrenergic tissue. Other examples of drug accumulation are well documented. For some drugs, the actual mechanism for drug accumulation may not be clearly understood.

In a few cases, the drug is irreversibly bound into a particular tissue. Irreversible binding of drug may occur when the drug or a reactive intermediate metabolite becomes covalently bound to a macromolecule within the cell, such as to a tissue protein. Many purine and pyrimidine drugs used in cancer chemotherapy are incorporated into nucleic acids, causing destruction of the cell.

Permeability of Cell and Capillary Membranes

Cell membranes vary in their permeability characteristics, depending on the tissue. For example, capillary membranes in the liver and kidneys are more permeable to transmembrane drug movement than capillaries in the brain. The sinusoidal capillaries of the liver are very permeable and allow the passage of large-molecular-weight molecules. In the brain and spinal cord, the capillary endothelial cells are surrounded by a layer of glial cells, which have tight intercellular junctions. This added layer of cells around the capillary membranes acts effectively to slow the rate of drug diffusion into the brain by acting as a thicker lipid barrier. This lipid barrier, which slows the diffusion and penetration of water-soluble and polar drugs into the brain and spinal cord, is called the *blood–brain barrier.*

Under certain pathophysiologic conditions, the permeability of cell membranes, including capillary cell membranes, may be altered. For example, burns will alter the permeability of skin and allow drugs and larger molecules to permeate inward or outward. In meningitis, which involves inflammation of the membranes of the spinal cord or brain, drug uptake into the brain will be enhanced.

The diameters of the capillaries are very small and the capillary membranes are very thin. The high blood flow within a capillary allows for intimate contact of the drug molecules with the cell membrane, providing for rapid drug diffusion. For capillaries that perfuse the brain and spinal cord, the layer of *glial* cells functions effectively to increase the thickness term h in Equation 10.1, thereby slowing the diffusion and penetration of water-soluble and polar drugs into the brain and spinal cord.

APPARENT VOLUME DISTRIBUTION

The concentration of drug in the plasma or tissues depends on the amount of drug systemically absorbed and the volume in which the drug is distributed. The *apparent volume of distribution,* V_D in a model, is used to estimate the extent of drug distribution in the body (see Chapters 3 and 4). Although the apparent volume of distribution does not represent a true anatomical, or physical volume, the V_D represents the result of dynamic drug distribution between the plasma and the tissues and accounts for the mass balance of the drug in the body. To illustrate the use of V_D, consider a drug dissolved in a simple solution. A volume term is needed to relate drug concentration in the system (or human body) to the amount of drug present in that system. The volume of the system may be estimated if the amount of drug added to the system and the drug concentration after equilibrium in the system are known.

$$\text{Volume (L)} = \frac{\text{amount (mg) of drug added to system}}{\text{drug concentration (mg/L) in system after equilibrium}} \quad \textbf{(10.3)}$$

Equation 10.3 describes the relationship of concentration, volume, and mass, as shown in Equation 10.4.

$$\text{Concentration (mg/L)} \times \text{volume (L)} = \text{mass (mg)} \quad \textbf{(10.4)}$$

Considerations in the Calculation of Volume of Distribution: A Simulated Example

The objective of this exercise is to calculate the fluid volume in each beaker and to compare the calculated volume to the real volume of water in the beaker. Assume that three beakers are each filled with 100 mL of aqueous fluid. Beaker 1 contains water only; beakers 2 and 3 each contain aqueous fluid and a small compartment filled with cultured cells. The cells in beaker 2 can bind the drug, while the cells in beaker 3 can metabolize the drug. The three beakers represent the following, respectively:

Beaker 1. Drug distribution in a fluid (water) compartment only, without drug binding and metabolism

Beaker 2. Drug distribution in a fluid compartment containing cell clusters that reversibly bind drugs

Beaker 3. Drug distribution in a fluid compartment containing cell clusters (similar to tissues *in vivo*) in which the drug may be metabolized and the metabolites bound to cells

Suppose 100 mg of drug is then added to each beaker (Fig. 10-7). After the fluid concentration of drug in each beaker is at equilibration, and the concentration of drug in the water (fluid) compartment has been sampled and assayed, the volume of water may be computed.

Case 1

The volume of water in beaker 1 is calculated from the amount of drug added (100 mg) and the equilibrated drug concentration using Equation 10.3. After equilibration, the drug concentration was measured to be 1 mg/mL.

Volume = 100 mg/1 mg/mL = 100 mL

The calculated volume in beaker 1 confirms that the system is a simple, homogeneous system and, in this case, represents the "true" fluid volume of the beaker.

Case 2

Beaker 2 contains cell clusters stuck to the bottom of the beaker. Binding of drug to the proteins of the cells occurs on the surface and within the cytoplasmic interior. This case represents a heterogeneous system consisting of a *well-stirred* fluid compartment and a tissue (cell). To determine the volume of this system, more information is needed than in Case 1:

1. The amount of drug dissolved in the fluid compartment must be determined. Because some of the drug will be bound within the cell compartment, the amount of drug in the fluid compartment will be less than the 100 mg placed in the beaker.
2. The amount of drug taken up by the cell cluster must be known to account for the entire amount of drug in the beaker. Therefore, both the cell and the fluid

Beaker 1   Beaker 2   Beaker 3

Fluid (water) compartment

Cell compartment

Figure 10-7. Experiment simulating drug distribution in the body. Three beakers each contain 100 mL of water (fluid compartment) and 100 mg of a water-soluble drug. Beakers 2 and 3 also contain 5 mL of cultured cell clusters.

compartments must be sampled and assayed to determine the drug concentration in each compartment.

3. The volume of the cell cluster must be determined.

Assume that the above measurements were made and that the following information was obtained:

- Drug concentration in fluid compartment = 0.5 mg/mL
- Drug concentration in cell cluster = 10 mg/mL
- Volume of cell cluster = 5 mL
- Amount of drug added = 100 mg
- Amount of drug taken up by the cell cluster = 10 mg/mL × 5 mL = 50 mg
- Amount of drug dissolved in fluid (water) compartment = 100 mg (total) − 50 mg (in cells) = 50 mg (in water)

Using the above information, the true volume of the fluid (water) compartment is calculated using Equation 10.3.

$$\text{Volume of fluid compartment} = \frac{50 \text{ mg}}{0.5 \text{ mg/mL}} = 100 \text{ mL}$$

The value of 100 mL agrees with the volume of fluid we put into the beaker.

If the tissue cells were not accessible for sampling as in the case of *in-vivo* drug administration, the volume of the fluid (water) compartment is calculated using Equation 10.3 assuming the system is homogenous and that 100 mg drug was added to the system

$$\text{Apparent volume} = \frac{100 \text{ mg}}{0.5 \text{ mg/mL}} = 200 \text{ mL}$$

The value of 200 mL is a substantial overestimation of the true volume (100 mL) of the system.

When a heterogeneous system is involved, the real or true volume of the system may not be accurately calculated by monitoring only one compartment. Therefore, an apparent volume of distribution is calculated and the infrastructure of the system is ignored. The term *apparent volume of distribution* refers to the lack of true volume characteristics. The apparent volume of distribution is used in pharmacokinetics because the tissue (cellular) compartments are not easily sampled and the true volume is not known. When the experiment in beaker 2 is performed with an equal volume of cultured cells that have different binding affinity for the drug, then the apparent volume of distribution is very much affected by the extent of cellular drug binding (Table 10.3).

As shown in Table 10.3, as the amount of drug in the cell compartment increases (column 3), the apparent V_D of the fluid compartment increases (column 6). Extensive cellular drug binding effectively pulls drug molecules out of the fluid compartment, decreases the drug concentration in the fluid compartment, and increases V_D. In biological systems, the quantity of cells, cell compartment volume, and extent of drug binding within the cells affect V_D. A large cell volume and/or extensive drug binding in the cells reduces the drug concentration in the fluid compartment and increases the apparent volume of distribution.

TABLE 10.3   Relationship of Volume of Distribution and Amount of Drug in Tissue (Cellular) Compartment[a]

TOTAL DRUG (mg)	VOLUME OF CELLS (mL)	DRUG IN CELLS (mg)	DRUG IN WATER (mg)	DRUG CONCENTRATION IN WATER (mg/mL)	V_D IN WATER (mL)
100	15	75	25	0.25	400
100	10	50	50	0.50	200
100	5	25	75	0.75	133
100	1	5	95	0.95	105

[a]For each condition, the true water (fluid) compartment is 100 mL. Apparent volume of distribution (V_D) is calculated according to Equation 10.3.

In this example, the fluid compartment is comparable to the *central compartment* and the cell compartment is analogous to the peripheral or *tissue compartment*. If the drug is distributed widely into the tissues or concentrates unevenly into the tissues, the V_D for a drug may exceed the physical volume of the body (about 70 L of total volume or 42 L of body water for a 70-kg subject). Besides cellular protein binding, partitioning of drug into lipid cellular components may greatly inflate V_D. Many drugs have oil/water partition coefficients above 10,000. These lipophilic drugs are mostly concentrated in the lipid phase of adipose tissue, resulting in a very low drug concentration in the extracellular water. Generally, drugs with very large V_D values have very low drug concentrations in plasma.

A large V_D is often interpreted as broad drug distribution for a drug, even though many other factors also lead to the calculation of a large apparent volume of distribution. A true V_D that exceeds the volume of the body is physically impossible. Only if the drug concentrations in both the tissue and plasma compartments are sampled, and the volumes of each compartment are clearly defined, can a true physical volume be calculated.

Case 3

The drug in the cell compartment in beaker 3 decreases due to undetected metabolism because the metabolite formed is bound to the inside the cells. Thus, the apparent volume of distribution is also greater than 100 mL. Any unknown source that decreases the drug concentration in the fluid compartment will increase the V_D, resulting in an overestimated apparent volume of distribution. This is illustrated with the experiment in beaker 3. In beaker 3, the cell cluster metabolizes the drug and binds the metabolite to the cells. Therefore, the drug is effectively removed from the fluid concentration. The data for this experiment (note that metabolite is expressed as equivalent intact drug) are as follows:

- Total drug placed in beaker = 100 mg
- Cell compartment:

  Drug concentration = 0.2 mg/mL
  Metabolite-bound concentration = 9.71 mg/mL
  Metabolite-free concentration = 0.29 mg/mL
  Cell volume = 5 mL

- Fluid (water) compartment:

    Drug concentration = 0.2 mg/mL
    Metabolite concentration = 0.29 mg/mL

To calculate the total amount of drug and metabolite in the cell compartment, Equation 10.3 is rearranged as shown:

   Total drug and metabolite in cells = 5 mL × (0.2 + 9.96 + 0.29 mg/mL) = 52.45 mg

Therefore, the total drug and metabolites in the fluid compartment is $100 - 52.45$ mg = 47.55 mg.

If only the intact drug is considered, V_D is calculated using Equation 10.3.

$$V_D = \frac{100 \text{ mg}}{0.2 \text{ mg/mL}} = 500 \text{ mL}$$

Considering that only 100 mL of water was placed into beaker 3, the calculated apparent volume of distribution of 500 mL is an overestimate of the true fluid volume of the system.

The following conclusions can be drawn from this beaker exercise:

1. Drug must be at equilibrium in the system before any drug concentration is measured. In nonequilibrium conditions, the sample removed from the system for drug assay does not represent all parts of the system.
2. Drug binding distorts the true physical volume of distribution when all components in the system are not properly sampled and assayed. Extravascular drug binding increases the apparent V_D.
3. Both intravascular and extravascular drug binding must be determined to calculate meaningful volumes of distribution.
4. The apparent V_D is essentially a measure of the relative extent of drug distribution outside the plasma compartment. Greater tissue drug binding and drug accumulation increases V_D, whereas greater plasma protein drug binding decreases the V_D distribution.
5. Undetected cellular drug metabolism increases V_D.
6. An apparent V_D larger than the combined volume of plasma and body water is indicative of (4) and (5), or both, above.
7. Although the V_D is not a true physiologic volume, the V_D is useful to relate the plasma drug concentration to the amount of drug in the body (Eq. 10.3). This relationship of the product of the drug concentration and volume to equal the total mass of drug is important in pharmacokinetics.

 PRACTICE PROBLEM

The amount of drug in the system calculated from V_D and the drug concentration in the fluid compartment is shown in Table 10.3. Calculate the amount of drug in the system using the true volume and the drug concentration in the fluid compartment.

Solution

In each case, the product of the drug concentration (column 5) times the apparent volume of distribution (column 6) yields 100 mg of drug, accurately accounting for the total amount of drug present in the system. For example, 0.25 mg/mL × 400 mL = 100 mg. Notice that the total amount of drug present cannot be determined using the true volume and the drug concentration (column 5).

The physiologic approach requires detailed information, including (1) cell drug concentration, (2) cell compartment volume, and (3) fluid compartment volume. Using the physiologic approach, the total amount of drug is equal to the amount of drug in the cell compartment and the amount of drug in the fluid compartment.

$$(15 \text{ mg/mL} \times 5 \text{ mL}) + (100 \text{ mL} \times 0.25 \text{ mg/mL}) = 100 \text{ mg}$$

The two approaches shown above each account correctly for the amount of drug present in the system. However, the second approach requires more information than is commonly available. The second approach does, however, make more physiologic sense. Most physiologic compartment spaces are not clearly defined for measuring drug concentrations.

Complex Biological Systems and V_D

The above example illustrates how the V_D represents the *apparent* volume into which a drug appears to distribute, whether into a beaker of fluid or the human body. The human body is a much more complex system than even a beaker of water containing drug metabolizing cells. Many components within cells, tissues, or organs can bind to or metabolize drug, thereby influencing the apparent V_D. Only free, unbound drug diffuses between the plasma and tissue fluids. The tissue fluid, in turn, equilibrates with the intracellular water inside the tissue cells. The tissue drug concentration is influenced by the partition coefficient (lipid/water affinity) of the drug and tissue protein drug binding. The distribution of drug in a biological system is illustrated by Figure 10-8.

Apparent Volume of Distribution

The apparent volume of distribution, in general relates the plasma drug concentration to the amount of drug present in the body. In classical compartment models, V_{DSS} is the volume of distribution determined at steady state when the drug concentration in the tissue compartment is at equilibrium with the drug concentration in the plasma compartment (Fig. 10-9, top). In a physiological system involving a drug distributed to a given tissue from the plasma fluid (Fig. 10-9, bottom), the two-compartment model is not assumed, and drug distribution from the plasma to a tissue is equilibrated by perfusion with arterial blood and returned by venous blood. The model parameter V_{app} is used to represent the apparent distribution volume in this model, which is different from V_{DSS} used in the compartment model. Similar to the apparent volume simulated in the beaker experiment

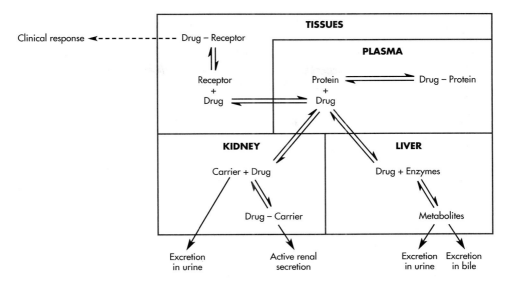

Figure 10-8.   Effect of reversible drug–protein binding on drug distribution and elimination. Drugs may bind reversibly with proteins. Free (nonbound) drugs penetrate cell membranes, distributing into various tissues including those tissues involved in drug elimination, such as kidney and liver. Active renal secretion, which is a carrier-mediated system, may have a greater affinity for free drug molecules compared to plasma proteins. In this case, active renal drug excretion allows for rapid drug excretion despite drug protein binding. If a drug is displaced from the plasma proteins, more free drug is available for distribution into tissues and interaction with the receptors responsible for the pharmacologic response. Moreover, more free drug is available for drug elimination.

in Equation 10.3, V_{app} is defined by Equation 10.5, and the amount of drug in the body is given by Equation 10.6.

$$V_{\text{app}} = \frac{D_{\text{B}}}{C_{\text{p}}} \tag{10.5}$$

$$D_{\text{B}} = V_{\text{p}}C_{\text{p}} + V_{\text{t}}C_{\text{t}} \tag{10.6}$$

where D_{B} is the amount of drug in the body, V_{p} is the plasma fluid volume, V_{t} is the tissue volume, C_{p} is the plasma drug concentration, and C_{t} is the tissue drug concentration.

For many protein-bound drugs, the ratio of $D_{\text{B}}/C_{\text{p}}$ is not constant over time, and this ratio depends on the nature of dissociation of the protein–drug complex and how the free drug is distributed; the ratio is best determined at steady state. Protein binding to tissue has an apparent effect of increasing the apparent volume of distribution. Several V_{D} terms were introduced in the classical compartment models (Chapter 4). However, protein binding was not introduced in those models.

Equation 10.6 describes the amount of drug in the body at any time point between a tissue and the plasma fluid. Instead of assuming the drug distributes to a hypothetical compartment, it was assumed that, after injection, the drug diffuses from the plasma to the extracellular fluid/water, where it further equilibrates with the given tissue. One or more tissue types may be added to the model if needed.

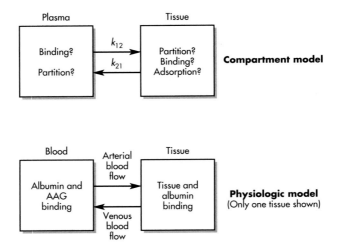

Figure 10-9.   A diagram showing **(top)** a two-compartment model approach to drug distribution; **(bottom)** a physiologic approach to drug distribution.

If the drug penetrates inside the cell, distribution into the intracellular water may occur. If the volume of body fluid and the protein level are known, this information may be incorporated into the model. Such a model may be more compatible with the physiology and anatomy of the human body.

When using pharmacokinetic parameters from the literature, it is important to note that most calculations of steady-state V_D involve some assumptions on how and where the drug distributes in the body; it could involve a physiologic or a compartmental approach.

For a drug that involves protein binding, some models assume that the drug distributes from the plasma water into extracellular tissue fluids, where the drug binds to extravascular proteins, resulting in a larger V_D due to extravascular protein binding. Unfortunately, drug binding and distribution to lipoid tissues are generally not distinquishable. If the pharmacokineticist suspects distribution to body lipids because the drug involved is very lipophilic, he or she may want to compare results simulated with different models before making a final conclusion.

Figure 10-10 lists the steady-state volume of distribution of 10 common drugs in ascending order. Most of these drugs follow multicompartment kinetics with various tissue distribution phases. The physiologic volumes of an ideal 70-kg subject are also plotted for comparison: (1) the plasma (3 L), (2) the extracellular fluid (15 L), and (3) the intracellular fluid (27 L). Drugs such as penicillin, cephalosporin, valproic acid, and furosemide are polar compounds that stay mostly within the plasma and extracellular fluids and therefore have a relatively low V_D.

In contrast, drugs with lower distribution to the extracellular water are more extensively distributed inside the tissues and tend to have a large V_D. An excessively high volume of distribution (greater than the body volume of 70 L) is due mostly to special tissue storage, tissue protein binding, carrier, or efflux system which removes drug from the plasma fluid. Digoxin, for example, is bound to myocardial membrane that has drug levels that are 60 and 130 times the serum drug level in

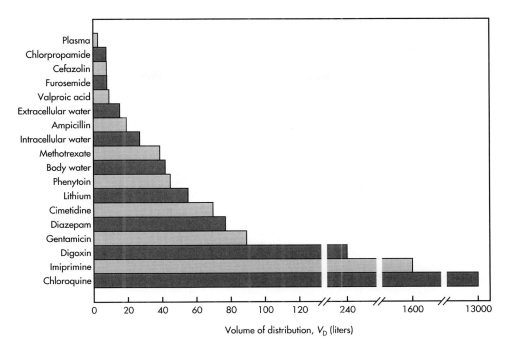

Figure 10-10. Lists of steady-state volumes of distribution of 10 common drugs in ascending order showing various factors affect V_D. Drugs with high V_D generally has high tissue affinity or low binding to serum albumin. Polar or hydrophilic drugs tend to have V_D similar to the volume of extracellular water.

adults and children, respectively (Park et al, 1982). The high tissue binding is responsible for the large steady-state volume of distribution (Chapter 4). The greater drug affinity also results in longer distribution α half-life in spite of the heart's great vascular blood perfusion. Imipramine is a drug that is highly protein bound and concentrated in the plasma, yet its favorable tissue partition and binding accounts for a large volume of distribution. Several tricyclic antidepressants (TCAs) also have large volumes of distribution due to tissue (CNS) penetration and binding.

PROTEIN BINDING OF DRUGS

Many drugs interact with plasma or tissue proteins or with other macromolecules, such as melanin and DNA, to form a *drug–macromolecule complex*. The formation of a drug protein complex is often named *drug–protein binding*. Drug–protein binding may be a reversible or an irreversible process. *Irreversible* drug–protein binding is usually a result of chemical activation of the drug, which then attaches strongly to the protein or macromolecule by covalent chemical bonding. Irreversible drug binding accounts for certain types of drug toxicity that may occur over a long time period, as in the case of chemical carcinogenesis, or within a relatively short time period, as in the case of drugs that form reactive chemical intermediates. For example, the hepatotoxicity of high doses of acetaminophen is due to the formation of reactive metabolite intermediates that interact with liver proteins.

Figure 10-11. Diagram showing that bound drugs will not diffuse across membrane but free drug will diffuse freely between the plasma and extracellular water.

Most drugs bind or complex with proteins by a reversible process. *Reversible drug–protein binding* implies that the drug binds the protein with weaker chemical bonds, such as hydrogen bonds or van der Waals forces. The amino acids that compose the protein chain have hydroxyl, carboxyl, or other sites available for reversible drug interactions.

Reversible drug–protein binding is of major interest in pharmacokinetics. The protein-bound drug is a large complex that cannot easily transverse cell or possibly even capillary membranes and therefore has a restricted distribution (Fig. 10-11). Moreover, the protein-bound drug is usually pharmacologically inactive. In contrast, the free or unbound drug crosses cell membranes and is therapeutically active. Studies that critically evaluate drug–protein binding are usually performed *in vitro* using a purified protein such as albumin. Methods for studying protein binding, including equilibrium dialysis and ultrafiltration, make use of a semipermeable membrane that separates the protein and protein-bound drug from the free or unbound drug (Table 10.4). By these *in-vitro* methods, the concentrations of bound drug, free drug, and total protein may be determined. Each method for the investigation of drug–protein binding *in vitro* has advantages and disadvantages in terms of cost, ease of measurement, time, instrumentation, and other considerations. Various experimental factors for the measurement of protein binding are listed in Table 10.5.

Drugs may bind to various macromolecular components in the blood, including albumin, α_1-acid glycoprotein, lipoproteins, immunoglobulins (IgG), and erythrocytes (RBC).

Albumin is a protein with a molecular weight of 65,000–69,000 Da that is synthesized in the liver and is the major component of plasma proteins responsible for reversible drug binding (Table 10.6). In the body, albumin is distributed in the plasma and in the extracellular fluids of skin, muscle, and various other tissues. Interstitial fluid albumin concentration is about 60% of that in the plasma. The elimination half-life of albumin is 17–18 days. Normally, albumin concentration is

TABLE 10.4   *Methods for Studying Drug–Protein Binding*

Equilibrium dialysis	Gel chromatography
Dynamic dialysis	Spectrophotometry
Diafiltration	Electrophoresis
Ultrafiltration	Optical rotatory dispersion and circulatory dichroism

TABLE 10.5 *Considerations in the Study of Drug–Protein Binding*

Equilibrium between bound and free drug must be maintained.

The method must be valid over a wide range of drug and protein concentrations.

Extraneous drug binding or drug adsorption onto the apparatus walls, membranes, or other components must be avoided or considered in the method.

Denaturation of the protein or contamination of the protein must be prevented.

The method must consider pH and ionic concentrations of the media and Donnan effects due to the protein.

The method should be capable of detecting both reversible and irreversible drug binding, including fast- and slow-phase associations and dissociations of drug and protein.

The method should not introduce interfering substances, such as organic solvents.

The results of the *in vitro* method should allow extrapolation to the *in vivo* situation.

Adapted with permission from Bridges and Wilson (1976).

maintained at a relatively constant level of 3.5–5.5% (weight per volume) or 4.5 mg/dL. Albumin is responsible for maintaining the osmotic pressure of the blood and for the transport of endogenous and exogenous substances. As a transport protein for endogenous substances, albumin complexes with free fatty acids (FFAs), bilirubin, various hormones (such as cortisone, aldosterone, and thyroxine), tryptophan, and other compounds. Many weak acidic (anionic) drugs bind to albumin by electrostatic and hydrophobic bonds. Weak acidic drugs such as salicylates, phenylbutazone, and penicillins are highly bound to albumin. However, the strength of the drug binding is different for each drug.

α_1-*Acid glycoprotein* (orosomucoid) is a globulin with a molecular weight of about 44,000 Da. The plasma concentration of α_1-acid glycoprotein is low (0.4–1%) and binds primarily basic (cationic) drugs such as propranolol, imipramine, and lidocaine. Globulins (α-, β-, γ-globulins) may be responsible for the plasma transport of certain endogenous substances such as corticosteroids. These globulins have a low capacity but high affinity for the binding of these endogenous substances.

Lipoproteins are macromolecular complexes of lipids and proteins and are classified according to their density and separation in the ultracentrifuge. The terms VLDL, LDL, and HDL are abbreviations for very-low-density, low-density, and high-density lipoproteins, respectively. Lipoproteins are responsible for the transport of plasma lipids to the liver and may be responsible for the binding of drugs if the albumin sites become saturated.

Erythrocytes, or red blood cells (RBCs), may bind both endogenous and exogenous compounds. RBCs consist of about 45% of the volume of the blood. Phenytoin, pentobarbital, and amobarbital are known to have a RBC/plasma water ratio of 4 to 2, indicating preferential binding of drug to the erythrocytes over plasma water.

TABLE 10.6 *Major Proteins to Which Drugs Bind in Plasma*

PROTEIN	MOLECULAR WEIGHT (Da)	NORMAL RANGE OF CONCENTRATIONS	
		(g/L)	(mol/L)
Albumin	65,000	35–50	$5–7.5 \times 10^{-4}$
α_1-Acid glycoprotein	44,000	0.4–1.0	$0.9–2.2 \times 10^{-5}$
Lipoproteins	200,000–3,400,000	Variable	

From Tozer (1984), with permission.

Penetration into RBC is dependent on the free concentration of the drug. In the case of phenytoin, RBC drug level increases linearly with an increase in the plasma-free drug concentration (Borondy et al, 1973). Increased drug binding to plasma albumin reduces RBC drug concentration. With most drugs, however, binding of drug to RBC generally does not significantly affect the volume of distribution, because the drug is often bound to albumin in the plasma water. Even though phenytoin has a great affinity for RBC, only about 25% of the blood drug concentration is present in the blood cells, and 75% is present in the plasma because the drug is also strongly bound to albumin. For drugs with strong erythrocyte binding, the hematocrit will influence the total amount of drug in the blood. For these drugs, the total whole-blood drug concentration should be measured.

Effect of Protein Binding on the Apparent Volume of Distribution

The extent of drug protein binding in the plasma or tissue affects V_D. Drugs that are highly bound to plasma proteins have a low fraction of free drug (f_u = unbound or free drug fraction) in the plasma water. The plasma protein-bound drug does not diffuse easily and is therefore less extensively distributed to tissues (Fig. 10-11). Drugs with low plasma protein binding have larger f_u, generally diffuse more easily into tissues, and have a greater volume of distributions. Since the apparent volume of distribution is influenced by lipid solubility in addition to protein binding, there are some exceptions to this rule. However, when several drugs are selected from a single family with close physical and lipid partition characteristics, the apparent volume of distribution may be explained by the relative degree of drug binding to tissue and plasma proteins.

The V_D of four cephalosporin antibiotics (Fig. 10-12) in humans and mice (Sawada et al, 1984) demonstrates that the differences in volume of distribution of cefazolin, cefotetan, moxalactam, and cefoperazone are due mostly to differences in

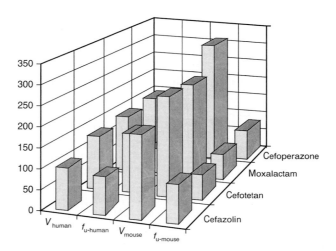

Figure 10-12. Plot of V_D of four cephalosporin antibiotics in humans and mice showing the relationship between the fraction of unbound drug (f_u) and the volume of distribution. (From Sawada et al, 1984.)

the degree of protein binding. For example, the fraction of unbound drug, f_u, in the plasma is the highest for cefoperazone in humans and mice, and the volume of distribution is also the highest among the four drugs in both humans and mice. Conversely, cefazolin has the lowest f_u in humans and is correlated with the lowest volume of distribution. Interestingly, the volume of distribution per kilogram in humans (V_{human}) is generally higher than that in mouse (V_{mouse}) because the fraction of unbound drug is also greater, resulting in a greater volume of distribution. Differences in V_D and $t_{1/2}$ among various species may be due to differences in drug–protein binding. An equation (see Eq. 10.12) relating quantitatively the effect of protein binding on apparent volume of distribution is derived in the next section.

Drugs such as furosemide, sulfisoxazole, tolbutamide, and warfarin are bound greater than 90% to plasma proteins and have a V_D value ranging from 7.7 to 11.2 L per 70-kg body weight (see Appendix E). Basic drugs such as imipramine, nortriptyline, and propranolol are extensively bound to both tissue and plasma proteins and have very large V_D values. Displacement of drugs from plasma proteins can affect the pharmacokinetics of a drug in several ways: (1) directly increase the free (unbound) drug concentration as a result of reduced binding in the blood; (2) increase the free drug concentration that reaches the receptor sites directly, causing a more intense pharmacodynamic (or toxic) response; (3) increase the free drug concentration, causing a transient increase in V_D and decreasing partly some of the increase in free plasma drug concentration; (4) increase the free drug concentration, resulting in more drug diffusion into tissues of eliminating organs, particularly the liver and kidney, resulting in a transient increase in drug elimination. The ultimate drug concentration reaching the target depends on one or more of these four factors dominating in the clinical situation. The effect of drug protein binding must be evaluated carefully before dosing changes are made (see below).

Effect of Changing Plasma Protein: An Example

The effect of increasing the plasma α_1-acid glycoprotein (AAG) level on drug penetration into tissues may be verified with cloned transgenic animals that have 8.6 times the normal α_1-acid glycoprotein levels. In an experiment investigating the activity of the tricyclic antidepressant drug imipramine, equal drug doses were administered to both normal and transgenic mouse. Since imipramine is highly bound to AAG, the steady-state imipramine serum level was greatly increased in the blood due to protein binding.

Imipramine serum level (transgenic mouse): 859 ng/mL
Imipramine serum level (normal mouse): 319.9 ng/mL
Imipramine brain level (transgenic mouse): 3862.6 ng/mL
Imipramine brain level (normal mouse): 7307.7 ng/mL

However, the imipramine concentration was greatly reduced in the brain tissue because of higher degree of binding to AAG in the serum, resulting in reduced drug penetration into the brain tissue. The volume of distribution of the drug was reported to be reduced. The antidepressant effect was observed to be lower in the transgenic mouse due to lower brain imipramine level. This experiment illustrates that high drug protein binding in the serum can reduce drug penetration to tissue receptors for some drugs (Holladay et al, 1996).

Another drug that is highly bound to AAG, saquinavir, is highly bound to AAG and has reduced free drug concentrations in transgenic mice that express elevated AAG (Holladay et al, 2001). In this study, the drug was bound to both albumin and AAG (2.1% to AAG versus 11.5% to albumin). Elevated AAG caused saquinavir's volume of distribution to be reduced in this study.

For a drug that distributes into the plasma and a given tissue in the body, the amount of drug bound may be found by Equation 10.7. Because drug may bind to both plasma and tissue proteins, the bound and unbound drug concentrations must be considered. At steady state, unbound drug in plasma and tissue are in equilibration.

$$D_B = V_p C_p + V_t C_t \tag{10.7}$$

$$C_u = C_{ut}$$

Alternatively,

$$C_p f_u = C_t f_{ut} \tag{10.8}$$

or

$$C_t = C_p \frac{f_u}{f_{ut}} \tag{10.9}$$

where all terms refer to steady-state condition: f_u is the unbound (free) drug fraction in the plasma, f_{ut} is the unbound drug fraction in the tissue, C_u is the unbound drug concentration in the plasma, and C_{ut} is the unbound drug concentration in the tissues. Substituting for C_t in Equation 10.7 using Equation 10.9 results in

$$D_B = V_p C_p + V_t \left[C_p \left(\frac{f_u}{f_{ut}} \right) \right] \tag{10.10}$$

Rearranging,

$$\frac{D_B}{C_p} = V_p + V_t \left(\frac{f_u}{f_{ut}} \right) \tag{10.11}$$

Because $D_B/C_p = V_{app}$, by substitution into Equation 10.11, V_{app} may be estimated by Equation 10.12:

$$V_{app} = V_p + V_t \left(\frac{f_u}{f_{ut}} \right) \tag{10.12}$$

Equation 10.12 relates the amount of drug in the body to plasma volume, tissue volume, and fraction of free plasma and tissue drug in the body. Equation 10.12 may be expanded to include several tissue organs with V_{ti} each with unbound tissue fraction f_{uti}.

$$V_{app} = V_p + \sum V_{ti} \left(\frac{f_u}{f_{uti}} \right)$$

where V_{ti} = tissue volume of the ith organ and f_{uti} = unbound fraction of the ith organ.

The following are important considerations in the calculation of V_{app}.

1. The volume of distribution is a constant only when the drug concentrations are in equilibrium between the plasma and tissue.
2. Values of f_u and f_{ut} are concentration dependent and must also be determined at equilibrium conditions.
3. Equation 10.12 shows that V_{app} is an indirect measure of drug binding in the tissues rather than a measurement of a true anatomic volume.
4. When f_u and f_{ut} are unity, Equation 10.12 is simplified to

$$\frac{D_B}{C_p} = V_p + V_t$$

When no drug binding occurs in tissue and plasma, the volume of distribution will not exceed the real anatomic volume. Only at steady state are the unbound plasma drug concentration, C_u, and the tissue drug concentration, C_{ut}, equal. At any other time, C_u may not equal to C_{ut}. The amount of drug in the body, D_B, cannot be calculated easily from V_{app} and C_p under nonequilibrium conditions. For simplicity, some models assume that the drug distributed to a tissue is approximated by the drug present in the fluid of that tissue. The tissue fluid volume is then represented by the volume of the extracellular/intracellular fluid, depending on drug penetration. Such a model fails to consider drug partition into fatty tissues/lipids, and simulates extravascular drug distribution based solely on protein binding.

In contrast, when the data are analyzed by the compartmental model, no specific binding interpretation is made. The analyst may interpret a large apparent volume due to either partition to fatty tissues or extravascular binding based on other observations. Compartment models are based on mass balance and focus on the amount of drug in each compartment and not on the tissue volume or tissue drug concentration. The tissue volume and drug concentrations are theoretical and do not necessarily reflect true physiologic values. Even the C_t may not be uniform in local tissues and under disease conditions.

PRACTICE PROBLEM

Drug A and drug B have V_{app} of 20 and 100 L, respectively. Both drugs have a V_p of 4 L and a V_t of 10 L, and they are 60% bound to plasma protein. What is the fraction of tissue binding of the two drugs? Assume that V_p is 4 L and V_t is 10 L.

Solution

Drug A
Applying Equation 10.12,

$$V_{app} = V_p + V_t\left(\frac{f_u}{f_{ut}}\right)$$

Because drug A is 60% bound, the drug is 40% free, or $f_u = 0.4$.

$$20 = 4 + 10\left(\frac{0.4}{f_{ut}}\right)$$

$$f_{ut} = \frac{4}{16} = 0.25$$

The fraction of drug bound to tissues is $1 - 0.25 = 0.75$ or 75%.

Drug B

$$100 = 4 + 10\left(\frac{0.4}{f_{ut}}\right)$$

$$f_{ut} = 0.042$$

The fraction of drug bound to tissues is $1 - 0.042 = 0.958 = 95.8\%$.

In this problem, the percent free (unbound) drug for drug A is 25% and the percent free drug for drug B is 4.2% in plasma fluid. Drug B is more highly bound to tissue, which results in a larger apparent volume of distribution. This approach assumes a pooled tissue group because it is not possible to identify physically the tissue group to which the drug is bound.

Equation 10.12 may explain the wide variation in the apparent volumes of distribution for drugs observed in the literature (Tables 10.7–10.9). Drugs in Table 10.7 have small apparent volumes of distribution due to plasma drug binding (less than 10 L when extrapolated to a 70-kg subject). Drugs in Table 10.8 show that, in general, as the fraction of unbound drug, f_u, in the plasma increases, the apparent volume increases. Reduced drug binding in the plasma results in increased free drug concentration, which diffuses into the extracellular water. Drugs showing exceptionally large volumes of distribution may have unusual tissue binding. Some drugs move into the interstitial fluid but are unable to diffuse across the cell membrane into the intracellular fluids, thereby reducing the volume of distribution.

TABLE 10.7   Relationship between Affinity for Serum Albumin and Volume of Distribution for Some Acidic Drugs

DRUG	PLASMA FRACTION BOUND (%)	AFFINITY CONSTANT (M^{-1})	V_D(L/kg)
Clofibric acid	97	300,000	0.09
Fluorophenindione	95	3,000,000	0.09
Phenylbutazone	99	230,000	0.09
Warfarin	97	230,000	0.13

From Houin (1985), with permission.

TABLE 10.8 Examples of Drugs for Which Diffusion Is Limited by Binding to Protein

DRUG	PLASMA FRACTION UNBOUND (%)	V_D (L/kg)
Carbenoxolone	1	0.10
Ibuprofen	1	0.14
Phenylbutazone	1	0.10
Naproxen	2	0.09
Fusidic acid	3	0.15
Clofibrate	3	0.09
Warfarin	3	0.10
Bumetanide	4	0.18
Dicloxacillin	4	0.29
Furosemide	4	0.20
Tolbutamide	4	0.14
Nalidixic acid	5	0.35
Cloxacillin	5	0.34
Sulfaphenazole	5	0.29
Chlorpropramide	8	0.20
Oxacillin	8	0.44
Nafcillin	10	0.63

From Houin (1985), with permission.

Drugs in Table 10.9 apparently do not obey the general binding rule, because their volumes of distribution are not related to plasma drug binding. These drugs have very large volumes of distribution and may have undiscovered tissue binding or tissue metabolism. Based on their pharmacologic activities, presumably all these drugs penetrate into the intracellular space.

RELATIONSHIP OF PLASMA DRUG–PROTEIN BINDING TO DISTRIBUTION AND ELIMINATION

In general, drugs that are highly bound to plasma protein have reduced overall drug clearance. For a drug that is metabolized mainly by the liver, binding to plasma proteins prevents the drug from entering the hepatocytes, resulting in reduced drug metabolism by the liver. In addition, molecularly bound drugs may not be available as substrates for liver enzymes, thereby further reducing the rate of metabolism.

Protein-bound drugs act as larger molecules that cannot diffuse easily through the capillary membranes in the glomeruli. The elimination half-lives of some drugs,

TABLE 10.9 Examples of Drugs for Which Tissue Distribution Is Apparently Independent of Plasma Protein Binding

DRUG	PLASMA FRACTION BOUND (%)	V_D (L/kg)
Desipramine	92	40
Imipramine	95	30
Nortriptyline	94	39
Vinblastine	70	35
Vincristine	70	11

From Houin (1985), with permission.

TABLE 10.10 Influence of Protein Binding on the Pharmacokinetics of Primarily Glomerular Filtrated Cephalosporins

	PROTEIN BOUND (%)	$t_{1/2}$ (hr)	RENAL CLEARANCE (mL/min/1.73 m^2)
Ceftriaxone	96	8.0	10
Cefoperazone	90	1.8	19
Cefotetan	85	3.3	28
Ceforanide	81	3.0	44
Cefazolin	70	1.7	56
Moxalactam	52	2.3	64
Cefsulodin	26	1.5	90
Ceftazidime	22	1.9	85
Cephaloridine	21	1.5	125

From Houin (1985), with permission.

such as the cephalosporins, which are excreted mainly by renal excretion, are generally increased when the percent of drug bound to plasma proteins increases (Table 10.10). The effect of serum protein binding on the renal clearance and elimination half-life on several tetracycline analogs is shown in Table 10.11. For example, doxycycline, which is 93% bound to serum proteins, has an elimination half-life of 15.1 hours, whereas oxytetracycline, which is 35.4% bound to serum proteins, has an elimination half-life of 9.2 hours. On the other hand, drug that is both extensively bound and actively secreted by the kidneys, such as penicillin, has a short elimination half-life, because active secretion takes preference in removing or stripping the drug from the proteins as the blood flows through the kidney.

Some cephalosporins are excreted by both renal and biliary secretion. The half-lives of drugs that are significantly excreted in the bile and do not correlate well with the extent of plasma protein binding.

Relationship between V_D and Drug Elimination Half-Life

Drug elimination is governed mainly by renal and other metabolic processes in the body. However, extensive drug distribution has the effect of diluting the drug in a large volume, making it harder for the kidney to filter the drug by glomerular filtration. Thus, the $t_{1/2}$ of the drug is prolonged if clearance (Cl) is constant and V_D is increased according to Equation 10.14. Cl is related to apparent volume of

TABLE 10.11 Comparison of Serum Protein Binding of Several Tetracycline Analogs with Their Half-Life in Serum Renal Clearance and Urinary Recovery after Intravenous Injection

TETRACYCLINE ANALOGS	SERUM BINDING (%)	HALF-LIFE (hr)	RENAL CLEARANCE (mL/min)	URINARY RECOVERY (%)
Oxytetracycline	35.4	9.2	98.6	70
Tetracycline	64.6	8.5	73.5	60
Demeclocycline	90.8	12.7	36.5	45
Doxycycline	93.0	15.1	16.0	45

distribution, V_D, and the elimination constant k, as shown in Equation 10.13 (see also Chapter 3).

$$Cl = kV_D \qquad \qquad \textbf{(10.13)}$$

$$t_{1/2} = 0.693\frac{V_D}{Cl} \qquad \qquad \textbf{(10.14)}$$

For a first-order process, Cl is the product of V_D and the elimination rate constant, k, according to Equation 10.13. The equation is derived for a given drug dose distributed in a single volume of body fluid without protein binding. The equation basically describes the empirical observation that a large clearance or large volume of distribution both leads to low plasma drug concentrations after a given dose. Mechanistically, a low plasma drug concentration may be due to (1) extensive distribution into tissues due to favorable lipophilicity, (2) extensive distribution into tissues due to protein binding in peripheral tissues, or (3) lack of drug plasma protein binding.

Two drug examples are selected to illustrate further the relationship between elimination half-life, clearance, and the volume of distribution. Although the kinetic relationship is straightforward, there is more than one way of explaining the observations.

 # CLINICAL EXAMPLES

Drug with a Large Volume of Distribution and a Long Elimination $t_{1/2}$

The macrolide antibiotic dirithromycin is extensively distributed in tissues, resulting in a large steady-state volume of distribution of about 800 L (range 504−1041 L). The elimination $t_{1/2}$ in humans is about 44 hours (range 16−65 hours). The drug has a relatively large total body clearance of 226−1040 mL/min (13.6−62.4 L/hr) and is given once daily. In this case, clearance is large due to a large V_D, whereas k is relatively small. In this case, Cl is large but the elimination half-life is longer because of the large V_D. Intuitively, the drug will take a long time to be removed when the drug is distributed extensively over a large volume; despite a relatively large clearance, $t_{1/2}$ accurately describes drug elimination alone.

Drug with a Small Volume of Distribution and a Long Elimination $t_{1/2}$

Tenoxicam is a nonsteroidal anti-inflammatory drug (Nilsen, 1994) that is about 99% bound in human plasma protein. The drug has low lipophilicity, is highly ionized (approximately 99%), and is distributed in blood. Because tenoxicam is very polar, the drug penetrates cell membranes slowly. The synovial fluid peak drug level is only one-third that of the plasma drug concentration and occurs 20 hours (range 10−34 hours) later than the peak plasma drug level. In addition, the drug is poorly distributed to body tissues and has an apparent volume of distribution, V_D, of 9.6 L (range 7.5−11.5 L). Tenoxicam has a low total plasma clearance of 0.106 L/hr

(0.079−0.142 L/hr) and an elimination half-life of 67 hours (range 49−81 hours), undoubtedly related to the extensive drug binding to plasma proteins.

According to Equation 10.13, drug clearance from the body is small if V_D is small and k is not too large. This relationship is consistent with a small Cl and a small V_D observed for tenoxicam. Equation 10.4, however, predicts that a small V_D would result in a small elimination $t_{1/2}$. In this case, the actual elimination half-life is long (67 hours) because the plasma tenoxicam clearance is so small that it dominates in Equation 10.4. The long elimination half-life of tenoxicam is better explained by restrictive drug clearance due to its binding to plasma protein, making it difficult for the drug to clear rapidly.

Clearance

Cl and V_D are regarded as independent model variables by some physiologic pharmacokineticists, based on Equation 10.14. Actually, Equation 10.13 and its equivalent, Equation 10.14, are rooted in classical pharmacokinetics. Initially, it may be difficult to understand why a drug such as dirithromycin, with a rapid clearance of 226−1040 mL/min, has a long half-life. In pharmacokinetics, the elimination constant $k = 0.0156 \text{ hr}^{-1}$ implies that 1/64 (ie, $0.0156 \text{ hr}^{-1} = 1/64$) of the drug is cleared per hour (a low efficiency elimination factor). From the elimination rate constant k, one can estimate that it takes 44 hours ($t_{1/2} = 44$ hours) to eliminate half the drug in the body, regardless of V_D. While $t_{1/2}$ is dependent on clearance and V_D as shown by Equation 10.4, clearance is clearly affected by the volume of distribution and by many variables of the drug in the biological system. In patients with ascites, clearance is increased but with no increase in half-life, reflecting the increase in volume of distribution in ascitic patients (Stoeckel et al, 1983).

Elimination of Protein-Bound Drug: Restrictive versus Nonrestrictive Elimination

When a drug is tightly bound to a protein, only the unbound drug is assumed to be metabolized; drugs belonging to this category are described as *restrictively eliminated*. On the other hand, some drugs may be eliminated even when they are protein bound; drugs in this category are described as *nonrestrictively eliminated*. When some drugs with different fractions of plasma protein binding are examined, the expected reduction in clearance is sometimes absent or very minor because some drugs are nonrestrictively cleared. The effect of protein binding on the kinetics of drug clearance in an organ system is discussed in detail in Chapter 11.

In practice, the molecular effect of protein binding on elimination is not always predictable. Drugs with restrictive elimination are recognized by very small plasma clearances and extensive plasma protein binding. The hepatic extraction ratios (ERs) for drugs that are restrictively eliminated are generally small, because of strong protein binding. Their hepatic extraction ratios are generally smaller than their unbound fractions in plasma (ie, $ER < f_u$). For example, phenylbutazone and the oxicams, including piroxicam, isoxicam, and tenoxicam, all have hepatic extraction ratios smaller than their unbound fraction in plasma (Verbeeck and

Wallace, 1994). The hepatic elimination for these drugs is therefore restrictive. A series of nonsteroid anti-inflammatory drugs (NSAIDs) were reported by the same authors to be nonrestrictive with the following characteristics: (1) drug elimination is exclusively hepatic, (2) bioavailability of the drug from an oral dosage form is complete, and (3) these drugs do not undergo extensive reversible biotransformation or enterohepatic circulation.

Propranolol is a drug that has low bioavailability with a hepatic extraction ratio, ER, of $0.7-0.9$. Propranolol is 89% bound, ie, 11% free (or $f_u = 0.11$) so that the ER $> f_u$. Thus, propranolol is considered to be *nonrestrictively* eliminated. The bioavailability of propranolol is very low because of the large first-pass effect, and its elimination half-life is relatively short. In contrast, diazepam is 98% bound ($f_u < 0.02$). Diazepam has a small ER of 0.1, because of extensive drug protein binding. Therefore, diazepam is considered *restrictively* eliminated. Diazepam has a long elimination half-life of 37 hours (Appendix E).

DETERMINANTS OF PROTEIN BINDING

Drug–protein binding is influenced by a number of important factors, including the following:

1. The drug
   - Physicochemical properties of the drug
   - Total concentration of the drug in the body

2. The protein
   - Quantity of protein available for drug–protein binding
   - Quality or physicochemical nature of the protein synthesized

3. The affinity between drug and protein
   - Includes the magnitude of the association constant

4. Drug interactions
   - Competition for the drug by other substances at a protein-binding site
   - Alteration of the protein by a substance that modifies the affinity of the drug for the protein; for example, aspirin acetylates lysine residues of albumin

5. The pathophysiologic condition of the patient
   - For example, drug–protein binding may be reduced in uremic patients and in patients with hepatic disease

Plasma drug concentrations are generally reported as the total drug concentration in the plasma, including both protein-bound drug and unbound (free) drug concentrations. Most literature values for the therapeutic effective drug concentrations refer to the total plasma or serum drug concentration. For therapeutic drug monitoring, the total plasma drug concentrations are generally used in the development of the appropriate drug dosage regimen for the patient. In the past, measurement of free drug concentration was not routinely performed in the laboratory. More recently, free drug concentrations may be measured quickly using ultrafiltration. Because of the high plasma protein binding of phenytoin and the narrow therapeutic index of the drug, more hospital laboratories are measuring both free and total phenytoin plasma levels.

KINETICS OF PROTEIN BINDING

The kinetics of reversible drug–protein binding for a protein with one simple binding site can be described by the *law of mass action*, as follows:

Protein + drug $\Leftrightarrow$ drug–protein–complex

or

$$[P] + [D] \Leftrightarrow [PD] \tag{10.15}$$

From Equation 10.15 and the law of mass action, an association constant, K_a, can be expressed as the ratio of the molar concentration of the products and the molar concentration of the reactants. This equation assumes only one-binding site per protein molecule.

$$K_a = \frac{[PD]}{[P][D]} \tag{10.16}$$

The extent of the drug–protein complex formed is dependent on the association binding constant K_a. The magnitude of K_a yields information on the degree of drug protein binding. Drugs strongly bound to protein have a very large K_a and exist mostly as the drug–protein complex. With such drugs, a large dose may be needed to obtain a reasonable therapeutic concentration of free drug.

Most kinetic studies *in vitro* use purified albumin as a standard protein source, because this protein is responsible for the major portion of plasma drug–protein binding. Experimentally, both the free drug $[D]$ and the protein-bound drug $[PD]$, as well as the total protein concentration $[P] + [PD]$, may be determined. To study the binding behavior of drugs, a determinable ratio r is defined, as follows:

$$r = \frac{\text{moles of drug bound}}{\text{total moles of protein}}$$

Because moles of drug bound is $[PD]$ and the total moles of protein is $[P] + [PD]$, this equation becomes

$$r = \frac{[PD]}{[PD] + [P]} \tag{10.17}$$

According to Equation 10.16, $[PD] = K_a[P][D]$; by substitution into Equation 10.17, the following expression is obtained:

$$r = \frac{K_a[P][D]}{K_a[P][D] + [P]}$$

$$r = \frac{K_a[D]}{1 + K_a[D]} \tag{10.18}$$

This equation describes the simplest situation, in which 1 mole of drug binds to 1 mole of protein in a 1:1 complex. This case assumes only one independent binding site for each molecule of drug. If there are n identical independent binding sites per protein molecule, then the following is used:

$$r = \frac{nK_a[D]}{1 + K_a[D]} \qquad (10.19)$$

In terms of K_d, which is $1/K_a$, Equation 10.19 reduces to

$$r = \frac{n[D]}{K_d + [D]} \qquad (10.20)$$

Protein molecules are quite large compared to drug molecules and may contain more than one type of binding site for the drug. If there is more than one type of binding site and the drug binds independently on each binding site with its own association constant, then Equation 10.20 expands to

$$r = \frac{n_1 K_1[P]}{1 + K_1[D]} + \frac{n_2 K_2[P]}{1 + K_2[D]} + \cdots \qquad (10.21)$$

where the numerical subscripts represent different types of binding sites, the K's represent the binding constants, and the n's represent the number of binding sites per molecule of albumin.

These equations assume that each drug molecule binds to the protein at an independent binding site, and the affinity of a drug for one binding site does not influence binding to other sites. In reality, drug–protein binding sometimes exhibits a phenomenon of *cooperativity*. For these drugs, the binding of the first drug molecule at one site on the protein molecule influences the successive binding of other drug molecules. The binding of oxygen to hemoglobin is an example of drug cooperativity.

Each method for the investigation of drug–protein binding *in vitro* has advantages and disadvantages in terms of cost, ease of measurement, time, instrumentation, and other considerations. Various experimental factors for the measurement of protein binding are listed in Table 10.10. Drug–protein binding kinetics yield valuable information concerning proper therapeutic use of the drug and predictions of possible drug interactions.

PRACTICAL FOCUS

1. How is r related to the fraction of drug bound (f_u), a term that is often of clinical interest?

Solution

r is the ratio of number of moles of drug bound/number of moles of albumin. r determines the extent to which the binding sites in albumin (or another protein) are occupied by the drug and the saturation drug concentration. f_u is based on the total concentration of drug and is used to determine the free drug concentration from the total plasma level. The value of f_u is often assumed to be fixed. However, f_u may change, especially with drugs that have therapeutic levels close to the K_d. (See examples on diazoxide.)

2. At maximum binding, the number of binding sites is n (see Eq. 10.21). The drug disopyramide has a $K_d = 1 \times 10^{-6}$ M/L. How close to saturation is the drug when the free drug concentration is 1×10^{-6} M/L?

Solution

Substitution for $[D] = 1 \times 10^{-6}$ M/L and $K_d = 1 \times 10^{-6}$ M/L in Equation 10.21 gives

$$r = \frac{n}{2}$$

When $n = 1$ and the unbound (free) drug concentration is equal to K_d, the protein binding of the drug is half-saturated. Interestingly, when $[D]$ is much greater than K_d, K_d is negligible in Equation 10.21, and $r = n$ (ie, r is independent of concentration or fully saturated).

When $K_d > [D]$, $[D]$ is negligible in the denominator of Equation 10.21, and r is dependent on $n/K_d[D]$, or $nK_a[D]$. In this case, the dissociation constant, K_d, is greater than the drug concentration, $[D]$, the number of sites bound is directly proportional to the number of binding sites, the association binding constant (also called the affinity constant), and the free drug concentration. This relationship also explains why a drug with a higher K_a may not necessarily have a higher percent of drug bound, because the number of binding sites, n, may be different from one drug to another.

DETERMINATION OF BINDING CONSTANTS AND BINDING SITES BY GRAPHIC METHODS

In-Vitro Methods (Known Protein Concentration)

A plot of the ratio of r (moles of drug bound per mole of protein) versus free drug concentration $[D]$ is shown in Figure 10-13. Equation 10.20 shows that as free drug concentration increases, the number of moles of drug bound per mole

Figure 10-13. Graphical representation of Equation 10.20, showing saturation of protein at high drug concentrations.

of protein becomes saturated and plateaus. Thus, drug protein binding resembles a *Langmuir* adsorption isotherm, which is also similar to adsorption of a drug to an adsorbent becoming saturated as the drug concentration increases. Because of nonlinearity in drug–protein binding, Equation 10.20 is rearranged for the estimation of n and K_a, using various graphic methods as discussed in the next section.

The values for the association constants and the number of binding sites are obtained by various graphic methods. The reciprocal of Equation 10.20 gives the following equation:

$$\frac{1}{r} = \frac{1 + K_a[D]}{n K_a[D]}$$

$$\frac{1}{r} = \frac{1}{n K_a[D]} + \frac{1}{n}$$

(10.22)

A graph of $1/r$ versus $1/[D]$ is called a *double reciprocal plot*. The y intercept is $1/n$ and the slope is $1/nK_a$. From this graph (Fig. 10-14), the number of binding sites may be determined from the y intercept, and the association constant may be determined from the slope, if the value for n is known.

If the graph of $1/r$ versus $1/[D]$ does not yield a straight line, then the drug–protein binding process is probably more complex. Equation 10.20 assumes one type of binding site and no interaction among the binding sites. Frequently, Equation 10.22 is used to estimate the number of binding sites and binding constants, using computerized iteration methods.

Another graphic technique called the *Scatchard plot*, is a rearrangement of Equation 10.20. The Scatchard plot spreads the data to give a better line for the estimation of the binding constants and binding sites. From Equation 10.20, we obtain

$$r = \frac{n K_a[D]}{1 + K_a[D]}$$

$$r + r K_a[D] = n K_a[D]$$

(10.23)

$$r = n K_a[D] - r K_a[D]$$

$$\frac{r}{D} = n K_a - r K_a$$

A graph constructed by plotting $r/[D]$ versus r yields a straight line with the intercepts and slope shown in Figures 10-15 and 10-16.

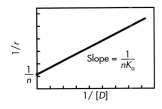

Figure 10-14. Hypothetical binding of drug to protein. The line was obtained with the double reciprocal equation.

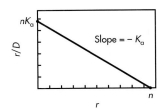

Figure 10-15. Hypothetical binding of drug to protein. The line was obtained with the Scatchard equation.

Figure 10-16. Graphic determination of number of binding sites and association constants for interaction of sulfonamides and phenylbutazone with albumin. (From Thorp, 1964, with permission.)

Some drug–protein binding data produce Scatchard graphs of curvilinear lines (Figs. 10-17 and 10-18). The curvilinear line represents the summation of two straight lines that collectively form the curve. The binding of salicylic acid to albumin is an example of this type of drug–protein binding in which there are at least two different, independent binding sites (n_1 and n_2), each with its own independent association constant (k_1 and k_2). Equation 10.21 best describes this type of drug–protein interaction.

Figure 10-18. Binding curves for salicylic acid to crystalline bovine serum albumin. Curve I, plot for one class, $n_1 = 0.72$, $k_1 = 25,000$. Curve II, plot for second class, $n_2 = 5.3$, $k_2 = 150$. Curve I + II, plot for both binding sites, sum of the above. (From Davison, 1971, with permission.)

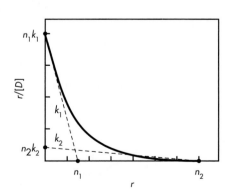

Figure 10-17. Hypothetical binding of drug to protein. The k's represent independent binding constants and the n's represent the number of binding sites per molecule of protein.

In-Vivo Methods (Unknown Protein Concentration)

Reciprocal and Scatchard plots cannot be used if the exact nature and amount of protein in the experimental system is unknown. The percent of drug bound is often used to describe the extent of drug–protein binding in the plasma. The fraction of drug bound, β, can be determined experimentally and is equal to the ratio of the concentration of bound drug, $[D_\beta]$, and the total drug concentration, $[D_T]$, in the plasma, as follows:

$$\beta = \frac{[D_\beta]}{[D_T]} \qquad (10.24)$$

The value of the association constant can be determined, even though the nature of the plasma proteins binding the drug is unknown, by rearranging Equation 10.24 into Equation 10.25:

$$r = \frac{[D_\beta]}{[P_T]} = \frac{nK_a[D]}{1 + K_a[D]} \qquad (10.25)$$

where $[D_\beta]$ is the bound drug concentration; $[D]$ is the free drug concentration; and $[P_T]$ is the total protein concentration. Rearrangement of this equation gives the following expression, which is analogous to the Scatchard equation:

$$\frac{[D_\beta]}{[D]} = nK_a[P_T] - K_a[D_\beta] \qquad (10.26)$$

Concentrations of both free and bound drug may be found experimentally, and a graph obtained by plotting $[D_\beta]/[D]$ versus $[D_\beta]$ will yield a straight line for which the slope is the association constant K_a. Equation 10.26 shows that the ratio of bound C_p to free C_p is influenced by the affinity constant, the protein concentration, $[P_T]$, which may change during disease states, and the drug concentration in the body.

The values for n and K_a give a general estimate of the affinity and binding capacity of the drug, as plasma contains a complex mixture of proteins. The drug–protein binding in plasma may be influenced by competing substances such as ions, free fatty acids, drug metabolites, and other drugs. Measurements of drug–protein binding should be obtained over a wide drug concentration range, because at low drug concentrations a high-affinity, low-capacity binding site might be missed or, at a higher drug concentration, saturation of protein-binding sites might occur.

Relationship between Protein Concentration and Drug Concentration in Drug–Protein Binding

The drug concentration, the protein concentration, and the association (affinity) constant, K_a, influence the fraction of drug bound (Eq. 10.24). With a constant concentration of protein, only a certain number of binding sites are available for a drug. At low drug concentrations, most of the drug may be bound to the protein, whereas at high drug concentrations, the protein-binding sites may become saturated, with a consequent rapid increase in the free drug concentrations (Fig. 10-19).

Figure 10-19.   Fraction of drug bound versus drug concentration at constant protein concentration.

To demonstrate the relationship of the drug concentration, protein concentration, and K_a, the following expression can be derived from Equations 10.24 and 10.25.

$$\beta = \frac{1}{1 + ([D]/n[P_T]) + (1/nK_a[P_T])} \tag{10.27}$$

From Equation 10.27, both the free drug concentration, $[D]$, and the total protein concentration, $[P_T]$, have important effects on the fraction of drug bound. Any factors that suddenly increase the fraction of free drug concentration in the plasma will cause a change in the pharmacokinetics of the drug.

Because protein binding is nonlinear in most cases, the percent of drug bound is dependent on the concentrations of both the drug and proteins in the plasma. In disease situations, the concentration of protein may vary, thus affecting the percent of drug bound. As the protein concentration increases, the percent of drug bound increases to a maximum. The shapes of the curves are determined by the association constant of the drug–protein complex and the drug concentration. The effect of protein concentration on drug binding is demonstrated in Figure 10-20.

CLINICAL SIGNIFICANCE OF DRUG–PROTEIN BINDING

Most drugs bind reversibly to plasma proteins to some extent. When the clinical significance of the fraction of drug bound is considered, it is important to know whether the study was performed using pharmacologic or therapeutic plasma drug concentrations. As mentioned previously, the fraction of drug bound can change with plasma drug concentration and dose of drug administered. In addition, the

Figure 10-20.   Effect of protein concentration on the percentage of drug bound. *A, B,* and *C* represent hypothetical drugs with respectively decreasing binding affinity.

TABLE 10.12   Factors That Decrease Plasma Protein Concentration

MECHANISM	DISEASE STATE
Decreased protein synthesis	Liver disease
Increased protein catabolism	Trauma, surgery
Distribution of albumin into extravascular space	Burns
Excessive elimination of protein	Renal disease

patient's plasma protein concentration should be considered. If a patient has a low plasma protein concentration, then, for any given dose of drug, the concentration of free (unbound) bioactive drug may be higher than anticipated. The plasma protein concentration is controlled by a number of variables, including (1) protein synthesis, (2) protein catabolism, (3) distribution of albumin between intravascular and extravascular space, and (4) excessive elimination of plasma protein, particularly albumin. A number of diseases, age, trauma, and related circumstances affect the plasma protein concentration (Tables 10.12–10.14).

TABLE 10.13   Physiologic and Pathologic Conditions Altering Protein Concentrations in Plasma[a]

	ALBUMIN	α_1-GLYCOPROTEIN	LIPOPROTEIN
Decreasing	Age (geriatric, neonate)	Fetal concentrations	Hyperthyroidism
	Bacterial pneumonia	Nephrotic syndrome	Injury
	Burns	Oral contraceptives	Liver disease?
	Cirrhosis of liver		Trauma
	Cystic fibrosis		
	GI disease		
	Histoplasmosis		
	Leprosy		
	Liver abscess		
	Malignant neoplasms		
	Malnutrition (severe)		
	Multiple myeloma		
	Nephrotic syndrome		
	Pancreatitis (acute)		
	Pregnancy		
	Renal failure		
	Surgery		
	Trauma		
Increasing	Benign tumor	Age (geriatric)	Diabetes
	Exercise	Celiac disease	Hypothyroidism
	Hypothyroidism	Crohn's disease	Liver disease?
	Neurological disease?	Injury	Nephrotic
	Neurosis	Myocardial infarction	syndrome
	Paranoia	Renal failure	
	Psychosis	Rheumatoid arthritis	
	Schizophrenia	Stress	
		Surgery	
		Trauma	

[a]In the conditions listed, the protein concentrations are altered, on average, by 30% or more, and in some cases by more than 100%.

From Tozer (1984), with permission.

TABLE 10.14   Protein Binding in Normal (Norm) Renal Function, End-Stage Renal Disease (ESRD), during Hemodialysis (HD), and in Nephrotic Syndrome (NS)

	NORM (% BOUND)	ESRD (% BOUND)	HD (% BOUND)	NS (% BOUND)
Azlocillin	28	25		
Bilirubin		Decreased		
Captopril	24	18		
Cefazolin	84	73	22	
Cefoxitin	73	20		
Chloramphenicol	53	45	30	
Chlorpromazine	98	98		
Clofibrate	96		89	
Clonidine	30	30		
Congo red		Decreased		
Dapsone		Normal		
Desipramine	80	Normal		
N-Desmethyldiazepam	98	94		
Desmethylimipramine	89	88		
Diazepam	99	94		
Diazoxide (30 μg/mL)	92	86	83	
(300 μg/mL)	77	72		
Dicloxacillin	96	91		
Diflunisal	88	56		39
Digitoxin	97	96	90	96
Digoxin	25		22	
Doxycycline	88	71		
Erythromycin	75	77		
Etomidate	75	57		
Fluorescein	86	Decreased		
Furosemid	96	94		93
Indomethacin		Normal		
Maprotiline	90	Normal		
β-Methyldigoxin	30		19	
Methyl orange		Decreased		
Methyl red		Decreased		
Morphine	35	31		
Nafcillin	88	81		
Naproxen	75	21		
Oxazepam	95	88		
Papaverine	97	94		
Penicillin G	72	36		
Pentobarbital	66	59		
Phenobarbital	55	Decreased		
Phenol red		Decreased		
Phenylbutazone	97	88		
Phenytoin	90	80	93	81
Pindolol	41	Normal		
Prazosin	95	92		
Prednisolone (50 mg)	74		65	64
(15 mg)	87	88		85
D-Propoxyphene	76	80		
Propranolol	88	89	90	
Quinidine	88	86	88	
Salicylate	94	85		
Sulfadiazine		Decreased		

(continued)

TABLE 10.14   Protein Binding in Normal (Norm) Renal Function, End-Stage Renal Disease (ESRD), during Hemodialysis (HD), and in Nephrotic Syndrome (NS) (*Continued*)

	NORM (% BOUND)	ESRD (% BOUND)	HD (% BOUND)	NS (% BOUND)
Sulfamethoxazole	74	50		
Sulfonamides		Decreased		
Strophantin	1		2	
Theophylline	60	Decreased		
Thiopental	72	44		
Thyroxine		Decreased		
Triamterene	81	61		
Trimethoprim	70	68		70
Tryptophan	75	Decreased		
D-Tubocurarine	44	41		
Valproic acid	85	Decreased		
Verapamil	90	Normal		
Warfarin	99	98		

From Keller et al (1984), with permission.

For example, liver disease results in a decrease in plasma albumin concentration due to decreased protein synthesis. In nephrotic syndrome, an accumulation of waste metabolites, such as urea and uric acid, as well as an accumulation of drug metabolites, may alter protein binding of drugs. Severe burns may cause an increased distribution of albumin into the extracellular fluid, resulting in a smaller plasma albumin concentration. In certain genetic diseases, the quality of the protein that is synthesized in the plasma may be altered due to a change in the amino acid sequence. Both chronic liver disease and renal disease, such as uremia, may cause an alteration in the quality of plasma protein synthesized. An alteration in the protein quality may be demonstrated by an alteration in the association constant or affinity of the drug for the protein.

When a highly protein-bound drug is displaced from binding by a second drug or agent, a sharp increase in the free drug concentration in the plasma may occur, leading to toxicity. For example, an increase in free warfarin level was responsible for an increase in bleeding when warfarin was co-administered with phenylbutazone, which competes for the same protein-binding site (O'Reilly, 1973; Udall, 1970; Koch-Weser and Sellers, 1971). Recently, studies and reviews have shown that the clinical significance of warfarin protein binding and its impact on bleeding are less prominent, adding other factors and explanations (Sands et al, 2002; Chan, 1995; Benet and Hoener, 2002).

Albumin has two known binding sites that share the binding of many drugs (MacKichan, 1992). Binding site I is shared by phenylbutazone, sulfonamides, phenytoin, and valproic acid. Binding site II is shared by the semisynthetic penicillins, probenecid, medium-chain fatty acids, and the benzodiazepines. Some drugs bind to both sites. Displacement occurs when a second drug is taken that competes for the same binding site in the protein as the initial drug.

Although it is generally assumed that binding sites are preformed, there is some evidence pointing to the *allosteric* nature of protein binding. This means that the binding of a drug modifies the conformation of protein in such a way that the drug binding influences the nature of binding of further molecules of the drug.

The binding of oxygen to hemoglobin is a well studied biochemical example in which the initial binding of other oxygen to the iron in the heme portion influences the binding of other oxygen molecules.

Effect of Displacement

Most studies on the kinetics of drug–protein binding consider binding to plasma proteins. However, certain drugs may also bind specific tissue proteins or other macromolecules, such as melanin or DNA.

Displacement of drugs from plasma or tissue binding will lead to an increased apparent volume of distribution and an increased half-life, but clearance will remain unaffected. If administered by multiple doses, the mean steady-state concentration will remain unchanged; however, the mean steady-state free drug level will be increased due to displacement. The therapeutic effect will therefore increase.

$$Cl = \frac{0.693 \ V_D}{t_{1/2}} \qquad\qquad (10.28)$$

Studies on the binding of drugs to intracellular components *in vivo* are more difficult to perform. However, recent studies have shown that drugs may also be displaced from tissue binding sites. For example, digoxin, a cardiac glycoside, binds strongly to the myocardial tissue of the heart. If patients who are on digoxin take quinidine, steady-state digoxin plasma levels increase, possibly due to displacement of the tissue-bound digoxin (Reifell et al, 1979).

Drug Distribution and Pharmacodynamics

The relationship of reversible drug–protein binding in the plasma and drug distribution and elimination is shown in Figure 10-8. A decrease in protein binding that results in increased free drug concentration will allow more drug to cross cell membranes and distribute into all tissues, as discussed above. More drug will therefore be available to interact at a receptor site to produce a more intense pharmacologic effect.

Clinically, the pharmacodynamic response is influenced by both the distribution of the drug and the concentration of the unbound drug fraction. The drug dose and the dosage form must be chosen to provide sufficiently high unbound drug concentrations so that an adequate amount of drug reaches the site of drug action (receptor). The onset of drug action depends on the rate of the free (unbound) drug that reaches the receptor and produces a *minimum effective concentration* (MEC) to produce a pharmacodynamic response (see Chapters 1 and 19). The onset time is often dependent on the rate of drug uptake and distribution to the receptor site. The intensity of a drug action depends on the total drug concentration of the receptor site and the number of receptors occupied by drug. To achieve a pharmacodynamic response with the initial (priming) dose, the amount (mass) of drug when dissolved in the volume of distribution must give a drug concentration ≥ MEC at the receptor site. Subsequent drug doses maintain the pharmacodynamic effect by sustaining the drug concentration at the receptor site. Subsequent doses are

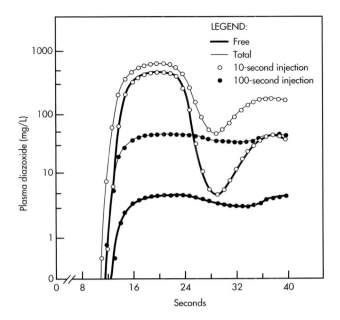

Figure 10-21. Calculated time course of total and free diazoxide concentrations in arterioles. (From Sellers and Koch-Weser, 1973, with permission.)

given at a dose rate (eg, 250 mg every 6 hours) that replaces drug loss from the receptor site, usually by elimination. However, redistributional factors may also contribute to the loss of drug from the receptor site.

A less understood aspect of protein binding is the effect of binding on the intensity and pharmacodynamics of the drug after intravenous administration. Rapid IV injection may increase the free drug concentration of some highly protein-bound drugs and therefore increase its intensity of action. Sellers and Koch-Weser (1973) reported a dramatic increase in hypotensive effect when diazoxide was injected rapidly IV in 10 seconds versus a slower injection of 100 seconds. Diazoxide was 9.1% and 20.6% free when the serum levels were 20 and 100 μg/mL, respectively. Figure 10-21 shows a transient high free diazoxide concentration that resulted after a rapid IV injection, causing maximum arterial dilation and hypotensive effect due to initial saturation of the protein-binding sites. In contrast, when diazoxide was injected more slowly over 100 seconds, free diazoxide serum level was low, due to binding and drug distribution. The slower injection of diazoxide produced a smaller fall in blood pressure, even though the total drug dose injected was the same. Although most drugs have linear binding at therapeutic dose, in some patients, free drug concentration can increase rapidly with rising drug concentration as binding sites become saturated. An example is illustrated in Figure 10-22 for lidocaine (MacKichan, 1992).

The nature of drug–drug and drug–metabolite interactions is also important in drug–protein binding. In this case, one drug may displace a second bound drug from the protein, causing a sudden increase in pharmacologic response due to an increase in free drug concentration.

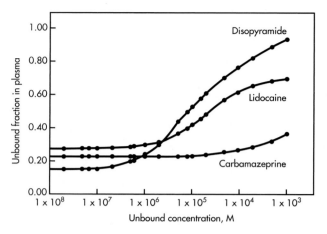

Figure 10-22. *Simulation showing changes in fraction of free (unbound) drug over various molar drug concentrations for three drugs with protein binding.*
(From MacKichan 1992.)

 # EXAMPLE

Compare the percent of change in free drug concentration when two drugs, A (95% bound) and B (50% bound), are displaced by 5% from their respective binding sites by the administration of another drug (Table 10.15). For a highly bound drug A, a displacement of 5% of free drug is actually a 100% increase in free drug level. For a weakly bound drug like drug B, a change of 5% in free concentration due to displacement would cause only a 10% increase in free drug level over the initially high (50%) free drug concentration. For a patient medicated with drug B, a 10% increase in free drug level would probably not affect the therapeutic outcome. However, a 100% increase in active drug, as occurs with drug A, might be toxic. Although this example is based on one drug displacing another drug, nutrients, physiologic products, and the waste products of metabolism may cause displacement from binding in a similar manner.

As illustrated by this example, displacement is most important with drugs that are more than 95% bound and have a narrow therapeutic index. Under normal circumstances, only a small proportion of the total drug is active. Consequently, a small displacement of bound drug causes a disproportionate increase in the free drug concentration, which may cause drug intoxication.

With drugs that are not as highly bound to plasma proteins, a small displacement from the protein causes a transient increase in the free drug concentration, which may cause a transient increase in pharmacologic activity. However, more free

TABLE 10.15 Comparison of Effects of 5% Displacement from Binding on Two Hypothetical Drugs

	BEFORE DISPLACEMENT	AFTER DISPLACEMENT	PERCENT INCREASE IN FREE DRUG
Drug A			
Percent drug bound	95	90	
Percent drug free	5	10	+100
Drug B			
Percent drug bound	50	45	
Percent drug free	50	55	+10

drug is available for both renal excretion and hepatic biotransformation, which may be demonstrated by a transient decreased elimination half-life. Drug displacement from protein by a second drug can occur by competition of the second drug for similar binding sites. Moreover, any alteration of the protein structure may also change the capacity of the protein to bind drugs. For example, aspirin acetylates the lysine residue of albumin, which changes the binding capacity of this protein for certain other anti-inflammatory drugs, such as phenylbutazone.

The displacement of endogenous substances from plasma proteins by drugs is usually of little consequence. Some hormones, such as thyroid and cortisol, are normally bound to specific plasma proteins. A small displacement of these hormones rarely causes problems because physiologic feedback control mechanisms take over. However, in infants, the displacement of bilirubin by drugs can cause mental retardation and even death, due to the difficulty of bilirubin elimination in newborns.

Finally, the binding of drugs to proteins can affect the duration of action of the drug. A drug that is extensively but reversibly bound to protein may have a long duration of action due to a depot effect of the drug–protein complex.

While a change in free drug concentration due to changing protein binding can potentially change the pharmacologic response of a drug, many drugs with a change in protein binding did not show a significant change in clinical effect (Benet and Hoener, 2002) as discussed in the next section. The important question to ask is: Will the increase in free drug concentration due to reduced binding elicit a rapid pharmacologic response before the temporary increase in free drug is diluted by a rapid distribution and/or elimination due to a greater fraction of free drug? Kruger and Figg (2001) observed that the angiogenesis activity of Suramin, an inhibitor of blood vessel proliferation, is greatly altered by protein binding. In biological assays with aorta rings of rats, the effect is measured *ex vivo* at the site directly, and the degree of protein binding was reported to be important. In the body, the pathways to reach the receptor, distribution, and elimination are factors that complicate the effect of a rise in free drug due to displacement from binding. In general, the outcome of a change in protein binding *in vivo* may be harder to measure depending on where the site of action is located. The onset of a drug, and its distribution half-life to the site of action, may need to be considered. In the next section, this subject is further discussed based on the recent concept of drug exposure. The concept of drug exposure is important because many vital organs and adverse reactions are related to their exposure to plasma drug concentration.

Protein Binding and Drug Exposure

The impact of protein binding on clinical drug efficacy and safety has long been recognized (Sellers E and Koch-Weser, 1976; Greenblatt et al, 1982) but has received renewed literature discussion recently (Sands et al, 2002; Chan, 1995; Benet and Hoener, 2002). Free plasma drug concentration is more relevant than total plasma drug concentration. However, when considering drug safety, how high and how long the free plasma drug level will be sustained are more important to a toxicokineticist. This is often measured by the AUC for the free drug concentration.

Based on the well-stirred venous equilibration model incorporating protein binding (Benet and Hoener, 2002), organ clearance for a drug (Cl) is expressed as

$$Cl = \frac{Q_{organ} f_u Cl_{int}}{Q_{organ} + f_u Cl_{int}} \tag{10.29}$$

For a low-extraction drug, where Q is blood flow, f_u is fraction of drug unchanged and Cl_{int} is intrinsic clearance, $Q_{organ} \gg f_u Cl_{int}$, the equation simplies to

$$Cl \approx f_u Cl_{int} \tag{10.30}$$

Clearance depends on f_u and intrinsic clearance. Intrinsic clearance is flow independent; whereas hepatic clearance, Cl_H is flow dependent for a high extraction drug.

Hepatic bioavailability of a drug, F_H, is expressed as

$$F_H = \frac{Q_H}{Q_H + f_u Cl_{int}} \tag{10.31}$$

Let F_{abs}, be the fraction of drug absorbed to the gut wall and F_G be the fraction that gets through the gut wall unchanged (ie, $F_{oral} = F_{abs} F_G F_H$). The systemic AUC after an oral dose is

$$AUC_{oral} = \frac{F_{abs} F_G \, Dose}{f_u Cl_{int}} \tag{10.32}$$

For an unbound drug, $AUC_{oral}^u = [f_u] AUC_{oral}$ (10.33)

When substituted for AUC_{oral} using Equation (10.32) into Equation (10.33), f_u cancels out, and the equation becomes

$$AUC_{oral}^u = \frac{F_{abs} F_G \, Dose}{Cl_{int}} \tag{10.34}$$

Equation (10.34) above shows that unbound drug exposure as measured by unbound plasma drug area under the curve is independent of f_u.

For a low-extraction drug, both IV and oral, changes in protein binding are generally not important. For a high-extraction drug after IV administration, changes in protein binding are clinically important whether metabolism is hepatic or nonhepatic. For a drug that is administered IV and is highly extracted by the liver ($Q_{organ} \ll f_u\, Cl_{int}$), AUC_{IV}^u or unbound drug systemic exposure is expressed by

$$AUC_{IV}^u = f_u\, AUC_{IV} \approx \frac{f_u \text{Dose}}{Q_H} \tag{10.35}$$

In this case, changes in binding may be clinically important, as shown by the change of f_u in Equation (10.35).

The derivation of Equation 10.33 into Equation 10.34 is dependent on the fact that f_u is constant as a function of t. If free drug concentration C_f is changing at various C_p, ie, concentration-dependent binding, then $C_f = F(t)$ is time dependent, and in fact, AUC will be nonlinear with dose and Equation 10.34 will be different for different doses (Chapter 9). Within therapeutic drug concentrations, the effect of changes in f_u is apparently not sufficient to change the efficacy of most drugs and is not of clinical concern. However, as more potent biological drugs with short elimination half-lives are used, plasma drug concentrations may potentially fall several-fold and f_u may change significantly at various plasma concentrations. An anatomic-physiologic approach to evaluate drug concentrations (Mather, 2001) may be helpful in understanding how drug efficacy and safety change in protein binding and clearances in local tissues (Chapter 12).

Clinical Examples

Protein concentration may change during some acute disease states. For example, plasma α_1-acid glycoprotein (AAG) levels in patients may increase due to the host's acute-phase response to infection, trauma, inflammatory processes, and some malignant diseases. The acute-phase response is a change in various plasma proteins that is observed within hours or days following the onset of infection or injury. The acute-phase changes may be also indicative of chronic disease (Kremer et al, 1988).

AAG binds to many basic drugs, and a change in AAG protein concentration can contribute to more fluctuation in free drug concentrations among patients during various stages of infection or disease. Amprenavir (Agenerase), a protease inhibitor of human immunodeficiency virus type 1 (HIV-1), is highly bound to human plasma proteins, mostly to AAG (approximately 90%). AAG levels are known to vary with infection, including HIV disease. Sadler et al (2001) showed a significant inverse linear relationship between AAG levels and amprenavir clearance as estimated by CL/F. Unbound, or free, amprenavir concentrations were not affected by AAG concentrations even though the apparent total drug clearance was increased. The intrinsic clearance of the drug was not changed. The authors cautioned that incorrect conclusions could be drawn about the pharmacokinetics of highly protein-bound drugs if AAG concentration is not included in the analysis.

In addition, race, age, and weight were also found to affect AAG levels. African-American subjects had significantly lower AAG concentrations than Caucasian subjects. AAG in African-Americans was 77.2 ± 13.8 mg/dL versus 90 ± 20.2 mg/dL in Caucasians, $p < 0.0001$. Pharmacokinetic analysis showed that AAG correlated significantly with age and race and was a significant predictor of amprenavir CL/F. Interestingly, in spite of a statistically significant difference in total plasma amprenavir level, a dose adjustment for racial differences was not indicated, because the investigators found the unbound amprenavir concentrations to be similar.

Protein binding can lead to *nonlinear* or *dose-dependent* kinetics. It was interesting to note that amprenavir *CL/F* was dose dependent in the analysis without AAG data, but that no dose dependence was observed when AAG concentration was considered in the analysis. The higher doses of amprenavir, which produce the greatest antiviral activity, resulted in the largest decrease in AAG concentration, which led to the greatest changes in total drug concentration.

In evaluating change in protein binding and its impact on free plasma drug, it is important to realize that protein changes or displacement often result in changes in free plasma drug concentration. Nonetheless, the free drug is not necessarily increasingly eliminated unless the change in free drug concentration facilitates metabolism, accompanied by a change in Cl_{int} (Cl_{int} measures the inherent capacity to metabolize the drug; see Chapter 11). For some drugs, the change in protein binding may be sufficiently compensated by a redistribution of the drug from one tissue to another within the body. In contrast, a change in drug protein binding accompanied by metabolism (Cl_{int}) will invariably result in an increased amount of drug needed to maintain a steady-state level because the total drug concentration is continuously being eliminated. The maintenance of an adequate therapeutic free drug level through re-equilibration is difficult in such a case.

MODELING DRUG DISTRIBUTION

Drug distribution may change in many disease and physiologic states, making it difficult to predict the concentration of drug that reaches the site of drug action (receptor). Pharmacokinetic models can be used to predict these pharmacokinetic changes due to changes in physiologic states. The model should consider free and bound drug equilibration and metabolism at the apparent site of action, and transient changes due to disease state (eg, pH change or impaired perfusion).

In pharmacokinetics, perfusion and rapid equilibration within a region form the basis for the *well-stirred models* that are used in many classical compartment models as well as some physiologic pharmacokinetic models. The concept of body or organ drug clearance both assume that uniform drug concentration is rapidly established within a given biological region (C_{organ} or C_{plasma}) at a given time point. The model also allows: (1) the mass of drug present in the region can be monitored by multiplying the concentration with its volume at a given time; and (2) the rate of drug elimination from the site can be calculated by the product of clearance times drug concentration.

Model simplicity using the well-stirred approach has advanced the concept of drug clearance and allowed practical drug concentration to be estimated based on body clearance and drug dose. The approach has generally provided more accurate dosing for many drugs for which drug action is determined mostly by steady-state concentration, and a transient change in concentration of short duration is not critical. However, caution should be exercised in equating model-predicted concentration to drug concentration at a given site in the body.

Arterial and Venous Differences in Drug Concentrations

Most pharmacokinetic studies are modeled based on blood samples drawn from various venous sites after either IV or oral dosing. Physiologists have long recognized the unique difference between arterial and venous blood. For example, arterial tension (pressure) of oxygen drives the distribution of oxygen to vital organs. Chiou (1989) and Mather (2001) have discussed the pharmacokinetic issues when differences in drug concentrations C_p in arterial and venous are observed. These reviewers question the validity of the assumption of the well-stirred condition or rapid mixing within the blood or plasma pool when there is gradual permeation into tissues in which the drug may then be metabolized. Indeed, some drug markers have shown that rapid mixing may not be typical, except when the drug is essentially confined to blood pool due to protein binding.

Differences ranging as high as several hundred-fold for griseofulvin due to differences in arterial and venous blood levels have been reported. Forty compounds have been shown to exhibit marked site dependence in plasma or blood concentration after dosing in both humans and animals. In some cases, differences are due mostly to large extraction of drug in poorly perfused local tissues, such as with nitroglycerin (3.8-fold arteriovenous difference) and procainamde (234% arteriovenous difference, venous being higher). The classical assumption in pharmacokinetics of rapid mixing within minutes in the entire blood circulation therefore may not be applicable to some drugs. Would the observed sampling differences result in significant difference between the AUCs between arterial and venous blood, or in prediction of toxicity or adverse effects of drugs? No such differences were observed in the reviews by Chiou and Mather, although the significance of these differences on drug therapy and toxicity has not been fully explored.

FREQUENTLY ASKED QUESTIONS

1. Do all drugs that bind proteins lead to clinically significant interactions?

2. What macromolecules participate in drug protein binding?

3. How does drug protein binding affect drug elimination?

4. How does a physical property, such as partition coefficient, affect drug distribution?

5. What are the factors to consider when adjusting the drug dose for a patient whose plasma protein concentration decreases to half that of normal?

6. How does one distinguish between the distribution phase and the elimination phase after an IV injection of a drug?

7. What are the causes of a long distribution half-life for a body organ if blood flow to the tissue is rapid?

8. How long does it take for a tissue organ to be fully equilibrated with the plasma? How long for a tissue organ to be half-equilibrated?

9. When a body organ is equilibrated with drug from the plasma, the drug concentration in that organ should be the same as that of the plasma. True or false?

10. What is the parameter that tells when half of the protein binding sites are occupied?

11. f_u is used to represent the fraction of free drug in the plasma (Eq. 10.30 and 10.33). Is f_u always a constant?

12. Can a protein-bound drug be metabolized?

13. Why are most of the plasma drug concentration data reported without indicating the sampling site when there is a substantial difference in arterial and venous blood drug concentrations for many drugs?

14. Does the drug concentration in the terminal phase of the curve show less dependency on site of sampling?

15. Why is a change in protein binding for many drugs now reported to be clinically not significant when it was previously thought to be important?

16. Would an identical free plasma drug AUC (or free drug exposure) be sufficient to demonstrate that both drug activity and toxicity are the same for a protein-bound drug?

LEARNING QUESTIONS

1. Why is the zone of inhibition in an antibiotic disc assay larger for the same drug concentration (10 μg/mL) in water than in serum? See Figure 10-23.

2. Determine the number of binding sites (n) and the association constant (K_a) from the following data using the Scatchard equation.

r	$(D \times 10^{-4}$ M$)$	r/D
0.40	0.33	
0.80	0.89	
1.20	2.00	
1.60	5.33	

Can n and K_a have fractional values? Why?

3. Discuss the clinical significance of drug protein binding on the following:

   a. Drug elimination

   b. Drug–drug interactions

   c. "Percent of drug-bound" data

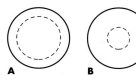

Figure 10-23. Antibiotic disc assay. **A.** Antibiotic in water (10 μg/mL). **B.** Antibiotic in serum (10 μg/mL).

d. Liver disease

e. Kidney disease

4. Vallner (1977) reviewed the binding of drugs to albumin or plasma proteins. The following data were reported:

Drug	Percent Drug Bound
Tetracycline	53
Gentamycin	70
Phenytoin	93
Morphine	38

Which drug listed above might be predicted to cause an adverse response due to the concurrent administration of a second drug such as sulfisoxazole (Gantrisin)? Why?

5. What are the main factors that determine the uptake and accumulation of a drug into tissues? Which tissues would have the most rapid drug uptake? Explain your answer.

6. As a result of edema, fluid may leave the capillary into the extracellular space. What effect does edema have on osmotic pressure in the blood and on drug diffusion into extracellular space?

7. Explain the effects of plasma drug–protein binding and tissue drug–protein binding on **(a)** the apparent volume of distribution and **(b)** drug elimination.

8. Naproxen (Naprosyn, Syntex) is a nonsteroidal anti-inflammatory drug (NSAID) that is highly bound to plasma proteins, >99%. Explain why the plasma concentration of free (unbound) naproxen increases in patients with chronic alcoholic liver disease and probably other forms of cirrhosis, whereas the total plasma drug concentration decreases.

9. Most literature references give an average value for the percentage of drug bound to plasma proteins.

   a. What factors influence the percentage of drug bound?

   b. How does renal disease affect the protein binding of drugs?

   c. How does hepatic disease affect the protein binding of drugs?

10. It is often assumed that linear binding occurs at therapeutic dose. What are the potential risks of this assumption?

11. When a drug is 99% bound, it means that there is a potential risk of saturation. True or false?

12. Adenosine is a drug used for termination of tachycardia. The $t_{1/2}$ after IV dose is only 20 to 30 seconds according to product information. Suggest a reason for such a short half-life based on your knowledge of drug distribution and elimination.

REFERENCES

Benet LZ, Hoener BA: Commentary: Changes in plasma protein binding have little clinical relevance. *Clin Pharm Ther* **71**:115–121, 2002

Borondy P, Dill WA, Chang T, et al: Effect of protein binding on the distribution of 5,5-diphenylhydantoin between plasma and red cells. *Ann N Y Acad Sci* **226:**293, 1973

Butler TC: The distribution of drugs. In LaDu BN, Mandel HG, Way EL (eds), *Fundamentals of Drug Metabolism and Disposition.* Baltimore, Williams & Wilkins, 1972

Chan TY: Adverse interactions between warfarin and nonsteroidal anti-inflammatory drugs: Mechanism, clinical significance, and avoidance. *Ann Pharmacother* **29:**1274–1283, 1995

Chien DS, Sandri RB, Tang-Liu DS: Systemic pharmacokinetics of acitretin, etretinate, isotretinoin, and acetylenic retinoids in guinea pigs. *Drug Metab Dispos* **20**(2):211–217, 1992

Chiou WL: The phenomenon and rationale of marked dependence of drug concentration on blood sampling site: Implication in pharmacokinetics, pharmacodynamics, toxicology and therapeutics (Part I). *Clin Pharmacokinet* **17**(3):175–199, 1989; Part II. *Clin Pharmacokinet* **17**(3):275–290, 1989

Davison C: Protein binding. In LaDu BN, Mandel HG, Way EL (eds), *Fundamentals of Drug Metabolism and Drug Disposition.* Baltimore, Williams & Wilkins, 1971

Goldstein A, Aronow L, Kalman SM: *Principles of Drug Action. The Basis of Pharmacology,* 2nd ed. New York, Wiley, 1974, p 166

Greenblatt DJ, Sellers EM, Koch-Weser J: Importance of protein binding for the interpretation of serum or plasma drug concentration. *J Clin Pharmacol* **22:**259–263, 1982

Holladay JW, Dewey MJ, Yoo SD: Steady state kinetics of imipramine in transgenic mice with elevated serum AAG levels. *Pharm Res* 1313, 1996

Holladay JW, Dewey MJ, Michniak BB, et al: Elevated alpha-1-acid glycoprotein reduces the volume of distribution and systemic clearance of saquinavir. *Drug Metab Dispos.* **29**(3):299–303, 2001

Houin G: Drug binding and apparent volume of distribution. In Tillement JP, Lindenlaub E (eds), *Protein Binding and Drug Transport.* Stuttgart, Schattauer, 1985

Keller F, Maiga M, Neumayer HH, et al: Pharmacokinetic effects of altered plasma protein binding of drugs in renal disease. *Eur J Drug Metab Pharmacokinet* **9:**275–282, 1984

Kremer JMH, Wilting J, Janssen LHM: Drug binding to human alpha-1-acid glycoprotein in health and disease. *Pharmacol Rev* **40:**1–47, 1988

Kruger EA, Figg WD: Protein binding alters the activity of Suramin, carboxyamidotriazole, and UCN-01 in an ex vivo rat aortic ring angiogenesis assay. *Clin Cancer Res* **7:**1867–1872, 2001

MacKichan JJ: Influence of protein binding. In Evans WE, Schentag JJ, Jusko WJ (eds), *Applied Pharmacokinetics—Principles of Drug Monitoring,* 3rd ed. Vancouver, WA, Applied Therapeutics, 1992, chap 5

Mather LE: Anatomical-physioloical approach in pharmacokinetics and pharmacodynamics. *Clin Pharacokinet* **40:**707–722, 2001

Nilsen OG: Clinical pharmacokinetics of tenoxicam. *Clin Pharmacokinet* **26**(1):16–43, 1994

O'Reilly RA: The binding of sodium warfarin to plasma albumin and its displacement by phenylbutazone. *Ann N Y Acad Sci* **226:**319–331, 1973

Park MK, Ludden T, Arom KV, et al: Myocardial vs serum concentration in infants and children. *J Dis Child* **136:**418–420, 1982

Reifell JA, Leahy EB, Drusin RE, et al: A previously unrecognized drug interaction between quinidine and digoxin. *Clin Cardiol* **2:**40–42, 1979

Sadler BM, Gillotin C, Lou Y, Stein DS: In vivo effect of alpha(1)-acid glycoprotein on pharmacokinetics of amprenavir, a human immunodeficiency virus protease inhibitor. *Antimicrob Agents Chemother* **45:**852–856, 2001

Sands CD, Chan ES, Welty TE: Revisiting the significance of warfarin protein-binding displacement interactions. *Ann Pharmacother* **36:**1642–1645, 2002

Sawada Y, Hanano M, Sugiyama Y, Iga T: Prediction of the disposition of b-lactam antibiotics in human from pharmacokinetic parameters in animals. *J Pharmacokinet Biopharm* **12:**241–261, 1984

Sellers EM, Koch-Weser J: Kinetics and clinical importance of displacement of warfarin from albumin by acidic drugs. *Ann N Y Acad Sci* **179:**213–223, 1971

Sellers EM, Koch-Weser J: Influence of intravenous injection rate on protein binding and vascular activity of diazoxide. *Ann N Y Acad Sci* **226:**214–224, 1973

Stoeckel K, Trueb V, Tuerk H: Minor changes in biological half-life of ceftriaxone in functionally anephric and liver diseased patients: Explanations and consequences. In Armengaud, Fernex (eds), *Long-Acting Cephalosporins: Ceftriaxone, Part 28. Proceedings of the 13th International Congress of Chemotherapy,* Vienna, 1983, pp 9–13

Thorp JM: The influence of plasma proteins on the action of drugs. In Binns TB (ed), *Absorption and Distribution of Drugs*. Baltimore, Williams & Wilkins, 1964

Tozer TN: Implications of altered plasma protein binding in disease states. In Benet LZ, Massoud N, Gambertoglio JG (eds), *Pharmacokinetic Basis for Drug Treatment*. New York, Raven, 1984

Udall JA: Drug interference with warfarin therapy. *Clin Med* 77:20, 1970

Vallner JJ: Binding of drugs by albumin and plasma proteins. *J Pharm Sci* **66**:447–465, 1977

Verbeeck RK, Wallace SM: Non-steroidal anti-inflammatory drugs: Restrictive or non-restrictive clearance? Arzneim-Forsch **44**:683–685 [Medline], (1994)

BIBLIOGRAPHY

Anton AH, Solomon HM (eds): Drug protein binding. *Ann N Y Acad Sci* **226**:1–362, 1973

Barza M, Samuelson T, Weinstein L: Penetration of antibiotics into fibrin loci in vivo, II. Comparison of nine antibiotics: Effect of dose and degree of protein binding. *J Infect Dis* **129**:66, 1974

Bergen T: Pharmacokinetic properties of the cephalosporins. *Drugs* **34**(suppl 2):89–104, 1987

Birke G, Liljedahl SO, Plantin LO, Wetterfors J: Albumin catabolism in burns and following surgical procedures. *Acta Chir Scand* **118**:353–366, 1959–1960

Bridges JW, Wilson AGE: Drug–serum protein interactions and their biological significance. In Bridges JW, Chasseaud LF (eds), *Progress in Drug Research*, vol 1. New York, Wiley, 1976

Coffey CJ, Bullock FJ, Schoenemann PT: Numerical solution of nonlinear pharmacokinetic equations: Effect of plasma protein binding on drug distribution and elimination. *J Pharm Sci* **60**:1623, 1971

D'Arcy PF, McElnay JC: Drug interactions involving the displacement of drugs from plasma protein and tissue binding sites. *Pharm Ther* **17**:211–220, 1982

Gibaldi M, Levy G, McNamara PJ: Effect of plasma protein and tissue binding on the biologic half-life of drugs. *Clin Pharmacol Ther* **24**:1–4, 1978

Gillette JR: Overview of drug-protein binding. *Ann N Y Acad Sci* **226**:6, 1973

Grainger-Rousseau TJ, McElnay JC, Collier PS: The influence of disease on plasma protein binding of drugs. *Int J Pharm* **54**:1–13, 1989

Hildebrandt P, Birch K, Mehlsen J: The relationship between the subcutaneous blood flow and the absorption of Lente type insulin. *Acta Endocrinol* **112**(suppl):275, 1986

Holladay JW, Dewey MJ, Yoo SD: Pharmacokinetics and antidepressant activity of fluoxetine in transgenic mice with elevated serum alpha-1-acid glycoprotein levels. *Drug Metab Dispos* **26**:20–24, 1998

Holladay JW, Dewey MJ, Yoo SD: Kinetic interaction between fluoxetine and imipramine as a function of elevated serum alpha-1-acid glycoprotein levels. *J Pharm Pharmacol* **50**:419–424, 1998

Jusko WJ: Pharmacokinetics in disease states changing protein binding. In Benet LZ (ed), *The Effects of Disease States on Drug Pharmacokinetics*. Washington, DC, American Pharmaceutical Association, 1976

Jusko WJ, Gretch M: Plasma and tissue protein binding of drugs in pharmacokinetics. *Drug Metab Rev* **5**:43–140, 1976

Koch-Wester J, Sellers EM: Binding of drugs to serum albumin. *N Engl J Med* **294**:311, 1976

Koch-Wester J, Sellers EM: Drug interactions with coumarin anticoagulants. *N Engl J Med* **285**:547–558, 1971

Kunin CM, Craig WA, Kornguth M, Monson R: Influence of binding on the pharmacologic activity of antibiotics. *Ann N Y Acad Sci* **226**:214–224, 1973

Levy R, Shand D (eds): Clinical implications of drug–protein binding. Proceedings of a symposium sponsored by Syva Company. *Clin Pharmacokinet* **9**(suppl 1), 1984

Limbert M, Siebert G: Serum protein binding and pharmacokinetics of cephalosporins. In Tillement JP, Lindenlaub E (eds), *Protein Binding and Drug Transport*. Stuttgart, Schattauer, 1985

MacKichan JJ: Pharmacokinetic consequences of drug displacement from blood and tissue proteins. *Clin Pharmacokinet* **9**(suppl 1):32–41, 1984

Meijer DKF, van der Sluijs P: Covalent and noncovalent protein binding of drugs: Implication for hepatic clearance, storage and cell-specific drug delivery. *Pharm Res* **6**:105–118, 1989

Meyer MC, Gutlman DE: The bindings of drugs by plasma proteins. *J Pharm Sci* **57**:895–918, 1968

Oie S: Drug distribution and binding. *J Clin Pharmacol* **26**:583–586, 1986

Pardridge WM: Recent advances in blood–brain barrier transport. *Annu Rev Pharmacol Toxicol* **26:**25–39, 1988

Rothschild MA, Oratz M, Schreiber SS: Albumin metabolism. *Gastroenterology* **64:**324–331, 1973

Rowland M: Plasma protein binding and therapeutic monitoring. *Ther Drug Monitor* **2:**29–37, 1980

Rowland M, Tozer TN: *Clinical Pharmacokinetics.* New York, Marcel Dekker, 1985, chap 25

Tillement JP, Houin G, Zini R, et al: The binding of drugs to blood plasma macromolecules: Recent advances and therapeutic significance. *Adv Drug Res* **13:**59–94, 1984

Tillement JP, Lhoste F, Guidicelli JF: Diseases and drug protein binding. *Clin Pharmacokinet* **3:**144–154, 1978

Tillement JP, Zini R, d'Athier P, Vassent G: Binding of certain acidic drugs to human albumin: Theoretical and practical estimation of fundamental parameters. *Eur J Clin Pharmacol* **7:**307–313, 1974

Upton RN: Regional pharmacokinetics, I. Physiological and physicochemical basis. *Biopharm Drug Dispos* **11:**647–662, 1990

Wandell M, Wilcox-Thole WL: Protein binding and free drug concentrations. In Mungall DR (ed), *Applied Clinical Pharmacokinetics.* New York, Raven, 1983, pp 17–48

Zini R, Riant P, Barre J, Tillement JP: Disease-induced variations in plasma protein levels. Implications for drug dosage regimens (Parts 1 and 2). *Clin Pharmacokinet* **19:**147–159, 218–229, 1990

11

HEPATIC ELIMINATION OF DRUGS

ROUTE OF DRUG ADMINISTRATION AND EXTRAHEPATIC DRUG METABOLISM

The decline in plasma concentrations after drug administration results from drug elimination or removal by the body. The elimination of most drugs from the body involves the processes of both metabolism (biotransformation) and renal excretion (see Chapter 6). For many drugs, the principal site of metabolism is the liver. However, other tissues or organs, especially those tissues associated with portals of drug entry into the body, may also be involved in drug metabolism. These sites include the lung, skin, gastrointestinal mucosal cells, microbiological flora in the distal portion of the ileum, and large intestine. The kidney may also be involved in certain drug metabolism reactions.

Knowledge of the fraction of the drug that is eliminated by metabolism and the fraction of drug that is eliminated by excretion is useful information that helps to predict whether a change in drug elimination is likely to be affected by renal disease, hepatic disease, or a drug–drug interaction. Drugs that are highly metabolized (such as phenytoin, theophylline, and lidocaine) demonstrate large intersubject variability in elimination half-lives and are dependent on the intrinsic activity of the biotransformation enzymes, which may be altered by genetic and environmental factors. Intersubject variability in elimination half-lives is less for drugs that are eliminated primarily by renal drug excretion. Renal drug excretion is highly dependent on the *glomerular filtration rate* (GFR). Since GFR is relatively constant among individuals with normal renal function, the elimination of drugs that are primarily excreted unchanged in the urine is less variable.

First-Order Elimination

The rate constant of elimination (k) is the sum of the first-order rate constant for metabolism (k_m) and the first-order rate constant for excretion (k_e):

$$k = k_e + k_m \tag{11.1}$$

In practice, the excretion rate constant (k_e) is easily evaluated for drugs that are primarily renally excreted. Nonrenal drug elimination is usually assumed to be due for the most part to hepatic metabolism, though metabolism or degradation can occur in any organ or tissue that contains metabolic enzymes or is in a degradative condition. Therefore, the rate constant for metabolism (k_m) is difficult to measure directly and is usually found from the difference between k and k_e.

$$k_m = k - k_e$$

A drug may be biotransformed to several metabolites (metabolite A, metabolite B, metabolite C, etc); thus, the metabolism rate constant (k_m) is the sum of the rate constants for the formation of each metabolite:

$$k_m = k_{mA} + k_{mB} + k_{mC} + \cdots + k_{mI} \tag{11.2}$$

The relationship in this equation assumes that the process of metabolism is first order and that the substrate (drug) concentration is very low. Drug concentrations at therapeutic plasma levels for most drugs are much lower than the Michaelis–Menten constant, K_M, and do not saturate the enzymes involved in metabolism. Nonlinear Michaelis–Menten kinetics must be used when drug concentrations saturate metabolic enzymes (see also Chapter 19).

Because these rates of elimination at low drug concentration are considered first-order processes, the percentage of total drug metabolized may be found by the following expression:

$$\% \text{ drug metabolized} = \frac{k_m}{k} \times 100 \tag{11.3}$$

Fraction of Drug Excreted Unchanged (f_e) and Fraction of Drug Metabolized ($1-f_e$)

For most drugs, the *fraction of dose eliminated unchanged* (f_e) and the fraction of dose eliminated as metabolites can be determined. For example, consider a drug that has two major metabolites and is also eliminated by renal excretion (Fig. 11-1). Assume that 100 μM of the drug were given to a patient and the drug was completely

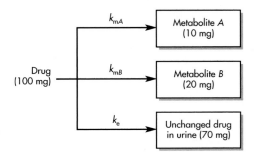

Figure 11-1. Model of a drug that has two major metabolites and is also eliminated by renal excretion.

absorbed (bioavailability factor $F = 1$). A complete (cumulative) urine collection was obtained, and the quantities in parentheses in Figure 11-1 indicate the amounts of each metabolite and unchanged drug that were recovered. The overall elimination half-life ($t_{1/2}$) for this drug was 2.0 hours ($k = 0.347\ \mathrm{hr}^{-1}$).

To determine the renal excretion rate constant, the following relationship is used:

$$\frac{k_e}{k} = \frac{\text{total dose excreted in urine}}{\text{total dose absorbed}} = \frac{D_u^{\infty}}{FD_0} \tag{11.4}$$

where D_u^{∞} is the total amount of unchanged drug recovered in the urine. In this example, k_e is found by proper substitution into Equation 11.4:

$$k_e = (0.347)\ \frac{70}{100} = 0.243\ \mathrm{hr}^{-1}$$

To find the percent of drug eliminated by renal excretion, the following approach may be used:

$$\% \text{ drug excretion} = \frac{k_e}{k} \times 100 = \frac{0.243}{0.347} \times 100 = 70\%$$

Alternatively, because 70 mg of unchanged drug was recovered from a total dose of 100 mg, the percent of drug excretion may be found by

$$\% \text{ drug excretion} = \frac{70}{100} \times 100 = 70\%$$

Therefore, the percent of drug metabolized is $100\% - 70\%$, or 30%.

For many drugs, the literature has approximate values for the fraction of drug (f_e) excreted unchanged in the urine. In this example, the value of k_e may be estimated from the literature values for the elimination half-life of the drug and f_e. Assuming that the elimination half-life of the drug is 2 hours and f_e is 0.7, then k_e is estimated by Equation 11.5.

$$k_e = f_e k \tag{11.5}$$

Because $t_{1/2}$ is 2 hours, k is $0.693/2\ \mathrm{hr} = 0.347\ \mathrm{hr}^{-1}$, and k_e is

$$k_e = (0.7)(0.347) = 0.243\ \mathrm{hr}^{-1}$$

PRACTICAL FOCUS

The percentages of drug excretion and metabolism are clinically useful information. If the renal excretion pathway becomes impaired, as in certain kidney disorders, then less drug will be excreted renally and hepatic metabolism may become the primary drug elimination route. The reverse is true if liver function declines. For example, if in the above situation renal excretion becomes totally impaired $(k_e \approx 0)$, the elimination $t_{1/2}$ can be determined as follows:

$$k = k_m + k_e$$

but

$$k_e \approx 0$$

Therefore,

$$k \approx k_m \approx 0.104 \, \text{hr}^{-1}$$

The new $t_{1/2}$ (after complete renal shutdown) is

$$t_{1/2} = \frac{0.693}{0.104} = 6.7 \, \text{hr}$$

In this example, renal impairment caused the drug elimination $t_{1/2}$ to be prolonged from 2 to 6.7 hours. Clinically, the dosage of this drug must be lowered to prevent the accumulation of toxic drug levels. Methods for adjusting the dose for renal impairment are discussed in Chapter 21.

HEPATIC CLEARANCE

The clearance concept may be applied to any organ and is used as a measure of drug elimination drug by the organ (see also Chapter 6). *Hepatic clearance* may be defined as the volume of blood that perfuses the liver and is cleared of drug per unit of time. As discussed in Chapter 6, total body clearance is composed of all the clearances in the body:

$$Cl_T = Cl_{nr} + Cl_r \tag{11.6}$$

where Cl_T is total body clearance, Cl_{nr} is nonrenal clearance (often equated with hepatic clearance, Cl_h), and Cl_r is renal clearance. Hepatic clearance (Cl_h) is also equal to total body clearance (Cl_T) minus renal clearance (Cl_R) assuming no other organ metabolism, as shown by rearranging Equation 11.6 to

$$Cl_h = Cl_T - Cl_R \tag{11.6a}$$

 # EXAMPLES

1. The total body clearance for a drug is 15 mL/min/kg. Renal clearance accounts for 10 mL/min/kg. What is the hepatic clearance for the drug?

Solution

Hepatic clearance $= 15 - 10 = 5\,\text{mL/min/kg}$

Sometimes the renal clearance is not known, in which case hepatic clearance and renal clearance may be calculated from the percent of intact drug recovered in the urine.

2. The total body clearance of a drug is 10 mL/min/kg. The renal clearance is not known. From a urinary drug excretion study, 60% of the drug is recovered intact and 40% is recovered as metabolites. What is the hepatic clearance for the drug, assuming that metabolism occurs in the liver?

Solution

Hepatic clearance $=$ total body clearance $\times (1 - f_e)$ $\qquad$ **(11.7)**

where $f_e =$ percent of intact drug recovered in the urine.

Hepatic clearance $= 10 \times (1 - 0.6) = 4\ \text{mL/min/kg}$

In this example, the metabolites are recovered completely and hepatic clearance may be obtained as total body clearance times the percent of dose recovered as metabolites. Often, the metabolites are not completely recovered, thus precluding the accuracy of this approach. In this case, hepatic clearance is estimated as the difference between body clearance and renal clearance.

Extrahepatic Metabolism

A few drugs (eg, nitroglycerin) are metabolized extensively outside the liver. This is known as *extrahepatic metabolism*. A simple way to assess extrahepatic metabolism is to calculate hepatic (metabolic) clearance of the drug.

 # EXAMPLES

1. Morphine clearance, Cl_T, for a 75-kg male patient is 1800 mL/min. After an oral dose, 4% of the drug is excreted unchanged in the urine ($f_e = 0.04$). The fraction of drug absorbed after an oral dose of morphine sulfate is 24% ($F = 0.24$). Hepatic blood flow is about 1500 mL/min. Does morphine have any extrahepatic metabolism?

Solution

Since $f_e = 0.04$, renal clearance $Cl_r = 0.04Cl_T$ and nonrenal clearance $Cl_{nr} = (1 - 0.04)\ Cl_T = 0.96Cl_T$. Therefore, $Cl_{nr} = 0.96 \times 1800\ \text{mL/min} = 1728\ \text{mL/min}$.

Since hepatic blood flow is about 1500 mL/min, the drug appears to be metabolized faster than the rate of hepatic blood flow. Thus, at least some of the drug must be metabolized outside the liver. The low fraction of drug absorbed after an oral dose indicates that much of the drug is metabolized before reaching the systemic circulation.

2. Flutamide (Eulexin, Schering), used to treat prostate cancer, is rapidly metabolized to an active metabolite, α-hydroxyflutamide in humans. The steady-state level is 51 ng/mL (range 24–78 ng/mL) after oral multiple doses of 250 mg of flutamide given 3 times daily or every 8 hours (manufacturer-supplied information). Calculate the total body clearance and hepatic clearance assuming that flutamide is 90% metabolized, and is completely (100%) absorbed.

Solution

From Chapters 6 and 8, total body clearance, Cl_T, can be calculated by

$$Cl_T = \frac{FD_0}{C_{av}^\infty \tau}$$

$$Cl_T = \frac{250 \times 1,000,000}{51 \times 8} = 6.127 \times 10^5 \text{ mL/hr} = 10,200 \text{ mL/min}$$

$$Cl_{nr} = 10,200 \text{ mL/min} \times 0.9 = 9180 \text{ mL/min}$$

The Cl_{nr} of flutamide is far greater than the rate of hepatic blood flow (about 1500 mL/min), indicating extensive extrahepatic clearance.

ENZYME KINETICS

The process of *biotransformation* or *metabolism* is the enzymatic conversion of a drug to a metabolite. In the body, the metabolic enzyme concentration is constant at a given site, and the drug (substrate) concentration may vary. When the drug concentration is low relative to the enzyme concentration, there are abundant enzymes to catalyze the reaction, and the rate of metabolism is a first-order process. Saturation of the enzyme occurs when the drug concentration is high, all the enzyme molecules become complexed with drug, and the reaction rate is at a maximum rate; the rate process then becomes a zero-order process (Fig. 11-2). The *maximum reaction rate* is known as V_{max}, and the substrate or drug concentration at which the reaction occurs at half the maximum rate corresponds to a composite parameter K_M. These two parameters determine the profile of a simple enzyme reaction rate at various drug concentrations. The relationship of these parameters is described by the *Michaelis–Menten* equation.

Enzyme kinetics generally considers that 1 mole of drug interacts with 1 mole of enzyme to form an enzyme–drug (ie, enzyme–substrate) intermediate. The enzyme–drug intermediate further reacts to yield a reaction product or a drug

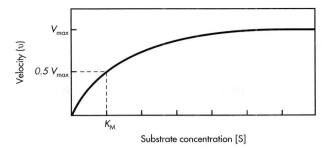

Figure 11-2. *Michaelis–Menten enzyme kinetics. The hyperbolic relationship between enzymatic reaction velocity and the drug substrate concentration is described by Michaelis–Menten enzyme kinetics. The K_M is the substrate concentration when the velocity of the reaction is at $0.5V_{max}$.*

metabolite (Fig. 11-3). The rate process for drug metabolism is described by the Michaelis–Menten equation (see Chapter 9), which assumes that the rate of an enzymatic reaction is dependent on the concentrations of both the enzyme and the drug and that an energetically favored drug–enzyme intermediate is initially formed, followed by the formation of the product and regeneration of the enzyme.

Each rate constant in Figure 11-3 is a first-order reaction rate constant. The following rates may be written:

Rate of intermediate $[ED]$ formation $= k_1[E][D]$

Rate of intermediate $[ED]$ decomposition $= k_2[ED] + k_3[ED]$

$$\frac{d[ED]}{dt} = k_1[E][D] - k_2[ED] - k_3[ED]$$

$$\frac{d[ED]}{dt} = k_1[E][D] - (k_2 + k_3)[ED]$$

(11.8)

By mass balance, the total enzyme concentration $[E_t]$ is the sum of the free enzyme concentration $[E]$ and the enzyme–drug intermediate concentration $[ED]$:

$$[E_t] = [E] + [ED]$$

(11.9)

Rearranging,

$$[E] = [E_t] - [ED]$$

(11.10)

Substituting for $[E]$ in Equation 11.8,

$$\frac{d[ED]}{dt} = k_1([E_t] - [ED])[D] - (k_2 + k_3)[ED]$$

(11.11)

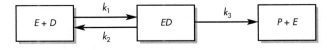

Figure 11-3. *$[D]$ = drug; $[E]$ = enzyme; $[ED]$ = drug–enzyme intermediate; $[P]$ = metabolite or product; k_1, k_2, and k_3 = first-order rate constants. Brackets denote concentration.*

At steady state, the concentration $[ED]$ is constant with respect to time, because the rate of formation of the drug–enzyme intermediate equals the rate of decomposition of the drug–enzyme intermediate. Thus, $d[ED]/dt = 0$, and

$$k_1[E_t][D] = [ED]\{k_1[D] + (k_2 + k_3)\} \tag{11.12}$$

$$[E_t][D] = [ED]\left([D] + \frac{k_2 + k_3}{k_1}\right) \tag{11.13}$$

Let

$$K_M = \frac{k_2 + k_3}{k_1} \tag{11.14}$$

$$[E_t][D] = [ED]([D] + K_M) \tag{11.15}$$

Solving for $[ED]$,

$$[ED] = \frac{[D][E_t]}{[D] + K_M} \tag{11.16}$$

Multiplying by k_3 on both sides,

$$\frac{k_3[E_t][D]}{[D] + K_M} = k_3[ED] \tag{11.17}$$

When all the enzyme is saturated (ie, all the enzyme is in the form of the ED intermediate) because of large drug concentration, the reaction is dependent on the availability of free enzyme, and the reaction proceeds at the maximum velocity, V_{max}.

$$V_{max} = k_3[E_t] \tag{11.18}$$

The *velocity* or rate (v) of the reaction is the rate for the formation of the product (metabolite), which is also the forward rate of decomposition of the ED intermediate (Fig. 11-3).

$$v = k_3[ED] \tag{11.19}$$

Therefore, the velocity of metabolism is given by the equation

$$v = \frac{V_{max}[D]}{[D] + K_M} \tag{11.20}$$

Equation 11.20 describes the rate of metabolite formation, or the Michaelis–Menten equation. The maximum velocity (V_{max}) corresponds to the rate when all of the available enzyme is in the form of the drug–enzyme (ED) intermediate. At V_{max}, the drug (substrate) concentration is in excess, and the forward reaction, $k_3[ED]$, is dependent on the availability of more free enzyme molecules.

The *Michaelis constant*, K_M, is defined as the substrate concentration when the velocity (v) of the reaction is equal to one-half the maximum velocity, or $0.5V_{max}$ (Fig. 11-2). The K_M is a useful parameter that reveals the concentration of the substrate at which the reaction occurs at half V_{max}. In general, for a drug with a large K_M, a higher concentration will be necessary before saturation is reached.

The Michaelis–Menten equation assumes that one drug molecule is catalyzed sequentially by one enzyme at a time. However, enzymes may catalyze more than one drug molecule (multiple sites) at a time, which may be demonstrated *in vitro*. In the body, drug may be eliminated by enzymatic reactions (metabolism) to one or more metabolites and by the excretion of the unchanged drug via the kidney. In Chapter 9, the Michaelis–Menton equation is used for modeling drug conversion in the body.

The relationship of the rate of metabolism to the drug concentration is a nonlinear, hyperbolic curve (Fig. 11-2). To estimate the parameters V_{max} and K_M, the reciprocal of the Michaelis–Menten equation is used to obtain a linear relationship.

$$\frac{1}{v} = \frac{K_M}{V_{max}} \frac{1}{[D]} + \frac{1}{V_{max}} \qquad \textbf{(11.21)}$$

Equation 11.21 is known as the *Lineweaver–Burk equation*, in which K_M and V_{max} may be estimated from a plot of $1/v$ versus $1/[D]$ (Fig. 11-4). Although the Lineweaver–Burk equation is widely used, other rearrangements of the Michaelis–Menten equation have been used to obtain more accurate estimates of V_{max} and K_M. In Chapter 9, drug concentration [D] is replaced by C, which represents drug concentration in the body.

Competitive enzyme inhibition

Noncompetitive enzyme inhibition

Uncompetitive enzyme inhibition

Figure 11-4. Lineweaver–Burk plots. The Lineweaver–Burk equation, which is the reciprocal of the Michaelis–Menten equation, is used to obtain estimates of V_{max} and K_M and to distinguish between various types of enzyme inhibition. [S] is the substrate concentration equal to [D] or drug concentration.

Kinetics of Enzyme Inhibition

Many compounds (eg, cimetidine) may inhibit the enzymes that metabolize other drugs in the body. An inhibitor may decrease the rate of drug metabolism by several different mechanisms. The inhibitor may combine with a cofactor such as $NADPH_2$ needed for enzyme activity, interact with the drug or substrate, or interact directly with the enzyme. Enzyme inhibition may be reversible or irreversible. The type of enzyme inhibition is usually classified by enzyme kinetic studies and observing changes in the K_M and V_{max} (Fig. 11-4).

In the case of *competitive enzyme inhibition,* the inhibitor and drug–substrate compete for the same active center on the enzyme. The drug and the inhibitor may have similar chemical structures. An increase in the drug (substrate) concentration may displace the inhibitor from the enzyme and partially or fully reverse the inhibition. Competitive enzyme inhibition is usually observed by a change in the K_M, but the V_{max} remains the same.

The equation for competitive inhibition is

$$v = \frac{V_{max}[D]}{[D] + K_M\{1 + [I]/k_i\}} \tag{11.22}$$

where $[I]$ is the inhibitor concentration and k_i is the inhibition constant, which is determined experimentally.

In *noncompetitive enzyme inhibition,* the inhibitor may inhibit the enzyme by combining at a site on the enzyme that is different from the active site (ie, an *allosteric site*). In this case, enzyme inhibition depends only on the inhibitor concentration. In noncompetitive enzyme inhibition, K_M is not altered, but V_{max} is lower. Noncompetitive enzyme inhibition cannot be reversed by increasing the drug concentration, because the inhibitor will interact strongly with the enzyme and will not be displaced by the drug.

For a noncompetitive reaction,

$$v = \frac{V_{max}[D]/\{1 + [I]/k_i\}}{[D] + K_M} \tag{11.23}$$

Other types of enzyme inhibition, such as mixed enzyme inhibition and enzyme uncompetitive inhibition, have been described by observing changes in K_M and V_{max}.

Metabolite Pharmacokinetics for Drugs That Follow a One-Compartment Model

The one-compartment model may be used to estimate simultaneously both metabolite formation and drug decline in the plasma. For example, a drug is given by intravenous bolus injection and the drug is metabolized by more than one parallel pathway (Fig. 11-5). Assume that both metabolites and parent drug concentrations follow linear (first-order) pharmacokinetics at therapeutic concentrations. The elimination rate constant and the volume of distribution for each metabolite and the parent drug are obtained from curve fitting of the plasma drug concentration–time

Figure 11-5. Parallel pathway for the metabolism of a drug to metabolite *A* and metabolite *B*. Each metabolite may be excreted and/or further metabolized.

and each metabolite concentration–time curves. If the metabolites are available, each metabolite should be administered IV separately, to verify the pharmacokinetic parameters independently.

The rate of elimination of the metabolite may be faster or slower than the rate of formation of the metabolite from the drug. Generally, metabolites such as glucuronide, sulfate, or glycine conjugates are more polar or more water soluble than the parent drug and will be eliminated more rapidly than the parent drug. Therefore, the rate of elimination of each of these metabolites is more rapid than the rate of formation. In contrast, if the drug is acetylated or metabolized to a less polar or less water-soluble metabolite, then the rate of elimination of the metabolite is slower than the rate of formation of the metabolite. In this case, metabolite accumulation will occur.

Compartment modeling of drug and metabolites is relatively simple and practical. The major shortcoming of compartment modeling is the lack of realistic physiologic information when compared to more sophisticated models that take into account spatial location of enzymes and flow dynamics. However, compartment models are useful for predicting drug and metabolite plasma levels.

For a drug given by IV bolus injection, the metabolite concentration may be predicted from the following equation:

$$C_{\mathrm{m}} = \frac{k_{\mathrm{f}} D_0}{V_{\mathrm{m}}(k_{\mathrm{f}} - k_{\mathrm{em}})}\left(e^{-k_{\mathrm{em}}t} - e^{-k_{\mathrm{f}}t}\right) \tag{11.24}$$

where C_{m} is the metabolite concentration in plasma, k_{em} is the metabolite elimination rate constant, k_{f} is the metabolite formation rate constant, V_{m} is the metabolite volume of distribution, D_0 is the dose of drug, and V_{D} is the apparent volume of distribution of drug. All rate constants are first order.

PRACTICE PROBLEM

A drug is eliminated primarily by biotransformation (metabolism) to a glucuronide conjugate and a sulfate conjugate. A single dose (100 mg) of the drug is given by IV bolus injection, and all elimination processes of the drug follow first-order kinetics. The V_{D} is 10 L and the elimination rate constant for the drug is 0.9 hr^{-1}. The rate constant (k_{f}) for the formation of the glucuronide conjugate is 0.6 hr^{-1}, and the rate constant for the formation of the sulfate conjugate is 0.2 hr^{-1}.

a. Predict the drug concentration 1 hour after the dose.

b. Predict the concentration of glucuronide and sulfate metabolites 1 hour after the dose, if the V_m for both metabolites is the same as for the parent drug and the k_{em} for both metabolites is 0.4 hr^{-1}. (*Note:* V_m and k_{em} usually differ between metabolites and parent drug.) In this example, V_m and k_{em} are assumed to be the same, so that the concentration of the two metabolites may be compared by examining the formation constants.

Solution

The plasma drug concentration 1 hour after the dose may be estimated using the following equation for a one-compartment-model, IV bolus administration:

$$C_p = C_p^0 e^{-kt} = \frac{D_0}{V_D} e^{-kt}$$

$$C_m = \frac{100}{10} e^{-(0.9)(1)} = 4.1\,mg/L$$

The plasma concentrations for the glucuronide and sulfate metabolites 1 hour postdose are estimated after substitution into Equation 11.24.

Glucuronide: $C_m = \dfrac{(0.6)(100)}{10(0.6 - 0.4)}(e^{-(0.4)(1)} - e^{-(0.6)(1)})$

$\qquad\qquad\quad C_m = 3.6\,mg/L$

Sulfate: $C_m = \dfrac{(0.2)(100)}{10(0.2 - 0.4)}(e^{-(0.4)(1)} - e^{-(0.2)(1)})$

$\qquad\qquad\quad C_m = 1.5\,mg/L$

After an IV bolus dose of a drug, the equation describing metabolite concentration formation and elimination by first-order processes is kinetically analogous to drug absorption after oral administration (Chapter 7). Simulated plasma concentration–time curves were generated using Equation 11.24 for the glucuronide and sulfate metabolites, respectively (Fig. 11-6). The rate constant

Figure 11-6. *Simulation showing an IV bolus with formation of two metabolites.*

for the formation of the glucuronide is faster than the rate constant for the formation of the sulfate. Therefore, the time for peak plasma glucuronide concentrations is shorter compared to the time for peak plasma sulfate conjugate concentrations. Equation 11.24 cannot be used if drug metabolism is nonlinear because of enzyme saturation (ie, if metabolism follows Michaelis–Menten kinetics).

Metabolite Pharmacokinetics for Drugs That Follow a Two-Compartment Model

Cephalothin is an antibiotic drug that is metabolized rapidly by hydrolysis in both humans and rabbits. The metabolite desacetylcephalothin has less antibiotic activity than the parent drug. In urine, 18–33% of the drug was recovered as desacetylcephalothin metabolite in a human. The time course of both the drug and the metabolite may be predicted after a given dose from the distribution kinetics of both the drug and the metabolite. Cephalothin follows a two-compartment model after IV bolus injection in a rabbit, whereas the desacetylcephalothin metabolite follows a one-compartment model (Fig. 11-7). After a single IV bolus dose of cephalothin (20 mg/kg) to a rabbit, cephalothin declines as a result of excretion and metabolism to desacetylcephalothin. The plasma levels of both cephalothin and desacetylcephalothin may be calculated using equations based on a model with linear metabolism and excretion.

The equations for cephalothin plasma and tissue levels are the same as those derived in Chapter 4 for a simple two-compartment model, except that the elimination constant k for the drug now consist of $k_e + k_f$, representing excretion and formation constant for metabolite, respectively.

$$C_p = D_0 \left[\frac{k_{21} - a}{V_p(b - a)} e^{-at} + \frac{k_{21} - b}{V_p(a - b)} e^{-bt} \right] \tag{11.25}$$

$$C_t = D_0 \left[\frac{k_{12}}{V_t(b - a)} e^{-at} + \frac{k_{12}}{V_t(a - b)} e^{-bt} \right] \tag{11.26}$$

$$a + b = k + k_{12} + k_{21} \tag{11.27}$$

$$ab = kk_{21} \tag{11.28}$$

$$k = k_f + k_e \tag{11.29}$$

Figure 11-7. Pharmacokinetic model of cephalothin and desacetylcephalothin (metabolite) after an IV bolus dose.

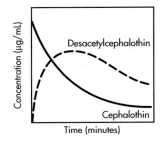

Figure 11-8. Formation of desacetylcephalothin from cephalothin in the rabbit after an IV bolus dose of cephalothin.

The equation for metabolite plasma concentration, C_m, is triexponential, with three preexponential coefficients (C_5, C_6, and C_7) calculated from the various kinetic constants, V_m, and the dose of the drug.

$$C_m = C_5 e^{-k_u t} + C_6 e^{-at} + C_7 e^{-bt} \tag{11.30}$$

$$C_5 = \frac{k_f D_0 k_{21} - k_f D_0 k_u}{V_m (b - k_u)(a - k_u)} \tag{11.31}$$

$$C_6 = \frac{k_f D_0 k_{21} - k_f D_0 a}{V_m (b - a)(k_u - a)} \tag{11.32}$$

$$C_7 = \frac{k_f D_0 k_{21} - k_f D_0 b}{V_m (k_u - b)(a - b)} \tag{11.33}$$

For example, after the IV administration of cephalothin to a rabbit, both metabolite and plasma cephalothin concentration may be fitted to Equations 11.25 and 11.30 simultaneously (Fig. 11-8), with the following parameters obtained using a regression computer program (all rate constants in min^{-1}).

$k_{12} = 0.052$	$k_{21} = 0.009$	$V_m = 285 \text{ mL/kg}$
$k_u = 0.079$	$k = 0.067$	$D_0 = 20 \text{ mg/kg}$
$k_f = 0.045$	$V_p = 548 \text{ mL/kg}$	$k_e = 0.022$

ANATOMY AND PHYSIOLOGY OF THE LIVER

The liver is the major organ responsible for drug metabolism. However, intestinal tissues, lung, kidney, and skin also contain appreciable amounts of biotransformation enzymes, as reflected by animal data (Table 11.1).

The liver is both a synthesizing and an excreting organ. The basic unit of liver is the liver lobule, which contains parenchymal cells, a network of interconnected lymph and blood vessels. The liver consists of large right and left lobes that merge in the middle. The liver is perfused by blood from the hepatic artery; in addition, the large hepatic portal vein that collects blood from various segments of the GI

TABLE 11.1 Distribution of Cytochrome P-450 and Glutathione S-Transferase in the Rat

TISSUE	CYT P-450[a]	GSH TRANSFERASE[b]
Liver	0.73	599
Lung	0.046	61
Kidney	0.135	88
Small intestine	0.042	103
Colon	0.016	—[c]
Skin	0.12	—[c]
Adrenal gland	0.5	308

[a]Cytochrome P-450, nmole/mg microsome protein.
[b]Glutathione S-transferase, nmole conjugate formed/min/mg cytosolic protein.
[c]Values not available.

Adapted from Wolf (1984), with permission.

tract also perfuses the liver (Fig. 11-9). The hepatic artery carries oxygen to the liver and accounts for about 25% of the liver blood supply. The hepatic portal vein carries nutrients to the liver and accounts for about 75% of liver blood flow. The terminal branches of the hepatic artery and portal vein fuse within the liver and mix with the large vascular capillaries known as *sinusoids* (Fig. 11-10). Blood leaves the liver via the hepatic vein, which empties into the vena cava (Fig. 11-9). The liver also secretes bile acids within the liver lobes, which flow through a network of channels and eventually empty into the common bile duct (Figs. 11-10 and 11-11).

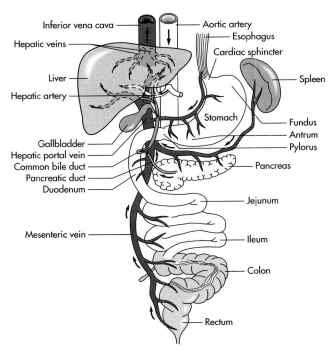

Figure 11-9. The large hepatic portal vein that collects blood from various segments of the GI tract also perfuses the liver.

Figure 11-10. *Intrahepatic distribution of the hepatic and portal veins.*

The common bile duct drains bile and biliary excretion products from both lobes into the gallbladder.

Sinusoids are blood vessels that form a large reservoir of blood, facilitating drug and nutrient removal before the blood enters the general circulation. The sinusoids are lined with endothelial cells, or *Kupffer cells.* Kupffer cells are phagocytic tissue macrophages that are part of the *reticuloendothelial system* (RES). Kupffer cells engulf worn-out red blood cells and foreign material.

Drug metabolism in the liver has been shown to be *flow* and *site dependent.* Some enzymes are reached only when blood flow travels from a given direction. The quantity of enzyme involved in metabolizing drug is not uniform throughout the liver. Consequently, changes in blood flow can greatly affect the fraction of drug metabolized. Clinically, hepatic diseases, such as cirrhosis, can cause tissue fibrosis, necrosis, and hepatic shunt, resulting in changing blood flow and changing bioavailability of drugs (see Chapter 21). For this reason, and in part because of genetic differences in enzyme levels among different subjects and environmental factors, the half-lives of drugs eliminated by drug metabolism are generally very variable.

A pharmacokinetic model simulating hepatic metabolism should involve several elements, including the heterogenicity of the liver, the hydrodynamics of hepatic

Figure 11-11. *Intrahepatic distribution of the hepatic artery, portal vein, and biliary ducts.* (From Lindner HH. *Clinical Anatomy.* Norwalk, CT, Appleton & Lange, 1989, with permission.)

blood flow, the nonlinear kinetics of drug metabolism, and any unusual or patho-logic condition of the subject. Most models in practical use are simple or incomplete models, however, because insufficient information is available about an individual patient. For example, the average hepatic blood flow is usually cited as 1.3–1.5 L/min. Actually, hepatic arterial blood flow and hepatic venous (portal) blood enter the liver at different flow rates, and their drug concentrations are different. It is possible that a toxic metabolite may be transiently higher in some liver tissues and not in others. The pharmacokinetic challenge is to build models that predict regional (organ) changes from easily accessible data, such as plasma drug concentration.

HEPATIC ENZYMES INVOLVED IN THE BIOTRANSFORMATION OF DRUGS

Mixed-Function Oxidases

The liver is the major site of drug metabolism, and the type of metabolism is based on the reaction involved. Oxidation, reduction, hydrolysis, and conjugation are the most common reactions, as discussed under phase I and phase II reactions in the next two sections. The enzymes responsible for oxidation and reduction of drugs (*xenobiotics*) and certain natural metabolites, such as steroids, are monoxygenase enzymes known as *mixed-function oxidases* (MFOs). The hepatic parenchymal cells contain MFOs in association with the *endoplasmic reticulum,* a network of lipopro-tein membranes within the cytoplasm and continuous with the cellular and nuclear membranes. If hepatic parenchymal cells are fragmented and differentially cen-trifuged in an ultracentrifuge, a microsomal fraction, or *microsome*, is obtained from the postmitochondrial supernatant. The microsomal fraction contains fragments of the endoplasmic reticulum.

The mixed-function oxidase enzymes are structural enzymes that constitute an electron-transport system that requires reduced NADPH (NADPH$_2$), molecular oxygen, cytochrome P-450, NADPH–cytochrome P-450 reductase, and phospho-lipid. The phospholipid is involved in the binding of the drug molecule to the cytochrome P-450 and coupling the NADPH–cytochrome P-450 reductase to the cytochrome P-450. Cytochrome P-450 is a heme protein with iron protoporphyrin IX as the prosthetic group. Cytochrome P-450 is the terminal component of an electron-transfer system in the endoplasmic reticulum and acts as both an oxygen- and a substrate-binding locus for drugs and endogenous substrates in conjunction with a flavoprotein reductase, NADPH–cytochrome P-450 reductase. Many lipid-soluble drugs bind to cytochrome P-450, resulting in oxidation (or reduction) of the drug. Cytochrome P-450 consists of closely related isoenzymes (*isozymes*) that differ somewhat in amino acid sequence and drug specificity (see Chapter 12). A general scheme for MFO drug oxidation is described in Figure 11-12.

DRUG BIOTRANSFORMATION REACTIONS

The hepatic biotransformation enzymes play an important role in the inactivation and subsequent elimination of drugs that are not easily cleared through the kidney.

Figure 11-12. Electron flow pathway in the microsomal drug-oxidizing system. (From Alvares and Pratt, 1990, with permission.)

For these drugs—theophylline, phenytoin, acetaminophen, and others—there is a direct relationship between the rate of drug metabolism (*biotransformation*) and the elimination half-life for the drug.

For most biotransformation reactions, the metabolite of the drug is more polar than the parent compound. The conversion of a drug to a more polar metabolite enables the drug to be eliminated more quickly than if the drug remained lipid soluble. A lipid-soluble drug crosses cell membranes and is easily reabsorbed by the renal tubular cells, exhibiting a consequent tendency to remain in the body. In contrast, the more polar metabolite does not cross cell membranes easily, is filtered through the glomerulus, is not readily reabsorbed, and is more rapidly excreted in the urine.

Both the nature of the drug and the route of administration may influence the type of drug metabolite formed. For example, isoproterenol given orally forms a sulfate conjugate in the gastrointestinal mucosal cells, whereas after IV administration, it forms the 3-O-methylated metabolite due to S-adenosylmethionine and catechol-O-methyltransferase. Azo drugs such as sulfasalazine are poorly absorbed after oral administration. However, the azo group of sulfasalazine is cleaved by the intestinal microflora, producing 5-aminosalicylic acid and sulfapyridine, which is absorbed in the lower bowel.

The biotransformation of drugs may be classified according to the pharmacologic activity of the metabolite or according to the biochemical mechanism for each biotransformation reaction. For most drugs, biotransformation results in the formation of a more polar metabolite that is pharmacologically inactive and is eliminated more rapidly than the parent drug (Table 11.2).

For some drugs the metabolite may be pharmacologically active or produce toxic effects. *Prodrugs* are inactive and must be biotransformed in the body to metabolites that have pharmacologic activity. Initially, prodrugs were discovered by serendipity, as in the case of prontosil, which is reduced to the antibacterial agent sulfanilamide. More recently, prodrugs have been intentionally designed to improve

TABLE 11.2   Biotransformation Reactions and Pharmacologic Activity of the Metabolite

REACTION	EXAMPLE
Active Drug to Inactive Metabolite	
Amphetamine Deamination →	Phenylacetone
Phenobarbital Hydroxylation →	Hydroxyphenobarbital
Active Drug to Active Metabolite	
Codeine Demethylation →	Morphine
Procainamide Acetylation →	N-acetylprocainamide
Phenylbutazone Hydroxylation →	Oxyphenbutazone
Inactive Drug to Active Metabolite	
Hetacillin Hydrolysis →	Ampicillin
Sulfasalazine Azoreduction →	Sulfapyridine + 5-aminosalicylic acid
Active Drug to Reactive Intermediate	
Acetaminophen Aromatic Hydroxylation →	Reactive metabolite (hepatic necrosis)
Benzo[a]pyrene Aromatic Hydroxylation →	Reactive metabolite (carcinogenic)

drug stability, increase systemic drug absorption, or to prolong the duration of activity. For example, the antiparkinsonian agent levodopa, crosses the blood–brain barrier and is then decarboxylated in the brain to L-dopamine, an active neurotransmitter. L-Dopamine does not easily penetrate the blood–brain barrier into the brain and therefore cannot be used as a therapeutic agent.

PATHWAYS OF DRUG BIOTRANSFORMATION

Pathways of drug biotransformation may be divided into two major groups of reactions, phase I and phase II reactions. *Phase I*, or *asynthetic reactions*, include oxidation, reduction, and hydrolysis. *Phase II*, or *synthetic* reactions, include conjugations. A partial list of these reactions is presented in Table 11.3. In addition, a

TABLE 11.3   Some Common Drug Biotransformation Reactions

PHASE I REACTIONS	PHASE II REACTIONS
Oxidation	Glucuronide conjugation
Aromatic hydroxylation	Ether glucuronide
Side chain hydroxylation	Ester glucuronide
N-, O-, and S-dealkylation	Amide glucuronide
Deamination	
Sulfoxidation, N-oxidation	Peptide conjugation
N-hydroxylation	
Reduction	Glycine conjugation (hippurate)
Azoreduction	
Nitroreduction	Methylation
Alcohol dehydrogenase	N-methylation
Hydrolysis	O-methylation
Ester hydrolysis	
Amide hydrolysis	Acetylation
	Sulfate conjugation
	Mercapturic acid synthesis

number of drugs that resemble natural biochemical molecules are able to utilize the metabolic pathways for normal body compounds. For example, isoproterenol is methylated by catechol O-methyl transferase (COMT), and amphetamine is deaminated by monamine oxidase (MAO). Both COMT and MAO are enzymes involved in the metabolism of noradrenaline.

Phase I Reactions

Usually, phase I biotransformation reactions occur first and introduce or expose a functional group on the drug molecules. For example, oxygen is introduced into the phenyl group on phenylbutazone by aromatic hydroxylation to form oxyphenbutazone, a more polar metabolite. Codeine is demethylated to form morphine. In addition, the hydrolysis of esters, such as aspirin or benzocaine, will yield more polar products, such as salicylic acid and p-aminobenzoic acid, respectively. For some compounds, such as acetaminophen, benzo[a]pyrene, and other drugs containing aromatic rings, reactive intermediates, such as epoxides, are formed during the hydroxylation reaction. These aromatic epoxides are highly reactive and will react with macromolecules, possibly causing liver necrosis (acetaminophen) or cancer (benzo[a]pyrene). The biotransformation of salicylic acid (Fig. 11-13) demonstrates the variety of possible metabolites that may be formed. It should be noted that salicylic acid is also conjugated directly (phase II reaction) without a preceding Phase I reaction.

Conjugation (Phase II) Reactions

Once a polar constituent is revealed or placed into the molecule, a phase II or conjugation reaction may occur. Common examples include the conjugation of salicyclic acid with glycine to form salicyluric acid or glucuronic acid to form salicylglucuronide (Fig. 11-13).

Figure 11-13. Biotransformation of salicylic acid.
(From Hucker et al, 1980, with permission.)

Conjugation reactions use conjugating reagents, which are derived from biochemical compounds involved in carbohydrate, fat, and protein metabolism. These reactions may include an active, high-energy form of the conjugating agent, such as uridine diphosphoglucuronic acid (UDPGA), acetyl CoA, 3′-phosphoadenosine-5′-phosphosulfate (PAPS), or S-adenosylmethionine (SAM), which, in the presence of the appropriate transferase enzyme, combines with the drug to form the conjugate. Conversely, the drug may be activated to a high-energy compound that then reacts with the conjugating agent in the presence of a transferase enzyme (Fig. 11-14). The major conjugation (phase II) reactions are listed in Tables 11.3 and 11.4.

Some of the conjugation reactions may have limited capacity at high drug concentrations, leading to nonlinear drug metabolism. In most cases, enzyme activity follows first-order kinetics with low drug (substrate) concentrations. At high doses, the drug concentration may rise above the Michaelis–Menten rate constant (K_M), and the reaction rate approaches zero order (V_{max}). Glucuronidation reactions have a high capacity and may demonstrate nonlinear (saturation) kinetics at very high drug concentrations. In contrast, glycine, sulfate, and glutathione conjugations show lesser capacity and demonstrate nonlinear kinetics at therapeutic drug concentrations (Caldwell, 1980). The limited capacity of certain conjugation pathways may be due to several factors, including (1) limited amount of the conjugate transferase, (2) limited ability to synthesize the active nucleotide intermediate, or (3) limited amount of conjugating agent, such as glycine.

In addition, the N-acetylated conjugation reaction shows genetic polymorphism: for certain drugs, the human population may be divided into fast and slow acetylators.

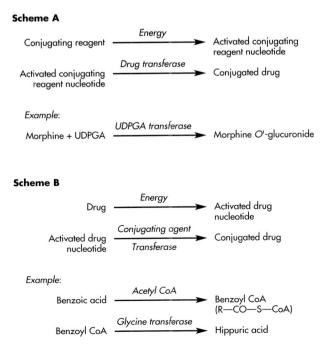

Scheme A

Conjugating reagent — *Energy* → Activated conjugating reagent nucleotide

Activated conjugating reagent nucleotide — *Drug transferase* → Conjugated drug

Example:

Morphine + UDPGA — *UDPGA transferase* → Morphine O′-glucuronide

Scheme B

Drug — *Energy* → Activated drug nucleotide

Activated drug nucleotide — *Conjugating agent* / *Transferase* → Conjugated drug

Example:

Benzoic acid — *Acetyl CoA* → Benzoyl CoA (R—CO—S—CoA)

Benzoyl CoA — *Glycine transferase* → Hippuric acid

Figure 11-14. General scheme for phase II reactions.

TABLE 11.4 Phase II Conjugation Reactions

CONJUGATION REACTION	CONJUGATING AGENT	HIGH-ENERGY INTERMEDIATE	FUNCTIONAL GROUPS COMBINED WITH
Glucuronidation	Glucuronic acid	UDPGA[a]	—OH, —COOH, —NH$_2$, SH
Sulfation	Sulfate	PAPS[b]	—OH, —NH$_2$
Amino acid conjugation	Glycine[c]	Coenzyme A thioesters	—COOH
Acetylation	Acetyl CoA	Acetyl CoA	—OH, —NH$_2$
Methylation	CH$_3$ from S-adenosylmethionine	S-adenosylmethionine	—OH, —NH$_2$
Glutathione (mercapturine acid conjugation)	Glutathione	Arene oxides, epoxides	Aryl halides, epoxides, arene oxides

[a]UDPGA = uridine diphosphoglucuronic acid.
[b]PAPS = 3′-phosphoadenosine-5′-phosphosulfate.
[c]Glycine conjugates are also known as hippurates.

Finally, some of these conjugation reactions may be diminished or defective in cases of inborn errors of metabolism.

Glucuronidation and sulfate conjugation are very common Phase II reactions that result in water-soluble metabolites being rapidly excreted in bile (for some high-molecular-weight glucuronides) and/or urine. Acetylation and mercapturic acid synthesis are conjugation reactions that are often implicated in the toxicity of the drug; they will now be discussed more fully.

Acetylation

The acetylation reaction is an important conjugation reaction for several reasons. First, the acetylated product is usually less polar than the parent drug. The acetylation of such drugs as sulfanilamide, sulfadiazine, and sulfisoxazole produces metabolites that are less water soluble and that in sufficient concentration precipitate in the kidney tubules, causing kidney damage and crystaluria. In addition, a less polar metabolite is reabsorbed in the renal tubule and has a longer elimination half-life. For example, procainamide (elimination half-life of 3 to 4 hours) has an acetylated metabolite, N-acetylprocainamide, which is biologically active and has an elimination half-life of 6 to 7 hours. Lastly, the N-acetyltransferase enzyme responsible for catalyzing the acetylation of isoniazid and other drugs demonstrates a genetic polymorphism. Two distinct subpopulations have been observed to inactivate isoniazid, including the "slow inactivators" and the "rapid inactivators" (Evans, 1968). Therefore, the former group may demonstrate an adverse effect of isoniazide, such as peripheral neuritis, due to the longer elimination half-life and accumulation of the drug.

Glutathione and Mercapturic Acid Conjugation

Glutathione (GSH) is a tripeptide of glutamyl-cysteine-glycine that is involved in many important biochemical reactions. GSH is important in the detoxification of reactive oxygen intermediates into nonreactive metabolites and is the main

Figure 11-15. Mercapturic acid conjugation.

intracellular molecule for protection of the cell against reactive electrophilic compounds. Through the nucleophilic sulfhydryl group of the cysteine residue, GSH reacts nonenzymatically and enzymatically via the enzyme glutathione S-transferase, with reactive electrophilic oxygen intermediates of certain drugs, particularly aromatic hydrocarbons formed during oxidative biotransformation. The resulting GSH conjugates are precursors for a group of drug conjugates known as mercapturic acid (N-acetylcysteine) derivatives. The formation of a mercapturic acid conjugate is shown in Figure 11-15.

The enzymatic formation of GSH conjugates is saturable. High doses of drugs such as acetaminophen (APAP) may form electrophilic intermediates and deplete GSH in the cell. The reactive intermediate covalently bonds to hepatic cellular macromolecules, resulting in cellular injury and necrosis. The suggested antidote for intoxication (overdose) of acetaminophen is the administration of N-acetylcysteine (Mucomyst), a drug molecule that contains available sulfhydryl (R—SH) groups.

Metabolism of Enantiomers

Many drugs are given as mixtures of stereoisomers. Each isomeric form may have different pharmacologic actions and different side effects. For example, the natural thyroid hormone is *l*-thyroxine; whereas the synthetic *d* enantiomer, *d*-thyroxine, lowers cholesterol but does not stimulate basal metabolic rate like the *l* form. Since enzymes as well as drug receptors demonstrate stereoselectivity, isomers of drugs may show differences in biotransformation and pharmacokinetics (Tucker and Lennard, 1990). With improved techniques for isolating mixtures of enantiomers,

TABLE 11.5 *Common Drug Enantiomers*

Atropine	Brompheniramine	Cocaine
Disopyramide	Doxylamine	Ephedrine
Propranolol	Nadolol	Verapamil
Tocainide	Propoxyphene	Morphine
Warfarin	Thyroxine	Flecainide
Ibuprofen	Atenolol	Subutamol
Metoprolol	Terbutaline	

many drugs are now available as pure enantiomers. The rate of drug metabolism and the extent of drug protein binding are often different for each stereoisomer. For example, (S)-(+)disopyramide is more highly bound in humans than (R)-(−)disopyramide. Carprofen, a nonsteroidal anti-inflammatory drug, also exists in both an S and an R configuration. The predominate activity lies in the S configuration. The clearance of the S-carprofen glucuronide through the kidney was found to be faster than that of the R form, 36 versus 26 mL/min (Iwakawa et al, 1989). A list of some common drugs with enantiomers is given in Table 11.5. A review (Ariens and Wuis, 1987) shows that of 475 semisynthetic drugs derived from natural sources, 469 were enantiomers, indicating that the biologic systems are very stereospecific.

The anticonvulsant drug mephenytoin is another example of a drug that exists as R and S enantiomers. Both enantiomers are metabolized by hydroxylation in humans (Wilkinson et al, 1989). After an oral dose of 300 mg of the racemic or mixed form, the plasma concentration of the S form in most subjects was only about 25% of that of the R form. The elimination half-life of the S form (2.13 hours) was much faster than that of the R form (76 hours) in these subjects (Fig. 11-16A). The severity of the sedative side effect of this drug was also less in subjects with rapid metabolism. Hydroxylation reduces the lipophilicity of the metabolite and may reduce the partition of the metabolite into the CNS. Interestingly, some subjects do not

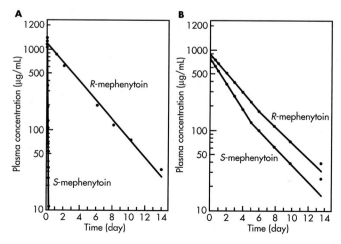

Figure 11-16. *Plasma level of mephenytoin after 300-mg oral dose of the recemic drug.* **A.** *Efficient metabolizer.* **B.** *Poor metabolizer. The plasma levels of the R and S form are different due to different rates of metabolism of the two isomers.*
(Adapted from Wilkinson et al, 1989, with permission.)

metabolize the S form of mephenytoin well, and the severity of sedation in these subjects was increased. The plasma level of the S form was much higher in these subjects (Fig. 11-16B). The variation in metabolic rate was attributed to genetically controlled enzymatic differences within the population.

Regioselectivity

In addition to stereoselectivity, biotransformation enzymes may also be regioselective. In this case, the enzymes catalyze a reaction that is specific for a particular region in the drug molecule. For example, isoproterenol is methylated via catechol-O-methyltransferase and S-adenosylmethionine primarily in the meta position, resulting in a 3-O-methylated metabolite. Very little methylation occurs at the hydroxyl group in the para position.

Species Differences in Hepatic Biotransformation Enzymes

The biotransformation activity of hepatic enzymes can be affected by a variety of factors (Table 11.6). During the early preclinical phase of drug development, drug metabolism studies attempt to identify the major metabolic pathways of a new drug through the use of animal models. For most drugs, different animal species may have different metabolic pathways. For example, amphetamine is mainly hydroxylated in rats, whereas in humans and dogs it is largely deaminated. In many cases, the rates of metabolism may differ among different animal species even though the biotransformation pathways are the same. In other cases, a specific pathway may be absent in a particular species. Generally, the researcher tries to find the best animal model that will be predictive of the metabolic profile in humans.

Variation of Biotransformation Enzymes

Variation in metabolism may be caused by a number of biologic and environmental variables (Table 11.6). *Pharmacogenetics* is the study of genetic differences in drug elimination (Chapter 12). For example, the N-acetylation of isoniazid has been found to be genetically determined, with at least two identifiable groups,

TABLE 11.6 *Sources of Variation in Intrinsic Clearance*

Genetic factors
    Genetic differences within population
    Racial differences among different populations
Environmental factors and drug interactions
    Enzyme induction
    Enzyme inhibition
Physiologic conditions
    Age
    Gender
    Diet/nutrition
    Pathophysiology
Drug dosage regimen
    Route of drug administration
    Dose dependent (nonlinear) pharmacokinetics

including rapid and slow acetylators (Evans et al, 1968). The difference is referred to as *genetic polymorphism*. Individuals with slow acetylation are prone to isoniazid-induced neurotoxicity. Procainamide and hydralazine are other drugs that are acetylated and demonstrate genetic polymorphism.

Another example of genetic differences in drug metabolism is glucose 6-phosphate-dehydrogenase deficiency, which is observed in approximately 10% of African Americans. A well-documented example of genetic polymorphism occurred with phenytoin (Wilkinson et al, 1989). Two phenotypes, EM (efficient metabolizer) and PM (poor metabolizer), were identified in the study population. The PM frequency in Caucasians was about 4% and among Japanese was about 16%. Variation in metabolic rate was also observed with mephobarbital. The incidence of side effects was higher in Japanese subjects, possibly due to a slower oxidative metabolism. Metabolism difference of propranolol due to genetic difference among Chinese populations was also reported (Lai et al, 1995). Some variations in metabolism may be also related to geographic differences rather than racial differences (Bertilsson, 1995).

Besides genetic influence, the basal level of enzyme activity may be altered by environmental factors and exposure to chemicals. Shorter theophylline elimination half-life due to smoking was observed in smoking subjects. Apparently, the aromatic hydrocarbons, such as benzpyrene, that are released during smoking stimulate the enzymes involved in theophylline metabolism. Young children are also known to eliminate theophylline more quickly. Phenobarbital is a potent inducer of a wider variety of hepatic enzymes. Polycyclic hydrocarbons such as 3-methylcholanthrene and benzpyrene also induce hepatic enzyme formation. These compounds are carcinogenic.

Hepatic enzyme activity may also be inhibited by a variety of agents including carbon monoxide, heavy metals, and certain imidazole drugs such as cimetidine. Enzyme inhibition by cimetidine may lead to higher plasma levels and longer elimination of co-administered phenytoin or theophylline. The physiologic condition of the host—including age, gender, nutrition, diet, and pathophysiology—also affects the level of hepatic enzyme activities.

Genetic Variation of Cytochrome P-450 (CYP) Isozymes

The most important enzymes accounting for variation in phase I metabolism of drugs is the cytochrome P-450 enzyme group, which exists in many forms among individuals because of genetic differences (May, 1994; Tucker, 1994; Parkinson, 1996; see also Chapter 12). Initially, the cytochrome P-450 enzymes were identified according to the substrate that was biotransformed. More recently, the genes encoding many of these enzymes have been identified. Multiforms of cytochrome P-450 are referred to as *isozymes,* and are classified into families (originally denoted by Roman numerals: I, II, III, etc) and subfamilies (denoted by A, B, C, etc) based on the similarity of the amino acid sequences of the isozymes. If an isozyme amino acid sequence is 60% similar or more, it is placed within a family. Within the family, isozymes with amino acid sequences of 70% or more similarity are placed into a subfamily, and an Arabic number follows for further classification.

The substrate specificities of the P-450 enzymes appear to be due to the nature of the amino acid residues, the size of the amino acid side chain, and the polarity and charge of the amino acids (Negishi et al, 1996). The individual gene is denoted by an Arabic number (last number) after the subfamily. For example, cytochrome P-450IA2 is involved in the oxidation of caffeine and cytochrome; P-450IID6 is involved in the oxidation of drugs, such as codeine, propranolol, and dextromethorphan. The well-known cytochrome P-450IID6 is responsible for debrisoquine metabolism among individuals showing genetic polymorphism. The vinca alkaloids used in cancer treatment have shown great inter- and intraindividual variabilities. P-450IIIA cytochromes are known to be involved in the metabolism of vindesine, vinblastine, and other vinca alkaloids (Rahmani and Zhou, 1993). Failing to recognize variations in drug clearance in cancer chemotherapy may result in greater toxicity or even therapeutic failure.

There are now at least eight families of cytochrome isozymes known in humans and animals. Cytochrome P-450 I–III (CYP 1–3) is best known for metabolizing clinically useful drugs in humans. Variation in isozyme distribution and content in the hepatocytes may affect intrinsic hepatic clearance of a drug. The levels and activities of the cytochrome P-450 isozymes differ among individuals as a result of genetic and environmental factors. Clinically, it is important to look for evidence of unusual metabolic profiles in patients before dosing. Pharmacokinetic experiments using a "marker" drug such as the antipyrine or dextromethorphan may be used to determine if the intrinsic hepatic clearance of the patient is significantly different from that of an average subject.

Nebert et al (1989) and Hansch and Zhang (1993) have reviewed the nomenclature of the P-450 family of enzymes. A new nomenclature starting with CYP as the root denoting cytochrome P-450, and an Arabic number now replaces the Roman numeral (Table 11.7). The CYP3A subfamily of CYP3 appears to be responsible for the metabolism of a large number of structurally diverse endogenous agents (eg, testosterone, cortisol, progesterone, estradiol) and xenobiotics (eg, nifedipine, lovastatin, midazolam, terfenadine, erythromycin).

The metabolism of debrisoquin is polymorphic in the population, with some individuals having extensive metabolism (EM) and other individuals having poor metabolism (PM). Those individuals who are PM lack functional CYP2D6 (P-450IID6). In EM individuals, quinidine will block CYP2D6 so that genotypic EM individuals appear to be phenotypic PM individuals (Caraco et al, 1996). Some drugs metabolized by CYP2D6 (P-450IID6) are codeine, flecainide, dextromethorphan, imipramine, and other cyclic antidepressants that undergo ring hydroxylation. The

TABLE 11.7   Comparison of P-450 Nomenclatures Currently in Use

P-450 GENE FAMILY/SUBFAMILY	NEW NOMENCLATURE
P-450I	CYP1
P-450IIA	CYP2A
P-450IIB	CYP2B
P-450IIC	CYP2C
P-450IID	CYP2D
P-450IIE	CYP2E
P-450III	CYP3
P-450IV	CYP4

Sources: Nebert et al (1989) and Hansch and Zhang (1993).

inability to metabolize substrates for CYP2D6 results in increased plasma concentrations of the parent drug in PM individuals.

Drug Interactions Involving Drug Metabolism

The enzymes involved in the metabolism of drugs may be altered by diet and the co-administration of other drugs and chemicals. *Enzyme induction* is a drug- or chemical-stimulated increase in enzyme activity, usually due to an increase in the amount of enzyme present. Enzyme induction usually requires some onset time for the synthesis of enzyme protein. For example, rifampin induction occurs within 2 days, while phenobarbital induction takes about 1 week to occur. Enzyme induction for carbmazepine begins after 3 to 5 days and is not complete for approximately 1 month or longer. Smoking can change the rate of metabolism of many cyclic antidepressant drugs (CAD) through enzyme induction (Toney and Ereshefsky, 1995). Agents that induce enzymes include aromatic hydrocarbons (such as benzopyrene, found in cigarette smoke), insecticides (such as chlordane), and drugs such as carbamazepine, rifampin, and phenobarbital (see also Chapter 20). *Enzyme inhibition* may be due to substrate competition or due to direct inhibition of drug-metabolizing enzymes, particularly one of several of the cytochrome P-450 enzymes. Many widely prescribed antidepressants generally known as selective serotonin reuptake inhibitors (SSRIs) have been reported to inhibit the CYP2D6 system, resulting in significantly elevated plasma concentration of co-administered psychotropic drugs. Fluoxetine causes a 10-fold decrease in the clearance of imipramine and desipramine because of its inhibitory effect on hydroxylation (Toney and Ereshefsky, 1995).

A few clinical examples of enzyme inhibitors and inducers are listed in Table 11.8. Diet also affects drug-metabolizing enzymes. For example, plasma theophylline concentrations and theophylline clearance in patients on a high-protein diet are lower than in subjects whose diets are high in carbohydrates. Sucrose or glucose plus fructose decrease the activity of mixed-function oxidases, an effect related to a slower metabolism rate and a prolongation in hexobarbital sleeping time in rats.

TABLE 11.8 Examples of Drug Interactions Affecting Mixed Function Oxidase Enzymes

INHIBITORS OF DRUG METABOLISM	EXAMPLE	RESULT
Acetaminophen	Ethanol	Increased hepatotoxicity in chronic alcoholics
Cimetidine	Warfarin	Prolongation of prothrombin time
Erythromycin	Carbamazepine	Decreased carbazepine clearance
Fluoxetine	Imipramine (IMI)	Decreased clearance of CAD
Fluoxetine	Desipramine (DMI)	Decreased clearance of CAD

INDUCERS OF DRUG METABOLISM	EXAMPLE	RESULT
Carbamazepine	Acetaminophen	Increased acetaminophen metabolism
Rifampin	Methadone	Increased methadone metabolism, may precipitate opiate withdrawal
Phenobarbital	Dexamethasone	Decreased dexamethasone elimination half-life
Rifampin	Prednisolone	Increased elimination of prednisolone

TABLE 11.9   Change in Drug Availability due to Oral Coadministration of Grapefruit Juice

DRUG	STUDY
Triazolam	Hukkinen et al, 1995
Midazolam	Kupferschmidt et al, 1995
Cyclosporine	Yee et al, 1995
Coumarin	Merket et al, 1994
Nisoldipine	Baily DG et al, 1993a
Felodipine	Baily DG et al, 1993b

Chronic administration of 5% glucose was suggested to affect sleeping time in subjects receiving barbiturates. A decreased intake of fatty acids may lead to decreased basal MFO activities (Campbell, 1977) and affect the rate of drug metabolism.

The protease inhibitor saquinavir mesylate (Invirase, Roche), has very low bioavailability—only about 4%. In studies conducted by Hoffmann-La Roche, the area under the curve (AUC) of saquinavir was increased to 150% when the volunteers took a 150-mL glass of grapefruit juice with the saquinavir, and then another 150-mL glass an hour later. Concentrated grapefruit juice increased the AUC up to 220%. Naringin, a bioflavonoid in grapefruit juice, was found to be at least partially responsible for the inhibition of the enzyme CYP3A4, present in the liver and the intestinal wall, which metabolizes saquinavir, resulting in an increase in its AUC. Ketoconazole and ranitidine (Zantac) may also increase the AUC of saquinavir by inhibition of the cytochrome P-450 enzymes. In contrast, rifampin greatly reduces the AUC of saquinavir, apparently due to enzymatic stimulation. Other drugs recently shown to have increased bioavailability when taken with grapefruit juice include several sedatives and the anticoagulant coumarin (Table 11.9). Increases in drug levels may be dangerous, and the pharmacokinetics of drugs with potential interactions should be closely monitored. More complete tabulations of the cytochrome P-450s are available (Flockhart, 2003; Parkinson, 1996; Cupp and Tracy, 1998); some examples are given in Table 11.10

For new drugs, the potential for drug metabolism/interaction is studied *in vitro* and/or *in vivo* by identifying whether the drug is a substrate for the common CYP450 subfamilies (FDA Guidance for Industry, 1999). Examples of substrates include, but are not limited to, (1) midazolam, buspirone, felodipine, simvastatin, or lovastatin for CYP3A4; (2) theophylline for CYP1A2; (3) S-warfarin for CYP2C9; and (4) desipramine for CYP2D6.

Other substrates mentioned for further study of a CYP3A4-interacting investigational drug include dihydropyridine calcium channel blockers and triazolobenzodiazepines. For CYP2D6 inhibiting, the investigational drug might include metoprolol.

Since metabolism usually occurs in the liver (some enzymes such as CYP3A4 are also important in gut metabolism), human liver microsomes provide a convenient way to study CYP450 metabolism. Microsomes are a subcellular fraction of tissue obtained by differential high-speed centrifugation. The key CYP450 enzymes are collected in the microsomal fraction. The CYP450 enzymes retain their activity for many years in microsomes or whole liver stored at low temperature. Hepatic microsomes can be obtained commercially, with or without prior phenotyping, for most important CYP450 enzymes. The cDNAs for the common CYP450s have been

TABLE 11.10   *Cytochrome P450 Isoforms and Examples*

CYP1A2	Substrates—amitriptyline, imipramine, theophylline (other enzymes also involved); induced by smoking
	Fluvoxamine, some quinolones and grapefruit juice are inhibitors
CYP2B6	Substrates—cyclophosphamide, methadone
CYP2C9	Metabolism of S-warfarin and tolbutamide by CYP2C9
	Substrates—NSAIDs—ibuprofen, diclofenac
CYP2C19	Omeprazole, S-mephenytoin, and Propranolol
	Diazepam (mixed), and imipramine (mixed)
	Inhibitors: cimetidine, fluoxetine, and ketoconazole.
CYP2D6	Many antidepressants, β-blockers are metabolized by CYP2D6
	SRIIs, cimetidine are inhibitors
	Substrates—amitriptyline, imipramine, fluoxetine, antipsychotics (haloperidol, thioridazine)
	Inhibitors—paroxetine, fluoxetine, sertraline, fluvoxamine, cimetidine, haloperidol
CYP2E1	Substrates—acetaminophen, ethanol, halothane
	Induced by INH and disulfiram
CYP3A4, 5, 6	CYP3A subfamilies are the most abundant cytochrome enzymes in humans and include many key therapeutic and miscellaneous groups:
	Ketoconazole, atorvastatin, lovastatin.
	Azithromycin, clarithromycins, amitriptyline
	Benzodiazepines—alprazolam, triazolam, midazolam
	Calcium blockers—verapamil, diltiazem
	Protease inhibitors—ritonavir, saquinavir, indinavir

Examples based on Flockardt (2003), Cupp and Tracy (1998), and Desta et al (2002).

cloned, and the recombinant human enzymatic proteins have been expressed in a variety of cells. These recombinant enzymes provides an excellent way to confirm results using microsomes. Pharmacokinetic endpoints recommended for assessment of the substrate are (1) exposure measures such as AUC, C_{max}, time to C_{max} (T_{max}), and others as appropriate; and (2) pharmacokinetic parameters such as clearance, volumes of distribution, and half-lives (FDA Guidance for Industry, 1999). For metabolism induction studies, *in-vivo* studies are more relied upon because enzyme induction may not be well predicted from *in-vitro* results. Considerations in drug-metabolizing/interaction studies include: (1) acute or chronic use of the substrate and/or interacting drug; (2) safety considerations, including whether a drug is likely to be an NTR (narrow therapeutic range) or non-NTR drug; (3) pharmacokinetic and pharmacodynamic characteristics of the substrate and interacting drugs; and (4) the need to assess induction as well as inhibition. The inhibiting/inducing drugs and the substrates should be dosed so that the exposures of both drugs are relevant to their clinical use.

FIRST-PASS EFFECTS

For some drugs, the route of administration affects the metabolic rate of the compound. For example, a drug given parenterally, transdermally, or by inhalation may distribute within the body prior to metabolism by the liver. In contrast, drugs given orally are normally absorbed in the duodenal segment of the small intestine and transported via the mesenteric vessels to the hepatic portal vein and then to the liver before entering the systemic circulation. Drugs that are highly metabolized by the liver or by the intestinal mucosal cells demonstrate poor systemic availability when given orally. This rapid metabolism of an orally administered drug before reaching the general circulation is termed *first-pass effect* or *presystemic elimination*.

Evidence of First-Pass Effects

First-pass effects may be suspected when there is a lack of parent (or intact) drug in the systemic circulation after oral administration. In such a case, the AUC for a drug given orally is less than the AUC for the same dose of drug given intravenously. From experimental findings in animals, first-pass effects may be assumed if the intact drug appears in a cannulated hepatic portal vein but not in general circulation.

For an orally administered drug that is chemically stable in the gastrointestinal tract and is 100% systemically absorbed ($F = 1$), the area under the plasma drug concentration curve, $AUC^{\infty}_{0,\,oral}$, should be the same when the same drug dose is given intravenously, $AUC^{\infty}_{0,\,IV}$. Therefore, the absolute bioavailability (F) may reveal evidence of drug being removed by the liver due to first-pass effects as follows:

$$F = \frac{[AUC]^{\infty}_{0,\,oral} / D_{0,\,oral}}{[AUC]^{\infty}_{0,\,IV} / D_{0,\,IV}} \tag{11.34}$$

For drugs that undergo first-pass effects $AUC^{\infty}_{0,\,oral}$ is smaller than $AUC^{\infty}_{0,\,IV}$ and $F < 1$. Drugs such as propranolol, morphine, and nitroglycerin have F values less than 1 because these drugs undergo significant first-pass effects.

Liver Extraction Ratio

Because there are many other reasons for a drug to have a reduced F value, the extent of first-pass effects is not very precisely measured from the F value. The liver extraction ratio (ER) provides a direct measurement of drug removal from the liver after oral administration of a drug.

$$ER = \frac{C_a - C_v}{C_a} \tag{11.35}$$

where C_a is the drug concentration in the blood entering the liver and C_v is the drug concentration leaving the liver.

Because C_a is usually greater than C_v, ER is usually less than 1. For example, for propranolol, ER or $[E]$ is about 0.7—that is, about 70% of the drug is actually removed by the liver before it is available for general distribution to the body. By contrast, if the drug is injected intravenously, most of the drug would be distributed before reaching the liver, and less of the drug would be metabolized.

Relationship between Absolute Bioavailability and Liver Extraction

Liver ER provides a measurement of liver extraction of a drug orally administered. Unfortunately, sampling of drug from the hepatic portal vein and artery is difficult and performed mainly in animals. Animal ER values may be quite different from those in humans. The following relationship between bioavailability and liver extraction enables a rough estimate of the extent of liver extraction:

$$F = 1 - ER - F'' \tag{11.36}$$

where F is the fraction of bioavailable drug, ER is the drug fraction extracted by the liver, and F'' is the fraction of drug removed by nonhepatic process.

If F'' is assumed to be negligible—that is, there is no loss of drug due to chemical degradation, gut metabolism, and incomplete absorption—ER may be estimated from

$$F = 1 - ER \tag{11.37}$$

After substitution of Equation 11.34 into Equation 11.37,

$$ER = 1 - \frac{[AUC]_{0, \text{oral}}^{\infty} / D_{0, \text{oral}}}{[AUC]_{0, \text{IV}}^{\infty} / D_{0, \text{IV}}} \tag{11.38}$$

ER is a rough estimation of liver extraction for a drug. Many other factors may alter this estimation: the size of the dose, the formulation of the drug, and the pathophysiologic condition of the patient all may affect the ER value obtained.

Liver ER provides valuable information in determining the oral dose of a drug when the intravenous dose is known. For example, propranolol requires a much higher oral dose compared to an IV dose to produce equivalent therapeutic blood levels, because of oral drug extraction by the liver. Because liver extraction is affected by blood flow to the liver, dosing of drug with extensive liver metabolism may produce erratic plasma drug levels. Formulation of this drug into an oral dosage form requires extensive, careful testing.

Estimation of Reduced Bioavailability due to Liver Metabolism and Variable Blood Flow

Blood flow to the liver plays an important role in the amount of drug metabolized after oral administration. Changes in blood flow to the liver may substantially alter the percentage of drug metabolized and therefore alter the percentage of bioavailable drug. The relationship between blood flow, hepatic clearance, and percent of drug bioavailable is

$$F' = 1 - \frac{Cl_h}{Q} = 1 - ER \tag{11.39}$$

where Cl_h is the hepatic clearance of the drug and Q is the effective hepatic blood flow. F' is the bioavailability factor obtained from estimates of liver blood flow and hepatic clearance, ER.

This equation provides a reasonable approach for evaluating the reduced bioavailability due to first-pass effect. The usual effective hepatic blood flow is 1.5 L/min, but it may vary from 1 to 2 L/min depending on diet, food intake, physical activity or drug intake (Rowland, 1973). For the drug propoxyphene hydrochloride, F' has been calculated from hepatic clearance (990 mL/min) and an assumed liver blood flow of 1.53 L/min:

$$F' = 1 - \frac{0.99}{1.53} = 0.35$$

The results, showing that 35% of the drug is systemically absorbed after liver extraction, are reasonable compared with the experimental values for propranolol.

Presystemic elimination or *first-pass effect* is a very important consideration for drugs that have a high extraction ratio (Table 11.11). Drugs with low extraction ratios, such as theophylline, have very little presystemic elimination, as demonstrated by complete systemic absorption after oral administration. In contrast, drugs with high extraction ratios have poor bioavailability when given orally. Therefore, the oral dose must be higher than the intravenous dose to achieve the same therapeutic response. In some cases, oral administration of a drug with high presystemic elimination, such as nitroglycerin, may be impractical due to very poor oral bioavailability, and thus a sublingual, transdermal, or nasal route of administration may be preferred.

Furthermore, if an oral drug product has slow dissolution characteristics or release rate, then more of the drug will be subject to first-pass effect compared to doses of drug given in a more bioavailable form (such as a solution). In addition, drugs with high presystemic elimination tend to demonstrate more variability in drug bioavailability between and within individuals. Finally, the quantity and quality of the metabolites formed may vary according to the route of drug administration, which may be clinically important if one or more of the metabolites has pharmacologic or toxic activity.

To overcome first-pass effect, the route of administration of the drug may be changed. For example, nitroglycerin may be given sublingually or topically, and xylocaine may be given parenterally to avoid the first-pass effects. Another way to overcome first-pass effects is to either enlarge the dose or change the drug product to a more rapidly absorbable dosage form. In either case, a large amount of drug is presented rapidly to the liver, and some of the drug will reach the general circulation in the intact state.

TABLE 11.11   Hepatic and Renal Extraction Ratios of Representative Drugs

EXTRACTION RATIOS		
LOW (<0.3)	**INTERMEDIATE (0.3–0.7)**	**HIGH (>0.7)**
HEPATIC EXTRACTION		
Amobarbital	Aspirin	Arabinosyl-cytosine
Antipyrine	Quinidine	Encainide
Chloramphenicol	Desipramine	Isoproterenol
Chlordiazepoxide	Nortriptyline	Meperidine
Diazepam		Morphine
Digitoxin		Nitroglycerin
Erythromycin		Pentazocine
Isoniazid		Propoxyphene
Phenobarbital		Propranolol
Phenylbutazone		Salicylamide
Phenytoin		Tocainide
Procainamide		Verapamil
Salicylic acid		
Theophylline		
Tolbutamide		
Warfarin		

From Rowland (1978), with permission, and Brouwer et al (1992).

Although Equation 11.39 seems to provide a convenient way of estimating the effect of liver blood flow on bioavailability, this estimation is actually more complicated. A change in liver blood flow may alter hepatic clearance and F'. A large blood flow may deliver enough drug to the liver to alter the rate of metabolism. In contrast, a small blood flow may decrease the delivery of drug to the liver and become the rate-limiting step for metabolism. The hepatic clearance of a drug is usually calculated from plasma drug data rather than whole-blood data. Significant nonlinearity may be the result of drug equilibration due to partitioning into the red blood cells.

 # EXAMPLES

1. A new propranolol 5-mg tablet was developed and tested in volunteers. The bioavailability of propranolol from the tablet was 70% compared to an oral solution of propranolol, and 21.6%, compared to an intravenous dose of propranolol. Calculate the relative and absolute bioavailability of the propranolol tablet. Comment on the feasibility of further improving the absolute bioavailability of the propranolol tablet.

Solution

The relative bioavailability of propranolol from the tablet compared to the solution is 70% or 0.7. The absolute bioailability, F, of propranolol from the tablet compared to the IV dose is 21.6%, or $F = 0.216$. From the table of ER values (Table 11.12), the ER for propranolol is 0.6 to 0.8. If the product is perfectly formulated, ie, the tablet dissolves completely and all the drug is released from the tablet, the fraction of drug absorbed after deducting for the fraction of drug extracted by the liver is

$$F' = 1 - ER$$
$$F' = 1 - 0.7 \qquad (\text{mean ER} = 0.7)$$
$$F' = 0.3$$

Thus, under normal conditions, total systemic absorption of propranolol from an oral tablet would be about 30% ($F = 0.3$). The measurement of relative bioavailability for propranolol is always performed against a reference standard given by the same route of administration and can have a value greater than 100%.

The following shows a method for calculating the absolute bioavailability from the relative bioavailability provided the ER is accurately known. Using the above example,

Absolute availability of the solution $= 1 - ER = 1 - 0.7 = 0.3 = 30\%$
Relative availability of the solution $= 100\%$

TABLE 11.12   Pharmacokinetic Classification of Drugs Eliminated Primarily by Hepatic Metabolism

DRUG CLASS	EXTRACTION RATIO (approx.)	PERCENT BOUND
Flow Limited		
Lidocaine	0.83	45–80[a]
Propranolol	0.6–0.8	93
Pethidine (meperidine)	0.60–0.95	60
Pentazocine	0.8	—
Propoxyphene	0.95	—
Nortriptyline	0.5	95
Morphine	0.5–0.75	35
Capacity Limited, Binding Sensitive		
Phenytoin	0.03	90
Diazepam	0.03	98
Tolbutamide	0.02	98
Warfarin	0.003	99
Chlorpromazine	0.22	91–99
Clindamycin	0.23	94
Quinidine	0.27	82
Digitoxin	0.005	97
Capacity Limited, Binding Insensitive		
Theophylline	0.09	59
Hexobarbital	0.16	—
Amobarbital	0.03	61
Antipyrine	0.07	10
Chloramphenicol	0.28	60–80
Thiopental	0.28	72
Acetaminophen	0.43	5[a]

[a]Concentration dependent in part.

From Blaschke (1977), with permission.

Absolute availability of the tablet $= x\%$
Relative availability of the tablet $= 70\%$

$$x = \frac{30 \times 70}{100} = 21\%$$

Therefore, this product has a theoretical absolute bioavailability of 21%. The small difference of calculated and actual (the difference between 21.6% and 21%) absolute bioavailability is due largely to liver extraction fluctuation. All calculations are performed with the assumption of linear pharmacokinetics, which is generally a good approximation. ER may deviate significantly with changes in blood flow or other factors.

2. Fluvastatin sodium (Lescol, Novartis) is a drug used to lower cholesterol. The absolute bioavailability after an oral dose is reported to be 19–29%. The drug is rapidly and completely absorbed (manufacturer's product information). What are the reasons for the low oral bioavailability in spite of reportedly good absorption? What is the extraction ratio of fluvastatin? (The absolute bioavailability, F, is 46%, according to values reported in the literature.)

Solution

Assuming the drug to be completely absorbed as reported, using Equation 11.37,

ER = 1 − 0.46 = 0.54

Thus, 54% of the drug is lost due to first-pass effect because of a relatively large extraction ratio. Since bioavailability is only 19–29%, there is probably some non-hepatic loss according to Equation 11.36. Fluvastatin sodium was reported to be extensively metabolized, with some drug excreted in feces.

Relationship between Blood Flow, Intrinsic Clearance, and Hepatic Clearance

Although Equation 11.39 seems to provide a convenient way of estimating the effect of liver blood flow on bioavailability, this estimation is actually more complicated. For example, factors that affect the hepatic clearance of a drug include (1) blood flow to the liver, (2) intrinsic clearance, and (3) the fraction of drug bound to protein.

A change in liver blood flow may alter hepatic clearance and F'. A large blood flow may deliver enough drug to the liver to alter the rate of metabolism. In contrast, a small blood flow may decrease the delivery of drug to the liver and become the rate-limiting step for metabolism. The hepatic clearance of a drug is usually calculated from plasma drug data rather than whole-blood data. Significant nonlinearity may be the result of drug equilibration due to partitioning into the red blood cells.

In experimental animals, the blood flow (Q) to the liver, the drug concentration in the artery (C_a), and the drug concentration in the vein (C_v) may be measured. As the arterial blood containing drug perfuses the liver, a certain portion of the drug is removed by metabolism and/or biliary excretion. Therefore, the drug concentration in the vein is less than the drug concentration in the artery. An extraction ratio may be expressed as 100% of the drug entering the liver less the relative concentration (C_v/C_a) of drug that is removed by the liver.

$$ER = \frac{C_a - C_v}{C_a} \tag{11.40}$$

The ER may vary from 0 to 1.0. An ER of 0.25 means that 25% of the drug was removed by the liver. If both the ER for the liver and the blood flow to the liver are known, then hepatic clearance may be calculated by the following expression:

$$Cl_h = \frac{Q\,(C_a - C_v)}{C_a} = Q \times ER \tag{11.41}$$

For some drugs (such as isoproterenol, lidocaine, and nitroglycerin), the extraction ratio is high (greater than 0.7), and the drug is removed by the liver almost as rapidly as the organ is perfused by blood in which the drug is contained. For drugs with very high extraction ratios, the rate of drug metabolism is sensitive to changes in hepatic blood flow. Thus, an increase in blood flow to the liver will increase the rate of drug removal by the organ. Propranolol, a β-adrenergic blocking agent, decreases hepatic blood flow by decreasing cardiac output. In such a case, the drug decreases its own clearance through the liver when given orally. Many drugs that demonstrate first-pass effects are drugs that have high extraction ratios with respect to the liver.

Intrinsic clearance (Cl_{int}) is used to describe the total ability of the liver to metabolize a drug in the absence of flow limitations, reflecting the inherent activities of the mixed-function oxidases and all other enzymes. Intrinsic clearance is a distinct characteristic of a particular drug, and as such, it reflects the inherent ability of the liver to metabolize the drug. Intrinsic clearance may be shown to be analogous to the ratio V_{max}/K_M for a drug that follows Michaelis–Menten kinetics. Hepatic clearance is a concept for characterizing drug elimination based on both blood flow and the intrinsic clearance of the liver, as shown in Equation 11.42.

$$Cl_h = Q \frac{Cl_{int}}{Q + Cl_{int}}$$ **(11.42)**

When the blood flow to the liver is constant, hepatic clearance is equal to the product of blood flow (Q) and the extraction ratio (ER) equation 11.41. However, the hepatic clearance of a drug is not constant. Hepatic clearance changes with blood flow (Fig. 11-17) and the intrinsic clearance of the drug, as described in Equation 11.42. For drugs with low extraction ratios (eg, theophylline, phenylbutazone, and procainamide), the hepatic clearance is less affected by hepatic blood flow. Instead, these drugs are more affected by the intrinsic activity of the mixed-function oxidases. Describing clearance in terms of all the factors in a physiologic model allow drug clearance to be estimated when physiologic or disease condition causes changes in blood flow or intrinsic enzyme activity. Smoking, for example, can increase the intrinsic clearance for the metabolism of many drugs.

Changes or alterations in mixed-function oxidase activity or biliary secretion can affect the intrinsic clearance and thus the rate of drug removal by the liver. Drugs

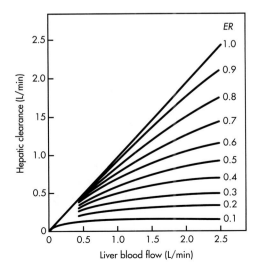

Figure 11-17. The relationship between liver blood flow and total hepatic clearance for drugs with varying extraction rates (*ER*).

that show low extraction ratios and are eliminated primarily by metabolism demonstrate marked variation in overall elimination half-lives within a given population. For example, the elimination half-life of theophylline varies from 3 to 9 hours. This variation in $t_{1/2}$ is thought to be due to genetic differences in intrinsic hepatic enzyme activity. Moreover, the elimination half-lives of these same drugs are also affected by enzyme induction, enzyme inhibition, age of the individual, nutritional, and pathologic factors.

Clearance may also be expressed as the rate of drug removal divided by plasma drug concentration:

$$Cl_h = \frac{\text{rate of drug removed by the liver}}{C_a} \tag{11.43}$$

Because the rate of drug removal by the liver is usually the rate of drug metabolism, Equation 11.43 may be expressed in terms of hepatic clearance and drug concentration entering the liver (C_a):

$$\text{Rate of liver drug metabolism} = Cl_h C_a \tag{11.44}$$

HEPATIC CLEARANCE OF A PROTEIN-BOUND DRUG: RESTRICTIVE AND NONRESTRICTIVE CLEARANCE FROM BINDING

It is generally assumed that protein-bound drugs are not easily metabolized (*restrictive clearance*), while free (unbound) drugs are subject to metabolism. Protein-bound drugs do not easily diffuse through cell membranes, while free drugs can reach the site of the mixed-function oxidase enzymes easily. Therefore, an increase in the free drug concentration in the blood will make more drug available for hepatic extraction. The concept is discussed under restrictive and nonrestrictive clearance (Gillette, 1973) of protein-bound drugs (see Chapter 10).

Most drugs are *restrictively* cleared—for example, diazepam, quinidine, tolbutamide, and warfarin. The clearance of these drugs is proportional to the fraction of unbound drug (f_u). However, some drugs, such as propranolol, morphine, and verapamil, are *nonrestrictively* extracted by the liver regardless of drug bound to protein or free. Kinetically, a drug is nonrestrictively cleared if its hepatic extraction ratio (ER) is greater than the fraction of free drug (f_u), and the rate of drug clearance is unchanged when the drug is displaced from binding. Mechanistically, the protein binding of a drug is a reversible process and for a nonrestrictively bound drug, the free drug gets "stripped" from the protein during the process of drug metabolism. The elimination half-life of a nonrestrictively cleared drug is not significantly affected by a change in the degree of protein binding. This is an analogous situation to a protein-bound drug that is actively secreted by the kidney.

For a drug with restrictive clearance, the relationship of blood flow, intrinsic clearance, and protein binding is

$$Cl_h = Q\left(\frac{f_u Cl'_{int}}{Q + f_u Cl'_{int}}\right) \tag{11.45}$$

where f_u is the fraction of drug unbound in the blood and Cl'_{int} is the intrinsic clearance of free drug. Equation 11.45 is derived by substituting $f_u Cl'_{int}$ for Cl_{int} in Equation 11.42.

From Equation 11.45, when Cl'_{int} is very small in comparison to hepatic blood flow (ie, $Q > Cl'_{int}$), then Equation 11.46 reduces to Equation 11.47.

$$Cl_h = \frac{Q f_u\, Cl'_{int}}{Q} \qquad\qquad (11.46)$$

$$Cl_h = f_u Cl'_{int} \qquad\qquad (11.47)$$

As shown in Equation 11.47, a change in Cl'_{int} or f_u will cause a proportional change in Cl_h for drugs with protein binding.

In the case where Cl'_{int} for a drug is very large in comparison to flow ($Cl'_{int} \gg Q$), Equation 11.48 reduces to Equation 11.49.

$$Cl_h = \frac{Q f_u\, Cl'_{int}}{f_u\, Cl'_{int}} \qquad\qquad (11.48)$$

$$Cl_h \approx Q \qquad\qquad (11.49)$$

Thus, for drugs with a very high Cl'_{int}, Cl_h is dependent on hepatic blood flow, and independent of protein binding.

For restrictively cleared drugs, change in binding generally alters drug clearance. For a drug with low hepatic extraction ratio and low plasma binding, clearance will increase, but not significantly, when the drug is displaced from binding. For a drug highly bound to plasma proteins (more than 90%), a displacement from these binding sites will significantly increase the free concentration of the drug, and clearance (both hepatic and renal clearance) will increase (Chapter 10). There are some drugs that are exceptional and show a paradoxical increase in hepatic clearance despite an increase in protein binding. In one case, increased binding to AAG (α, acid glycoprotein) was found to concentrate drug in the liver, leading to an increased rate of metabolism because the drug was nonrestrictively cleared in the liver.

Effect of Changing Intrinsic Clearance and/or Blood Flow on Hepatic Extraction and Elimination Half-Life after IV and Oral Dosing

The effects of altered hepatic intrinsic clearance and liver blood flow on the blood level–time curve have been described by Wilkinson and Shand (1975) after both IV and oral dosing (Figs. 11-18 and 11-19). These illustrations show how changes in intrinsic clearance and blood flow affect the elimination half-life, first-pass effects, and bioavailability of the drug as represented by the area under the curve.

Effect of Changing Intrinsic Clearance
For drugs with low ER, the effect of doubling Cl_{int} (see Fig. 11-18) from 0.167 to 0.334 L/min increases both the extraction ratio (ER) and clearance (Cl) of the

Figure 11-18. The effect of increasing hepatic total intrinsic clearance (Cl_{int}) on the total blood concentration–time curves after intravenous (upper panels) and oral (lower panels) administration of equal doses of two totally metabolized drugs. The left panels refer to a drug with an initial Cl_{int} equivalent to an extraction ratio of 0.1 at a liver blood flow of 1.5 L/min and the right panels to one with an initial extraction ratio of 0.9. The AUCs after oral administration are inversely proportional to Cl_{int}.
(From Wilkinson and Shand, 1975, with permission.)

drug, leading to a steeper slope (dotted line) or shorter $t_{1/2}$. The elimination half-life decreases about 50% due to the increase in intrinsic clearance. Figure 11-18 (bottom left) shows the change in drug concentrations after oral administration when Cl_{int} doubles. In this case, there is a decrease in both AUC and $t_{1/2}$ (dashed line) due the increase in clearance of the drug.

For drugs with high ER, the effect of doubling Cl_{int} (see Fig. 11-18) from 13.70 to 27.00 L/min increases both the extraction ratio and clearance only moderately, leading to a slightly steeper slope. The elimination half-life decreases only marginally. Figure 11-18 (bottom right) shows the change in drug levels after oral administration. Some decrease in AUC is observed and the $t_{1/2}$ is shortened moderately.

The elimination half-life of a drug with a low extraction ratio is decreased significantly by an increase in hepatic enzyme activity. In contrast, the elimination half-life of a drug with a high extraction ratio is not markedly affected by an increase

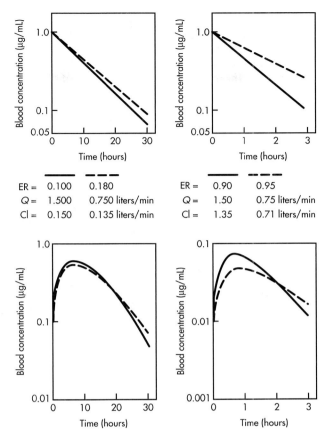

Figure 11-19. Effects of decreasing liver blood flow in the total blood concentration–time curves after intravenous (upper panels) and oral (lower panels) administration of equal doses of two totally metabolized drugs. The left panels refer to a drug with a total intrinsic clearance equivalent to an extraction ratio of 0.1 when blood flow equals 1.5 L/min, and the right panels to a drug with an intrinsic clearance equivalent to an extraction ratio of 0.9. (From Wilkinson and Shand, 1975, with permission.)

in hepatic enzyme activity because enzyme activity is already quite high. In both cases, an orally administered drug with a higher extraction ratio results in a greater first-pass effect as shown by a reduction in the AUC (Fig. 11-18).

Effect of Changing Blood Flow on Drugs with High or Low Extraction Ratio

Drug clearance and elimination half-life are both affected by changing blood flow to the liver. For drugs with low extraction ($E = 0.1$), a decrease in hepatic blood flow from normal (1.5 L/min) to one-half decreases clearance only slightly, and blood level is slightly higher (Fig. 11-19, top left, dashed line). In contrast, for a drug with high extraction ratio ($E = 0.9$), decreasing the blood flow to one-half of normal greatly decreases clearance, and the blood level is much higher (Fig. 11-19, top right, dashed line).

Alterations in hepatic blood flow significantly affect the elimination of drugs with high extraction ratios (eg, propranolol) and have very little effect on the elimination of drugs with low extraction ratios (eg, theophylline). For drugs with low extraction ratios, any concentration of drug in the blood that perfuses the liver is more than the liver can eliminate. Consequently, small changes in hepatic blood flow do not affect the removal rate of such drugs. In contrast, drugs with high extraction ratios are removed from the blood as rapidly as they are presented to the liver. If the blood flow to the liver decreases, then the elimination of these drugs is prolonged. Therefore, drugs with high extraction ratios are considered to be *flow dependent*. A number of drugs have been investigated and classified according to their extraction by the liver, as shown in Table 11.12. The relationship between hepatic clearance and blood flow for drugs with different extraction ratio is shown in Figure 11-19.

Effect of Changing Protein Binding on Hepatic Clearance

The effect of protein binding on hepatic clearance is often difficult to quantitate precisely, because it is not always known whether the bound drug is restrictively or nonrestrictively cleared. For example, animal tissue levels of imipramine, a nonrestrictively cleared drug, was shown to change as the degree of plasma protein binding changes (see Chapter 10). As discussed, drug protein binding is not a factor in hepatic clearance for drugs that have high extraction ratios. These drugs are considered to be *flow limited*. In contrast, drugs that have low extraction ratios may be affected by plasma protein binding depending on the fraction of drug bound. For a drug that has a low extraction ratio and is less than 75–80% bound, small changes in protein binding will not produce significant changes in hepatic clearance. These drugs are considered *capacity-limited, binding-insensitive drugs* (Blaschke, 1977) and are listed in Table 11.12. Drugs that are highly bound to plasma protein but with low extraction ratios are considered *capacity limited and binding sensitive,* because a small displacement in the protein binding of these drugs will cause a very large increase in the free drug concentration. These drugs are good examples of restrictively cleared drugs. A large increase in free drug concentration will cause an increase in the rate of drug metabolism, resulting in an overall increase in hepatic clearance. Figure 11-20 illustrates the relationship of protein binding, blood flow, and extraction.

BILIARY EXCRETION OF DRUGS

The biliary system of the liver is an important system for the secretion of bile and the excretion of drugs. Anatomically, the intrahepatic bile ducts join outside the liver to form the common hepatic duct (Fig. 11-21). The bile that enters the gallbladder becomes highly concentrated. The hepatic duct, containing hepatic bile, joins the cystic duct that drains the gallbladder to form the common bile duct. The common bile duct then empties into the duodenum. Bile consists primarily of water, bile salts, bile pigments, electrolytes, and, to a lesser extent, cholesterol and fatty acids. The hepatic cells lining the bile canaliculi are responsible for the production of bile. The production of bile appears to be an active secretion process. Separate active biliary secretion processes have been reported for organic anions, organic cations, and for polar, uncharged molecules.

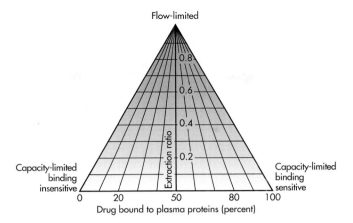

Figure 11-20. This diagram illustrates the way in which two pharmacokinetic parameters (hepatic extraction ratio and percent plasma protein binding) are used to assign a drug into one of three classes of hepatic clearance (flow limited; capacity limited, binding sensitive; and capacity limited, binding insensitive). Any drug metabolized by the liver can be plotted on the triangular graph, but the classification is important only for those eliminated primarily by hepatic processes. The closer a drug falls to a corner of the triangle (shaded areas), the more likely it is to have the characteristic changes in disposition in liver disease as described for the three drug classes in the text. (From Blaschke, 1977, with permission.)

Drugs that are excreted mainly in the bile have molecular weights in excess of 500. Drugs with molecular weights between 300 and 500 are excreted both in urine and in bile. For these drugs, a decrease in one excretory route results in a compensatory increase in excretion via the other route. Compounds with molecular weights of less than 300 are excreted almost exclusively via the kidneys into urine.

In addition to relatively high molecular weight, drugs excreted into bile usually require a strongly polar group. Many drugs excreted into bile are metabolites, very often glucuronide conjugates. Most metabolites are more polar than the parent drug. In addition, the formation of a glucuronide increases the molecular weight of the compound by nearly 200, as well as increasing the polarity.

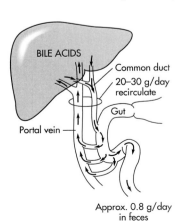

Figure 11-21. Enterohepatic recirculation of bile acids and drug. (From Dow, 1963.)

TABLE 11.13   Examples of Drugs Undergoing Enterohepatic Circulation and Biliary Excretion

Enterohepatic Circulation

Imipramine
Indomethacin
Morphine
Pregnenolone

Biliary Excretion (intact or as metabolites)

Cefamandole	Fluvastatin
Cefoperazone	Lovastatin
Chloramphenicol	Moxalactam
Diazepam	Practolol
Digoxin	Spironolactone
Doxorubicin	Testosterone
Doxycycline	Tetracycline
Estradiol	Vincristine

Drugs excreted into the bile include the digitalis glycosides, bile salts, choles-terol, steroids, and indomethacin (Table 11.13). Compounds that enhance bile production stimulate the biliary excretion of drugs normally eliminated by this route. Furthermore, phenobarbital, which induces many mixed-function oxidase activities, may stimulate the biliary excretion of drugs by two mechanisms: by an increase in the formation of the glucuronide metabolite and by an increase in bile flow. In contrast, compounds that decrease bile flow or pathophysiologic con-ditions that cause cholestasis decrease biliary drug excretion. The route of ad-ministration may also influence the amount of the drug excreted into bile. For example, drugs given orally may be extracted by the liver into the bile to a greater extent than the same drugs given intravenously.

Estimation of Biliary Clearance

The rate of drug elimination may be measured by monitoring the amount of drug secreted into the GI perfusate using a special intubation technique that blocks off a segment of the gut with an inflating balloon. In animals, bile duct cannulation allows both the volume of the bile and the concentration of drug in the bile to be measured directly.

Assuming an average bile flow of 0.5–0.8 mL/min in humans, biliary clearance can be calculated if the bile concentration, C_{bile}, is known.

$$Cl_{biliary} = \frac{\text{bile flow} \times C_{bile}}{C_p} \qquad (11.50)$$

Alternatively, using the perfusion technique, the amount of drug eliminated in bile is determined from the GI perfusate, and $Cl_{biliary}$ may be calculated without the bile flow rate, as follows.

$$Cl_{biliary} = \frac{\text{amount of drug secreted from bile per minute}}{C_p} \qquad (11.51)$$

To avoid any complication of unabsorbed drug in the feces, the drug should be given by parenteral administration (eg, IV) during biliary determination experiments. The amount of drug in the GI perfusate recovered periodically may be determined. The extent of biliary elimination of digoxin has been determined in humans using this approach.

Enterohepatic Circulation

A drug or its metabolite is secreted into bile and upon contraction of the gallbladder is excreted into the duodenum via the common bile duct. Subsequently, the drug or its metabolite may be excreted into the feces or the drug may be reabsorbed and become systemically available. The cycle in which the drug is absorbed, excreted into the bile, and reabsorbed is known as *enterohepatic circulation*. Some drugs excreted as a glucuronide conjugate become hydrolyzed in the gut back to the parent drug by the action of a β-glucuronidase enzyme present in the intestinal bacteria. In this case, the parent drug becomes available for reabsorption.

Significance of Biliary Excretion

When a drug appears in the feces after oral administration, it is difficult to determine whether this presence of drug is due to biliary excretion or incomplete absorption. If the drug is given parenterally and then observed in the feces, one can assess that some of the drug was excreted in the bile. Because drug secretion into bile is an active process, this process can be saturated with high drug concentrations. Moreover, other drugs may compete for the same carrier system.

Enterohepatic circulation after a single dose of drug is not as important as after multiple doses or a very high dose of drug. With a large dose or multiple doses, a larger amount of drug is secreted in the bile, from which drug is then reabsorbed. This reabsorption process may affect the absorption and elimination rate constants. Furthermore, the biliary secretion process may become saturated, thus altering the plasma level–time curve.

Drugs that undergo enterohepatic circulation sometimes show a small secondary peak in the plasma drug–concentration curve. The first peak occurs as the drug in the GI tract is depleted; a small secondary peak then emerges as biliary-excreted drug is reabsorbed. In experimental studies involving animals, bile duct cannulation provides a means of estimating the amount of drug excreted through the bile. In humans, a less accurate estimation of biliary excretion may be made from the recovery of drug excreted through the feces. However, if the drug were given orally, some of the fecal drug excretion could represent unabsorbed drug.

CLINICAL EXAMPLE

Leflunomide, an immunomodulator for rheumatoid arthritis, is metabolized to a major active metabolite and several minor metabolites. Approximately 48% of the dose is eliminated in the feces due to high biliary excretion. The active metabolite is slowly eliminated from the plasma. In the case of serious adverse toxicity, the manufacture recommends giving orally, cholestyramine or activated charcoal to bind the active metabolite in the GI tract to prevent its reabsorption and to facilitate its elimination. The use of cholestyramine or activated charcoal reduces the plasma levels of the active metabolite by approximately 40% in 24 hrs and by about 50% in 48 hrs.

FREQUENTLY ASKED QUESTIONS

1. Why do we use the term *hepatic drug clearance* to describe drug metabolism in the liver?
2. Please explain why many drugs with significant metabolism often have variable bioavailability.
3. The metabolism of some drugs is affected more than others when there is a change in protein binding. Why?
4. Give some examples that explain why the metabolic pharmacokinetics of drugs are important in patient care.

LEARNING QUESTIONS

1. A drug fitting a one-compartment model was found to be eliminated from the plasma by the following pathways with the corresponding elimination rate constants.

   Metabolism: $k_m = 0.200 \text{ hr}^{-1}$

   Kidney excretion: $k_e = 0.250 \text{ hr}^{-1}$

   Biliary excretion: $k_b = 0.150 \text{ hr}^{-1}$

   a. What is the elimination half-life of this drug?

   b. What would be the half-life of this drug if biliary secretion were completely blocked?

   c. What would be the half-life of this drug if drug excretion through the kidney were completely impaired?

   d. If drug-metabolizing enzymes were induced so that the rate of metabolism of this drug doubled, what would be the new elimination half-life?

2. A new broad-spectrum antibiotic was administered by rapid intravenous injection to a 50-kg woman at a dose of 3 mg/kg. The apparent volume of

distribution of this drug was equivalent to 5% of body weight. The elimination half-life for this drug is 2 hours.

a. If 90% of the unchanged drug was recovered in the urine, what is the renal excretion rate constant?

b. Which is more important for the elimination of the drugs, renal excretion or biotransformation? Why?

3. Explain briefly:

a. Why does a drug that has a high extraction ratio (eg, propranolol) demonstrate greater differences between individuals after oral administration than after intravenous administration?

b. Why does a drug with a low hepatic extraction ratio (eg, theophylline) demonstrate greater differences between individuals after hepatic enzyme induction than a drug with a high hepatic extraction ratio?

4. A drug is being screened for antihypertensive activity. After oral administration, the onset time is 0.5–1 hour. However, after intravenous administration, the onset time is 6–8 hours.

a. What reasons would you give for the differences in the onset times for oral and intravenous drug administration?

b. Devise an experiment that would prove the validity of your reasoning.

5. Calculate the hepatic clearance for a drug with an intrinsic clearance of 40 mL/min in a normal adult patient whose hepatic blood flow is 1.5 L/min.

a. If the patient develops congestive heart failure that reduces hepatic blood flow to 1.0 L/min but does not affect the intrinsic clearance, what is the hepatic drug clearance in this patient?

b. If the patient is concurrently receiving medication, such as phenobarbital, which increases the Cl_{int} to 90 mL/min but does not alter the hepatic blood flow (1.5 L/min), what is the hepatic clearance for the drug in this patient?

6. Calculate the hepatic clearance for a drug with an intrinsic clearance of 12 L/min in a normal adult patient whose hepatic blood flow is 1.5 L/min. If this same patient develops congestive heart failure that reduces his hepatic blood flow to 1.0 L/min but does not affect intrinsic clearance, what is the hepatic drug clearance in this patient?

a. Calculate the extraction ratio for the liver in this patient before and after congestive heart failure develops.

b. From the above information, estimate the fraction of bioavailable drug, assuming the drug is given orally and absorption is complete.

7. Why do elimination half-lives of drugs eliminated primarily by hepatic biotransformation demonstrate greater intersubject variability than those drugs eliminated primarily by glomerular filtration?

8. A new drug demonstrates high presystemic elimination when taken orally. From which of the following drug products would the drug be most bioavailable? Why?

a. Aqueous solution

b. Suspension

c. Capsule (hard gelatin)

d. Tablet

e. Sustained release

9. For a drug that demonstrated presystemic elimination, would you expect qualitative and/or quantitative differences in the formation of metabolites from this drug given orally compared to intravenous injection? Why?

10. The bioavailability of propranolol is 26%. Propranolol is 87% bound to plasma proteins and has an elimination half-life of 3.9 hours. The apparent volume of distribution of propranolol is 4.3 L/kg. Less than 0.5% of the unchanged drug is excreted in the urine.

   a. Calculate the hepatic clearance for propranolol in an adult male patient (43 years old, 80 kg).

   b. Assuming the hepatic blood flow is 1500 mL/min, estimate the hepatic extraction ratio for propranolol.

   c. Explain why hepatic clearance is more important than renal clearance for the elimination of propranolol.

   d. What would be the effect of hepatic disease such as cirrhosis on the (1) bioavailability of propranolol and (2) hepatic clearance of propranolol?

   e. Explain how a change in (1) hepatic blood flow, (2) intrinsic clearance, or (3) plasma protein binding would affect hepatic clearance of propranolol.

   f. What is meant by first-pass effects? From the data above, why is propranolol a drug with first-pass effects?

11. The following pharmacokinetic information for erythromycin was reported by Gilman et al 1990, p. 1679):

   Bioavailability: 35%

   Urinary excretion: 12%

   Bound in plasma: 84%

   Volume of distribution: 0.78 L/kg

   Elimination half-life: 1.6 hours

   An adult male patient (41 years old, 81 kg) was prescribed 250 mg of erythromycin base every 6 hours for 10 days. From the data above, calculate the following:

   a. Total body clearance

   b. Renal clearance

   c. Hepatic clearance

12. Why would you expect hepatic clearance of theophylline in identical twins to be less variable compared to hepatic clearance in fraternal twins?

13. Which of the following statements describe(s) correctly the properties of a drug that follows nonlinear or capacity-limited pharmacokinetics?

   a. The elimination half-life will remain constant when the dose changes.

   b. The area under the plasma curve (AUC) will increase proportionately with an increase in dose.

c. The rate of drug elimination $= C_p \times K_M$.

d. At maximum saturation of the enzyme by the substrate, the reaction velocity is at V_{max}.

e. At very low substrate concentrations, the reaction rate approximates a zero-order rate.

14. The V_{max} for metabolizing a drug is 10 μm/hr. The rate of metabolism (v) is 5 μm/hr when drug concentration is 4 μm. Which of the following statements is/are true?

a. K_M is 5 μm for this drug.

b. K_M cannot be determined from the information given.

c. K_M is 4 μm for this drug.

15. Which of the following statements is/are true regarding the pharmacokinetics of diazepam (98% protein bound) and propranolol (87% protein bound)?

a. Diazepam has a long elimination half-life due to its lack of metabolism and its extensive plasma protein binding.

b. Propranolol is a drug with high protein binding but unrestricted (unaffected) metabolic clearance.

c. Diazepam exhibits low hepatic extraction.

16. The hepatic intrinsic clearance of two drugs are as follows:

Drug A: 1300 mL/min

Drug B: 26 mL/min

Which drug is likely to show the greatest increase in hepatic clearance when hepatic blood flow is increased from 1 L/min to 1.5 mL/min? Which drug will likely be blood-flow limited?

REFERENCES

Alvares AP, Pratt WB: Pathways of drug metabolism. In Pratt WB, Taylor P (eds): *Principles of Drug Action*, 3rd ed. New York, Churchill Livingstone, 1990, chap 5

Ariens EJ, Wuis EW: Commentary: Bias in pharmacokinetics and clinical pharmacology. *Clin Pharm Ther* **42**:361–363, 1987

Baily DG, Arnold JMO, Munoz C, Spence JD: Grapefruit juice–felodipine interaction: Mechanism, predictability, and effect of naringin. *Clin Pharm Ther* **53**:637–642, 1993b

Baily DG, Arnold JMO, Strong HA, Munoz C, Spence JD: Effect of grapefruit juice and naringin on nisoldipine pharmacokinetics. *Clin Pharm Ther* **54**:589–593, 1993a

Bertilsson L: Geographic/interracial differences in polymorphic drug oxidation. *Clin Pharmacokinet* **29**(4):192–209, 1995

Blaschke TF: Protein binding and kinetics of drugs in liver diseases. *Clin Pharmacokinet* **2**:32–44, 1977

Brosen K: Recent developments in hepatic drug oxidation. *Clin Pharmacokinet* **18**:220, 1990

Brouwer KL, Dukes GE, Powell JR: Influence of liver function on drug disposition. Applied pharmacokinetics. In Evans WE, Schentag JJ, Jusko WJ, et al (eds); *Principles of Therapeutic Drug Monitoring*. Vancouver, WA, Applied Therapeutics, 1992, chap 6

Caldwell J: Conjugation reactions. In Jenner P, Testa B (eds), *Concepts in Drug Metabolism*. New York, Marcel Dekker, 1980, chap 4

Campbell TC: Nutrition and drug-metabolizing enzymes. *Clin Pharm Ther* **22**:699–706, 1977

Caraco Y, Sheller J, Wood AJJ: Pharmacogenetic determination of the effects of codeine and prediction of drug interactions. *J Pharmacol Exp Ther* **278**:1165–1174, 1996

Cupp MJ, Tracy TS: Cytochrome P-450: New nomenclature and clinical implications. *Am Family Physician*, January 1, 1998 (http://www.aafp.org/afp/980101ap/cupp.html).

Desta Z, Xiaox, Shin JG, et al: Clinical significance of the cytochrome P450 2C19 genetic polymorphism. *Clin Pharmacokinet* **41**(12):913–958, 2002

Dow P: *Handbook of Physiology*, vol 2, Circulation. Washington, DC, American Physiology Society, 1963, p 1406

Evans DAP: Genetic variations in the acetylation of isoniazid and other drugs. Ann N Y Acad Sci **151**:723, 1968

Evans DAP, Manley KA, McKusik VC: Genetic control of isoniazid metabolism in man. *Br Med J* **2**:485, 1968

FDA Guidance for Industry: *Drug Metabolism/Drug Interaction Studies in the Drug Development Process: Studies in vitro*, issued 4/1997

FDA Guidance for Industry: *In Vivo Drug Metabolism/Drug Interaction Studies—Study Design, Data Analysis, and Recommendations for Dosing and Labeling*, issued 11/24/1999 (www.fda.gov/cder/guidance.htm)

Flockhart: http://medicine.iupui.edu/flockhart/ Drug interaction table maintained by David Flockhart. Division of clinical pharmacology, Indiana University

Gilman AG, Rall TW, Nies AS, Taylor (eds): *Goodman and Gilman's The Pharmacological Basis of Therapeutics*, 8th ed. Elmsford, NY, Pergamon Press, 1990

Gray H: *Anatomy of the Human Body*, 30th ed. Philadelphia, Lea & Febiger, 1985, p 1495

Hansch C, Zhang L: Quantitative structure-activity relationships of cytochrome P-450. *Drug Metab Rev* **25**:1–48, 1993

Harder S, Baas H, Rietbrock S: Concentration effect relationship of levodopa in patients with Parkinson's disease. *Clin Pharmacokinet* **29**:243–256, 1995

Hucker HB, Kwan KC, Duggan DE: Pharmacokinetics and metabolism of nonsteroidal antiinflammatory agents. In Bridges JW, Chasseaud LF (eds), *Progress in Drug Research*, vol 5. New York, Wiley, 1980, chap 3

Hukkinen SK, Varhe A, Olkkola KT, Neuvonen PJ: Plasma concentrations of triazolam are increased by concomitant ingestion of grapefruit juice. *Clin Pharm Ther* **58**:127–131, 1995

Iwakawa S, Suganuma T, Lee S, et al: Direct determination of diastereomeric carprofen glucuronides in human plasma and urine and preliminary measurements of stereoselective metabolic and renal elimination after oral administration of carprofen in man. *Drug Metab Disp* **17**:414–419, 1989

Kupferschmidt HH, Ha HR, Ziegler WH, Meier PJ, Krahenbuhl S: Interaction between grapefruit juice and midazolam in humans. *Clin Pharm Ther* **58**:20–28, 1995

Lai ML, Wang SL, Lai MD, Lin ET, Tse M, Huang JD: Propranolol disposition in Chinese subjects of different CYT2D6 genotypes. *Clin Pharm Ther* **58**:264–268, 1995

Levy RH, Boddy AV: Stereoselectivity in pharmacokinetics: A general theory. *Pharm Res* **8**:551–556, 1991

Lanctot KL, Naranjo CA: Comparison of the Bayesian approach and a simple algorithm for assessment of adverse drug events. *Clin Pharm Ther* **58**:692–698, 1995

Lindner HH: *Clinical Anatomy*. Norwalk, CT, Appleton & Lange, 1989

May GD: Genetic differences in drug disposition. *J Clin Pharmacol* **34**:881–897, 1994

Merkel U, Sigusch H, Hoffmann A: Grapefruit juice inhibits 7-hydroxylation of coumarin in healthy volunteers. *Eur J Clin Pharm* **46**:175–177, 1994

Nebert DW, Nelson DR, Adesnik M, et al: The P-450 superfamily: Updated listing of all genes and recommended nomenclature for the chromosomal loci. *DNA* **8**:1, 1989

Negishi M, Tomohide U, Darden TA, Sueyoshi T, Pedersen LG: Structural flexibility and functional versatility of mammalian P-450 enzymes. *FASEB J* **10**:683–689, 1996

Parkinson A: Biotransformation of xenobiotics. In Klaassen, CD (ed), *Casarett & Doull's Toxicology*, 5th ed. McGraw-Hill, New York, 1996, chap 6

Rahmani R, Zhou XJ: Pharmacokinetics and metabolism of vinca alkaloids. *Cancer Surv* **17**:269–281, 1993

Rowland M: Drug administration and regimens. In Melmon K, Morelli HF (eds), *Clinical Pharmacology*. New York, Macmillan, 1978

Rowland M: Effect of some physiologic factors on bioavailability of oral dosage forms. In Swarbrick J (ed), *Current Concepts in the Pharmaceutical Sciences: Dosage Form Design and Bioavailability.* Philadelphia, Lea & Febiger, 1973, chap 6

Toney GB, Ereshefsky L: Cyclic antidepressants. In Schumacher GE (ed), *Therapeutic Drug Monitoring.* Norwalk, CT, Appleton & Lange, 1995, chap 13

Tucker GT: Clinical implications of genetic polymorphism in drug metabolism. *J Pharm Pharmacol* **46**(suppl):417–424, 1994

Tucker GT, Lennard MS: Enantiomer-specific pharmacokinetics. *Pharmacol Ther* **45**:309–329, 1990

Wilkinson GR, Guengerich FP, Branch RA: Genetic polymorphism of S-mephenytoin hydroxylation. *Pharmacol Ther* **43**:53–76, 1989

Wilkinson GR, Shand DG: A physiological approach to hepatic drug clearance. *Clin Pharmacol Ther* **18**:377–390, 1975

Wolf CR: Distribution and regulation of drug-metabolizing enzymes in mammalian tissues. In Caldwell J, Paulson GD (eds), *Foreign Compound Metabolism.* London, Taylor & Francis, 1984

Yee GC, Stanley DL, Pessa LJ, et al: Effect of grapefruit juice on blood cyclosporin concentration. *Lancet* **345**:955–956, 1995

BIBLIOGRAPHY

Anders MW: *Bioactivation of Foreign Compounds.* New York, Academic Press, 1985

Balant LP, McAinsh JM: Use of metabolite data in the evaluation of pharmacokinetics and drug action. In Jenner P, Testa B (eds), *Concepts in Drug Metabolism.* New York, Marcel Dekker, 1980, chap 7

Benet LZ: Effect of route of administration and distribution on drug action. *J Pharm Biopharm* **6**:559–585, 1978

Brown C (ed): Chirality in Drug Design and Synthesis: Racemic Therapeutics—Problems All Along the Line (EJ Ariens), New York, Academic Press, 1990

Ducharme MP, Warbasse LH, Edwards DJ: Disposition of intravenous and oral cyclosporine after administration with grapefruit juice. *Clin Pharm Ther* **57**:485–491, 1995

Geroge CF, Shand DG, Renwick AG (eds): *Presystemic Drug Elimination.* Boston, Butterworth, 1982

Gibaldi M, Perrier D: Route of administration and disposition. *Drug Metab Rev* **3**:185–199, 1974

Gibson GG, Skett P: *Introduction to Drug Metabolism,* 2nd ed. New York, Chapman & Hall, 1994

Glocklin VC: General considerations for studies of the metabolism of drugs and other chemicals. *Drug Metab Rev* **13**:929–939, 1982

Gorrod JW, Damani LA: *Biological Oxidation of Nitrogen in Organic Molecules: Chemistry, Toxicology and Pharmacology.* Deerfield Beach, FL, Ellis Horwood, 1985

Hildebrandt A, Estabrook RW: Evidence for the participation of cytochrome b5 in hepatic microsomal mixed-function oxidation reactions. *Arch Biochem Biophys* **143**:66–79, 1971

Houston JB: Drug metabolite kinetics. *Pharmacol Ther* **15**:521–552, 1982

Jakoby WB: *Enzymatic Basis of Detoxification.* New York, Academic Press, 1980

Jenner P, Testa B: *Concepts in Drug Metabolism.* New York, Marcel Dekker, 1980–1981

Kaplan SA, Jack ML: Physiologic and metabolic variables in bioavailability studies. In Garrett ER, Hirtz JL (eds), *Drug Fate and Metabolism,* vol 3. New York, Marcel Dekker, 1979

LaDu BL, Mandel HG, Way EL: *Fundamentals of Drug Metabolism and Drug Disposition.* Baltimore, Williams & Wilkins, 1971

Levine WG: Biliary excretion of drugs and other xenobiotics. *Prog Drug Res* **25**:361–420, 1981

Morris ME, Pang KS: Competition between two enzymes for substrate removal in liver: Modulating effects due to substrate recruitment of hepatocyte activity. *J Pharm Biopharm* **15**:473–496, 1987

Nies AS, Shand DG, Wilkinson GR: Altered hepatic blood flow and drug disposition. *Clin Pharmacokinet* **1**:135–156, 1976

Pang KS, Rowland M: Hepatic clearance of drugs, 1. Theoretical considerations of a "well-stirred" model and a "parallel tube" model. Influence of hepatic blood flow, plasma, and blood cell binding and the hepatocellular enzymatic activity on hepatic drug clearance. *J Pharmacokinet Biopharmacol* **5**:625, 1977

Perrier D, Gibaldi M: Clearance and biologic half-life as indices of intrinsic hepatic metabolism. *J Pharmacol Exp Therapeut,* **191**:17–24, 1974

Plaa GL: The enterohepatic circulation. In Gillette JR, Mitchell JR (eds), *Concepts in Biochemical Pharmacology*. New York, Springer-Verlag, 1975, chap 63

Pratt WB, Taylor P: *Principles of Drug Action: The Basis of Pharmacology*, 3rd ed. New York, Churchill Livingstone, 1990

Roberts MS, Donaldson JD, Rowland M: Models of hepatic elimination: Comparison of stochastic models to describe residence time distributions and to predict the influence of drug distribution, enzyme heterogeneity, and systemic recycling on hepatic elimination. *J Pharm Biopharm* **16**:41–83, 1988

Routledge PA, Shand DG: Presystemic drug elimination. *Annu Rev Pharmacol Toxicol* **19**:447–468, 1979

Semple HA, Tam YK, Coutts RT: A computer simulation of the food effect: Transient changes in hepatic blood flow and Michaelis–Menten parameters as mediators of hepatic first-pass metabolism and bioavailability of propranolol. *Biopharm Drug Disp* **11**:61–76, 1990

Shand DG, Kornhauser DM, Wilkinson GR: Effects of route administration and blood flow on hepatic drug elimination. *J Pharmacol Exp Therapeut*, **195**:425–432, 1975

Stoltenborg JK, Puglisi CV, Rubio F, Vane FM: High performance liquid chromatographic determination of stereoselective disposition of carprofen in humans. *J Pharm Sci* **70**:1207–1212, 1981

Testa B, Jenner B: *Drug Metabolism: Chemical and Biochemical Aspects*. New York, Marcel Dekker, 1976

Venot A, Walter E, Lecourtier Y, et al: Structural identifiability of "first-pass" models. *J Pharm Biopharm* **15**:179–189, 1987

Wilkinson GR: Pharmacodynamics of drug disposition: Hemodynamic considerations. *Annu Rev Pharmacol* **15**:11–27, 1975

Wilkinson GR: Pharmacodynamics in disease states modifying body perfusion. In Benet LZ (ed), *The Effect of Disease States on Drug Pharmacokinetics*. Washington, DC, American Pharmaceutical Association, 1976

Wilkinson GR, Rawlins MD: *Drug Metabolism and Disposition: Considerations in Clinical Pharmacology*. Boston, MTP Press, 1985

Williams RT: Hepatic metabolism of drugs. *Gut* **13**:579–585, 1972

12

PHARMACOGENETICS

The genetic basis underlying variation in drug response among individuals has become evident with the introduction of modern analytical methods for the analysis of gene sequence and expression. *Pharmacogenetics* is the study of how genes affect the way people respond to drug therapy. The goal of pharmacogenetics is to individualize drug therapy to a person's unique genetic makeup. The environment, diet, age, lifestyle, and state of health can influence a person's response to medicine. An understanding of an individual's genetic makeup is thought to be the key to creating personalized drugs with greater efficacy and safety (Pillips et al, 2001; Mancinelli et al, 2000). Pharmacogenetics is an established discipline that studies the genetic basis of interindividual variability in the response to drug therapy, and allows for individualization of drug therapy. In contrast, *pharmacokinetics* provides a means for estimating pharmacokinetic parameters of the drug in various population subgroups and then applying the information to drug therapy for the average patient.

A closely related, and considered by some to be an equivalent or overlapping field, is pharmacogenomics. *Pharmacogenomics* involves study of the role of genes and their genetic variations (DNA, RNA level) in the molecular basis of disease, and therefore, the resulting pharmacologic impact of drugs on that disease. Pharmacogenetics and pharmacogenomics are both important disciplines involved in the study of genes that code for drug-metabolizing enzymes (Chapter 11), drug receptors (Chapter 19), drug transporters, and ion channels or efflux systems (Chapter 13). Many of the above are new factors involved in determining how genetic variation contributes to variation in the response to drugs, including the ultimate fate of the drug and its ability to exert a therapeutic response without undue side effects.

Application of pharmacogenetics to pharmacokinetics and pharmacodynamics helps the development of models that predict an individual's risk to an adverse drug event and therapeutic response. With some drugs, pharmacogenetics allows the recognition of subgroups with different genetic makeup that results in alterations in drug receptors and the pharmacodynamic response to drugs. Understanding the genetic and molecular differences in disease etiology and drug mechanism produce insight on how a patient will respond to a given drug. For example, the monoclonal antibody Herceptin was designed to treat a subset of breast cancer patients who

355

overexpress the HER-2 (human epidermal growth factor receptor-2) gene. Patients who lack HER-2 overexpression are considered to be nonresponders to Herceptin therapy. In the past, such differences would be apparent only after a trial-and-error period. This genetic knowledge improves our ability to select or design the proper drug for individuals suffering from a disease with a varying range of molecular defects.

Pharmacogenetics can provide justification for individualized dosing for many drugs known to be highly variable in their effects. The outcome of disease, resistance to treatment, and adverse reactions are increasingly recognized as an interaction of the individual's genes and the environment. Dominic Kwiatkowski, of the Wellcome Trust Center for Human Genetics, recently reviewed the role of genes in human susceptibility to infection (Kwiatkowski, 2000). He predicted that recent advances in genetics and high-throughput genotyping technology will make it feasible within the next decade to screen the whole genome for genetic factors that determine susceptibility to HIV and AIDS, malaria, and tuberculosis. Kwiatkowski listed many genes and their encoded proteins that play roles in immunity and disease fighting. Examples include genes with alleles that affect susceptibility to hepatitis B, HIV, and other known infections. Besides host factors, progress has been even faster for genes of microbes that play roles in efflux of drugs out of the system, a principal factor for antibiotic resistance in many pathogens. The subject of drug pumps in microbes has been reviewed by Borges-Walmsley and Walmsley (2001).

Pharmacogenetics (PGt), or pharmacogenomics (PGx), a more modern term preferred by some researchers, has been the subject of discussion by industry and regulatory agencies. These groups tried to generate a consensus on how and to what extent should PGx or PGt information be applied to improve drug therapy and safety of both old and new drugs (Lesko and Woodcock, 2002).

This chapter will focus on variations in drug response due to pharmacogenetics. However, variation in drug response is also in large part due to nongenetic factors, as listed on Table 12-1.

EXAMPLE OF POLYMORPHISMS

Interindividual differences in response to drug therapy due to differences in acetylation of drugs is a well-studied example of genetic polymorphism. Patients' ability to metabolize certain drugs such as hydralazine, procainamide, and isoniazid can be categorized as either "fast acetylators," "normal acetylators," or "slow acetylators." Acetylation status is dependent on the patient's genetic composition, which determines the activity of the acetylation enzyme N-acetyltransferase. Acetylation status determines whether a patient is dosed with a correspondingly higher or lower dose compared to "normal acetylators."

Although acetylation status is well known in the medical community, other metabolic or pharmacologic variations have been poorly understood until recently. Genetic variations are well known in bacteria and other microorganisms because the rapid changes in these organisms are easily observed. In humans, mutations and related changes occur to different degrees in thousands of proteins and other macromolecules.

TABLE 12.1   Pharmacogenetic and Nongenetic Influences on Variations in Disease and Drug Therapy[a]

	VARIANT TYPE	EXAMPLE
Genetic influences	(PK)	Drug metabolism—Polymorphism in many cytochrome P-450 family enzymes (CYPs) and others in Table 12.2
	(PK)	P-glycoprotein or other drug transporter (difference in genetic expression)
	Drug receptor (PD)	Variation in receptor number, affinity, or response to drug
	Indirect drug response (PD)	Inherited differences in coagulation may predispose women to deep vein thrombosis when taking oral contraceptives
		Variations in SCNA receptor predisposes patients to drug-induced arrhythmia (Makita et al, 2002)
Nongenetic[a] influences	Environmental (PK, PD, or disease prognosis)	Cigarette smoking—enzyme induction
		Exposure to mutagenic agents and occupational or environmental hazards
		Geographic differences
		▪ Climate (ultraviolet light on skin tumor)
		▪ Diet[b] (effect of diet, including grapefruit, and influence on GI enzymes and drug absorption)
		▪ Drinking water (dissolved minerals and effect on health)
		▪ Nutrients or supplements[c]
Mixed covariates[d]	Gender, age, body weight/surface (PK/PD)	Male, female
		Infant, young adult, or geriatric patient
	Pathophysiology (PK/PD)	Renal, hepatic, cardiovascular, or other disease
	Drug–drug interactions (PK/PD)	Metabolic, binding, or PD interactions

[a]Environmental factors may switch on genes, and the nongenetic category may not be absolute. The two primary independent variables in life processes are genetics and environment.
[b]Examples of diet: Atkins diet, vegetarian, diabetic, and other hospital diets, etc. Foods rich in carbohydrates/protein may have an effect on urinary pH and affect renal tubular drug reabsorption. Diet can also affect PK drug absorption; certain groups lack or have abundant GI enzymes, lactase, etc (even though it might be genetic rather than adaptive, arguably).
[c]Examples of nutrients include vitamins, antioxidants, fortified fruit drinks, and supplements taken regularly, other than meals.
[d]Some genetic/environmental outcomes may become a covariate for a new pharmacogenetic response.

Some examples partially adapted from Evans and McLeod (2003).

Polymorphisms or genetic variations with a frequency of greater than 1% of the population, or *mutations,* in less than 1% of the population, in genetic sequences can affect patient therapeutic response or metabolism of a given drug (Meyer, 2000). However, many alleles encoding different drug receptors are being discovered and studied with increasing frequency. Pharmacokinetic parameters now known to be influenced by genetic differences include drug bioavailability, distribution, metabolism and tissue binding. Our understanding of the impact of these genetic differences on clinical pharmacokinetics and pharmacodynamics are in their infancy.

Polymorphism in cytochrome isozymes is well known in drug metabolism, and the corresponding allele genes involved have been widely studied and are fairly well understood clinically at this time. Genetic tests are available to screen polymorphisms for cytochrome P-450 drug-metabolizing enzymes in an individual. Prior knowledge of an individual's metabolic capability can reduce the risk of adverse drug reactions because dose regimens may be adjusted according to an individual patient's metabolic capability. The types of genetic mutations affecting metabolic enzymes are illustrated in Figure 12-1.

Genetic polymorphism within a specific genotype may occur with different frequencies depending on racial or population factors, which evolved from selective geographic, regional, and ethnic factors. The probability of carrying a specific allele is therefore different in different subjects depending on whether the dominating factor is geographic or ethnic. In practice, genetic polymorphisms with higher frequencies are more important because they are likely to affect more people. However, some rare mutations are important because they cause extreme medical consequences or may be fatal for the individual.

Using genetic polymorphism considerations, drugs may be developed that have less intersubject variation in pharmacodynamic response and less risk of an adverse event. In addition, doses for patients can be based on their metabolic capacity by using the frequency of genotypes of "poor metabolizers" or "ultrarapid metabolizers." Molecular studies in pharmacogenetics began with cloning of CYP2D6 and now have been extended to more than two dozen drug-metabolizing enzymes and several drug transport systems (Meyer, 2000). The most important isozymes with genetic polymorphism involved in drug metabolism are shown in Figure 12-2.

Figure 12-1. Plot of frequency of all drug metabolism phenotypes found in population versus enzyme activity or drug clearance. The left panel indicates mutations leading to almost complete loss of enzyme activity (note serious causes such as gene deletion or transcription failure); the right panel depicts mutations leading to altered but not complete loss of enzyme activity. (*Note:* SNP promoters may "switch on/off" and are responsible for individual variations in drug metabolism. The width of the bell-shaped curve shows the spread of enzymatic activity that corresponds to drug clearance.) (Adapted from M. Relling, personal communication, as reprinted in Evans and Johnson, 2001, with permission.)

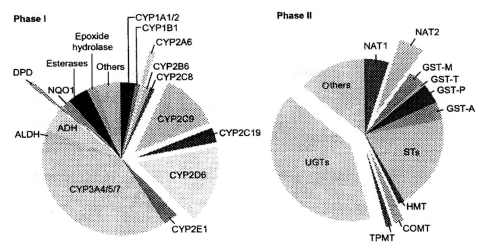

Figure 12-2. Most drug-metabolizing enzymes exhibit clinically relevant genetic polymorphisms. Essentially all of the major human enzymes responsible for modification of functional groups [classified as phase I reactions (**left**)] or conjugation with endogenous substituents [classified as phase II reactions (**right**)] exhibit common polymorphisms at the genomic level; those enzyme polymorphisms that have already been associated with changes in drug effects are separated from the corresponding pie charts. The percentage of phase I and phase II metabolism of drugs that each enzyme contributes is estimated by the relative size of each section of the corresponding chart. ADH, alcohol dehydrogenase; ALDH, aldehyde dehydrogenase; CYP, cytochrome P-450; DPD, dihydropyrimidine dehydrogenase; NQO1, NADPH: quinone oxidoreductase or DT diaphorase; COMT, catechol *O*-methyltransferase; GST, glutathione *S*-transferase; HMT, histamine methyltransferase; NAT, *N*-acetyltransferase; STs, sulfotransferases; TPMT, thiopurine methyltransferase; UGTs, uridine 5′-triphosphate glucuronosyltransferases.
(From Evans and Relling, 1999, with permission.)

Recognition of the genotypes associated with drug disposition and metabolism and the ability to obtain a "specific pharmacogenetic profile" for the patient will individualize drug therapy and reduce drug interactions (Evans and Relling, 1999; Roses, 2000, 2001). To realize this lofty objective, pharmacogenomics research aims to elucidate these *polygenic* (multiple-gene) determinants of drug effects. The interplay of genetic polymorphism with interindividual differences in pharmacokinetics and pharmacodynamics is well reviewed (Evans and Johnson, 2001; McLeod and Evans, 2001). The ultimate goal is to provide new strategies for optimizing drug efficacy and toxicity based on each patient's genetic determinants.

PHARMACOGENOMICS

Pharmacogenomics developed rapidly as a result of advances in molecular genetics and genomics. High-throughput tests such as microarray technology allow many human genes and their sequences to be probed or detected rapidly. The previously held notion of the *monogenic* nature of disease (one gene causing one disorder) is yielding to the concept of *polygenic* disorders, by which several, or even dozens, of genes may be differentially expressed compared to normal, healthy tissue

(Clark et al, 2002). As such new information arises, new challenges and opportunities also emerge for novel drug development.

The coordinated goal to sequence the 30,000 or more human genes via the Human Genome Project has also fueled progress in pharmacogenomics. Many new genes or gene products are emerging from the Human Genome Project as new potential drug targets. These new targets may be receptors, membrane proteins, enzymes, or ion channels that may be directly or indirectly involved in disease pathogenesis. While these newly discovered receptors or target enzymes can be exploited as new drug targets, polymorphic variations of those genes must be considered when developing new drugs that target these proteins.

Specific genetic codes are known for thousands of proteins and endogenous substances that support normal cellular functions. The genetic information is coded in the two helical strands of DNA. DNA consists of four basic nitrogenous substance or bases (C, cytosine; A, adenine; T, thymine; and G, guanine), which combine with deoxyribose and phosphate to form the respective nucleotides. The four nucleotides are combined in unique sequences for each gene. Genes are coded in a special region or *locus* in the DNA.

A change or mutation in gene sequence may or may not result in chronically reduced or increased level or activity of a protein or an essential enzyme. In some cases, such changes result in an exaggerated or reduced therapeutic response to a drug. The cell is *homozygous* if the genetic sequences occupying the locus are the same on the maternal and paternal chromosome; if they are different, the cell is *heterozygous*. When more than one alternative forms of a gene exists, they are referred to as *alleles* of the gene. The identity of the alleles carried by an individual at a given gene locus is referred to as the *genotype*. Alleles that vary by a single nucleotide change can now be characterized rapidly at the DNA level by *single-nucleotide polymorphism* (SNP) screening. The physical effect observed as a result of genotype difference is referred to as *phenotype*. Genes are considered functionally *polymorphic* when allelic variants exist stably in the population and their gene products exhibit altered activity in relation to the *wild type* ("normal"). Ideally, variation in drug response can be predicted by monitoring changes in phenotype or genotype for a single patient or a group of patients.

To determine whether a patient is a rapid or slow metabolizer, the patient is given a known substrate for that enzyme and the patient's intrinsic clearance (Chapter 11) is measured. Traditionally, intersubject variation in metabolism has been investigated by this method followed by *in-vitro* verification of enzyme level. Alternatively, it is possible to determine metabolic-status genotype directly from subjects' DNA. The latter approach is more definitive and offers much insight during drug development into how genes affect the metabolism of drugs. Many drugs have been elucidated with both approaches. In practice, fragments of DNA samples are compared based on SNPs. If the SNP and its functional activity are known, the probable individual drug response can be predicted.

In the future, rapid sequencing and SNPs will play a major role in detecting unusual variations in heritable clinical phenotypes of drug response. SNPs occur in about one of every 100–1500 base pairs (bp) between two unrelated individuals. Any two individuals may differ by 0.1% of their more than 3 billion base pairs. Common or informative SNPs are those that occur at frequencies of greater than 1% (Meyer, 2000). Once a large number of these SNPs and their frequencies in different populations are known, they can be used to correlate a patient's genetic "fingerprint" and the patient's probable individual drug response.

SNPs in coding regions of genes (about 30,000–100,000 per genome) cause variations in amino acid and protein function. SNPs in gene regulatory regions can cause differences in protein expression that may affect drug response. SNP profiles of individuals may be analyzed to determine disease susceptibility as well as predisposition to pharmacogenetic considerations in drug efficacy or toxicity.

ADVERSE DRUG REACTIONS ATTRIBUTED TO GENETIC DIFFERENCES

Variations in drug pharmacokinetics and pharmacodynamics are due largely to genetic polymorphism in genes involved in drug metabolism, absorption, disposition, and disease pathogenesis. As early as the 1950s, researchers realized that some adverse drug reactions were caused by genetically determined variations in enzyme activity. More recently, a review of the pharmacogenetic literature showed that a sizable portion of ADRs (~30%) involved in drug therapy implicated genetic polymorphism of drug metabolism by CYP2D6 (Sadee, 2002). For example, prolonged muscle relaxation in some subjects after receiving a cholinergic drug was explained by an inherited deficiency of a plasma cholinesterase. Hemolysis caused by antimalarial drugs is recognized as being caused by inherited variants of glucose 6-phosphate dehydrogenase. Slow metabolism of isoniazid in some patients (acetylation of isoniazid) has been found to be the cause of peripheral neuropathy caused by this drug.

More recently, adverse drug reactions of debrisoquin have led to the discovery of the genetic polymorphism of the drug-metabolizing enzyme, debrisoquin hydroxylase CYP2D6. The same isozyme deficiency causes more nausea, diplopia, and blurred vision after dosing of the antiarrhythmic drug sparteine in deficient patients. It is important to determine whether the variation in ADR is truly genetic or due to other factors. A method used to distinguish hereditary and environmental components of variability is the comparison of monozygotic and dizygotic twins, or pharmacokinetically by repeated drug administration and comparison of the variability of the responses within and between individuals. Many examples of genetic polymorphism affecting drug response/side effect are listed in Table 12.2.

GENETIC POLYMORPHISM IN DRUG METABOLISM: CYTOCHROME P-450 ISOZYMES

CYP2D6

CYP2D6 (Chapter 11) is a large isozyme family that affects metabolism of many drugs. CYP2D6 is highly polymorphic. More than 70 variant alleles of the CYP2D6 locus have been reported. The metabolism of the tricyclic antidepressants amitriptyline, clomipramine, desipramine, imipramine, nortriptyline, and the tetracyclic compounds maprotiline and mianserin is influenced by the CYP2D6 polymorphism to various degrees. Genetic polymorphism of CYP2D6 was first investigated with debrisoquine (Gonzalez et al, 1988). Poor metabolizers often carry two nonfunctional alleles of this gene, resulting in reduced drug clearance.

TABLE 12.2   Clinically Important Genetic Polymorphisms of Drug Metabolism That Influence Drug Response

ENZYME/RECEPTOR	FREQUENCY OF POLYMORPHISM	DRUG	DRUG EFFECT/SIDE EFFECT
CYP2C9	14–28% (heterozygotes) 0.2–1% (homozygotes)	Warfarin Tolbutamide Phenytoin Glipizide Losartan	Hemorrhage Hypoglycemia Phenytoin toxicity Hypoglycemia Decreased antihypertensive effect
CYP2D6	5–10% (poor metabolizers)	Antiarrhythmics	Proarrhythmic and other toxic effects Toxicity in poor metabolizers
	1–10% (ultrarapid metabolizers)	Antidepressants	Inefficacy in ultrarapid metabolizers
		Antipsychotics	Tardive dyskinesia
		Opioids	Inefficacy of codeine as analgesic, narcotic side effects, dependence
		Beta-adrenoceptor antagonists	Increased—blockade
CYP2C19	3–6% (whites) 8–23% (Asians)	Omeprazole	Higher cure rates when given with clarithromycin
		Diazepam	Prolonged sedation
Dihydropyrimidine dehydrogenase	0.1%	Fluorouracil	Myelotoxicity, Neurotoxicity
Plasma pseudo-cholinesterase	1.5%	Succinylcholine	Prolonged apnea
N-acetyltransferase	40–70% (whites) 10–20% (Asians)	Sulphonamides Amonafide	Hypersensitivity Mylelotoxicity (rapid acetylators)
		Procainamide, hydralazine, isoniazid	Drug-induced lupus erythematosus
Thiopurine Methyltransferase	0.3%	Mercaptopurine, thioguanine, azothioprine	Myelotoxicity
UDP-glucuronosyl-transferase	10–15%	Irinotecan	Diarrhea, myelosuppression
ACE		Enalapril, lisinapril captopril	Renoprotective effect, cardiac indexes, blood pressure
Potassium channels		Quinidine	Drug-induced QT syndrome
HERG		Cisapride	Drug-induced torsade de pointes
KvLQT1		Terfenadine Disopyramide	Drug-induced long-QT syndrome
HKCNE2		Meflaquine Clarithromycin	Drug-induced arrhythmia

From Meyer (2000) with permission, adapted partly from Evans and Relling (1999).

Since about 10% of the population are poor CYP2D6 metabolizers, CYP2D6 drug candidates are often dropped from further development by researchers in favor of others (Sadee, 2002). Poor metabolizers have increased plasma concentrations of tricyclic antidepressants when given recommended doses of the drug. Adverse effects may occur more frequently in poor metabolizers and may be misinterpreted as symptoms of depression and may further lead to erroneous increases in the dose. When determining CYP2D6 metabolic status (slow versus fast metabolizers) in patients on tricyclic antidepressants, co-administration of other CYP2D6 substrates such as serotonin-selective reuptake inhibitors may result in erroneously concluding poor CYP2D6 metabolic status.

In contrast, ultrarapid metabolizers have relatively fast drug metabolism due to the presence of more enzyme or increased enzyme activity. Patients in this group are prone to therapeutic failure due to the resulting subtherapeutic drug concentrations when "normal" doses are given. Pharmacogenomic studies have revealed that some fast metabolizers of CYP2D6 are the result of gene duplication among different racial groups. Depending on the population studied, 5–20% of patients can be classified as either rapid or poor metabolizers.

Polymorphic drug metabolism is found in a large number of drugs used in psychiatric patients. Retrospective analysis of psychiatric patients treated with substrates of CYP2D6 strongly indicate that genotyping can improve the likelihood of preventing adverse drug reactions, and decrease the costs of therapy.

The polymorphic O-demethylation of codeine is of clinical importance when this drug is given as an analgesic. About 10% of codeine is O-demethylated by CYP2D6 to morphine, and this conversion is deficient in poor metabolizers. Poor metabolizers therefore experience no analgestic effects of codeine.

CYP1A2

Another isozyme, CYP1A2, which metabolizes 5% of randomly selected drugs, may also be considered during development, since up to 15% of a patient population can be classified as poor metabolizers, according to Sadee (2002). Fluvoxamine is a substrate and potent inhibitor of CYP1A2, causing important interactions with drugs such as amitriptyline, clomipramine, imipramine, clozapine, and theophylline that are partly metabolized by this cytochrome P-450 enzyme.

CYP2C9

Still another example of a clinically important drug metabolism polymorphism is the association of variant alleles of CYP2C9 with the requirement for lower warfarin dose. In a retrospective study of a population from an anticoagulant clinic, the CYP2C9 alleles associated with decreased enzyme activity (*2 and *3) were found to be overrepresented in patients stabilized on low doses of warfarin. These patients had an increase incidence of major and minor hemorrhage.

CYP2C19

The 4'-hydroxylation of the (S)-enantiomer of mephenytoin is catalyzed by CYP2C19. The polymorphic enzyme has a poor metabolizer (PM) frequency of about 3% in Caucasians, 15–25% among Asians, and 4–7% among Black Africans

(Dahl, 2002). The major defective allele responsible for the PM phenotype is CYP2C19***2,** which is found among 13% and 32% of Caucasians and Asians, respectively. A second allele, CYP2C19***3,** is found mostly among Asians and rarely in Caucasians.

Interestingly, few polymorphisms are reported for the isozyme subfamily CYP3A. This isozyme is involved in the metabolism of endogenous steroid and testosterone. Mutations of this vital enzyme may not be compatible with life.

Not all therapeutic variations and side effects result from genetic differences in the receptor or drug metabolism. Drug response (including therapeutic and unintended side effects) is influenced by many direct and indirect factors, including modifying effects from environmental factors on the disease process and drug disposition. As a result, some researchers are unsure whether prescribing drugs based on a pharmacogenetic profile will significantly reduce side effects for most drugs, since many side effects and therapeutic failures may be the result of incorrect diagnosis or failure to account for other influencing variables such as the nature and severity of the disease, the individual's age and race, organ function, concomitant therapy, drug interactions, and concomitant illnesses.

GENETIC POLYMORPHISM IN DRUG TRANSPORT: P-GLYCOPROTEIN AND MULTIDRUG RESISTANCE

Transporter pharmacogenetics is a rapidly developing field that is concerned with drug uptake and efflux into or through tissues. Significant problems in the clinical application of drugs result from poor or variable oral drug bioavailability, and high intra- and interindividual variation in pharmacokinetics. Several membrane transporter proteins are involved in the absorption of drugs from the intestinal tract into the body, into nonintestinal tissues, or into specific target sites of action (Borst et al, 2000).

Drug efflux is an important cause of drug resistance in certain types of cells. In cytotoxic chemotherapy for several human cancerous diseases, drugs are generally very effective, but in the case of *intrinsic* or *acquired multidrug resistance*, usually highly effective antineoplastic compounds, eg, vincristine, vinblastine, daunorubicin, or doxorubicin, fail to produce cures. One of the major causes of such multidrug resistance is the appearance of special integral membrane proteins, the *P-glycoprotein multidrug transporter*, or MDR1 (Sharom et al, 1999), which is one of the major causes of low drug level in targeted cells. P-glycoprotein is discussed in Chapter 13.

The multidrug resistance-associated proteins (MRPs) are members of the ATP-binding cassette (ABC) superfamily with six members currently, of which MRP1, MRP2, and MRP3 are commonly known to affect drug disposition. MRP1 is ubiquitous in the body. Substrates for MRP1 include glutathione, glucuronide, and sulfate. MRP1 is expressed basolaterally in the intestine, although its role in extruding drugs out of the enterocytes is still uncertain. There is some substrate overlap between MRP1 and apically located P-glycoprotein. The amino acid homology between MDR1 and P-glycoprotein was reported to be 15% in some cell lines (see Chapter 13).

GENETIC POLYMORPHISM IN DRUG TARGETS

In the future, proteins involved in disease will become identified as important biomarkers for pharmacodynamic studies. Genomics has led to the development of proteonomics, which involves the study of biologically interesting proteins and their variants. Proteins can be used as probes for drug discovery or as biomarkers for drug safety, such as cell surface proteins (eg, COX-2, D-2R), intracellular proteins (eg, troponin I), and secreted proteins (eg, MCP-l).

The physiologic response of the body to a drug is generally the result of interaction of the drug at a specific target site in the body. It is estimated that about 50% of drugs act on membrane receptors, about 30% act on enyzmes, and about 5% act on ion channels (Meyer, 2000). Many of the genes encoding these target proteins exhibit polymorphisms that may alter drug response. Clinically relevant examples of polymorphism leading to variable responses are listed in Table 12.3. For example, the β-2-adrenergic receptor, and its common mutation of Arg→Gly at amino acid 16, greatly reduces the bronchodilator response of albuterol (Ligget, 2000). In addition, mutations in the angiotensin-converting enzyme (ACE) gene have been proposed to account for variations in the response to ACE inhibitors. Another study has shown that a combination of two mutations in the gene encoding a high-affinity sulphonylurea receptor leads to a 40% reduction in the insulin response to tolbutamide (Hansen et al, 1998). The response to clozapine in patients with schizophrenia appears to involve genetic polymorphisms in the 5-hydroxytryptamine (serotonin) receptor, HTR2A. Finally, mutations in five genes involved in the cardiac ion channels affect the risk of drug-induced long-QT syndrome (Priori et al, 1999), a potential cause of sudden cardiac death in young individuals without structural heart disease. The prevalence of long-QT syndrome is about 1 in 10,000. All five genes code for membrane ion channels affecting sodium or potassium transport and are influenced by antiarrhythmics and other drugs (Evans and Relling, 1999).

The systematic identification and functional analysis of human genes is changing the study of disease processes and drug development. Pharmacogenetics enable clinicians to make reliable assessments of an individual's risk of acquiring a particular disease, be more specific in targeting drugs, and account for individual variation of therapeutic response and toxicity of drugs. Mutant alleles at a single gene locus are the best studied individual risk factors for adverse drug reactions, including the genes

TABLE 12.3 Clinically Important Genetic Polymorphisms of Drug Targets and Drug Transporters

GENE	FREQUENCY	DRUG	DRUG EFFECT
Multidrug resistance gene (MDR1)	24%	Digoxin	Increased concentrations of digoxin in plasma
Beta-2 adrenergic receptor gene (2AR)	37%	Albuterol	Decreased response to Beta-2 adrenergic agonists
Sulphonylurea receptor gene (SUR1)	2–3%	Tolbutamide	Decreased insulin response
Five genes coding for cardiac ion channels	1–2%	Antiarrhythmics, terfenadine, many other drugs	Sudden cardiac death due to long-QT syndrome

From Meyer (2000), with permission.

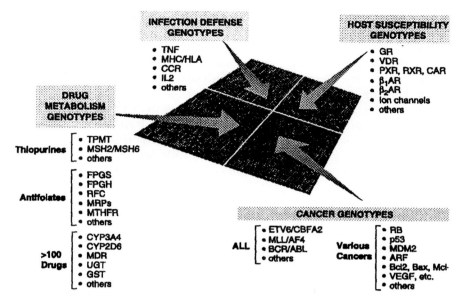

Figure 12-3. Molecular diagnostics of pharmacogenomic traits. DNA arrays are being made for automated, high-throughput detection of functionally important mutations in genes that are important determinants of drug effects, such as drug-metabolizing enzymes, drug targets (receptors), disease pathogenesis, and other polymorphic genes that influence an individual's susceptibility to drug toxicities or environmental exposures (such as pathogens, carcinogens, and others). This figure exemplifies components of a potential diagnostic DNA array for genes that could influence a patient's response to chemotherapy for acute lymphoblastic leukemia, including genes that determine drug metabolism, disease sensitivity, and the risk of adverse effects of treatment (cardiovascular or endocrine toxicities, infections, etc).
(From Evans and Relling, 1999, with permission.)

for N-acetyltransferase, thiopurine methyltransferase, dihydropyrimidine dehydrogenase, and the cytochrome P-450 isozymes. Genotyping can predict phenotype extremes in these situations and identify metabolic status in individual patients. Genomics is providing the information and technology needed to analyze the complex multifactorial situations involved in drug therapy (Fig. 12-3). Awareness of inherited variations of drug response can lead to dose adjustment on the basis of the patient's genetic makeup and provides a promising approach to reducing adverse drug reactions (Evans and Johnson, 2001; Roses, 2000). Dahl (2002) has reviewed the issues involving pharmacogenomics and the prescribing of antipsychotic drugs.

PHARMACOKINETICS/PHARMACODYNAMICS (PK/PD) CONSIDERATIONS AND PHARMACOGENETICS/PHARMACOGENOMICS (PGt/PGx)

The study of drug interactions and PGt/PGx has revealed that many unexpected pharmacodynamic responses and pharmacokinetic variations among individuals during drug therapy involve genetic factors. These genetic factors contribute to variation at many levels, including drug transport, metabolism, and interaction at the receptor site.

Applying genetics to study interindividual variations in drug response may greatly improve drug therapy. Understanding and monitoring the underlying pharmacogenetic factors will allow physicians to optimize efficacy and minimize side effects. The labeling of many new drugs now contains more information on drug interactions and metabolism based on our understanding of PGt/PGx. PGt/PGx is influencing the study of pharmacokinetics and pharmacodynamics. Population pharmacokinetics has already assimilated some of these changes by enriching what are often simple or even empirical PK/PD models to simulate the quantitative aspect of drug distribution and drug action.

Models that will predict dosing and an individual's drug clearance more accurately will require more details concerning the individual patient's genetic profile, demographic and pathologic information, as well as the drug's PK profile. If one of the patient's parents is homozygous for a specific isozyme that metabolizes the drug, how would that information be linked to a clearance prediction for the patient? Recognizing the allele that predisposes the patient to a severe adverse reaction or toxic plasma concentration may allow the dose to be reduced or the drug avoided entirely. Similarly, if a patient is known to be a nonresponder due to genetic variation, that information can be used to select an alternate drug *a priori*.

In Chapter 20, a mixed-effects model is described that takes into account the effect of enzyme induction due to concomitant administration of a drug that induces enzyme. Should new models be developed, or will an extension of some of the mixed-effect models suffice? Advances in PGt will no doubt stimulate developments in PK and PD.

The successful application of genetic screening tests to identify patients with specific risks in drug response or drug toxicity depends on many factors. Large amounts of relevant genetic information must be monitored. Robust, high-throughput, high-positive and low-negative predictive tests must be developed and implemented. Such an endeavor will also involve considerable training, adaptation, and acceptance of the new technology by physicians and other health care personnel. With genetic diagnostic tests becoming more common and affordable, it is expected that individual drug dosing will become more accurate and ultimately result in vast improvements in therapeutic response and better drug tolerance. Researchers have high expectations that the use of diagnostic DNA microarrays or gene chips will simplify and expand testing and have clinical applications in diagnosis, disease prevention, drug selection, and dose calculation. The challenge to pharmacokinetics is to integrate all the relevant information into a model that is accurate and simple enough for practical application.

FREQUENTLY ASKED QUESTIONS

1. In genetic polymorphism of CY2C9, the frequency of polymorphism is much higher in heterocytes (14–28 %) than in homocytes (0.2–1%). Why?
2. How do drug efflux transporters affect the rate and extent of drug absorption and the bioavailability of a drug?

3. Which human ABC-transport protein may influence the activation of transcription factors such as PXR in the liver, and which nuclear hormone receptors regulate drug detoxification genes?

4. How is biliary excretion affected if genetic expression of a transport protein is enhanced?

5. Without pharmacogenetic profiling of subjects, what are the chances of a subject with an unusually high expression of P-glycoprotein to be interpreted as a "statistical outliner" in a bioavailability study due to more rapid efflux that results in lower drug levels compared with other subjects? Is deviation from the mean a rational valid reason for data exclusion?

6. Should exclusion criteria based on pharmacogenomics be used in designing protocol for pharmacokinetics or clinical studies? In other words, minimize variation (prevent monkey wrench) and increase power in bioequivalence studies?

7. Often, the most likely functions are employed to minimize deviations from the data when pharmacokinetic parameters are estimated by iteration within a group. These parameters are estimated for an average individual such that most subjects resemble the mean within a group. However, for a subject with the unusual allele, the underlying genetic factors contribute parameter differences that are the result of genetic expression. How useful are the parameters obtained from a classical pharmacokinetic model that does not incorporate parameters accounting for genomic determinants? (*Note:* An attempt to force data fitting the mean would seriously err for a few individuals, ie, fit most subjects well, but err badly for the few, on the basis of minimization of the sum of squared deviations.)

8. What are the differences between pharmacogenetics and pharmacogenomics? There are many but no uniformly accepted definition. The two terms are regarded as similar by some and different by others. The latter term is preferred by more recent investigators. It is regarded by some to be more focused on the deployment of high-throughput technologies, besides its applications in drug therapy and drug discovery.

REFERENCES

Borges-Walmsley MI, Walmsley AR: The structure and function of drug Pumps. *Trends Microbiol* **9**(2):71–79, 2001

Borst P, Evers R, Kool M, et al: A family of drug transporters: the multi-drug resistance-associated proteins. *J Natl Cancer Inst* **92**:1295–302, 2000

Clark EA, Golub TR, Lander ES, Hynes RO: Genomic analysis of metastasis reveals an essential role for RhoC. *Nature* **406**(6795):532–535, 2000

Dahl, ML: Cytochrome P450—Phenotyping/genotyping in patients receiving antipsychotics: Useful aid to prescribing? *Clin Pharmacokinet* **41**:453–470, 2002

Doherty MM, Charman WN: The mucosa of the small intestine: How clinically relevant as an organ of drug metabolism? *Clin Pharmacokinet* **41**(4):235–253, 2002

Evans WE, Johnson JA: Pharmacogenomics: The inherited basis for interindividual differences in drug response. *Annu Rev Genom Hum Genet* **2**:9–39, 2001

Evans WE, McLeod HL: Pharmacogenomics—Drug disposition, drug targets and side effects. *N Engl J Med* **348**:538–549, 2003

Evans WE, Relling MV: Pharmacogenomics: Translating functional genomics into rational therapeutics. *Science* **286:**487–491, 1999

Gonzalez FJ, Skoda RC, et al. Characterization of the common genetic defect in humans deficient in debrisoquine metabolism. *Nature* **331:**442–446, 1988

Hansen T, Echwald SM, Hansen L, et al. Decreased tolbutamide-stimulated insulin secretion in healthy subjects with sequence variants in the high-affinity sulfonyurea receptor gene. *Diabetes* **47:**598–605, 1998

Kwiatkowski D: Clinical review: Science, medicine, and the future—Susceptibility to infection *Br Med J* **321:**1061–1065, 2000

Lesko LJ, Woodcock J: Pharmacogenomic-guided drug development: Regulatory perspective. *Pharmacogenom J* **2:**20–24, 2002

Ligget SB: The pharmacogenetics of beta2-adrenergic receptors: Relevance to asthma. *J Allergy Clin Immunol* **105:**487–492, 2000

Makita N, Horie M, Nakamura T, et al. Drug-induced long-QT syndrome associated with a subclinical SCN5A mutation. *Circulation,* **106:** 1269–74, 2002

Mancinelli L , Cronin M, Sadée W: Pharmacogenomics: The promise of personalized medicine. *AAPS PharmSci* **2**(1):Article 4, 2000 (www.aapspharmsci.org)

McLeod HL and Evans WE: Pharmacogenomics: Unlocking the human genome for better drug therapy, *Annu. Rev. Pharmacol. Toxicol.* **41:**101-21, 2001.

Meyer UA. Genotype or phenotype: the definition of a pharmacogenetic polymorphism. *Pharmacogenetics* **1:**66–67 1991

Meyer UA: Pharmacogenetics and adverse drug reactions. *Lancet* **356:**1167–1171, 2000

Pillips KA et al: Potential role of pharmacogenetics in reducing adverse drug reactions—A systematic review. *JAMA* **286:**2270, 2001

Priori SG, Barhanin J, Hauer RN, et al: Genetic and molecular basis of cardiac arrhythmias: Impact on clinical management, Parts I and II. *Circulation* **99:**518–528, 1999

Roses AD: Pharmacogenetics and future drug development and delivery. *Lancet* **355:**1355–1361, 2000

Roses AD: Pharmacogenetics. *Hum Mol Genet* **10:**2261–2267, 2001

Sadee W: Pharmacogenomics: The implemention phase. *AAPS News Lett* 2002

Sharom FJ et al: Interaction of the P-glycoprotein multidrug transporter (MDR1) with high affinity peptide chemosensitizers in isolated membranes, reconstituted systems, and intact cells. *Biochem Pharmacol* **58:**571–586, 1999

Workshop on Pharmacogenetics/Pharmacogenomics in Drug Development and Regulatory Decision-Making. Sponsored by FDA, PhRMA, Preclinical Safety Committee (DrugSafe) and Pharmacogenetics Working Group (PWG) at University of Maryland, Rockville. MD, May 16–17, 2002

BIBLIOGRAPHY

Arranz MJ, Munro J, Sham P, et al: Meta-analysis of studies on genetic variation in 5-HT2A receptors and clozapine response. *Schizophr Res* **32:**93–99, 1998

Hoffmeyer S, Burk O, von Richter O, et al: Functional polymorphisms of the human multi-drug resistance gene: Multiple sequence variations and correlation of one allele with P-glycoprotein expression and activity in vivo. *Proc Natl Acad Sci USA* **97:**3473–3478, 2000

Human Genome Project: www.ornl.gov/hgmis/medicine/pharma.html. The U.S. Human Genome Project is a 13-year effort coordinated by the U.S. Department of Energy and the National Institutes of Health.

Kidd RS, Straughn AB, Meyer MC, Blaisdell J, Goldstein JA, Dalton JT: Pharmacokinetics of chlorpheniramine, phenytoin, glipizide and nifedipine in an individual homozygous for the CYP2C9*3 allele. *Pharmacogenetics* **9:**71–80, 1999

Liu R, Siemiarczuk A, Sharom, FJ: Intrinsic fluorescence of the P-glycoprotein multidrug transporter: Sensitivity of tryptophan residues to binding of drugs and nucleotides. *Biochemistry* **39**(48):14927–14938, 2000

Miners JP, Birkett DJ: Cytochrome P4502C9: An enzyme of major importance in human drug metabolism. *Br J Clin Pharmacol* **45:**525–538, 1998

Navis G, van der Kleij FG, de Zeeuw D, de Jong PE: Angiotensin-converting enzyme gene I/D polymorphism and renal disease. *J Mol Med* **77:**781–791, 1999

PharmGKB: www.pharmgkb.org PharmGKB is an integrated resource about how variation in human genes leads to variation in response to drugs.

Raimundo S, Fischer J, Eichelbaum M, Griese E-U, Schwab M, Zanger UM: Elucidation of the genetic basis of the common "intermediate metabolizer" phenotype for drug oxidation by CYP2D6. *Pharmacogenetics* **10:**1–5, 2000

Synold TW, Dussault I, Forman BM: The orphan nuclear receptor SXR coordinately regulates drug metabolism and efflux. *Nature Med* **7**(5), 2001

13

PHYSIOLOGIC FACTORS RELATED TO DRUG ABSORPTION

The systemic absorption of a drug is dependent on (1) the physicochemical properties of the drug, (2) the nature of the drug product, and (3) the anatomy and physiology of the drug absorption site. All of these considerations are important in the manufacture and biopharmaceutic evaluation of drug products (Chapter 14). Proper drug product selection requires a thorough understanding of the physiologic and pathologic factors affecting drug absorption to assure therapeutic efficacy and to avoid potential drug–drug and drug–nutrient interactions. This chapter will focus on the anatomic and physiologic considerations for the systemic absorption of a drug.

ROUTE OF DRUG ADMINISTRATION

Drugs may be given by parenteral, enteral, inhalation, transdermal (percutaneous), or intranasal route for systemic absorption. Each route of drug administration has certain advantages and disadvantages. Some characteristics of the more common routes of drug administration are listed in Table 13.1. The systemic availability and onset of drug action are affected by blood flow to the administration site, the physicochemical characteristics of the drug and the drug product, and by any pathophysiologic condition at the absorption site.

Many drugs are not administered orally because of drug instability in the gastrointestinal tract or drug degradation by the digestive enzymes in the intestine. For example, erythropoietin and human growth hormone (somatrophin) are administered intramuscularly, and insulin is administered subcutaneously or intramuscularly, because of the potential for degradation of these drugs in the stomach or intestine. Biotechnology products (Chapter 18) are often too labile to be administered orally and therefore are usually given parenterally. Drug absorption after subcutaneous injection is slower than intravenous injection. Pathophysiologic

TABLE 13.1   Common Routes of Drug Administration

ROUTE	BIOAVAILABILITY	ADVANTAGES	DISADVANTAGES
Parenteral Routes			
Intravenous bolus (IV)	Complete (100%) systemic drug absorption. Rate of bioavailability considered instantaneous.	Drug is given for immediate effect.	Increased chance for adverse reaction. Possible anaphylaxis.
Intravenous infusion (IV inf)	Complete (100%) systemic drug absorption. Rate of drug absorption controlled by infusion rate.	Plasma drug levels more precisely controlled. May inject large fluid volumes. May use drugs with poor lipid solubility and/or irritating drugs.	Requires skill in insertion of infusion set. Tissue damage at site of injection (infiltration, necrosis, or sterile abscess).
Intramuscular injection (IM)	Rapid from aqueous solution. Slow absorption from non-aqueous (oil) solutions.	Easier to inject than intravenous injection. Larger volumes may be used compared to subcutaneous solutions.	Irritating drugs may be very painful. Different rates of absorption depending on muscle group injected and blood flow.
Subcutaneous injection (SC)	Prompt from aqueous solution. Slow absorption from repository formulations.	Generally, used for insulin injection.	Rate of drug absorption depends on blood flow and injection volume.
Enteral Routes			
Buccal or sublingual (SL)	Rapid absorption from lipid-soluble drugs.	No "first-pass" effects.	Some drugs may be swallowed. Not for most drugs or drugs with high doses.
Oral (PO)	Absorption may vary. Generally, slower absorption rate compared to IV bolus or IM injection.	Safest and easiest route of drug administration. May use immediate-release and modified-release drug products.	Some drugs may have erratic absorption, be unstable in the gastointestinal tract, or be metabolized by liver prior to systemic absorption.
Rectal (PR)	Absorption may vary from suppository. More reliable absorption from enema (solution).	Useful when patient cannot swallow medication. Used for local and systemic effects.	Absorption may be erratic. Suppository may migrate to different position. Some patient discomfort.
Other Routes			
Transdermal	Slow absorption, rate may vary. Increased absorption with occlusive dressing.	Transdermal delivery system (patch) is easy to use. Used for lipid-soluble drugs with low dose and low MW.	Some irritation by patch or drug. Permeability of skin variable with condition, anatomic site, age, and gender. Type of cream or ointment base affects drug release and absorption.
Inhalation and intranasal	Rapid absorption. Total dose absorbed is variable.	May be used for local or systemic effects.	Particle size of drug determines anatomic placement in respiratory tract. May stimulate cough reflex. Some drug may be swallowed.

conditions such as burns will increase the permeability of drugs across the skin compared with normal intact skin.

When a drug is administered by an extravascular route of administration (eg, oral, topical, intranasal, inhalation, rectal), the drug must first be absorbed into the systemic circulation and then diffuse or be transported to the site of action before eliciting biological and therapeutic activity. The general principles and kinetics of absorption from these extravascular sites follow the same principles as oral dosing, although the physiology of the site of administration differs.

NATURE OF CELL MEMBRANES

Many drugs administered by extravascular routes are intended for local effect. Other drugs are designed to be absorbed from the site of administration into the systemic circulation. For systemic drug absorption, the drug must cross cellular membranes. After oral administration, drug molecules must cross the intestinal epithelium by going either through or between the epithelial cells to reach the systemic circulation. The permeability of a drug at the absorption site into the systemic circulation is intimately related to the molecular structure of the drug and to the physical and biochemical properties of the cell membranes. Once in the plasma, the drug may have to cross biological membranes to reach the site of action. Therefore, biological membranes potentially pose a significant barrier to drug delivery.

Transcellular absorption is the process of drug movement across a cell. Some polar molecules may not be able to traverse the cell membrane but, instead, go through gaps or *tight junctions* between cells, a process known as *paracellular drug absorption.* Figure 13-1 shows the difference between the two processes. Some drugs are probably absorbed by a mixed mechanism involving one or more processes.

Membranes are major structures in cells, surrounding the entire cell (plasma membrane) and acting as a boundary between the cell and the interstitial fluid. In addition, membranes enclose most of the cell organelles (eg, the mitochondrion membrane). Functionally, cell membranes are semipermeable partitions that act as selective barriers to the passage of molecules. Water, some selected small molecules, and lipid-soluble molecules pass through such membranes, whereas highly charged molecules and large molecules, such as proteins and protein-bound drugs, do not.

The transmembrane movement of drugs is influenced by the composition and structure of the plasma membranes. Cell membranes are generally thin, approximately 70 to 100 Å in thickness. Cell membranes are composed primarily of phospholipids in the form of a bilayer interdispersed with carbohydrates and protein groups. There are several theories as to the structure of the cell membrane. The *lipid bilayer* or *unit membrane theory,* originally proposed by Davson and Danielli (1952), considers the plasma membrane to be composed of two layers of phospholipid between two surface layers of proteins, with the hydrophilic "head" groups of the phospholipids facing the protein layers and the hydrophobic "tail" groups of the phospholipids aligned in the interior. The lipid bilayer theory explains the observation that lipid-soluble drugs tend to penetrate cell membranes more easily than polar molecules. However, the bilayer cell membrane structure does not account for the diffusion of water, small-molecular-weight molecules such as urea, and certain charged ions.

Figure 13-1. Summary of intestinal epithelial transporters. Transporters shown by square and oval shapes demonstrate active and facilitated transporters, respectively. Names of cloned transporters are shown with square or oval shapes. In the case of active transporter, arrows in the same direction represent symport of substance and the driving force. Arrows going in the reverse direction mean the antiport.
(From Tsuji and Tamai, 1996, with permission.)

The *fluid mosaic model*, proposed by Singer and Nicolson (1972), explains the transcellular diffusion of polar molecules. According to this model, the cell membrane consists of globular proteins embedded in a dynamic fluid, lipid bilayer matrix (Fig. 13-2). These proteins provide a pathway for the selective transfer of certain polar molecules and charged ions through the lipid barrier. As shown in

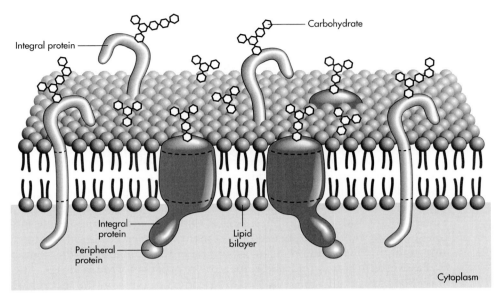

Figure 13-2.   Model of the plasma membrane including proteins and carbohydrates as well as lipids. Integral proteins are embedded in the lipid bilayer; peripheral proteins are merely associated with the membrane surface. The carbohydrate consists of monosaccharides, or simple sugars, strung together in chains attached to proteins (forming glycoproteins) or to lipids (forming glycolipids). The asymmetry of the membrane is manifested in several ways. Carbohydrates are always on the exterior surface and peripheral proteins are almost always on the cytoplasmic, or inner, surface. The two lipid monolayers include different proportions of the various kinds of lipid molecule. Most important, each species of integral protein has a definite orientation, which is the same for every molecule of that species. (From Lodish and Rothman, 1979, with permission.)

Figure 13-2, transmembrane proteins are interdispersed throughout the membrane. Two types of pores of about 10 nm and 50 to 70 nm were inferred to be present in membranes based on capillary membrane transport studies (Pratt and Taylor, 1990). These small pores provide a channel through which water, ions, and dissolved solutes such as urea may move across the membrane.

PASSAGE OF DRUGS ACROSS CELL MEMBRANES

Passive Diffusion

Theoretically, a lipophilic drug may pass through the cell or go around it. If the drug has a low molecular weight and is lipophilic, the lipid cell membrane is not a barrier to drug diffusion and absorption. *Passive diffusion* is the process by which molecules spontaneously diffuse from a region of higher concentration to a region of lower concentration. This process is *passive* because no external energy is expended. In Figure 13-3, drug molecules move forward and back across a membrane. If the two sides have the same drug concentration, forward-moving drug molecules are balanced by molecules moving back, resulting in no net transfer of drug. When one side is higher in drug concentration, at any given time, the number of

Figure 13-3. Passive diffusion of molecules. Molecules in solution diffuse randomly in all directions. As molecules diffuse from left to right and vice versa (small arrows), a net diffusion from the high-concentration side to the low-concentration side results. This results in a net flux (J) to the right side. Flux is measured in mass per unit area (eg, mg/cm²).

forward-moving drug molecules will be higher than the number of backward-moving molecules; the net result will be a transfer of molecules to the alternate side, as indicated in the figure by the big arrow. The rate of transfer is called *flux,* and is represented by a vector to show its direction in space. The tendency of molecules to move in all directions is natural, because molecules possess kinetic energy and constantly collide with one another in space. Only left and right molecule movements are shown in Figure 13-3, because movement of molecules in other directions will not result in concentration changes because of the limitation of the container wall.

Passive diffusion is the major absorption process for most drugs. The driving force for passive diffusion is higher drug concentrations on the mucosal side compared to the blood. According to *Fick's law of diffusion,* drug molecules diffuse from a region of high drug concentration to a region of low drug concentration.

$$\frac{dQ}{dt} = \frac{DAK}{h}(C_{\mathrm{GI}} - C_{\mathrm{p}}) \tag{13.1}$$

where dQ/dt = rate of diffusion, D = diffusion coefficient, K = lipid water partition coefficient of drug in the biologic membrane that controls drug permeation, A = surface area of membrane; h = membrane thickness, and $C_{\mathrm{GI}} - C_{\mathrm{p}}$ = difference between the concentrations of drug in the gastrointestinal tract and in the plasma.

Because the drug distributes rapidly into a large volume after entering the blood, the concentration of drug in the blood initially will be quite low with respect to the concentration at the site of drug absorption. For example, a drug is usually given in milligram doses, whereas plasma concentrations are often in the microgram-per-milliliter or nanogram-per-milliliter range. If the drug is given orally, then $C_{\mathrm{GI}} \gg C_{\mathrm{p}}$ and a large concentration gradient is maintained, thus driving drug molecules into the plasma from the gastrointestinal tract.

Given Fick's law of diffusion, several other factors can be seen to influence the rate of passive diffusion of drugs. For example, the degree of lipid solubility of the drug influences the rate of drug absorption. The partition coefficient, K, represents the lipid–water partitioning of a drug across the hypothetical membrane in the mucosa. Drugs that are more lipid soluble have a larger value of K. The surface area, A, of the membrane also influences the rate of absorption. Drugs may be absorbed from most areas of the gastrointestinal tract. However, the duodenal area of the small intestine shows the most rapid drug absorption, due to such anatomic features as villi and microvilli, which provide a large surface area. These villi are less abundant in other areas of the gastrointestinal tract.

The thickness of the hypothetical model membrane, h, is a constant for any particular absorption site. Drugs usually diffuse very rapidly through capillary plasma membranes in the vascular compartments, in contrast to diffusion through plasma membranes of capillaries in the brain. In the brain, the capillaries are densely lined with glial cells, so a drug diffuses slowly into the brain as if a thick lipid membrane existed. The term *blood–brain barrier* is used to describe the poor diffusion of water-soluble molecules across capillary plasma membranes into the brain. However, in certain disease states such as meningitis these membranes may be disrupted or become more permeable to drug diffusion.

The diffusion coefficient, D, is a constant for each drug and is defined as the amount of a drug that diffuses across a membrane of a given unit area per unit time when the concentration gradient is unity. The dimensions of D are area per unit time—for example, cm^2/sec.

Because D, A, K, and h are constants under usual conditions for absorption, a combined constant P or permeability coefficient may be defined.

$$P = \frac{DAK}{h} \tag{13.2}$$

Furthermore, in Equation 13.1 the drug concentration in the plasma, C_p, is extremely small compared to the drug concentration in the gastrointestinal tract, C_{GI}. If C_p is negligible and P is substituted into Equation 13.1, the following relationship for Fick's law is obtained:

$$\frac{dQ}{dt} = P(C_{GI}) \tag{13.3}$$

Equation 13.3 is an expression for a first-order process. In practice, the extravascular absorption of most drugs tends to be a first-order absorption process. Moreover, because of the large concentration gradient between C_{GI} and C_p, the rate of drug absorption is usually more rapid than the rate of drug elimination.

Many drugs have both lipophilic and hydrophilic chemical substituents. Those drugs that are more lipid soluble tend to traverse cell membranes more easily than less lipid-soluble or more water-soluble molecules. For drugs that act as weak electrolytes, such as weak acids and bases, the extent of ionization influences the rate of drug transport. The ionized species of the drug contains a charge and is more water soluble than the nonionized species of the drug, which is more lipid soluble. The extent of ionization of a weak electrolyte will depend on both the pK_a of the drug and the pH of the medium in which the drug is dissolved. *Henderson and Hasselbalch* used the following expressions pertaining to weak acids and weak bases to describe the relationship between pK_a and pH:

For weak acids,

$$\text{Ratio} = \frac{[\text{salt}]}{[\text{acid}]} = \frac{[A^-]}{[HA]} = 10^{(pH-pK_a)} \tag{13.4}$$

For weak bases,

$$\text{Ratio} = \frac{[\text{base}]}{[\text{salt}]} = \frac{[RNH_2]}{[RNH_3^+]} = 10^{(pH-pK_a)} \tag{13.5}$$

With Equations 13.4 and 13.5, the proportion of free acid or free base existing as the nonionized species may be determined at any given pH, assuming the pK_a for the drug is known. For example, at a plasma pH of 7.4, salicylic acid ($pK_a = 3.0$) exists mostly in its ionized or water-soluble form, as shown below:

$$\text{Ratio} = \frac{[\text{salt}]}{[\text{acid}]} = 10^{(7.4-3.0)}$$

$$\log \frac{[\text{salt}]}{[\text{acid}]} = 7.4 - 3.0 = 4.4$$

$$\frac{[\text{salt}]}{[\text{acid}]} = 2.51 \times 10^4$$

In a simple system, the total drug concentration on either side of a membrane should be the same at equilibrium, assuming Fick's law of diffusion is the only distribution factor involved. For diffusible drugs, such as nonelectrolyte drugs or drugs that do not ionize, the drug concentrations on either side of the membrane are the same at equilibrium. However, for electrolyte drugs or drugs that ionize, the total drug concentrations on either side of the membrane are not equal at equilibrium if the pH of the medium differs on respective sides of the membrane. For example, consider the concentration of salicylic acid ($pK_a = 3.0$) in the stomach (pH 1.2) as opposed to its concentration in the plasma (pH 7.4) (Fig. 13-4). According to the Henderson–Hasselbalch equation (Eq. 13.4) for weak acids, at pH 7.4 and at pH 1.2, salicylic acid exists in the ratios that follow.

In the plasma, at pH 7.4:

$$\text{Ratio} = \frac{(\text{RCOO}^-)}{(\text{RCOOH})} = 2.51 \times 10^4$$

In gastric juice, at pH 1.2:

$$\text{Ratio} = \frac{(\text{RCOO}^-)}{(\text{RCOOH})} = 10^{(1.2-3.0)} = 1.58 \times 10^{-2}$$

The total drug concentration on either side of the membrane is determined as shown in Table 13.2.

Thus, the pH affects distribution of salicylic acid (RCOOH) and its salt (RCOO$^-$) across cell membranes. It is assumed that the acid, RCOOH, is freely permeable and the salt, RCOO$^-$, is not permeable across the cell membrane. In this example the total concentration of salicylic acid at equilibrium is approximately 25,000 times greater in the plasma than in the stomach (Table 13.2). These calculations can also be applied to weak bases, using Equation 13.5.

Figure 13-4. *Model for the distribution of an orally administered weak electrolyte drug such as salicylic acid.*

TABLE 13.2 Relative Concentrations of Salicylic Acid as Affected by pH

DRUG	GASTRIC JUICE (pH 1.2)	PLASMA (pH 7.4)
RCOOH	1.0000	1
RCOO$^-$	0.0158	25100
Total drug concentration	1.0158	25101

According to the *pH–partition hypothesis*, if the pH on one side of a cell membrane differs from the pH on the other side of the membrane, then (1) the drug (weak acid or base) will ionize to different degrees on respective sides of the membrane; (2) the total drug concentrations (ionized plus nonionized drug) on either side of the membrane will be unequal; and (3) the compartment in which the drug is more highly ionized will contain the greater total drug concentration. For these reasons, a weak acid (such as salicylic acid) will be rapidly absorbed from the stomach (pH 1.2), whereas a weak base (such as quinidine) will be poorly absorbed from the stomach.

Another factor that can influence drug concentrations on either side of a membrane is a particular *affinity* of the drug for a tissue component, which prevents the drug from moving freely back across the cell membrane. For example, a drug such as dicumarol binds to plasma protein, and digoxin binds to tissue protein. In each case, the protein-bound drug does not move freely across the cell membrane. Drugs such as chlordane are very lipid soluble and will partition into adipose (fat) tissue. In addition, a drug such as tetracycline might form a complex with calcium in the bones and teeth. Finally, a drug may concentrate in a tissue due to a specific uptake or active transport process. Such processes have been demonstrated for iodide in thyroid tissue, potassium in the intracellular water, and certain catecholamines into adrenergic storage sites. Such drugs may have a higher total drug concentration on the side where binding occurs, yet the free drug concentration that diffuses across cell membranes will be the same on both sides of the membrane.

Instead of diffusing into the cell, drugs can also diffuse into the spaces around the cell as an absorption mechanism. In *paracellular drug absorption,* drug molecules smaller than 500 MW diffuse into the tight junctions, or spaces between intestinal epithelial cells.

Carrier-Mediated Transport

Theoretically, a lipophilic drug may pass through the cell or go around it. If the drug has a low molecular weight and is lipophilic, the lipid cell membrane is not a barrier to drug diffusion and absorption. In the intestine, drugs and other molecules can go through the intestinal epithelial cells by either diffusion or a carrier-mediated mechanism. Numerous specialized carrier-mediated transport systems are present in the body, especially in the intestine for the absorption of ions and nutrients required by the body.

Active Transport

Active transport is a carrier-mediated transmembrane process that plays an important role in the gastrointestinal absorption and in renal and biliary secretion of many drugs and metabolites. A few lipid-insoluble drugs that resemble natural physiologic metabolites (such as 5-fluorouracil) are absorbed from the gastrointestinal tract by

Figure 13-5.   Hypothetical carrier-mediated transport process.

this process. Active transport is characterized by the transport of drug against a concentration gradient—that is, from regions of low drug concentrations to regions of high concentrations. Therefore, this is an energy-consuming system. In addition, active transport is a specialized process requiring a carrier that binds the drug to form a carrier–drug complex that shuttles the drug across the membrane and then dissociates the drug on the other side of the membrane (Fig. 13-5).

The carrier molecule may be highly selective for the drug molecule. If the drug structurally resembles a natural substrate that is actively transported, then it is likely to be actively transported by the same carrier mechanism. Therefore, drugs of similar structure may compete for sites of adsorption on the carrier. Furthermore, because only a fixed number of carrier molecules are available, all the binding sites on the carrier may become saturated if the drug concentration gets very high. A comparison between the rate of drug absorption and the concentration of drug at the absorption site is shown in Figure 13-6. Notice that for a drug absorbed by passive diffusion, the rate of absorption increases in a linear relationship to drug concentration. In contrast, when a drug is absorbed by a carrier-mediated process, the rate of drug absorption increases with drug concentration until the carrier molecules are completely saturated. At higher drug concentrations, the rate of drug absorption remains constant, or zero order.

Facilitated Diffusion

Facilitated diffusion is also a carrier-mediated transport system, differing from active transport in that the drug moves along a concentration gradient (ie, moves from a region of high drug concentration to a region of low drug concentration). Therefore, this system does not require energy input. However, because this system is carrier mediated, it is saturable and structurally selective for the drug and shows competition kinetics for drugs of similar structure. In terms of drug absorption, facilitated diffusion seems to play a very minor role.

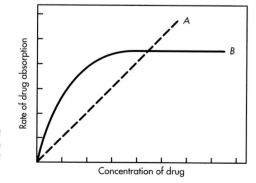

Figure 13-6. Comparison of the rates of drug absorption of a drug absorbed by passive diffusion (line A) and a drug absorbed by a carrier-mediated system (line B).

TABLE 13.3   Intestine Transporters and Examples of Drugs Transported

TRANSPORTER	EXAMPLES	
Amino acid transporter	Gabapentin	D-Cycloserine
	Methyldopa	Baclofen
	L-dopa	
Oligopeptide transporter	Cefadroxil	Cephradine
	Cefixime	Ceftibuten
	Cephalexin	Captopril
	Lisinopril	Thrombin inhibitor
Phosphate transporter	Fostomycin	Foscarnet
Bile acid transporter	S3744	
Glucose transporter	p-Nitrophenyl-β-D-glucopyranoside	
P-glycoprotein efflux	Etoposide	Vinblastine
	Cyclosporin A	
Monocarboxylic acid transporter	Salicylic acid	Benzoic acid
	Pravastatin	

Adapted from Tsuji and Tamai (1996).

Carrier-Mediated Intestinal Transport

Various carrier-mediated systems (transporters) are present at the intestinal brush border and basolateral membrane for the absorption of specific ions and nutrients essential for the body (Tsuji and Tamal, 1996). Many drugs are absorbed by these carriers because of the structural similarity to natural substrates (Table 13.3). A transmembrane protein, P-glycoprotein (Pgp), has been identified in the intestine. Pgp appears to reduce apparent intestinal epithelial cell permeability from lumen to blood for various lipophilic or cytotoxic drugs and is discussed in more detail below. Other transporters are also present in the intestines (Tsuji and Tamal, 1996). For example, many oral cephalosporins are absorbed through the amino acid transporter. Cefazolin, a parenteral-only cephalosporin, is not available orally because it cannot be absorbed to a significant degree through this mechanism.

Vesicular Transport

Vesicular transport is the process of engulfing particles or dissolved materials by the cell. Pinocytosis and phagocytosis are forms of vesicular transport that differ by the type of material ingested. *Pinocytosis* refers to the engulfment of small solutes or fluid, whereas *phagocytosis* refers to the engulfment of larger particles or macromolecules, generally by macrophages. *Endocytosis* and *exocytosis* are the processes of moving specific macromolecules into and out of a cell, respectively.

During pinocytosis or phagocytosis, the cell membrane invaginates to surround the material and then engulfs the material, incorporating it into the cell (Fig. 13-7). Subsequently, the cell membrane containing the material forms a vesicle or vacuole within the cell. Vesicular transport is the proposed process for the absorption of orally administered Sabin polio vaccine and various large proteins.

An example of exocytosis is the transport of a protein such as insulin from insulin-producing cells of the pancreas into the extracellular space. The insulin molecules are first packaged into intracellular vesicles, which then fuse with the plasma membrane to release the insulin outside the cell.

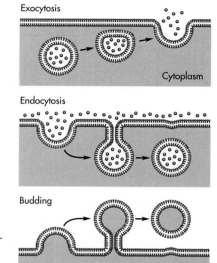

Figure 13-7.   Diagram showing exocytosis and endocytosis.
(From Alberts et al, 1988, with permission.)

Pore (Convective) Transport

Very small molecules (such as urea, water, and sugars) are able to cross cell membranes rapidly, as if the membrane contained channels or pores. Although such pores have never been directly observed by microscopy, the model of drug permeation through aqueous pores is used to explain renal excretion of drugs and the uptake of drugs into the liver.

A certain type of protein called a *transport protein* may form an open channel across the lipid membrane of the cell (Fig. 13-1). Small molecules including drugs move through the channel by diffusion more rapidly than at other parts of the membrane.

Ion-Pair Formation

Strong electrolyte drugs are highly ionized or charged molecules, such as quaternary nitrogen compounds with extreme pK_a values. Strong electrolyte drugs maintain their charge at all physiologic pH values and penetrate membranes poorly. When the ionized drug is linked up with an oppositely charged ion, an *ion pair* is formed in which the overall charge of the pair is neutral. This neutral drug complex diffuses more easily across the membrane. For example, the formation of ion pairs to facilitate drug absorption has been demonstrated for propranolol, a basic drug that forms an ion pair with oleic acid, and quinine, which forms ion pair with hexylsalicylate (Nienbert, 1989).

An interesting application of ion pairs is the complexation of amphotericin B and DSPG (disteroylphosphatidylglycerol) in some amphotericin B/liposome products. Ion pairing may transiently alter distribution, reduce high plasma free drug concentration, and reduce renal toxicity.

ORAL DRUG ABSORPTION

The oral route of administration is the most common and popular route of drug dosing. The oral dosage form must be designed to account for extreme pH ranges, the presence or absence of food, degradative enzymes, varying drug permeability in the different regions of the intestine, and motility of the gastrointestinal tract. In this chapter we will discuss intestinal variables that affect absorption; dosage-form considerations will be discussed in Chapters 14–17.

Anatomic and Physiologic Considerations

The normal physiologic processes of the alimentary canal may be affected by diet, contents of the gastrointestinal (GI) tract, hormones, the visceral nervous system, disease, and drugs. Thus, drugs given by the enteral route for systemic absorption may be affected by the anatomy, physiologic functions, and contents of the alimentary tract. Moreover, the physical, chemical, and pharmacologic properties of the drug itself will also affect its own absorption from the alimentary canal.

The *enteral system* consists of the alimentary canal from the mouth to the anus (Fig. 13-8). The major physiologic processes that occur in the GI system are secretion, digestion, and absorption. Secretion includes the transport of fluid, electrolytes, peptides, and proteins into the lumen of the alimentary canal. Enzymes in saliva and pancreatic secretions are also involved in the digestion of carbohydrates and

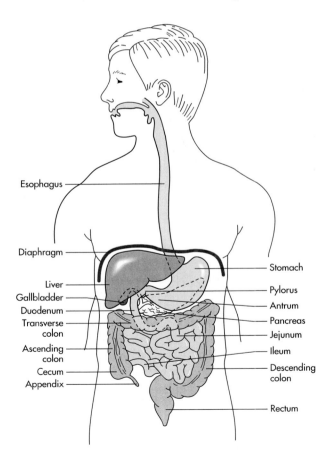

Figure 13-8. Gastrointestinal tract.

proteins. Other secretions, such as mucus, protect the linings of the lumen of the GI tract. Digestion is the breakdown of food constituents into smaller structures in preparation for absorption. Food constituents are mostly absorbed in the proximal area (duodenum) of the small intestine. The process of absorption is the entry of constituents from the lumen of the gut into the body. Absorption may be considered as the net result of both lumen-to-blood and blood-to-lumen transport movements.

Drugs administered orally pass through various parts of the enteral canal, including the oral cavity, esophagus, and various parts of the gastrointestinal tract. Residues eventually exit the body through the anus. The total transit time, including gastric emptying, small intestinal transit, and colonic transit, ranges from 0.4 to 5 days (Kirwan and Smith, 1974). The most important site for drug absorption is the small intestine. Small intestine transit time (SITT) ranges from 3 to 4 hours for most healthy subjects. If absorption is not completed by the time a drug leaves the small intestine, absorption may be erratic or incomplete. The small intestine is normally filled with digestive juices and liquids, keeping the lumen contents fluid. In contrast, the fluid in the colon is reabsorbed, and the lumenal content in the colon is either semisolid or solid, making further drug dissolution erratic and difficult. The lack of the solubilizing effect of the chyme and digestive fluid contributes to a less favorable environment for drug absorption.

Oral Cavity

Saliva is the main secretion of the oral cavity, and it has a pH of about 7. Saliva contains ptyalin (salivary amylase), which digests starches. Mucin, a glycoprotein that lubricates food, is also secreted and may interact with drugs. About 1500 mL of saliva is secreted per day.

Esophagus

The esophagus connects the pharynx and the cardiac orifice of the stomach. The pH of the fluids in the esophagus is between 5 and 6. The lower part of the esophagus ends with the esophageal sphincter, which prevents acid reflux from the stomach. Tablets or capsules may lodge in this area, causing local irritation. Very little drug dissolution occurs in the esophagus.

Stomach

The stomach is innervated by the vagus nerve. However, local nerve plexus, hormones, mechanoreceptors sensitive to the stretch of the GI wall, and chemoreceptors control the regulation of gastric secretions, including acid and stomach emptying. The fasting pH of the stomach is about 2 to 6. In the presence of food, the stomach pH is about 1.5 to 2, due to hydrochloric acid secreted by parietal cells. Stomach acid secretion is stimulated by gastrin and histamine. Gastrin is released from G cells, mainly in the antral mucosa and also in the duodenum. Gastrin release is regulated by stomach distention (swelling) and the presence of peptides and amino acids. A substance called intrinsic factor for vitamin B-12 absorption and various gastric enzymes, such as pepsin, which initiates protein digestion, are secreted into the gastric lumen to initiate digestion.

Basic drugs are solubilized rapidly in the presence of stomach acid. Mixing is intense and pressurized in the antral part of the stomach, a process of breaking down large food particles described as *antral milling*. Food and liquid are emptied by opening the pyloric sphincter into the duodenum. Stomach emptying is influenced by the food content and osmolality. Fatty acids and mono- and diglycerides delay gastric emptying (Hunt and Knox, 1968). High-density foods generally are emptied from the stomach more slowly. The relation of gastric emptying time to drug absorption is discussed more fully in the next section.

Duodenum

A common duct from the pancreas and the gallbladder enters into the duodenum. The duodenal pH is about 6 to 6.5, because of the presence of bicarbonate that neutralizes the acidic chyme emptied from the stomach. The pH is optimum for enzymatic digestion of protein and peptide food. Pancreatic juice containing enzymes is secreted into the duodenum from the bile duct. Trypsin, chymotrypsin, and carboxypeptidase are involved in the hydrolysis of proteins into amino acids. Amylase is involved in the digestion of carbohydrates. Pancreatic lipase secretion hydrolyzes fats into fatty acid. The complex fluid medium in the duodenum helps to dissolve many drugs with limited aqueous solubility.

The duodenum is a site where many ester prodrugs are hydrolyzed during absorption. The presence of proteolytic enzymes also makes many protein drugs unstable in the duodenum, preventing adequate absorption.

Jejunum

The jejunum is the middle portion of the small intestine, between the duodenum and the ileum. Digestion of protein and carbohydrates continues after addition of pancreatic juice and bile in the duodenum. This portion of the small intestine generally has fewer contractions than the duodenum and is preferred for *in-vivo* drug absorption studies.

Ileum

The ileum is the terminal part of the small intestine. This site has fewer contractions than the duodenum and may be blocked off by catheters with an inflatable balloon and perfused for drug absorption studies. The pH is about 7, with the distal part as high as 8. Due to the presence of bicarbonate secretion, acid drugs will dissolve. Bile secretion helps to dissolve fats and hydrophobic drugs. The ileocecal valve separates the small intestine from the colon.

Colon

The colon lacks villi and has limited drug absorption also, because of the more viscous and semisolid nature of the lumen contents. The colon is lined with mucin that functions as lubricant and protectant. The pH in this region is 5.5 to 7 (Shareef et al, 2003). A few drugs, such as theophylline and metoprolol, are absorbed in this region. Drugs that are absorbed well in this region are good candidates for an oral sustained-release dosage form. The colon contains both aerobic and anaerobic microorganisms that may metabolize some drugs. For example, L-dopa and lactulose are metabolized by enteric bacteria. Crohn's disease affects the colon and thickens the bowel wall. The microflora also become more anaerobic. Absorption of clindamycin and propranolol are increased, whereas other drugs have reduced absorption with this disease (Rubinstein et al, 1988).

Rectum

The rectum is about 15 cm long, ending at the anus. In the absence of fecal material, the rectum has a small amount of fluid (approximately 2 mL) with a pH about 7. The rectum is perfused by the superior, middle, and inferior hemorrhoidal veins. The inferior hemorrhoidal vein (closest to the anal sphincter) and the middle hemorrhoidal vein feed into the vena cava and back to the heart. The superior hemorrhoidal vein joins the mesenteric circulation, which feeds into the hepatic portal vein and then to the liver.

Drug absorption after rectal administration may be variable, depending on the placement of the suppository or drug solution within the rectum. A portion of the drug dose may be absorbed via the lower hemorrhoidal veins, from which the drug feeds directly into the systemic circulation; some drugs may be absorbed via the superior hemorrhoidal vein, which feeds into the mesenteric veins to the hepatic portal vein to the liver, and be metabolized before systemic absorption.

Drug Absorption in the Gastrointestinal Tract

Drugs may be absorbed by passive diffusion from all parts of the alimentary canal including sublingual, buccal, GI, and rectal absorption. For most drugs, the optimum site for drug absorption after oral administration is the upper portion of the small intestine or duodenum region. The unique anatomy of the duodenum provides an immense surface area for the drug to diffuse passively (Fig. 13-9). The large surface area of the duodenum is due to the presence of valvelike folds in the mucous membrane on which are small projections known as *villi*. These villi contain even smaller projections known as *microvilli*, forming a brush border. In addition, the duodenal region is highly perfused with a network of capillaries, which helps to maintain a concentration gradient from the intestinal lumen and plasma circulation.

Gastrointestinal Motility

Once a drug is given orally, the exact location and/or environment of the drug product within the GI tract is difficult to discern. GI motility tends to move the drug through the alimentary canal, so the drug may not stay at the absorption site. For drugs given orally, an anatomic absorption window may exist within the GI tract in which the drug is efficiently absorbed. Drugs contained in a non-biodegradable controlled-release dosage form must be completely released into this absorption window to be absorbed before the movement of the dosage form into the large bowel.

The transit time of the drug in the GI tract depends on the physiochemical and pharmacologic properties of the drug, the type of dosage form, and various physiologic factors. Physiologic movement of the drug within the GI tract depends on whether the alimentary canal contains recently ingested food (digestive or fed state) or is in the fasted or interdigestive state (Fig. 13-10). During the fasted or interdigestive state, alternating cycles of activity known as the *migrating motor complex* (MMC) act as a propulsive movement that empties the upper GI tract to the cecum. Initially, the alimentary canal is quiescent. Then, irregular contractions followed by regular contractions with high amplitude (housekeeper waves) push any residual contents distally or farther down the alimentary canal.

STRUCTURE	INCREASE IN SURFACE AREA (relative to cylinder)	SURFACE AREA (sq cm)
Area of simple cylinder	1	3300
Folds of Kerckring (valvulae conninventes)	3	10,000
Villi	30	100,000
Microvilli	600	2,000,000

Figure 13-9.   Three mechanisms for increasing surface area of the small intestine. The increase in surface area is due to folds of Kerkring, villi, and microvilli.
(From Wilson, 1962, with permission.)

In the fed state, the migrating motor complex is replaced by irregular contractions, which have the effect of mixing intestinal contents and advancing the intestinal stream toward the colon in short segments (Table 13.4). The pylorus and ileocecal valves prevent regurgitation or movement of food from the distal to the proximal direction.

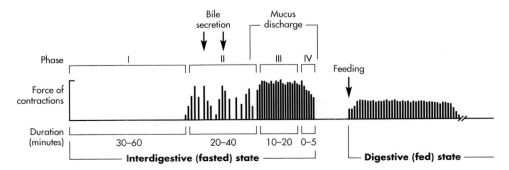

Figure 13-10.   A pictorial representation of the typical motility patterns in the interdigestive (fasted) and digestive (fed) state.
(From Rubinstein et al, 1988, with permission.)

TABLE 13.4 *Characteristics of the Motility Patterns in the Fasted Dog*

PHASE	DURATION	CHARACTERISTICS
Fasted State		
I	30–60 min	Quiescence.
II	20–40 min	• Irregular contractions.
		• Medium amplitude but can be as high as phase III.
		• Bile secretion begins.
		• Onset of gastric discharge of administered fluid of small volume usually occurs before that of particle discharge.
		• Onset of particle and mucus discharge may occur during the latter part of phase II.
III	5–15 min	• Regular contractions (4–5 contractions/min) with high amplitude.
		• Mucus discharge continues.
		• Particle discharge continues.
IV	0–5 min	• Irregular contractions.
		• Medium descending amplitude.
		• Sometimes absent.
Fed State		
One phase only	As long as food is present in the stomach	• Regular, frequent contractions.
		• Amplitude is lower than phase III.
		• 4–5 Contractions/min.

From Rubinstein et al (1988), with permission.

Gastric Emptying Time

Anatomically, a swallowed drug rapidly reaches the stomach. Eventually, the stomach empties its contents into the small intestine. Because the duodenum has the greatest capacity for the absorption of drugs from the GI tract, a delay in the gastric emptying time for the drug to reach the duodenum will slow the rate and possibly the extent of drug absorption, thereby prolonging the onset time for the drug. Some drugs, such as penicillin, are unstable in acid and decompose if stomach emptying is delayed. Other drugs, such as aspirin, may irritate the gastric mucosa during prolonged contact.

A number of factors affect gastric emptying time (Table 13.5). Some factors that tend to delay gastric emptying include consumption of meals high in fat, cold beverages, and anticholinergic drugs (Burks et al, 1985; Rubinstein et al, 1988). Liquids and small particles less than 1 mm are generally not retained in the stomach. These small particles are believed to be emptied due to a slightly higher basal pressure in the stomach over the duodenum. Different constituents of a meal empty from the stomach at different rates. Feldman and associates (1984) observed that 10 oz of liquid soft drink, scrambled egg (digestible solid), and a radio-opaque marker (undigestible solid) were 50% emptied from the stomach in 30 minutes, 154 minutes, and 3 to 4 hours, respectively. Thus, liquids are generally emptied faster than digested solids from the stomach (Fig. 13-11).

Large particles, including tablets and capsules, are delayed from emptying for 3 to 6 hours by the presence of food in the stomach. Indigestible solids empty very slowly, probably during the interdigestive phase, a phase in which food is not present and the stomach is less motile but periodically empties its content due to housekeeper wave contraction (Fig. 13-12).

TABLE 13.5 Factors Influencing Gastric Emptying

FACTOR	INFLUENCE ON GASTRIC EMPTYING
1. Volume	The larger the starting volume, the greater the initial rate of emptying, after this initial period, the larger the original volume, the slower the rate of emptying.
2. Type of meal	
Fatty acids	Reduction in rate of emptying is in direct proportion to their concentration and carbon chain length; little difference is detected from acetic to octanoic acids; major inhibitory influence is seen in chain lengths greater than 10 carbons (decanoic to stearic acids).
Triglycerides	Reduction in rate of emptying; unsaturated triglycerides are more effective than saturated ones; the most effective in reducing emptying rate were linseed and olive oils.
Carbohydrates	Reduction in rate emptying, primarily as a result of osmotic pressure; inhibition of emptying increases as concentration increases.
Amino acids	Reduction in rate of emptying to an extent directly dependent upon concentration, probably as a result of osmotic pressure.
3. Osmotic pressure	Reduction in rate of emptying to an extent dependent upon concentration for salts and nonelectrolytes: rate of emptying may increase at lower concentrations and then decrease at higher concentrations.
4. Physical state of gastric contents	Solutions or suspensions of small particles empty more rapidly than do chunks of material that must be reduced in size prior to emptying.
5. Chemicals	
Acids	Reduction in rate of emptying dependent upon concentration and molecular weight of the acid; lower molecular weight acids are more effective than those of higher molecular weight (in order of decreasing effectiveness: HCl, acetic, lactic, tartaric, citric acids).
Alkali (NaHCO$_3$)	Increased rate of emptying at low concentrations (1%), and decreased rate at higher concentrations (5%).
6. Drugs	
Anticholinergics	Reduction in rate of emptying.
Narcotic analgesics	Reduction in rate of emptying.
Metoclopramide	Increase in rate of emptying.
Ethanol	Reduction in rate of emptying.
7. Miscellaneous	
Body position	Rate of emptying is reduced in a patient lying on left side.
Viscosity	Rate of emptying is greater for less viscous solutions.
Emotional states	Aggressive or stressful emotional states increase stomach contractions and emptying rate; depression reduces stomach contraction and emptying.
Bile salts	Rate of emptying is reduced.
Disease states	Rate of emptying is reduced in some diabetics and in patients with local pyloric lesions (duodenal or pyloric ulcers; pyloric stenosis) and hypothyroidism; gastric emptying rate is increased in hyperthyroidism.
Exercise	Vigorous exercise reduces emptying rate.
Gastric surgery	Gastric emptying difficulties can be a serious problem after surgery.

From Mayersohn (1979), with permission.

Intestinal Motility

Normal peristaltic movements mix the contents of the duodenum, bringing the drug particles into intimate contact with the intestinal mucosal cells. The drug must have a sufficient time (*residence time*) at the absorption site for optimum absorption. In the case of high motility in the intestinal tract, as in diarrhea, the drug has a very brief residence time and less opportunity for adequate absorption.

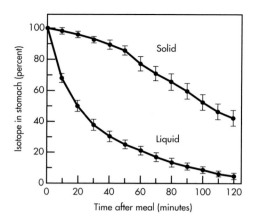

Figure 13-11. Gastric emptying of a group of normal subjects using the dual-isotope method. The mean and 1 SE of the fraction of isotope remaining in the stomach are depicted at various time intervals after ingestion of the meal. Note the exponential nature of liquid emptying and the linear process of solid emptying.
(From Minami and McCallum, 1984, with permission.)

The average normal small intestine transit time (SITT) was about 7 hours in early studies using indirect methods based on the detection of hydrogen after an oral dose of lactulose (fermentation of lactulose by colon bacteria yields hydrogen in the breath). Newer studies using gamma scintigraphy have shown SITT to be about 3 to 4 hours. Thus a drug may take about 4 to 8 hours to pass through the stomach and small intestine during the fasting state. During the fed state, SITT may take 8 to 12 hours. For modified-release or controlled-dosage forms, which slowly release the drug over an extended period of time, the dosage form must stay within a certain segment of the intestinal tract so that the drug contents are released and absorbed before loss of the dosage form in the feces. Intestinal transit is discussed further in relation to the design of sustained-release products in Chapter 17.

In one study reported by Shareef et al, 2003, utilizing a radioopaque marker, mean mouth-to-anus transit time was 53.3 hours. The mean colon transit time was 35 hours, with 11.3 hours for the right (ascending transverse portion), 11.4 hours for the left (descending and portion of the transverse), and 12.4 hours for the rectosigmoid colon. Dietary fiber has the greatest effect on colonic transit. Dietary fiber increases fecal weight, partly by retaining water and partly by increasing bacterial mass (Shareef et al, 2003).

Perfusion of the Gastrointestinal Tract

The blood flow to the GI tract is important in carrying absorbed drug to the systemic circulation. A large network of capillaries and lymphatic vessels perfuse the duodenal region and peritoneum. The splanchnic circulation receives about 28% of the cardiac output and is increased after meals. Once the drug is absorbed from

Figure 13-12. Motor activity responsible for gastric emptying of indigestible solids. Migrating myoelectric complex (MMC), usually initiated at proximal stomach or lower esophageal sphincter, and contractions during phase 3 sweep indigestible solids through open pylorus.
(From Minami and McCallum, 1984, with permission.)

the small intestine, it enters via the mesenteric vessels to the hepatic-portal vein and the liver prior to reaching the systemic circulation. Any decrease in mesenteric blood flow, as in the case of congestive heart failure, will decrease the rate of drug removal from the intestinal tract, thereby reducing the rate of drug bioavailability (Benet et al, 1976).

The role of the lymphatic circulation in drug absorption is well established. Drugs are absorbed through the lacteal or lymphatic vessels under the microvilli. Absorption of drugs through the lymphatic system bypasses the first-pass effect due to liver metabolism, because drug absorption through the hepatic-portal vein is avoided. The lymphatics are important in the absorption of dietary lipids and may be partially responsible for the absorption for some lipophilic drugs. Many poorly water-soluble drugs are soluble in oil and lipids, which may dissolve in chylomicrons and be absorbed systemically via the lymphatic system. Bleomycin or aclarubicin were prepared in chylomicrons to improve oral absorption through the lymphatic system (Yoshikawa et al, 1983, 1989).

Effect of Food on Gastrointestinal Drug Absorption

The presence of food in the GI tract can affect the bioavailability of the drug from an oral drug product (Table 13.6). Digested foods contain amino acids, fatty acids, and many nutrients that may affect intestinal pH and solubility of drugs. The effects of food are not always predictable and can have clinically significant consequences. Some effects of food on the bioavailability of a drug from a drug product include (U.S. Food and Drug Administration, Guidance for Industry, December 2002):

TABLE 13.6   Drugs With Absorption Reduced, Delayed, Increased, or Not Affected by the Presence of Food

REDUCED	DELAYED	INCREASED	NOT AFFECTED
Amoxicillin	Acetaminophen	Canrenone	Cephradine
Ampicillin	Amoxicillin	Dicoumarol	Chlorpropamide
Aspirin	Aspirin	Griseofulvin	Digoxin (elixir)
Demethylchlortetracycline	Cefaclor	Hydralazine	Glibenclamide
Ethanol	Cephalexin	Hydrochlorothiazide	Glipizide
Isoniazid	Cephradine	Metoprolol	Melperone
Levodopa	Digoxin (solid)	Oxazepam	Metronidazole
Furosemide	Nitrofurantoin	Phenytoin	Penicillin V (acid)
Methacycline	Potassium ion	Propoxyphene	Prednisone
Oxytetracycline	Sulfadiazine	Propranolol	Propylthiouracil
Penicillin G	Sulfadimethoxine	Metaxalone	Theophylline
Penicillin V (K)	Sulfanilamide		
Penicillin V (Ca)	Sulfisoxazole	**Slightly Increased**	
Penicillin V (acid)		Hetacillin	
Phenacetin			
Phenethicillin			
Phenylmercaptomethyl-penicillin			
Pivampicillin			
Propantheline			
Rifampin			
Tetracycline			
Slightly Reduced			
Doxycycline			

From Welling (1980), with permission.

- Delay in gastric emptying
- Stimulation of bile flow
- A change in the pH of the GI tract
- An increase in splanchnic blood flow
- A change luminal metabolism of the drug substance
- Physical or chemical interaction of the meal with the drug product or drug substance

Food effects on bioavailability are generally greatest when the drug product is administered shortly after a meal is ingested. The nutrient and caloric contents of the meal, the meal volume, and the meal temperature can cause physiologic changes in the GI tract in a way that affects drug product transit time, luminal dissolution, drug permeability, and systemic availability. In general, meals that are high in total calories and fat content are more likely to affect GI physiology and thereby result in a larger effect on the bioavailability of a drug substance or drug product. The FDA recommends the use of high-calorie and high-fat meals to study the effect of food on the bioavailability and bioequivalence of drug products. (FDA Guidance for Industry.)

The absorption of some antibiotics, such as penicillin and tetracycline, is decreased with food; whereas other drugs, particularly lipid-soluble drugs such as griseofulvin and metazalone, are better absorbed when given with food containing a high fat content (Fig. 13-13). The presence of food in the GI lumen stimulates the flow of bile. Bile contains bile acids, which are surfactants involved in the digestion and solubilization of fats, and also increases the solubility of fat-soluble drugs through micelle formation. For some basic drugs (eg, cinnarizine) with limited aqueous solubility, the presence of food in the stomach stimulates hydrochloric acid secretion, which lowers the pH, causing more rapid dissolution of the drug and better absorption. Absorption of this basic drug is reduced when gastric acid secretion is reduced (Ogata et al, 1986).

Most drugs should be taken with a full glass (approximately 8 fluid ounces) of water to ensure that drugs will wash down the esophagus. Generally, the bioavail-

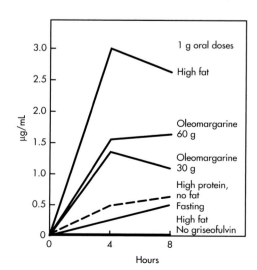

Figure 13-13. A comparison of the effects of different types of food intake on the serum griseofulvin levels following a 1.0-g oral dose.
(From Crounse, 1961, with permission.)

Figure 13-14. Mean plasma or serum drug levels in healthy, fasting human volunteers ($n = 6$ in each case) who received single oral doses of aspirin (650-mg) tablets, erythromycin stearate (500-mg) tablets, amoxicillin (500-mg) capsules, and theophylline (260-mg) tablets, together with large and small accompanying volumes of water.
(From Welling, 1980, with permission.)

ability of drugs is better in patients in the fasted state and with a large volume of water (Fig. 13-14). The solubility of many drugs is limited, and sufficient fluid is necessary for dissolution of the drug. Some patients may be on several drugs that are dosed frequently for months. These patients are often nauseous and are reluctant to take a lot of fluid. For example, HIV patients with active viral counts may be on an AZT or DDI combination with one or more of the protease inhibitors, Invirase (Hoffmann-La Roche), Crixivan (Merck), or Norvir (Abbott). These HIV treatments appear to be better than any previous treatments but depend on patient compliance in taking up to 12 to 15 pills daily for weeks. Any complications affecting drug absorption can influence the outcome of these therapies. With antibiotics, unabsorbed drug may influence the GI flora. For drugs that cause GI disturbances, residual drug dose in the GI tract can potentially aggravate the incidence of diarrhea.

Some drugs, such as erythromycin, iron salts, aspirin, and nonsteroidal antiinflammatory agents (NSAIDs), are irritating to the GI mucosa and are given with food to reduce this irritation. For these drugs, the rate of absorption may be reduced in the presence of food, but the extent of absorption may be the same and the efficacy of the drug is retained.

The GI transit time for enteric-coated and nondisintegrating drug products may also be affected by the presence of food. Enteric-coated tablets may stay in the stomach for a longer period of time because food delays stomach emptying. Thus, the enteric-coated tablet does not reach the duodenum rapidly, delaying drug release and systemic drug absorption. In contrast, since enteric-coated beads or microparticles disperse in the stomach, stomach emptying of the particles is less affected by food, and these preparations demonstrate more consistent drug absorption from the duodenum. The presence of food may delay stomach emptying of enteric-coated tablets or nondisintegrating dosage forms for several hours. Fine granules (smaller than 1 to 2 mm in size) and tablets that disintegrate are not significantly delayed from emptying from the stomach in the presence of food.

Food can also affect the integrity of the dosage form, causing an alteration in the release rate of the drug. For example, theophylline bioavailability from Theo-24 controlled-release tablets is much more rapid when given to a subject in the fed rather than fasted state because of dosage form failures, known as dose-dumping. (Fig. 13-15.)

Food may enhance the absorption of a drug beyond 2 hours after meals. For example, the timing of a fatty meal on the absorption of cefpodoxime proxetil was studied in 20 healthy adults (Borin et al, 1995). The area under the plasma concentration–time curve and peak drug concentration were significantly higher after administration of cefpodoxime proxetil tablets with a meal and 2 hours after a meal relative to dosing under fasted conditions or 1 hour before a meal. The time to peak concentration was not affected by food, which suggests that food increased the extent but not the rate of drug absorption. These results indicate that absorption of cefpodoxime proxetil is enhanced with food or if the drug is taken closely after a heavy meal.

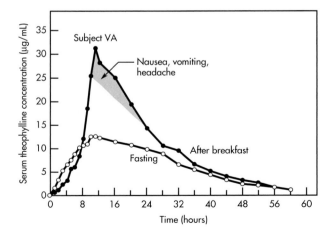

Figure 13-15. Theophylline serum concentrations in an individual subject after a single 1500-mg dose of Theo-24 taken during fasting and after breakfast. The shaded area indicates the period during which this patient experienced nausea, repeated vomiting, or severe throbbing headache. The pattern of drug release during the food regimen is consistent with "dose dumping." (From Hendeles et al, 1985, with permission.)

Timing of drug administration in relation to meals is often important. Pharmacists regularly advise patients to take a medication either 1 hour before or 2 hours after meals to avoid any delay in drug absorption. Since fatty foods may delay stomach emptying time beyond 2 hours, patients who have just eaten a heavy, fatty meal should take these drugs 3 hours or more after the meal, whenever possible. Products that are used to curb stomach acid secretion are usually taken before meals, in anticipation of acid secretion stimulated by food. Famotidine (Pepcid), and cimetidine (Tagamet) are taken before meals to curb excessive acid production.

Fluid volume tends to distend the stomach and speed up stomach emptying; however, large volume of nutrients with high caloric content supersedes that faster rate and delays stomach emptying time. Reduction in drug absorption may be caused by several factors. For example, tetracycline hydrochloride absorption is reduced by milk and food that contains calcium, due to tetracycline chelation. However, significant reduction in absorption may simply be the result of reduced dissolution due to increased pH. Co-administration of sodium bicarbonate raises the stomach pH and reduces tetracycline dissolution and absorption (Barr et al, 1971).

Ticlopidine (Ticlid) is an antiplatelet agent that is commonly used to prevent thromboembolic disorders. Ticlopidine has enhanced absorption after a meal. The absorption of ticlopidine was compared in subjects who received either an antacid or food or were in a control group (fasting). Subjects who received ticlopidine 30 minutes after a fatty meal had an average of 20% increase in plasma concentration over fasting subjects, whereas antacid reduced ticlopidine plasma concentration by approximately the same amount. There was a higher gastrointestinal complaint in the fasting group. Many other drugs have reduced gastrointestinal side effects when taken with food. The decreased gastrointestinal side effects associated with food consumption may greatly improve tolerance and compliance in patients.

Double-Peak Phenomenon

Some drugs, such as ranitidine, cimetidine, and dipyridamole, after oral administration produce a blood concentration curve consisting of two peaks (Fig. 13-16). This double-peak phenomenon is generally observed after the administration of a single dose to fasted patients. The rationale for the double-peak phenomenon has been attributed to variability in stomach emptying, variable intestinal motility, presence of food, enterohepatic recycling, or failure of a tablet dosage form.

The double-peak phenomenon observed for cimetidine (Oberle and Amidon, 1987) may be due to variability in stomach emptying and intestinal flow rates during the entire absorption process after a single dose. For many drugs, very little absorption occurs in the stomach. For a drug with high water solubility, dissolution of the drug occurs in the stomach, and partial emptying of the drug into the duodenum will result in the first absorption peak. A delay in stomach emptying results in a second absorption peak as the remainder of the dose is emptied into the duodenum.

In contrast, ranitidine (Miller, 1984) produces a double peak after both oral or parenteral (IV bolus) administration. Ranitidine is apparently concentrated in the bile within the gallbladder from the general circulation after IV administration. When stimulated by food, the gallbladder contracts and bile containing drug is released into the small intestine. The drug is then reabsorbed and recycled (enterohepatic recycling).

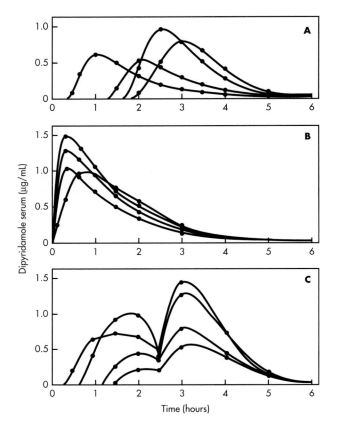

Figure 13-16. Serum concentrations of dipyridamole in three groups of four volunteers each. **A.** After taking 25 mg as tablet intact. **B.** As crushed tablet. **C.** As tablet intact 2 hours before lunch. (From Mellinger and Bohorfoush, 1966, with permission.)

Tablet integrity may also be a factor in the production of a double-peak phenomenon. Mellinger and Bohorfoush (1966) compared a whole tablet or a crushed tablet of dipyridamole in volunteers and showed that a tablet that does not disintegrate or incompletely disintegrates may have delayed gastric emptying, resulting in a second absorption peak.

METHODS FOR STUDYING FACTORS THAT AFFECT DRUG ABSORPTION

Gamma Scintigraphy to Study Site of Drug Release

Gamma scintigraphy is a technique commonly used to track drug dosage form movement from one region to another within the GI tract after oral administration. Gamma scintigraphy also has many research applications and is widely used for formulation studies, such as the mechanism of drug release from a hydrophilic matrix tablet (Abrahamsson et al, 1998). Generally a nonabsorbable radionuclide that emits gamma rays is included as marker in the formulation. In some studies, two radiolabels may be used for simultaneous detection of liquid and solid phases. One approach is to use labeled technesium (Tc^{99m}) in a capsule matrix to study how a drug is absorbed. The image of the capsule breaking up in the stomach or the GI tract is monitored using a gamma camera. Simultaneously, blood levels or urinary excretion of the drug may be measured. This study can be used to correlate residence time of the drug in a given region after capsule breakup to drug absorption. The same technique is used to study drug absorption mechanisms in different regions of the GI tract before a drug is formulated for extended release.

Gamma scintigraphy has been used to study the effect of transit time on the absorption of theophylline (Sournac et al, 1988). *In-vitro* drug release characteristics were correlated with total gastrointestinal transit time. The results showed a significant correlation between the *in-vitro* release of theophylline and the percent of the total amount of theophylline absorbed *in-vivo*. This study illustrates the importance of gamma scintigraphy for the development of specialized drug dosage forms.

Markers to Study Effect of Gastric and GI Transit Time on Absorption

Many useful agents are available that may be used as tools to study absorption and understand the mechanism of the absorptive process. For example, mannitol has a concentration-dependent effect on small intestinal transit. Adkin et al (1995) showed that small concentrations of mannitol included in a pharmaceutical formulation could lead to reduced uptake of any drug absorbed exclusively from the small intestine. No significant differences between the gastric emptying times of the four solutions of different concentrations tested were observed.

Similarly, Hebden et al (1999) demonstrated that codeine slowed GI transit, decreased stool water content, and diminished drug absorption when compared to controls. The results indicated that stool water content may be an important determinant in colonic drug absorption. In contrast, the sugar lactulose accelerated GI transit, increased stool water content, and enhanced drug absorption from the distal gut. Quinine absorption was greater when given with lactulose compared to no lactulose.

Riley et al (1992) studied the effects of gastric emptying and GI transit on the absorption of several drug solutions (furosemide, atenolol, hydrochlorothiazide, and salicylic acid) in healthy subjects. These drugs may potentially be absorbed differently at various sites in the GI system. Subjects were given 20 mg oral metoclopramide or 60 mg oral codeine phosphate to slow gastric emptying. The study showed that gastric emptying affects the absorption of salicylic acid, but not that of furosemide, hydrochlorothiazide or atenolol. *In-vivo* experiments are needed to determine the effect of changing transit time on drug absorption.

Remote Drug Delivery Capsules (RDDCs)

Drug absorption *in-vivo* may be studied either directly by an intubation technique that directly takes samples from the GI tract, or remotely with a special device, such as the Heidelberg capsule. The *Heidelberg capsule* (Baine 1999) is a device used to determine the pH of the stomach. The capsule contains a pH sensor and a miniature radio transmitter (invented by H. G. Noeller and used at Heidelberg University in Germany decades ago). The capsule is about 2 cm × 0.8 cm and can transmit data to the outside after the device is swallowed and tethered to the stomach. Other, newer telemetric methods may be used to take pictures of various regions of the GI tract.

An interesting *remote drug delivery capsule* (RDDC) with electronic controls for noninvasive regional drug absorption study was recently reported by Parr et al (1999). This device was used to study absorption of ranitidine hydrochloride solution in 12 healthy male volunteers. Mean gastric emptying of the RDDC was 1.50 hours, and total small intestine transit was 4.79 hours. The capsule was retrieved from the feces at 30.25 hours. The onset of ranitidine serum levels depended on the time of capsule activation and the site of drug release.

Osmotic Pump Systems

The osmotic pump system is a drug product that contains a small hole from which dissolved drug is released (pumped out) at a rate determined by the rate of entrance of water from the GI tract across a semipermeable membrane due to osmotic pressure (Chapter 17). The drug is either mixed with an osmotic agent or is located in a reservoir. Osmotic pump systems may be used to study drug absorption in different parts of the GI tract because the rate of drug release is constant (zero order) and generally not altered by the environment of the gastrointestinal tract. The constant rate of drug release provides relatively constant blood concentrations.

In-Vivo GI Perfusion Studies

In the past, segments of guinea pig or rat ileums were cut and used to study drug absorption; however, we now know that many of the isolated preparations were not viable shortly after removal, making the absorption data collected either invalid or difficult to evaluate. In addition, the differences among species make it difficult to extrapolate animal data to humans.

GI perfusion is an *in-vivo* method used to study absorption and permeability of a drug in various segments of the GI tract. A tube is inserted from the mouth or anus and placed in a specific section of the GI tract. A drug solution is infused from the tube at a fixed rate, resulting in drug perfusion of the desired GI region. The jejunal site is peristaltically less active than the duodenum, making it easier to intubate, and therefore it is often chosen for perfusion studies. Perfusion studies in other sites such as the duodenum, ileum, and even the colon have also been performed by gastroenterologists and pharmaceutical scientists.

Lennernas et al (1992, 1995) have applied perfusion techniques in humans to study permeability in the small intestine and the rectum. These methods yield direct absorption information in various segments of the GI tract. The regional jejunal perfusion method was reported to have great potential for mechanistic evaluations of drug absorption.

Intestinal Permeability to Drugs

Drugs that are completely absorbed ($F > 90\%$) after oral administration generally demonstrate high permeability in models *in-vitro*. Previously, poor drug absorption was mostly attributed to poor dissolution, slow diffusion, degradation, or poor intestinal permeation. Modern technology has shown that poor or variable oral drug bioavailability among individuals is also the result of individual genetic differences in intestinal absorption (Chapter 12). Interindividual differences in membrane proteins, ion channels, transporters, and antiporters (such as P-glycoprotein, P-gp) that mediate directional transport of drugs and their metabolites across biological membranes can change the extent of drug absorption, or even transport to the site of action elsewhere in the body. It is now clear that the behavior of drugs in the body is the result of an intricate interplay between these nuclear hormone receptors, drug transporters, and the drug-metabolizing systems. This insight provides another explanation for erratic drug absorption beyond poor formulation and first-pass metabolism.

Alternative methods to study intestinal drug permeability include *in-vivo* or *in-situ* intestinal perfusion in a suitable animal model (eg, rats), and/or *in-vitro* permeability methods using excised intestinal tissues, or monolayers of suitable epithelial cells such as Caco-2 cells. In addition, the physicochemical characterization of a drug substance (eg, oil/water partition coefficient) provides useful information to predict a drug's permeability.

Caco-2 Cells for in-Vitro Permeability Studies

Although *in-vivo* studies yield much definitive information about drug permeability in humans, they are tedious and costly to perform. The *Caco-2* cell line is a human colon adenocarcinoma cell line that differentiates in culture and resembles the epithelial lining of the human small intestine. The permeability of the cellular monolayer may vary with the stage of cell growth and the cultivation method used. However, under controlled condition, using monolayers of Caco-2 cells, the permeability of a drug may be determined. Caco-2 cells can also be used to study interactions of drugs with the transporter P-glycoprotein discussed below.

Drug permeability using the Caco-2 cell line has been suggested as an *in-vitro* method for passively transported drugs. In some cases, the drug permeability may appear to be low due to efflux of drugs via membrane transporters such as P-glycoprotein (P-gp). Permeability studies using the Caco-2 cell line have been suggested as a method for classifying the permeability of a drug according to the Biopharmaceutics Classification System, BCS (Tolle-Sander and Polli, 2001; U.S. FDA, Guidance 2003, August 2002). The main purpose of the BCS classification is to classify a drug as having high or low permeability as a predictor of systemic drug absorption from the GI tract (see Chapter 15).

Drug Transporters

Several transport proteins are expressed in the intestinal epithelial cells. Although some transporters facilitate absorption, other transporters, such as P-glycoprotein may effectively inhibit drug absorption. P-gp, an energy-dependent, membrane-bound protein, is an *efflux transporter* that mediates the secretion of compounds from inside the cell back out into the intestinal lumen, thereby limiting overall absorption. Thus, drug absorption may be reduced or increased by the presence or absence of efflux proteins. The role of efflux proteins is generally believed to be a defense mechanism for the body to excrete and reduce drug accumulation.

P-glycoprotein is expressed also in other tissues such as the blood–brain barrier, liver, and kidney, where it limits drug penetration into the brain, mediates biliary drug secretion, and renal tubular drug secretion, respectively. Efflux pumps are present throughout the body and are involved in transport of a diverse group of hydrophobic drugs, natural products, and peptides. Many drugs and chemotherapeutic agents, such as cyclosporin A, verapamil, terfenadine, fexofenadine, and most HIV-1 protease inhibitors are substrates of P-gp (see Chapter 12). In addition, individual genetic differences in intestinal absorption may be the result of genetic differences in P-gp and other transporters.

CLINICAL EXAMPLES

Multidrug resistance (MDR) to cancer cells has been linked to efflux transporter proteins such as P-gp that either exclude or extrude chemotherapeutic agents from the cells (Sauna et al, 2001). Paclitaxel (Taxol) is an example of coordinated metabolism, efflux, and triggering of hormone nuclear receptor to induce efflux protein (Figure 13.17). P-gp (see MDR1 in Fig. 13-1) is responsible for 85% of paclitaxel excretion back into the GI tract (Synold et al, 2001). Paclitaxel induces the steroid xenobiotic receptor SXR (also known as PXR), which in turn activates MDR1 transcription and P-gp expression, resulting in even further excretion of paclitaxel into the intestinal fluid. Paclitaxel also induces CYP 3A4 and CYP2C8 transcription, resulting in increased paclitaxel metabolism. Thus, in response to

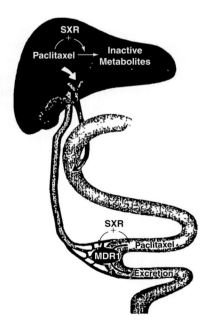

Figure 13.17 *Mechanism of coordinated efflux and metabolism of paclitaxel by SXR.*
(From Synold T et al, 2001, with permission.)

a xenobiotic challenge, SXR can induce both a first line of defense (intestinal excretion) and a backup system (hepatic drug inactivation) that limits exposure to potentially toxic compounds. In contrast to paclitaxel, docetaxel is a closely related antineoplastic agent that does not activate SXR but has a much better absorption profile.

Mutations of other transporters, particularly those involved in reuptake of serotonin, dopamine, and gamma-aminobutyric acid (GABA) are presently being studied with regard to clinically relevant changes in drug response. Pharmacogenetic variability in these transporters is an important consideration in patient dosing. When therapeutic failures occur, the following questions should be asked: (1) Is the drug a substrate for P-gp and/or CYP3A4? (2) Is the drug being co-administered with anything that inhibits either P-gp and/or CYP3A4? For example, grapefruit juice and many drugs can affect drug metabolism and oral absorption.

EFFECT OF DISEASE STATES ON DRUG ABSORPTION

Drug absorption may be affected by any disease that causes changes in (1) intestinal blood flow, (2) gastrointestinal motility, (3) changes in stomach emptying time, (4) gastric pH that affects drug solubility, (5) intestinal pH that affects the extent of ionization, (6) the permeability of the gut wall, (7) bile secretion, (8) digestive enzyme secretion, or (9) alteration of normal GI flora. Some factors may dominate, while other factors sometimes cancel the effects of each other. Pharmacokinetic studies comparing subjects with and without the disease are generally necessary to establish the effect of the disease on drug absorption. Several clinical examples are given below.

Patients in an advanced stage of *Parkinson's disease* may have difficulty swallowing and greatly diminished gastrointestinal motility. A case was reported in which the patient could not be controlled with regular oral levodopa medication because of poor absorption. Infusion of oral levodopa solution using a j-tube gave adequate control of his symptoms. The patient was subsequently placed on this mode of therapy.

Patients on tricyclic antidepressants (imiprimine, amitriptyline, and nortriptyline) and antipsychotic drugs (phenothiazines) with anticholinergic side effects may have reduced gastrointestinal motility or even intestinal obstructions. Delays in drug absorption, especially with slow-release products, have occurred.

Achlorhydric patients may not have adequate production of acids in the stomach; stomach HCl is essential for solubilizing insoluble free bases. Many weak-base drugs that cannot form soluble salts will remain undissolved in the stomach when there is no hydrochloric acid present and are therefore unabsorbed. Salt forms of these drugs cannot be prepared because the free base readily precipitates out due to the weak basicity.

Dapsone, itraconazole, and ketoconazole may also be less well absorbed in the presence of achlorhydria. In patients with acid reflux disorders, proton pump inhibitors, such as omeprazole, render the stomach achlorhydric, which may also affect drug absorption. Co-administering orange juice, colas, or other acidic beverages can facilitate the absorption of some medications requiring an acidic environment.

HIV-AIDS patients are prone to a number of gastrointestinal (GI) disturbances, such as increased gastric transit time, diarrhea, and achlorhydria. Rapid gastric transit time and diarrhea can alter the absorption of orally administered drugs. Achlorhydria may or may not decrease absorption, depending on the acidity needed for absorption of a specific drug. Indinavir, for example, requires a normal acidic environment for absorption. The therapeutic window of indinavir is extremely narrow, so optimal serum concentrations are critical for this drug to be efficacious.

Congestive heart failure (CHF) *patients* with persistent edema have reduced splanchnic blood flow and develop edema in the bowel wall. In addition, intestinal motility is slowed. The reduced blood flow to the intestine and reduced intestinal motility results in a decrease in drug absorption. For example, furosemide (Lasix), a commonly used loop diuretic, has erratic and reduced oral absorption in patients with CHF and a delay in the onset of action.

Crohn's disease is an inflammatory disease of the distal small intestine and colon. The disease is accompanied by regions of thickening of the bowel wall, overgrowth of anaerobic bacteria, and sometimes obstruction and deterioration of the bowel. The effect on drug absorption is unpredictable, although impaired absorption may potentially occur because of reduced surface area and thicker gut wall for diffusion. For example, higher plasma propranolol concentration has been observed in patients with Crohn's disease after oral administration of propranolol. Alpha-1-acid glycoprotein level is increased in Crohn's disease patients. Higher alpha-1-acid glycoprotein may affect the protein binding and distribution of propranolol in the body and result in higher plasma concentration.

Celiac disease is an inflammatory disease affecting mostly the proximal small intestine. Celiac disease is caused by sensitization to gluten, a viscous protein found in cereals. Patients with celiac disease generally have an increased rate of stomach emptying and increased permeability of the small intestine. Cephalexin absorption appears to be increased in celiac disease, although it is not possible to make general predictions about these patients. Other intestinal conditions that may potentially affect drug absorption include corrective surgery involving peptic ulcer, antrectomy with gastroduodenostomy, and selective vagotomy.

Drugs That Affect Absorption of Other Drugs

Anticholinergic drugs in general may reduce stomach acid secretion. Propantheline bromide is an anticholinergic drug that may slow stomach emptying and motility of the small intestine. Tricyclic antidepressants and phenothiazines also have anticholinergic side effects that may cause slower peristalsis in the GI tract. Slower stomach emptying may cause delay in drug absorption.

Metoclopramide is a drug that stimulates stomach contraction, relaxes the pyloric sphincter, and, in general, increases intestinal peristalsis, which may reduce the effective time for the absorption of some drugs and thereby reduce the peak drug concentration and the time to reach peak drug concentration. For example, digoxin absorption from a tablet is reduced by metoclopramide but increased by an anticholinergic drug, such as propantheline bromide. Allowing more time in the stomach for the tablet to dissolve generally helps with the dissolution and absorption of a poorly soluble drug, but would not be helpful for a drug that is not soluble in stomach acid.

Antacids should not be given with cimetidine, because antacids may reduce drug absorption. Antacids containing aluminum, calcium, or magnesium may complex with drugs such as tetracycline, ciprofloxacin, and indinavir, resulting in a decrease in drug absorption. To avoid this interaction, antacids should be taken 2 hours before or 6 hours after drug administration. As mentioned, proton pump inhibitors, such as omeprazole, render the stomach achlorhydric, which may also affect drug absorption.

Cholestyramine is a nonabsorbable ion-exchange resin for the treatment of hyperlipemia. Cholestyramine adsorbs warfarin, thyroxine, and loperamide, similar to activated charcoal, thereby reducing absorption of these drugs.

Absorption of calcium in the duodenum is an active process facilitated by vitamin D, with calcium absorption as much as four times more than that in vitamin D deficiency states. It is believed that a calcium-binding protein, which increases after vitamin D administration, binds calcium in the intestinal cell and transfers it out of the base of the cell to the blood circulation.

Nutrients That Interfere with Drug Absorption

Many nutrients substantially interfere with the absorption or metabolism of drugs in the body (Anderson, 1988; Kirk, 1995). The effect of food on bioavailability was discussed earlier. Oral drug–nutrient interactions are often drug specific and can result in either an increase or decrease in drug absorption.

Absorption of water-soluble vitamins, such as vitamin B-12 and folic acid, are aided by special absorption mechanisms. Vitamin B-12 absorption is facilitated by intrinsic factors in the stomach, where it forms a complex with the factor and is carried in the intestinal stream to the ileum, where it binds to a specific receptor. Vitamin B-12 then ultimately disassociates from the complex and is absorbed.

Grapefruit juice often increases bioavailability, as observed by an increase in plasma levels of many drugs that are substrates for cytochrome P450 (CYP) 3A4 (see Chapter 11). Grapefruit juice contains various flavonoids such as naringin that inhibits certain cytochrome P-450 enzymes involved in drug metabolism. In this case, the observed increase in the plasma drug blood levels is due to decreased presystemic elimination in the GI tract and/or liver. Indirectly, the amount of drug absorbed systemically from the drug product is increased. Grapefruit juice can also block drug efflux by inhibiting P-gp for some drugs.

MISCELLANEOUS ROUTES OF DRUG ADMINISTRATION

For systemic drug absorption, the oral route is the easiest, safest, and most popular route of drug administration. Increasingly popular nonparenteral alternatives to oral drug delivery for systemic drug absorption include nasal, inhalation, and transdermal drug delivery. Nasal, inhalation, and topical drug delivery may also be used for local drug action.

Nasal Drug Delivery

Nasal drug delivery may be used for either local or systemic effects. Because the nasal region is richly supplied with blood vessels, nasal administration is also useful for systemic drug delivery. However, the total surface area in the nasal cavity is relatively small, retention time in the nasal cavity is generally short, and some drug may be swallowed. These factors may limit the nose's capacity for systemic delivery of drugs requiring large doses. Surfactants are often used to increase systemic penetration, although the effect of chronic drug exposure on the integrity of nasal membranes must also be considered. In general, a drug must be sufficiently lipophilic to cross the membranes of the nasal epithelium in order to be absorbed. Small molecules with balanced lipophilic and hydrophilic properties tend to be absorbed more easily. This observation poses a challenge for nasal delivery of larger molecules such as proteins and peptides, which would benefit from delivery routes that avoid the degradative environment of the intestine. Dosage forms intended for nasal drug delivery include nasal drops, nasal sprays, aerosols, and nebulizers (Su and Campanale, 1985).

Depending on the metabolic, absorption, and chemical profile of the drug, some drugs are rapidly absorbed through the nasal membrane and can deliver rapid therapeutic effect. Various hormones and insulin have been tested for intranasal delivery. In some cases the objective is to improve availability, and in other cases it is to reduce side effects. Vasopressin and oxytocin are older examples of drugs marketed as intranasal products. In addition, many opioids are known to be rapidly absorbed from the nasal passages and can deliver systemic levels of the drug almost as rapidly as an intravenous injection (Dale et al, 2002). A common problem with nasal drug delivery is the challenge of developing a formulation with nonirritating ingredients. Many surfactants that facilitate absorption tend to be moderately or very irritating to the nasal mucosa.

Intranasal corticosteroids for treatment of allergic and perennial rhinitis have become more popular since intranasal delivery is believed to reduce the total dose of corticosteroid required. A lower dose also leads to minimization of side effects such as growth suppression. This logic has led to many second-generation corticosteroids such as beclomethasone dipropionate, budesonide, flunisolide, fluticasone propionate, mometasone furoate, and triamcinolone acetonide that are being considered for intranasal delivery (Szefler, 2002). However, the potential for growth suppression in children varies. In one study, beclomethasone dipropionate reduced growth in children, but mometasone furoate nasal spray used for 1 year showed no signs of growth suppression. Overall, the second-generation corticosteroid by nasal delivery have been concluded to cause minimal systemic side effects (Szefler, 2002).

Inhalation Drug Delivery

Inhalation drug delivery may also be used for local or systemic drug effects. The lung has a potential absorption surface of some 70 m^2, a much larger surface than the small intestine or nasal passages. When a substance is inhaled, it is exposed to membranes of the mouth or nose, pharynx, trachea, bronchi, bronchioles, alveolar sacs, and alveoli. The lungs and their associated airways are designed to remove foreign matter from the highly absorptive peripheral lung surfaces via mucociliary clearance. However, if compounds such as aerosolized drug can reach the peripheral region of the lung, absorption can be very efficient.

Particle (droplet) size and velocity of application control the extent to which inhaled substances penetrate into airway spaces. Optimum size for deep airway penetration of drug particles is 3 to 5 μm. Large particles tend to deposit in upper airways, whereas very small molecules (<3 μm) are exhaled before absorption can occur. Most inhalation devices deliver approximately 10% of the administered dose to the lower respiratory tract. A number of devices such as spacers (to reduce turbulence and improve deep inhalation) have been developed to increase lung delivery. An *in-vitro* device useful to measure the particle size emitted from an aerosol or a mechanically produced fine mist is the cascade impacter.

Topical and Transdermal Drug Delivery

Topical drug delivery is generally used for local drug effects. Drug may be applied as an ointment or cream to the skin or various mucous membranes such as intravaginally. Even though the objective is to obtain a local drug effect, some of the drug may be absorbed systemically. For transdermal drug delivery the drug is incorporated into a transdermal therapeutic system or patch, but it may be incorporated into an ointment as well (Chapter 14). Transdermal drug delivery is generally for systemic drug absorption. The advantages of transdermal delivery include continuous release of drug over a period of time, low presystemic clearance, and good patient compliance.

Other routes of drug administration are discussed elsewhere and in Chapter 14.

FREQUENTLY ASKED QUESTIONS

1. What is an "absorption window"?
2. Why are some drugs absorbed better with food and others are retarded by food?
3. If a drug is administered orally as a solution, does it mean that all of the drug will be systemically absorbed?
4. What is the biggest biological factor that contributes to delay in drug absorption?

LEARNING QUESTIONS

1. A recent bioavailability study in adult human volunteers demonstrated that after the administration of a single enteric-coated aspirin granule product given with a meal, the plasma drug levels resembled the kinetics of a sustained-release

drug product. In contrast, when the product was given to fasted subjects, the plasma drug levels resembled the kinetics of an immediate-release drug product. Give a plausible explanation for this observation.

2. The aqueous solubility of a weak-base drug is poor. In an intubation (intestinal perfusion) study, the drug was not absorbed beyond the jejunum. Which of the following would be the correct strategy to improve drug absorption from the intestinal tract?

   a. Give the drug as a suspension and recommend that the suspension be taken on an empty stomach.

   b. Give the drug as a hydrochloride salt.

   c. Give the drug with milk.

   d. Give the drug as a suppository.

3. What is the primary reason that protein drugs such as insulin are not given orally for systemic absorption?

4. Which of the following statements are true regarding an acidic drug with a pK_a of 4?

   a. The drug is more soluble in the stomach when food is present.

   b. The drug is more soluble in the duodenum than in the stomach.

   c. The drug is more soluble when dissociated.

5. Which region of the gastrointestinal tract is most populated by bacteria? What types of drugs might affect the gastrointestinal flora?

6. Discuss methods by which the first-pass effect (presystemic absorption) may be circumvented.

7. Misoprostol (Cytotec, GD Searle) is a synthetic prostaglandin E1 analog. According to the manufacturer, the following information was obtained when misoprostol was taken with an antacid or high-fat breakfast:

Condition	C_{max} (pg/mL)	AUC_{0-24} hr (pg hr/mL)	t_{max} (min)
Fasting	811 ± 317^a	417 ± 135	14 ± 8
With antacid	689 ± 315	349 ± 108^b	20 ± 14
With high-fat breakfast	303 ± 176^b	373 ± 111	64 ± 79^b

[a] Results are expressed as the mean ± SD (standard deviation).
[b] Comparisons with fasting results statistically significant, $p < 0.05$.

What is the effect of antacid and high-fat breakfast on the bioavailability of misoprostol? Comment on how these factors affect the rate and extent of systemic drug absorption.

REFERENCES

Abrahamsson B, Alpsten M, Bake B, et al: Drug absorption from nifedipine hydrophilic matrix extended release (er) tablet—Comparison with an osmotic pump tablet and effect of food, *J Controlled Release* (Netherlands), **52**:301–310, 1998

Adkin DA, Davis SS, Sparrow RA, et al: Effect of different concentrations of mannitol in solution on small intestinal transit: Implications for drug absorption, *Pharm Res* **12**:393–396, 1995

Alberts B, Bray D, Lewis J, et al: *Molecular Biology of the Cell.* New York, Garland, 1988

Anderson KE: Influences of diet and nutrition on clinical pharmacokinetics. *Clin Pharm* **14**:325–346, 1988

Barr WH, Adir J, Garrettson L: Decrease in tetracycline absorption in man by sodium bicarbonate. *Clin Pharmacol Ther* **12**:779–784, 1971

Barrie S: Heidelberg pH capsule gastric analysis. In *Textbook of Natural Medicine*, 2nd ed, JE Pizzorno, MT Murray (Eds) London: Churchill Livingstone, 1999, chap 16

Benet LZ, Greither A, Meister W: Gastrointestinal absorption of drugs in patients with cardiac failure. In Benet LZ (ed), *The Effect of Disease States on Drug Pharmacokinetics.* Washington, DC, American Pharmaceutical Association, 1976, chap 3

Borin MT, Driver MR, Forbes KK: Effect of timing of food on absorption of cefpodoxime proxetil. *J Clin Pharmacol* **35**(5):505–509, 1995

Burks TF, Galligan JJ, Porreca F, Barber WD: Regulation of gastric emptying. *Fed Proc* **44**:2897–2901, 1985

Crounse RG: Human pharmacology of griseofulvin: The effect of fat intake on gastrointestinal absorption. *J Invest Dermatol* **37**:529–533, 1961

Dale O, Hoffer C, Sheffels P, Kharasch ED: Disposition of nasal, intravenous, and oral methadone in healthy volunteers. *Clin Pharmacol Therapeut* **72**:536–545, 2002

Davson H, Danielli JF: *The Permeability of Natural Membranes.* Cambridge, UK, Cambridge University Press, 1952

Doherty MM, Charman WN: The mucosa of the small intestine: How clinically relevant as an organ of drug metabolism? *Clin Pharmacokinet* **41**(4):235–253, 2002

Feldman M, Smith HJ, Simon TR: Gastric emptying of solid radio-opaque markers: Studies in healthy and diabetic patients. *Gastroenterology* **87**:895–902, 1984

Hebden JM, et al: Stool water content and colonic drug absorption: contrasting effects of lactulose and codeine. *Pharm Res* **16**:1254–1259, 1999

Hendeles L, Weinberger M, Milavetz G, et al: Food induced dumping from "once-a-day" theophylline product as cause of theophylline toxicity. *Chest* **87**:758–785, 1985

Hunt JN, Knox M: Regulation of gastric emptying. In Code CF (ed), *Handbook of Physiology. Section 6: Alimentary Canal.* Washington, DC, American Physiological Society, 1968, pp 1917–1935

Kirk JK: Significant drug-nutrient interactions. *Am Fam Physician* **51**:1175–1182, 1185, 1995

Kirwan WO, Smith AN: Gastrointestinal transit estimated by an isotope capsule. *Scand J Gastroenterol* **9**:763–766, 1974

Lennernas H, Ahrenstedt O, Hallgren R, et al: Regional jejunal perfusion, a new in vivo approach to study oral drug absorption in man. *Pharm Res* **9**:1243–1251, 1992

Lennernas H, Falgerholm U, Raab Y, et al: Regional rectal perfusion: New in vivo approach to study rectal drug absorption in man. *Pharm Res* **12**:426–432, 1995

Lodish HF, Rothman JE: The assembly of cell membranes. *Sci Am* **240**:48–63, 1979

Mayersohn M: Physiological factors that modify systemic drug availability and pharmacologic response in clinical practice. In Blanchard J, Sawchuk RJ, Brodie BB (eds), *Principles and Perspectives in Drug Bioavailability.* Basel, Karger, 1979, chap 8

Mellinger TJ, Bohorfoush JG: Blood levels of dipyridamole (Persantin) in humans. *Arch Int Pharmacodynam Ther* **163**:465–480, 1966

Miller R: Pharmacokinetics and bioavailability of ranitidine in humans. *J Pharm Sci* **73**:1376–1379, 1984

Minami H, McCallum RW: The physiology and pathophysiology of gastric emptying in humans. *Gastroenterology* **86**:1592–1610, 1984

Nienbert R: Ion pair transport across membranes. *Pharm Res* **6**:743–747, 1989

Oberle RL, Amidon GL: The influence of variable gastric emptying and intestinal transit rates on the plasma level curve of cimetidine: An explanation for the double-peak phenomenon. *J Pharmacokinet Biopharmacol* **15**:529–544, 1987

Ogata H, Aoyagi N, Kaniwa N, et al: Gastric acidity dependent bioavailability of cinnarizine from two commercial capsules in healthy volunteers. *Int J Pharm* **29**:113–120, 1986

Parr AF, Sandefer EP, Wissel P, et al: Evaluation of the feasibility and use of a prototype remote drug delivery capsule (RDDC) for noninvasive regional drug absorption studies in the GI tract of man and beagle dog. *Pharm Res* **16**:266–271, 1999

Pratt P, Taylor P (eds): *Principles of Drug Action: The Basis of Pharmacology*, 3rd ed. New York, Churchill Livingstone, 1990, p 241

Rubinstein A, Li VHK, Robinson JR: Gastrointestinal–physiological variables affecting performance of oral sustained release dosage forms. In Yacobi A, Halperin-Walega E (eds), *Oral Sustained Release Formulations: Design and Evaluation.* New York, Pergamon, 1988, chap 6

Riley SA, Sutcliffe F, Kim M, et al: Influence of gastrointestinal transit on drug absorption in healthy volunteers. *Br J Clin Pharm* **34**:32–39, 1992

Sauna ZE, Smith MM, Muller M, Kerr KM, Ambudkar SV: The mechanism of action of multidrug resistance linked P-glycoprotein. *J Bioenerget Biomembranes* **33**:481–491, 2001

Shareef MA, Ahuja A, Ahmad FJ, Raghava S: Colonic drug delivery: An updated review. *AAPS PharmSci* **5**:161–186, 2003

Singer SJ, Nicolson GL: The fluid mosaic model of the structure of cell membranes. *Science* **175**:720–731, 1972

Sournac S, Maublant JC, Aiache JM, et al: Scintigraphic study of the gastrointestinal transit and correlations with the drug absorption kinetics of a sustained release theophylline tablet. Part 1. Administration in fasting state. *J. Controlled Release* **7**:139–146, 1988

Su KSE, Campanale KM: Nasal drug delivery systems requirements, development and evaluations. In Chien YW (ed), *Transnasal Systemic Medications.* Amsterdam, Elsevier Scientific, 1985, pp 139–159

Synold TW, Dussault I, Forman BM: The orphan nuclear receptor SXR coordinately regulates drug metabolism and efflux. *Nature Med* **7**(5), 584–590, 2001.

Szefler SJ: Pharmacokinetics of intranasal corticosteroids. *J Allergy Clin Immunol* **108**:S26–S31, 2002

Tolle-Sander S, Polli JE: Method considerations for Caco-2 permeability assessment in the biopharmaceutics classification system. *Pharmacopoeial Forum* **28**:164–172, 2002

Tsuji A, Tamai I: Carrier-mediated intestinal transport of drugs. *Pharm Res* **13**(7):963–977, 1996

U.S. Food and Drug Administration: *FDA Guidance for Industry: Waiver of In Vivo Bioavailability and Bioequivalence Studies for Immediate-Release Solid Oral Dosage Forms Based on a Biopharmaceutics Classification System,* August 2002

U.S. Food and Drug Administration: *FDA Guidance for Industry: Food-Effect Bioavailability and Fed Bioequivalence Studies,* December 2002

Welling PG: Drug bioavailability and its clinical significance. In Bridges KW, Chasseaud LF (eds), *Progress in Drug Metabolism, Vol 4.* London, Wiley, 1980, chap 3

Wilson TH: *Intestinal Absorption.* Philadelphia, Saunders, 1962

Yoshikawa H, Muranishi S, Sugihira N, Seaki H: Mechanism of transfer of bleomycin into lymphatics by bifunctional delivery system via lumen of small intestine. *Chem Pharm Bull* **31**:1726–1732, 1983

Yoshikawa H, Nakao Y, Takada K, et al: Targeted and sustained delivery of aclarubicin to lymphatics by lactic acid oligomer microsphere in rat. *Chem Pharm Bull* **37**:802–804, 1989

BIBLIOGRAPHY

Berge S, Bighley L, Monkhouse D: Pharmaceutical salts. *J Pharm Sci* **66**:1–19, 1977

Blanchard J: Gastrointestinal absorption, II. Formulation factors affecting bioavailability. *Am J Pharm* **150**:132–151, 1978

Davenport HW: *Physiology of the Digestive Tract,* 5th ed. Chicago, Year Book, 1982

Evans DF, Pye G, Bramley R, et al: Measurement of gastrointestinal pH profiles in normal ambulant human subjects. *Gut* **29**:1035–1041, 1988

Eye IS: A review of the physiology of the gastrointestinal tract in relation to radiation doses from radioactive materials. *Health Physics* **12**:131–161, 1966

Houston JB, Wood SG: Gastrointestinal absorption of drugs and other xenobiotics. In Bridges JW, Chasseaud LF (eds), *Progress in Drug Metabolism, Vol 4.* London, Wiley, 1980, chap 2

Leesman GD, Sinko PJ, Amidon GL: Stimulation of oral drug absorption: Gastric emptying and gastrointestinal motility. In Welling PW, Tse FLS (eds), *Pharmacokinetics: Regulatory, Industry, Academic Perspectives.* New York, Marcel Dekker, 1988, chap 6

Mackowiak PA: The normal microbial flora. *N Engl J Med* **307**:83–93, 1982

Martonosi AN (ed): *Membranes and Transport,* vol 1. New York, Plenum, 1982

McElnay JC: Buccal absorption of drugs. In Swarbick J, Boylan JC (eds), *Encyclopedia of Pharmaceutical Technology,* vol 2. New York, Marcel Dekker, 1990, pp 189–211

Palin K: Lipids and oral drug delivery. *Pharma Int* Nov, 272–275, 1985

Palin K, Whalley D, Wilson C, et al: Determination of gastric-emptying profiles in the rat: Influence of oil structure and volume. *Int J Pharm* **12:**315–322, 1982

Welling PG: Interactions affecting drug absorption. *Clin Pharmacokinet* **9:**404–434, 1984

Welling PG: Dosage route, bioavailability and clinical efficacy. In Welling PW, Tse FLS (eds), *Pharmacokinetics: Regulatory, Industry, Academic Perspectives.* New York, Marcel Dekker, 1988, chap 3

Welling PG: Absorption of drugs. In Swarbrick J, Boylan JC (eds), *Encyclopedia of Pharmaceutical Technology.* New York, Marcel Dekker, 2002, pp 8–22

Wilson TH: *Intestinal Absorption.* Philadelphia, Saunders, 1962

14

BIOPHARMACEUTIC CONSIDERATIONS IN DRUG PRODUCT DESIGN

Drugs are not generally given as pure chemical drug substances but are formulated into finished dosage forms (drug products), such as tablets, capsules, ointments, etc, before being administered to patients for therapy. Formulated drug products usually include the active drug substance and selected ingredients (*excipients*) that make up the dosage form. Drug products are designed to deliver drug for local or systemic effects. Common drug products include liquids, tablets, capsules, injectables, suppositories, transdermal systems, and topical products such as creams and ointments. The design and formulation of drug products requires a thorough understanding of the biopharmaceutic principles of drug delivery.

Biopharmaceutics is the study of the *in-vitro* impact of the physicochemical properties of drugs and drug products on drug delivery to the body under normal or pathologic conditions. A primary concern in biopharmaceutics is the bioavailability of drugs. *Bioavailability* refers to the measurement of the rate and extent of active drug that becomes available at the site of action. Because the systemic blood circulation delivers therapeutically active drug to the tissues and to the site of action of the drug, changes in bioavailability affect changes in the pharmacodynamics and toxicity of a drug. The aim of biopharmaceutics is to adjust the delivery of drug from the drug product in such a manner as to provide optimal therapeutic activity and safety for the patient.

Biopharmaceutic studies allow for the rational design of drug products based on (1) the physical and chemical properties of the drug substance; (2) the route of drug administration, including the anatomic and physiologic nature of the application site (eg, oral, topical, injectable, implant, transdermal patch, etc); and (4) desired pharmacodynamic effect (eg, immediate or prolonged activity); (5) toxicologic properties of the drug; (6) safety of excipients; and (7) effect of excipients and dosage form on drug delivery. For example, some drugs are intended for topical or local therapeutic action at the site of administration. For these drugs, systemic absorption is undesirable. Drugs intended for local activity are designed to have a direct pharmacodynamic action without affecting other body organs. These drugs may be applied topically to the skin, nose, eye, mucous membranes, buccal cavity, throat, or rectum. A drug intended for local activity may be given intravaginally, into the urethral tract, intranasally, into the ear, on the eye, or orally. Examples of drugs used for local action include anti-infectives, antifungals, local anesthetics, antacids, astringents, vasoconstrictors, antihistamines, and corticosteroids. However, some systemic drug absorption may occur with drugs used for local activity.

Each route of drug application presents special biopharmaceutic considerations in drug product design. For example, the design of a vaginal tablet formulation for the treatment of a fungal infection must use ingredients compatible with vaginal anatomy and physiology. An eye medication may require special biopharmaceutic considerations, including appropriate pH, isotonicity, sterility, local irritation to the cornea, draining by tears, and concern for systemic drug absorption.

For a drug administered by an extravascular route (eg, intramuscular injection), local irritation, drug dissolution, and drug absorption from the intramuscular site are some of the factors that must be considered. The systemic absorption of a drug from an extravascular site is influenced by the anatomic and physiologic properties of the site and the physicochemical properties of the drug and the drug product. If the drug is given by an intravascular route (eg, IV administration), systemic drug absorption is considered complete or 100% bioavailable, because the drug is placed directly into the general circulation.

In some cases, a drug product is designed so that it may be used in conjunction with a specialized medical device or packaging component. For example, a drug solution or suspension may be formulated to work with a nebulizer or metered-dose inhaler for administration into the lungs. Both the physical characteristics of the nebulizer and the formulation of the drug product can influence the droplet particles and the spray pattern that the patient receives upon inhalation of the drug product.

By choosing the route of drug administration carefully and properly designing the drug product, the bioavailability of the active drug can be varied from rapid and complete absorption to a slow, sustained rate of absorption or even virtually no absorption, depending on the therapeutic objective. Once the drug is systemically absorbed, normal physiologic processes for distribution and elimination occur, which usually are not influenced by the specific formulation of the drug. The rate of drug release from the product and the rate and extent of drug absorption are important in determining the distribution, onset, intensity, and duration of drug action.

Biopharmaceutic considerations often determine the ultimate dose and dosage form of a drug product. For example, the dosage for a drug intended for local activity, such as a topical drug product (eg, ointment), is often expressed in concentration or as percentage of the active drug in the formulation (eg, 0.5% hydrocortisone ointment). The amount of drug applied is not specified because the concentration of the drug at the active site relates to the pharmacodynamic action. However, biopharmaceutic studies must be performed to ensure that the drug product does not irritate, cause an allergic response, or allow significant systemic drug absorption. In contrast, the dosage of a drug intended for systemic absorption is given on the basis of mass, such as milligrams or grams. In this case, dosage is based on the amount of drug that is absorbed systemically and dissolved in an apparent volume of distribution to produce a desired drug concentration at the target site. The therapeutic dose may be based on the weight or surface area of the patient, to account for the differences in the apparent volume of distribution. Thus, doses are expressed as mass per unit of body weight (mg/kg) or mass per unit of body surface area (mg/m^2). For many commercial drug products, the dose is determined on average body weights and may be available in several dose strengths, such as 10-mg, 5-mg, and 2.5-mg tablets, to accommodate differences in body weight and possibly to titrate the dose in the patient.

RATE-LIMITING STEPS IN DRUG ABSORPTION

Systemic drug absorption from a drug product consists of a succession of rate processes (Fig. 14-1). For solid oral, immediate-release drug products (eg, tablets, capsules), the rate processes include (1) disintegration of the drug product and subsequent release of the drug, (2) dissolution of the drug in an aqueous environment, and (3) absorption across cell membranes into the systemic circulation. In the process of drug disintegration, dissolution, and absorption, the rate at which drug reaches the circulatory system is determined by the slowest step in the sequence. The slowest step in a series of kinetic processes is called the *rate-limiting step*. Except for controlled-release products, disintegration of a solid oral drug product is usually more rapid than drug dissolution and drug absorption. For drugs that have very poor aqueous solubility, the rate at which the drug dissolves (*dissolution*) is often the slowest step and therefore exerts a rate-limiting effect on drug bioavailability. In contrast, for a drug that has a high aqueous solubility, the dissolution rate is rapid, and the rate at which the drug crosses or permeates cell membranes is the slowest or rate-limiting step.

PHARMACEUTIC FACTORS AFFECTING DRUG BIOAVAILABILITY

Considerations in the design of a drug product that will deliver active drug with the desired bioavailability characteristics include (1) the type of drug product (eg, solution, suspension, suppository), (2) the nature of the excipients in the drug product, (3) the physicochemical properties of the drug molecule, and (4) the route of drug administration.

Figure 14-1.   Rate processes of drug bioavailability.

Disintegration

For immediate-release, solid oral dosage forms, the drug product must disintegrate into small particles and release the drug. To monitor uniform tablet disintegration, the *United States Pharmacopeia* (USP) has established an official disintegration test. Solid drug products exempted from disintegration tests include troches, tablets that are intended to be chewed, and drug products intended for sustained release or prolonged or repeat action.

The process of disintegration does not imply complete dissolution of the tablet and/or the drug. Complete disintegration is defined by the USP (27th edition, 2004) as "that state in which any residue of the tablet, except fragments of insoluble coating, remaining on the screen of the test apparatus in the soft mass have no palpably firm core." The official apparatus for the disintegration test and procedure is described in the USP. Separate specifications are given for drug products that are designed not to disintegrate. These products include troches, chewable tablets, and modified-release drug products.

Although disintegration tests allow for precise measurement of the formation of fragments, granules, or aggregates from solid dosage forms, no information is obtained from these tests on the rate of dissolution of the active drug. However, there has been some interest in using only the disintegration test and no dissolution test for drug products that meet the Biopharmaceutical Classification System (BCS) for highly soluble and highly permeable drugs (chapter 15). In general, the disintegration test serves as a component in the overall quality control of tablet manufacture.

Dissolution and Solubility

Dissolution is the process by which a solid drug substance becomes dissolved in a solvent. *Solubility* is the mass of solute that dissolves in a specific mass or volume of solvent at a given temperature (eg, 1 g of NaCl dissolves in 2.786 mL of water at 25°C). Solubility is a static property; wheareas dissolution is a dynamic property. In biologic systems, drug dissolution in an aqueous medium is an important prior condition for systemic absorption. The rate at which drugs with poor aqueous solubility dissolve from an intact or disintegrated solid dosage form in the gastrointestinal tract often controls the rate of systemic absorption of the drug. Thus, dissolution tests may be used to predict bioavailability and may be used to discriminate formulation factors that affect drug bioavailability. The dissolution test is required for all U.S. Food and Drug Administration (FDA)-approved solid oral drug products.

Noyes and Whitney (1897) and other investigators studied the rate of dissolution of solid drugs. According to their observations, the steps in dissolution include the process of drug dissolution at the surface of the solid particle, thus forming a saturated solution around the particle. The dissolved drug in the saturated solution, known as the *stagnant layer*, diffuses to the bulk of the solvent from regions of high drug concentration to regions of low drug concentration (Fig. 14-2).

The overall rate of drug dissolution may be described by the *Noyes–Whitney equation* (Eq. 14.1),

$$\frac{dC}{dt} = \frac{DA}{h}(C_S - C) \tag{14.1}$$

Figure 14-2.   Dissolution of a solid drug particle in a solvent. (C_s = concentration of drug in the stagnant layer, C = concentration of drug in the bulk solvent.)

where dC/dt = rate of drug dissolution at time t, D = diffusion rate constant, A = surface area of the particle, C_S = concentration of drug (equal to solubility of drug) in the stagnant layer, C = concentration of drug in the bulk solvent, and h = thickness of the stagnant layer. The rate of dissolution, dC/dt, is the rate of drug dissolved per time expressed as concentration change in the dissolution fluid.

The Noyes–Whitney equation shows that dissolution in a flask may be influenced by the physicochemical characteristics of the drug, the formulation, and the solvent. Drug in the body, particularly in the gastrointestinal tract, is considered to be dissolving in an aqueous environment. Permeation of drug across the gut wall (a model lipid membrane) is affected by the ability of the drug to diffuse (D) and to partition between the lipid membrane. A favorable partition coefficient ($K_{oil/water}$) will facilitate drug absorption.

In addition to these factors, the temperature of the medium and the agitation rate also affect the rate of drug dissolution. *In vivo*, the temperature is maintained at a constant 37°C, and the agitation (primarily peristaltic movements in the gastrointestinal tract) is reasonably constant. In contrast, *in-vitro* studies of dissolution kinetics require maintenance of constant temperature and agitation. Temperature is generally kept at 37°C, and the agitation or stirring rate is held to a specified rpm (revolutions per minute). An increase in temperature will increase the kinetic energy of the molecules and increase the diffusion constant, D. Moreover, an increase in agitation of the solvent medium will reduce the thickness, h, of the stagnant layer, allowing for more rapid drug dissolution.

Factors that affect drug dissolution of a solid oral dosage form include (1) the physical and chemical nature of the active drug substance, (2) the nature of the excipients, and (3) the method of manufacture.

PHYSICOCHEMICAL NATURE OF THE DRUG

In addition to their effect on dissolution kinetics, the physical and chemical properties of the drug substance as well as the excipients are important considerations in the design of a drug product (Table 14.1). For example, intravenous solutions are difficult to prepare with drugs that have poor aqueous solubility. Drugs that are physically or chemically unstable may require special excipients, coatings, or manufacturing processes to protect the drug from degradation. The potent pharmacodynamic activity of drugs such as estrogens and other hormones, penicillin antibiotics, cancer chemotherapeutic agents, and others, may cause adverse reactions

TABLE 14.1 *Physicochemical Properties for Consideration in Drug Product Design*

pK$_a$ and pH profile	Necessary for optimum stability and solubility of the final product.
Particle size	May affect the solubility of the drug and therefore the dissolution rate of the product.
Polymorphism	The ability of a drug to exist in various crystal forms may change the solubility of the drug. Also, the stability of each form is important, because polymorphs may convert from one form to another.
Hygroscopicity	Moisture absorption may affect the physical structure as well as stability of the product.
Partition coefficient	May give some indication of the relative affinity of the drug for oil and water. A drug that has high affinity for oil may have poor release and dissolution from the drug product.
Excipient interaction	The compatibility of the excipients with the drug and sometimes trace elements in excipients may affect the stability of the product. It is important to have specifications of all raw materials.
pH stability profile	The stability of solutions is often affected by the pH of the vehicle; furthermore, because the pH in the stomach and gut is different, knowledge of the stability profile would help to avoid or prevent degradation of the product during storage or after administration.

to personnel who are exposed to these drugs during manufacture and also presents a problem.

Solubility, pH, and Drug Absorption

The *solubility–pH profile* is a plot of the solubility of the drug at various physiologic pH values. In designing oral dosage forms, the formulator must consider that the natural pH environment of the gastrointestinal tract varies from acidic in the stomach to slightly alkaline in the small intestine. A basic drug is more soluble in an acidic medium, forming a soluble salt. Conversely, an acid drug is more soluble in the intestine, forming a soluble salt at the more alkaline pH. The solubility–pH profile gives a rough estimation of the completeness of dissolution for a dose of a drug in the stomach or in the small intestine. Solubility may be improved with the addition of an acidic or basic excipient. Solubilization of aspirin, for example, may be increased by the addition of an alkaline buffer. In the formulation of controlled-release drugs, buffering agents may be added to slow or modify the release rate of a fast-dissolving drug. To be effective, however, the controlled-release drug product must be a nondisintegrating dosage form. The buffering agent is released slowly rather than rapidly, so that the drug does not dissolve immediately in the surrounding gastrointestinal fluid.

Stability, pH, and Drug Absorption

The *stability–pH profile* is a plot of the reaction rate constant for drug degradation versus pH. If drug decomposition occurs by acid or base catalysis, some prediction of degradation of the drug in the gastrointestinal tract may be made. For example, erythromycin has a pH-dependent stability profile. In acidic medium, as in the stomach, erythromycin decomposition occurs rapidly, whereas in neutral or alkaline pH, the drug is relatively stable. Consequently, erythromycin tablets are enteric coated to protect against acid degradation in the stomach. This information also led subsequently to the preparation of a less water-soluble erythromycin salt that is more stable in the stomach. The dissolution rate of erythromycin powder varied from 100% dissolved in 1 hour to less than 40% dissolved in 1 hour. The slow-dissolving raw drug material (active pharmaceutical ingredient) also resulted in slow-dissolving drug products. Therefore, the dissolution of powdered raw drug material is a very useful *in-vitro* method for predicting bioavailability problems of the erythromycin product in the body.

Particle Size and Drug Absorption

The effective surface area of a drug is increased enormously by a reduction in the particle size. Because dissolution takes place at the surface of the solute (drug), the greater the surface area, the more rapid is the rate of drug dissolution. The geometric shape of the particle also affects the surface area, and, during dissolution, the surface is constantly changing. In dissolution calculations, the solute particle is usually assumed to have retained its geometric shape.

Particle size and particle size distribution studies are important for drugs that have low water solubility. Many drugs are very active intravenously but are not very effective when given orally, because of poor oral absorption. Griseofulvin, nitrofurantoin, and many steroids are drugs with low aqueous solubility; reduction of the particle size by milling to a micronized form has improved the oral absorption of these drugs. Smaller particle size results in an increase in the total surface area of the particles, enhances water penetration into the particles, and increases the dissolution rate. For poorly soluble drugs, a disintegrant may be added to the formulation to ensure rapid disintegration of the tablet and release of the particles. The addition of surface-active agents may increase wetting as well as solubility of these drugs.

Polymorphism, Solvates, and Drug Absorption

Polymorphism refers to the arrangement of a drug substance in various crystal forms or polymorphs. In recent years the term polymorph has been used frequently to describe polymorphs, solvates, amorphous forms, and desolvated solvates. *Amorphous forms* are noncrystalline forms, *solvates* are forms that contain a solvent (solvate) or water (hydrate), and *desolvated* solvates are forms that are made by removing the solvent from the solvate.

Polymorphs have the same chemical structure but different physical properties, such as solubility, density, hardness, and compression characteristics. Some polymorphic crystals have much lower aqueous solubility than the amorphous forms, causing a product to be incompletely absorbed. Chloramphenicol, for example, has several crystal forms, and when given orally as a suspension, the drug concentration in the body was found to be dependent on the percent of β-polymorph in the suspension. The β form is more soluble and better absorbed (see Fig. 14-3). In general, the crystal form that has the lowest free energy is the most stable polymorph. A drug that exists as an amorphous form (noncrystalline form) generally dissolves more rapidly than the same drug in a more structurally rigid crystalline form. Some polymorphs are *metastable* and may convert to a more stable form over time. A change in crystal form may cause problems in manufacturing the product. For example, a change in the crystal structure of the drug may cause cracking in a tablet or even prevent a granulation from being compressed into a tablet.

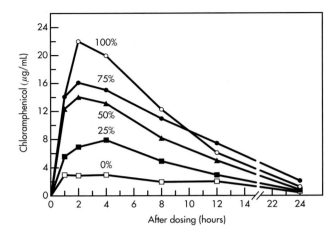

Figure 14-3. Comparison of mean blood serum levels obtained with chloramphenicol palmitate suspensions containing varying ratios of α and β polymorphs, following single oral dose equivalent to 1.5 g chloramphenicol. Percentage polymorph β in the suspension.
(From Aguiar et al, 1967, with permission.)

Re-formulation of a product may be necessary if a new crystal form of a drug is used. Some drugs interact with solvent during preparation to form a crystal called a *solvate.* Water may form special crystals with drugs called *hydrates;* for example, erythromycin hydrates have quite different solubility compared to the anhydrous form of the drug (Fig. 14-4). Ampicillin trihydrate, on the other hand, was reported to be less absorbed than the anhydrous form of ampicillin because of faster dissolution of the latter.

FORMULATION FACTORS AFFECTING DRUG DISSOLUTION

Excipients are added to a formulation to provide certain functional properties to the drug and dosage form. Some of these functional properties of the excipients

Figure 14-4. Dissolution behavior of erythromycin dihydrate, monohydrate, and anhydrate in phosphate buffer (pH 7.5) at 37°C.
(From Allen et al, 1978, with permission.)

TABLE 14.2   Common Excipients Used in Solid Drug Products

EXCIPIENT	PROPERTY IN DOSAGE FORM
Lactose	Diluent
Dibasic calcium phosphate	Diluent
Starch	Disintegrant, diluent
Microcrystalline cellulose	Disintegrant, diluent
Magnesium stearate	Lubricant
Stearic acid	Lubricant
Hydrogenated vegetable oil	Lubricant
Talc	Lubricant
Sucrose (solution)	Granulating agent
Polyvinyl pyrrolidone (solution)	Granulating agent
Hydroxypropylmethylcellulose	Tablet-coating agent
Titinium dioxide	Combined with dye as colored coating
Methylcellulose	Coating or granulating agent
Cellulose acetate phthalate	Enteric coating agent

are used to improve the compressibility of the active drug, stabilize the drug against degradation, decrease gastric irritation, control the rate of drug absorption from the absorption site, increase drug bioavailability, etc. Some of the excipients used in the manufacture of solid and liquid drug products are listed in Tables 14.2 and 14.3.

Excipients in the drug product may also affect the dissolution kinetics of the drug, either by altering the medium in which the drug is dissolving or by reacting with the drug itself. Some of the more common manufacturing problems that affect dissolution are listed in Table 14.2. Other excipients include suspending agents that increase the viscosity of the drug vehicle and thereby diminish the rate of drug dissolution from suspensions. Tablet lubricants, such as magnesium stearate, may repel water and reduce dissolution when used in large quantities. Coatings, particularly shellac, will crosslink upon aging and decrease the dissolution rate. However, surfactants may affect drug dissolution in an unpredictable fashion. Low concentrations of surfactants decrease the surface tension and increase the rate of drug dissolution, whereas higher surfactants concentrations tend to form micelles

TABLE 14.3   Common Excipients Used in Oral Liquid Drug Products

EXCIPIENT	PROPERTY IN DOSAGE FORM
Sodium carboxymethylcellulose	Suspending agent
Tragacanth	Suspending agent
Sodium alginate	Suspending agent
Xanthan gum	Thixotropic suspending agent
Veegum	Thixotropic suspending agent
Sorbitol	Sweetener
Alcohol	Solubilizing agent, preservative
Propylene glycol	Solubilizing agent
Methyl, propylparaben	Preservative
Sucrose	Sweetener
Polysorbates	Surfactant
Sesame oil	For emulsion vehicle
Corn Oil	For emulsion vehicle

with the drug and thus decrease the dissolution rate. Large drug particles have a smaller surface area and dissolve more slowly than smaller particles. High compression of tablets without sufficient disintegrant may cause poor disintegration of a compressed tablet.

Some excipients, such as sodium bicarbonate, may change the pH of the medium surrounding the active drug substance. Aspirin, a weak acid when formulated with sodium bicarbonate, will form a water-soluble salt in an alkaline medium, in which the drug rapidly dissolves. The term for this process is *dissolution in a reactive medium.* The solid drug dissolves rapidly in the reactive solvent surrounding the solid particle. However, as the dissolved drug molecules diffuse outward into the bulk solvent, the drug may precipitate out of solution with a very fine particle size. These small particles have enormous collective surface area, dispersing and redissolving readily for more rapid absorption upon contact with the mucosal surface.

Excipients in a formulation may interact directly with the drug to form a water-soluble or water-insoluble complex. For example, if tetracycline is formulated with calcium carbonate, an insoluble complex of calcium tetracycline is formed that has a slow rate of dissolution and poor absorption.

Excipients may be added intentionally to the formulation to enhance the rate and extent of drug absorption or to delay or slow the rate of drug absorption (Table 14.4). For example, excipients that increase the aqueous solubility of the drug generally increase the rate of dissolution and drug absorption. Excipients may increase the retention time of the drug in the gastrointestinal tract and therefore increase the total amount of drug absorbed. Excipients may act as carriers to increase drug diffusion across the intestinal wall. In contrast, many excipients may retard drug dissolution and thus reduce drug absorption.

Common excipients found in oral drug products are listed in Table 14.2 and Table 14.3. Excipients should be pharmacodynamically inert. However, excipients may change the functionality of the drug substance and the bioavailability of the drug from the dosage form. For solid oral dosage forms such as compressed tablets, excipients may include (1) a diluent (eg, lactose), (2) a disintegrant (eg, starch), (3) a lubricant (eg, magnesium stearate), and (4) other components such as binding and stabilizing agents. If used improperly in a formulation, the rate and extent

TABLE 14.4   Effect of Excipients on the Pharmacokinetic Parameters of Oral Drug Products[a]

EXCIPIENTS	EXAMPLE	k_a	T_{MAX}	AUC
Disintegrants	Avicel, Explotab	↑	↓	↑ /—
Lubricants	Talc, hydrogenated vegetable oil	↓	↑	↓ /—
Coating agent	Hydroxypropylmethyl cellulose	—	—	—
Enteric coat	Cellulose acetate phthalate	↓	↑	↓ /—
Sustained-release agents	Methylcellulose, ethylcellulose	↓	↑	↓ /—
Sustained-release agents (waxy agents)	Castorwax, Carbowax	↓	↑	↓ /—
Sustained-release agents (gum/viscous)	Veegum, Keltrol	↓	↑	↓ /—

[a]This may be concentration and drug dependent. ↑ = Increase, ↓ = decrease, — = no effect, k_a = absorption rate constant, t_{max} = time for peak drug concentration in plasma, AUC = area under the plasma drug concentration–time curve.

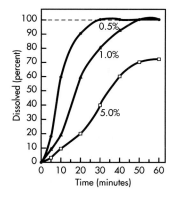

Figure 14-5. Effect of lubricant on drug dissolution. Percentage of magnesium stearate in formulation.

of drug absorption may be affected. For example, Figure 14-5 shows that an excessive quantity of magnesium stearate (a hydrophobic lubricant) in the formulation may retard drug dissolution and slow the rate of drug absorption. The total amount of drug absorbed may also be reduced (Fig. 14-6). To prevent this problem, the lubricant level should be decreased or a different lubricant selected. Sometimes, increasing the amount of disintegrant may overcome the retarding effect of lubricants on dissolution. However, with some poorly soluble drugs an increase in disintegrant level has little or no effect on drug dissolution because the fine drug particles are not wetted. The influence of some common ingredients on drug absorption parameters is summarized in Table 14.4. These are general trends for typical preparations.

DISSOLUTION AND DRUG RELEASE TESTING

Dissolution and drug release tests are *in-vitro* tests that measure the rate and extent of dissolution or release of the drug substance from a drug product, usually in an aqueous medium under specified conditions. The dissolution test is an important quality control procedure for the drug product and is often linked to product performance *in vivo*. *In-vitro* drug dissolution studies are most often used for monitoring drug product stability and manufacturing process control. The USP-NF (United States Pharmacopeia) sets standards for dissolution and drug release tests of most drug products. Ideally, the dissolution method used for a particular drug product *in vitro* relates to the bioavailability of the drug *in vivo* (see

Figure 14-6. Effect of lubricant on drug absorption. Percentage of magnesium stearate in formulation. Incomplete drug absorption occurs for formulation with 5% magnesium stearate.

in-vitro–in-vivo correlation, below). In addition, the dissolution method should be able to discriminate changes in formulation of the drug product. Furthermore, dissolution and drug release tests are important quality control components for the manufacture of the drug product. As a quality control test, dissolution and drug release testing may be used for:

- Batch-to-batch drug release uniformity
- Stability
- Scale-up and postapproval changes (SUPAC)
- Predicting *in-vivo* performance

Often, the dissolution test is a valuable tool in formulation development. A suitable dissolution method may uncover a formulation problem with the drug product that could result in a bioavailability problem. Each dissolution method is specific for the drug product and its formulation. The dissolution test should be able to distinguish between acceptable and unacceptable drug formulations as observed by different drug dissolution rates under the same experimental conditions. A suitable dissolution test should be able to reflect changes in the formulation, manufacturing process, and physical and chemical characteristics of the drug, such as particle size, polymorphs, and surface area (Gray et al, 2001). The dissolution test is a major requirement for scale-up and postapproval changes, SUPAC (see Chapter 16). After a change is made in a formulation, the manufacturer should assess the potential effect of the change on bioequivalence, which usually includes multipoint and/or multimedia dissolution profiling and, if necessary, an *in-vivo* bioequivalence study.

Dissolution Conditions

The development of an appropriate dissolution test requires the investigator to try different agitation rates, different media (including volume and pH of medium), and different kinds of dissolution apparatus (Table 14-5). The current USP-NF

TABLE 14.5 Conditions That May Affect Drug Dissolution and Release

Drug substance
  Particle size
  Polymorph
  Surface area
  Chemical stability in dissolution media
Formulation of drug product
  Excipients (lubricants, suspending agents, etc)
Medium
  Volume
  pH
  Molarity
  Co-solvents, added enzymes/surfactants
Temperature of medium
Apparatus
Hydrodynamics
  Agitation rate
  Shape of dissolution vessel
  Placement of tablet in vessel
  Sinkers (for floating products and products that stick to side of vessel)

TABLE 14.6   Dissolution of Erythromycin Stearate Bulk Drug and Corresponding Tablets

Curve No.	PERCENT DISSOLUTION AFTER 1.0 hr		
	Bulk Drug	500-mg Tablet	250-mg Tablet
4	49	44	
6	72	70	
7	75	70	
—	78	—	80
8	82	75	
9	92	85	

From Philip and Daly (1983), with permission.

(United States Pharmacopeia) lists officially recognized dissolution apparatus. Once a suitable dissolution test is obtained, acceptable dissolution criteria are developed for the drug product and its formulation. These criteria or dissolution specifications (eg, percent of drug dissolved in 30 minutes) are used to investigate formulation problems. For example, Philip and Daly (1983) devised a method using pH 6.6 phosphate buffer as the dissolution medium instead of 0.1 N HCL to avoid instability of the antibiotic drug erythromycin. Using the USP paddle method at 50 rpm and a temperature of 22°C, the dissolution of the various erythromycin tablets was shown to vary with the source of the bulk active drug (as shown in Table 14.6 and Fig. 14-7).

Visual observations of the dissolution and disintegration behavior of the drug product are important and should be recorded. Dissolution and disintegration patterns can indicate manufacturing variables. These observations are particularly useful during method development and formulation optimization.

The size and shape of the dissolution vessel may affect the rate and extent of dissolution. For example, dissolution vessels range in size from several milliliters to several liters. The shape may be round-bottomed or flat, so the tablet might lie in

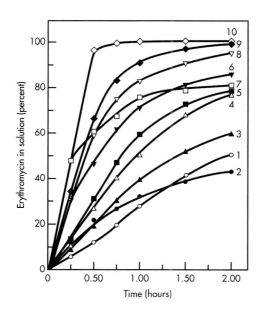

Figure 14-7.   Dissolution profile of various lots of erythromycin stearate as a function of time (0.05 M, pH 6.6 phosphate buffer).
(From Philip and Daly, 1983, with permission.)

a different position in different experiments. The usual volume of the medium is 500–1000 mL. Drugs that are poorly water soluble may require use of a very-large-capacity vessel (up to 2000 mL) to observe significant dissolution. In some cases, 1% sodium lauryl sulfate (SLS) may be used as the dissolution medium for water-insoluble drugs. *Sink conditions* is a term referring to an excess volume of medium that allows the solid drug to dissolve continuously. If the drug solution becomes saturated, no further net drug dissolution will take place. According to the USP-NF, "the quantity of medium used should be not less than 3 times that required to form a saturated solution of the drug substance."

The amount of agitation and the nature of the stirrer affect hydrodynamics of the system, thereby affecting the dissolution rate. Stirring rates must be controlled, and specifications differ between drug products. Low stirring rates (50–75 rpm) are more discriminating of formulation factors affecting dissolution than higher stirring rates. However, higher dissolution rate may be needed for some special formulations in order to obtain reproducible dissolution rates. Suspensions that contain viscous or thickening agents may settle into a diffusion-controlled "cone-shape" region in the flask when stirring rate is too slow. The temperature of the dissolution medium must be controlled, and variations in temperature must be avoided. Most dissolution tests are performed at 37°C. However, for transdermal drug products, the recommended temperature is 32°C.

The nature of the dissolution medium will also affect the dissolution test. The solubility of the drug must be considered, as well as the total amount of drug in the dosage form. The dissolution medium should not be saturated by the drug (ie, sink conditions are maintained). Usually, a volume of medium larger than the amount of solvent needed to completely dissolve the drug is used in the dissolution test. Which medium is best is a matter of considerable controversy. The dissolution medium in many USP dissolution tests is deaerated water or, if substantiated by the solubility characteristics of the drug or formulation, a buffered aqueous solution (typically pH 4–8) or dilute HCl may be used. The significance of deaeration of the medium should be determined. Various investigators have used 0.1 N HCl, phosphate buffer, simulated gastric juice, water, and simulated intestinal juice, depending on the nature of the drug product and the location in the gastrointestinal tract where the drug is expected to dissolve.

The design of the dissolution apparatus, along with the factors described above, has a marked effect on the outcome of the dissolution test. No single apparatus and test can be used for all drug products. Each drug product must be tested individually with the dissolution test that best correlates to *in-vivo* bioavailability.

Usually, the report on the dissolution test will state that a certain percentage of the labeled amount of drug product must dissolve within a specified period of time. In practice, the absolute amount of drug in the drug product may vary from tablet to tablet. Therefore, a number of tablets from each lot are usually tested to get a representative dissolution rate for the product.

COMPENDIAL METHODS OF DISSOLUTION

The USP-NF provides several official methods for carrying out dissolution tests of tablets, capsules and other special products such as transdermal preparations.

TABLE 14.7   Dissolution Apparatus

APPARATUS[a]	NAME	DRUG PRODUCT
Apparatus 1	Rotating basket	Tablets
Apparatus 2	Paddle	Tablets, capsules, modified drug products, suspensions
Apparatus 3	Reciprocating cylinder	Extended-release drug products
Apparatus 4	Flow cell	Drug products containing low-water-soluble drugs
Apparatus 5	Paddle over disk	Transdermal drug products
Apparatus 6	Cylinder	Transdermal drug products
Apparatus 7	Reciprocating disk	Extended-release drug products
Rotating bottle	(Non-USP-NF)	Extended-release drug products (beads)
Diffusion cell (Franz)	(Non-USP-NF)	Ointments, creams, transdermal drug products

[a]Apparatus 1–7 refer to compendial dissolution apparatus in USP-NF.

Tablets are grouped into uncoated, plain-coated, and enteric-coated tablets. The selection of a particular method for a drug is usually specified in the monograph for a particular drug product. Buccal and sublingual tablets are tested applying the uncoated tablet procedure. Table 14.7 lists various types of dissolution apparatus and the type of drug products that is often used with the apparatus. For Apparatus 1 and 2, low rotational speeds affect the reproducibility of the hydrodynamics; whereas at high rotational speeds, turbulence may occur. Dissolution profiles that show the drug dissolving too slowly or too rapidly may justify increasing or decreasing the rotational speed (Gray et al, 2001).

Rotating Basket Method (Apparatus 1)

The rotating basket apparatus (Apparatus 1) consists of a cylindrical basket held by a motor shaft. The basket holds the sample and rotates in a round flask containing the dissolution medium. The entire flask is immersed in a constant-temperature bath set at 37°C. The rotating speed and the position of the basket must meet specific requirements set forth in the current USP. The most common rotating speed for the basket method is 100 rpm. Dissolution calibration standards are available to make sure that these mechanical and operating requirements are met. Calibration tablets containing prednisone are made specially for dissolution tests requiring disintegrating tablets, whereas salicylic acid calibration tablets are used as a standard for nondisintegrating tablets. Apparatus 1 is generally preferred for capsules and for dosage forms that tend to float or disintegrate slowly.

Paddle Method (Apparatus 2)

The paddle apparatus (Apparatus 2) consists of a special, coated paddle that minimizes turbulence due to stirring (Fig. 14-8). The paddle is attached vertically to a variable-speed motor that rotates at a controlled speed. The tablet or capsule is placed into the round-bottom dissolution flask, which minimizes turbulence of the dissolution medium. The apparatus is housed in a constant-temperature water bath maintained at 37°C, similar to the rotating-basket method. The position and alignment of the paddle are specified in the USP. The paddle method is very sensitive to tilting. Improper alignment may drastically affect the dissolution results with some drug products. The same set of dissolution calibration standards is used to

Figure 14-8.   Typical setup for performing the USP dissolution test with the Distek 2000. The system is equipped with a height adjustment ring for easy adjustment of paddle height. (Drawing courtesy of Distek inc, Somerset, NJ.)

check the equipment before tests are run. The most common operating speeds for Apparatus 2 are 50 rpm for solid oral dosage forms and 25 rpm for suspensions. Apparatus 2 is generally preferred for tablets. A *sinker,* such as a few turns of platinum wire, may be used to prevent a capsule or tablet from floating. A sinker may also be used for film-coated tablets that stick to the vessel walls or to help position the tablet or capsule under the paddle (Gray et al, 2001). The sinker should not alter the dissolution characteristics of the dosage form.

Reciprocating Cylinder Method (Apparatus 3)

The reciprocating cylinder apparatus (Apparatus 3) consists of a set of cylindrical, flat-bottomed glass vessels equipped with reciprocating cylinders for dissolution testing of extended-release products, particularly bead-type modified-release dosage forms. Six units are tested, and the dissolution medium is maintained at 37°C.

Flow-through-Cell Method (Apparatus 4)

The flow-through-cell apparatus (Apparatus 4) consists of a reservoir for the dissolution medium and a pump that forces dissolution medium through the cell holding the test sample. Flow rate ranges from 4 to 16 mL/min. Six samples are tested during the dissolution testing, and the medium is maintained at 37°C. Apparatus 4 may be used for modified-release dosage forms that contain active ingredients having very limited solubility.

There are many variations of this method. Essentially, the sample is held in a fixed position while the dissolution medium is pumped through the sample holder, thus dissolving the drug. Laminar flow of the medium is achieved by using a pulseless pump. Peristaltic or centrifugal pumps are not recommended. The flow rate is usually maintained between 10 and 100 mL/min. The dissolution medium may be fresh or recirculated. In the case of fresh medium, the dissolution rate at any moment may be obtained, whereas in the official paddle or basket method, cumulative dissolution rates are monitored. A major advantage of the flow-through method is the easy maintenance of a sink condition for dissolution. A large volume of dissolution medium may also be used, and the mode of operation is easily adapted to automated equipment.

Paddle-over-Disk Method (Apparatus 5)

The USP-NF also lists a paddle-over-disk method for testing the release of drugs from transdermal products. The apparatus (Apparatus 5) consists of a sample holder or disk assembly that holds the product. The entire preparation is placed in a dissolution flask filled with specified medium maintained at 32°C. The paddle is placed directly over the disk assembly. Samples are drawn midway between the surface of the dissolution medium and the top of the paddle blade at specified times. Similar to dissolution testing with capsules and tablets, six units are tested during each run. Acceptance criteria are stated in the individual drug monographs.

Cylinder Method (Apparatus 6)

The cylinder method (Apparatus 6) for testing transdermal preparation is modified from the basket method (Apparatus 1). In place of the basket, a stainless steel cylinder is used to hold the sample. The sample is mounted onto cuprophan (an inert porous cellulosic material) and the entire system adheres to the cylinder. Testing is maintained at 32°C. Samples are drawn midway between the surface of the dissolution medium and the top of the rotating cylinder for analysis.

Reciprocating Disk Method (Apparatus 7)

In the reciprocating disk method for testing transdermal products, a motor drive assembly (Apparatus 7) is used to reciprocate the system vertically, and the samples are placed on disk-shaped holders using cuprophan supports. The test is also carried out at 32°C, and reciprocating frequency is about 30 cycles per minute. The acceptance criteria are listed in the individual drug monographs.

Methods for Testing Enteric-Coated Products

USP-NF lists two methods (Method A and Method B) for testing enteric-coated products. The latest revision of the USP-NF should be consulted for complete details of the methods.

Both methods require that the dissolution test be performed in the apparatus specified in the drug monograph (usually Apparatus 2 or Apparatus 1). The product is first tested with 0.1 N HCl for 2 hours and then changed to pH 6.8 buffer medium. The buffer stage generally runs for 45 minutes or for the time specified in the monograph. The objective is that no significant dissolution occurs in the acid phase (less than 10% for any sample unit), and a specified percentage of drug must be released in the buffer phase. Specifications are set in the individual drug monographs.

MEETING DISSOLUTION REQUIREMENTS

Dissolution test times and specifications are usually established on the basis of an evaluation of dissolution profile data. The dissolution test time points should be selected to characterize adequately the ascending and plateau phases of the dissolution curve. USP-NF sets dissolution requirements for many products (Table 14.8). The requirements apply to both the basket and the paddle methods. The amount of drug dissolved within a given time period (Q) is expressed as a percentage of label content. The Q is generally specified in the monograph for a drug product to pass the dissolution test. Three stages (S_1, S_2, and S_3) of testing are allowed by USP-NF. Initially, six tablets or capsules are tested for the dissolution test. If the dissolution test fails to meet the criteria for S_1, then six more units are tested. Dissolution testing continues until the dissolution criteria are met or until the three stages are exhausted (Table 14.8).

For many products the passing value for Q is set at 75% in 45 minutes. Some products require a Q of 85% in 30 minutes, others 75% in 60 minutes. For a new drug product, setting the dissolution specification requires a thorough consideration of the physical and chemical properties of the drug. In addition to the consideration that the dissolution test must ensure consistent bioavailability of the

TABLE 14.8 *Dissolution Acceptance*

STAGE	NUMBER TESTED	ACCEPTANCE CRITERIA
S_1	6	Each unit is not less than $Q + 5\%$
S_2	6	Average of 12 units ($S_1 + S_2$) is equal to or greater than Q, and no unit is less than $Q - 15\%$
S_3	12	Average of 24 units ($S_1 + S_2 + S_3$) is equal to or greater than Q, not more than 2 units are less than $Q - 15\%$, and no unit is less than $Q - 25\%$

Adapted with permission from United States Pharmacopeia.

product, the test must provide for variation in manufacturing and testing variables so that a product may not be improperly rejected (Hofer and Gray, 2003).

ALTERNATIVE METHODS OF DISSOLUTION TESTING

Rotating Bottle Method

The rotating bottle method was suggested in NF-XIII (National Formulary) but has become less popular since. The rotating bottle method was used mainly for controlled-release beads. For this purpose the dissolution medium may be easily changed, such as from artificial gastric juice to artificial intestinal juice. The equipment consists of a rotating rack that holds the sample drug products in bottles. The bottles are capped tightly and rotated in a 37°C temperature bath. At various times, the samples are removed from the bottle, decanted through a 40-mesh screen, and the residues are assayed. To the remaining drug residues within the bottles are added an equal volume of fresh medium and the dissolution test is continued. A dissolution test with pH 1.2 medium for 1 hour, pH 2.5 medium for the next 1 hour, followed by pH 4.5 medium for 1.5 hours, pH 7.0 medium for 1.5 hours, and pH 7.5 medium for 2 hours was recommended to simulate condition of the gastrointestinal tract. The main disadvantage is that this procedure is manual and tedious. Moreover, it is not known if the rotating bottle procedure results in a better *in-vitro–in-vivo* correlation (see below) for drugs.

Intrinsic Dissolution Method

Most methods for dissolution deal with a finished drug product. Sometimes a new drug or substance may be tested for dissolution without the effect of excipients or the fabrication effect of processing. The dissolution of a drug powder by maintaining a constant surface area is called *intrinsic dissolution*. Intrinsic dissolution is usually expressed as $mg/cm^2/min$. In one method, the basket method is adapted to test dissolution of powder by placing the powder in a disk attached with a clipper to the bottom of the basket.

Peristalsis Method

The peristalsis method attempts to simulate the hydrodynamic conditions of the gastrointestinal tract in an *in-vitro* dissolution device. The apparatus consists of a rigid plastic cylindrical tubing fitted with a septum and rubber stoppers at both ends. The dissolution chamber consists of a space between the septum and the lower stopper. The apparatus is placed in a beaker containing the dissolution medium. The dissolution medium is pumped with peristaltic action through the dosage form.

Diffusion Cells

Static and flow-through diffusion cells are commercially available to characterize *in-vitro* drug release and drug permeation kinetics from a topical drug product (eg,

Figure 14-9. The Franz diffusion cell.
(Courtesy of Hanson Research Corporation [www.hansonresearch.com/vert_diffusion_cell.htm], with permission.)

ointment, cream) or transdermal drug product. The *Franz diffusion cell* is a static diffusion system that is used for characterizing drug permeation through a skin model (Fig. 14.9). The source of skin may be human cadaver skin or animal skin (eg, hairless mouse skin). Anatomically, each skin site (eg, abdomen, arm) has different drug permeation qualities. The skin is mounted on the Franz diffusion cell system. The drug product (eg, ointment) is placed on the skin surface and the drug permeates across the skin into a receptor fluid compartment that may be sampled at various times. The Franz diffusion cell system is useful for comparing *in-vitro* drug release profiles and skin permeation characteristics to aid in selecting an appropriate formulation that has optimum drug delivery.

PROBLEMS OF VARIABLE CONTROL IN DISSOLUTION TESTING

Various equipment and operating variables are associated with dissolution testing. Depending on the particular dosage form involved, the variables may or may not exert a pronounced effect on the rate of dissolution of the drug or drug product. Variations of 25% or more may occur with the same type of equipment and procedure. The centering and alignment of the paddle is critical in the paddle method. Turbulence can create increased agitation, resulting in a higher dissolution rate. Wobbling and tilting due to worn equipment should be avoided. The basket method is less sensitive to the tilting effect. However, the basket method is more sensitive to clogging due to gummy materials. Pieces of small particles can also clog up the basket screen and create a local non-sink condition for dissolution. Furthermore, dissolved gas in the medium may form air bubbles on the surface of the dosage form unit and can affect dissolution in both the basket and paddle methods.

The interpretation of dissolution data is probably the most difficult job for the pharmacist. In the absence of *in-vivo* data, it is generally impossible to make valid conclusions about bioavailability from the dissolution data alone. The use of various testing methods makes it even more difficult to interpret dissolution results, because there is no simple correlation among dissolution results obtained with various methods. For many drug products, the dissolution rates are higher with the paddle method. Dissolution results at 50 rpm with the paddle method may be equivalent to dissolution at 100 rpm with the basket method. In a study of sustained-release theophylline tablets compressed at various degrees of hardness, Cameron et al (1983) found that, at 50 rpm, dissolution with the paddle method was faster than that of the basket method for tablets of 4.0-kg hardness. However, with tablets of 6.8-kg hardness, similar dissolution profiles were obtained at 125 rpm for the basket and paddle methods over a period of 6 hours. With both methods, increased dissolution rates were observed as the rates were increased. Apparently, the composition of the formulation as well as the process variables in manufacturing may both be important. No simple correlation can be made for dissolution results obtained with different methods.

In a comparison of the paddle and basket methods in evaluating a sustained-release pseudoephedrine–guaifenesin preparation, Masih et al (1983) found that the paddle method was more discriminating in demonstrating dissolution differences among drug products. At 100 rpm, the basket method failed to pick up formulation differences detected by the paddle method.

In the absence of *in-vivo* data, the selection of the dissolution method is based on the type of drug product to be tested. For example, a low-density preparation may be poorly wetted in the basket method. A gummy preparation may clog up the basket screen; therefore the paddle method is preferred. A floating dosage form (eg, suppository) may be placed in a stainless steel coil (sinker) so that the dosage form remains at the bottom of the dissolution flask. For many drugs, a satisfactory dissolution test may be obtained with more than one method by optimizing the testing conditions.

IN-VITRO–IN-VIVO CORRELATION

In-vitro–in-vivo correlation (IVIVC) establishes a relationship between a biological property of the drug (such as pharmacodynamic effect or plasma drug concentration) and a physicochemical property of the drug product containing the drug substance, such as dissolution rate (Leeson, 2002). In order to have an IVIVC, some property of the drug release from the drug product *in vitro*, under specified conditions, must relate to *in-vivo* drug performance. Dissolution tests should discriminate formulation factors that may affect bioavailability of the drug (see Chapter 15). In some cases, dissolution tests for immediate-release solid oral drug products may be overdiscriminating and a clinically acceptable product might perform poorly in the dissolution test. When a proper dissolution method is chosen, the rate of dissolution of the product may be correlated to the rate of absorption of the drug into the body. Well-defined *in-vitro–in-vivo* correlations have been reported for modified-release drug products (Chapter 17) but have been more difficult to predict for immediate-release drug products. An IVIVC should be evaluated to demonstrate that predictability of *in-vivo* performance of a drug product from its *in-vitro* dissolution characteristics is maintained over a range of *in-vitro* dissolution release rates and manufacturing changes. The *in-vitro* dissolution characteristics are dependent on the physical properties of the active pharmaceutical ingredient (API), the drug formulation, the hydrodynamics of the dissolution apparatus, and the dissolution medium. IVIVC may be useful for establishing upper and lower dissolution specifications for a solid oral dosage form.

For multisource drug products such as brand-name drug products and marketed generic drug products containing the same active drug, USP-NF may list multiple dissolution tests, one for each product. For example, USP-NF includes 10 separate dissolution tests for theophylline extended-release capsules that are labeled for dosing every 12 hours. USP-NF has separate and distinct dissolution test requirements for two different phenytoin sodium capsules. For extended-release phenytoin sodium capsules, USP-NF states that "not more than 35%, between 30% and 70% and not less than 85% of the labeled amount of $C_{15}H_{11}N_2NaO_2$ in the Extended Capsules dissolves in 30 minutes, 60 minutes, and 120 minutes, respectively, under the specified dissolution conditions." In contrast, about tolerances for "Prompt Phenytoin Sodium Capsules," USP states "not less than 85% of the labeled amount of $C_{15}H_{11}N_2NaO_2$ in the Prompt Capsules dissolves in 30 minutes."

It is important to note that multisource, pharmaceutically equivalent drug products may not be bioequivalent even if these drug products meet the same USP-NF monograph specifications. In the United States, only FDA-approved generic, bioequivalent drug products that meet the requirements for therapeutic equivalence may be interchanged. These generic drug products are listed in the FDA publication, Approved Drug Products with Therapeutic Equivalence Evaluations, also known as the Orange Book (www.fda.gov/cder/ob/default.htm). Bioequivalent drug products are discussed in Chapter 13.

Biopharmaceutic Drug Classification System

The Biopharmaceutic Drug Classification system, BCS, discussed more fully in Chapter 15, is a predictive approach to relate certain physicochemical characteristics of a drug substance and drug product to *in-vivo* bioavailability. The BCS is not a direct *in-vitro–in-vivo* correlation. For example, the drug substance from an immediate-release oral drug product would tend to be rapidly and mostly absorbed if the drug substance and drug product meet the criteria for BCS Class I drugs. A BCS Class I drug product contains a highly soluble drug substance that is highly permeable and from which the drug rapidly dissolves from the drug product (FDA Guidance for Industry, 2000). Since predictability is a major function of IVIVC, any system that predicts *in-vivo* performance from *in-vitro* data may be considered an IVIVC (Leeson, 2002).

Dissolution Rate versus Absorption Rate

If dissolution of the drug is rate limiting, a faster dissolution rate may result in a faster rate of appearance of the drug in the plasma. It may be possible to establish a correlation between rate of dissolution and rate of absorption of the drug.

The absorption rate is usually more difficult to determine than peak absorption time. Therefore, the absorption time may be used in correlating dissolution data to absorption data. In the analysis of *in-vitro–in-vivo* drug correlation, rapid drug dissolution may be distinguished from the slower drug absorption by observation of the absorption time for the preparation. The absorption time refers to the time for a constant amount of drug to be absorbed. In one study involving three sustained-release aspirin products (Levy et al, 1965), the dissolution time for the preparations were linearly correlated to the absorption times

Figure 14-10. An example of correlation between time required for a given amount of drug to be absorbed and time required for the same amount of drug to be dissolved *in vitro* for three sustained-release aspirin products.
(From Wood, 1966, with permission.)

(Fig. 14-10). The results from this study demonstrated that aspirin was rapidly absorbed and was very much dependent on the dissolution rate for absorption.

Percent of Drug Dissolved versus Percent of Drug Absorbed

If a drug is absorbed completely after dissolution, a linear correlation may be obtained by comparing the percentage of drug absorbed to the percentage of drug dissolved. In choosing the dissolution method, one must consider the appropriate dissolution medium and use a slow dissolution stirring rate so that *in-vivo* dissolution is approximated.

Aspirin is absorbed rapidly, and a slight change in formulation may be reflected in a change in the amount and rate of drug absorption during the period of observation (Figs. 14-10 and 14-11). If the drug is absorbed slowly, which occurs when

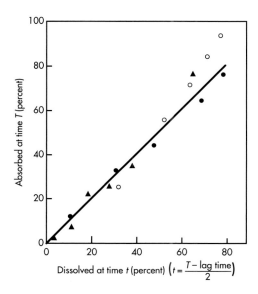

Figure 14-11. An example of continuous *in-vivo–in-vitro* correlation of aspirin.
(From Levy et al, 1965, with permission.)

absorption is the rate-limiting step, a difference in dissolution rate of the product may not be observed. In this case, the drug would be absorbed very slowly independent of the dissolution rate.

Maximum Plasma Concentrations versus Percent of Drug Dissolved *in-Vitro*

When different drug formulations are tested for dissolution, a poorly formulated drug may not be completely dissolved and released, resulting in lower plasma drug concentrations. The percentage of drug released at any time interval will be greater for the more bioavailable drug product. When such drug products are tested *in-vivo*, the peak drug serum concentration will be higher for the drug product that shows the highest percent of drug dissolved. An example of *in-vitro–in-vivo* correlation for 100-mg phenytoin sodium capsules is shown in Figure 14-12. Several products were tested (Shah et al, 1983). A linear correlation was observed between the maximum drug concentration in the body and the percent of drug dissolved *in-vitro*.

The dissolution study on the phenytoin sodium products (Shah et al, 1983) showed that the fastest dissolution rate was product C, for which about 100% of the labeled contents dissolved in the test (Fig. 14-13). Interestingly, these products also show the shortest time to reach peak concentration (t_{max}). The t_{max} is dependent on the absorption rate constant. In this case, the fastest absorption would also result in the shortest t_{max} (see Chapter 9).

Serum Drug Concentration versus Percent of Drug Dissolved

In a study on aspirin absorption, the serum concentration of aspirin was correlated to the percent of drug dissolved using an *in-vitro* dissolution method (Wood, 1966). The dissolution medium was simulated gastric juice. Because aspirin is rapidly absorbed from the stomach, the dissolution of the drug is the rate-limiting step, and

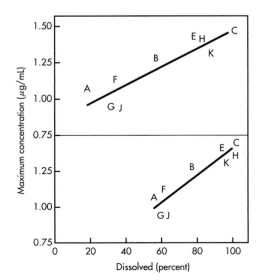

Figure 14-12. *In-vitro–in-vivo* correlation between C_{max} and percent drug dissolved. Top, 30 min (slope = 0.06, r = 0.902, p < 0.001). Bottom, 60 min (slope = 0.10, r = 0.940, p < 0.001.) (Letters on graph indicate different products.)
(From Shah et al, 1983, with permission.)

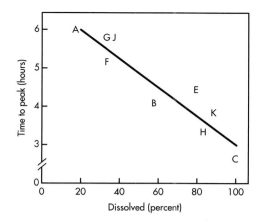

Figure 14-13. *In-vitro–in-vivo* correlation between t_{max} and percent drug dissolved in 30 minutes by basket method. Letters on graph indicate different products.
(From Shah et al, 1983, with permission.)

various formulations with different dissolution rates will cause differences in the serum concentration of aspirin by minutes (Fig. 14-14).

Failure of Correlation of *in-Vitro* Dissolution to *in-Vivo* Absorption

Although there are many published examples of drugs with dissolution data that correlate well with drug absorption in the body, there are also many examples indicating poor correlation of dissolution to drug absorption. There are also instances where a drug has failed the dissolution test and yet is well absorbed. The problem of no correlation between bioavailability and dissolution may be due to the complexity of drug absorption and the weakness of the dissolution design. For example, a product that involves fatty components may be subjected to longer retention in the gastrointestinal tract. The effect of digestive enzymes may also play an important role in the dissolution of the drug *in vivo*. These factors may not be

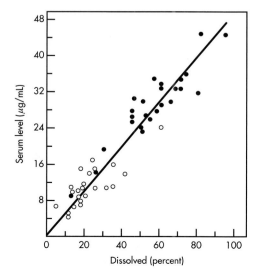

Figure 14-14. Example of *in-vivo–in-vitro* two-point correlation between 10-minute serum level and percent dissolved at 1.2 minutes (O) and the 20-minute serum level and percent dissolved 4.2 minutes (●).
(From Wood, 1966, with permission.)

Figure 14-15. *Dissolution profile of two quinidine gluconate sustained release products in different dissolution media. Each data point is the mean of 12 tablets. (● = product BE, O = product BO-1.) (From Prasad et al, 1983, with permission.)*

adequately simulated with a simple dissolution medium. An excellent example showing the importance of dissolution design is shown in Figure 14-15. Dissolution tests using four different dissolution media were performed for two quinidine gluconate sustained-release tablets (Prasad et al, 1983). Brand BE was known to be bioavailable, whereas product BO-1 was known to be incompletely absorbed. It is interesting to see that using acid medium as well as acid followed by pH 7.4 buffer did not distinguish the two products well, whereas using water or pH 5.4 buffer as dissolution medium clearly distinguished the "good" product from the one that was not completely available. In this case, the use of an acid medium is consistent with the physiologic condition in the stomach, but this procedure would be misleading as a quality control tool. It is important that any new dissolution test be carefully researched before being adopted as a method for predicting drug absorption.

BIOPHARMACEUTIC CONSIDERATIONS

Some of the major biopharmaceutic considerations in the design of a drug product are given in Table 14.9. The prime considerations in the design of a drug product are safety and efficacy. The drug product must effectively deliver the active drug at an appropriate rate and amount to the target receptor site so that the intended therapeutic effect is achieved. The finished dosage form should not produce any additional side effects or discomfort due to the drug and/or excipients. Ideally, all excipients in the drug product should be inactive ingredients alone or in combination in the final dosage form.

TABLE 14.9   Biopharmaceutic Considerations in Drug Product Design

Pharmacodynamic considerations	Patient considerations
Therapeutic objective	Compliance and acceptability of drug product
Toxic effects	Cost
Adverse reactions	Manufacturing considerations
Drug considerations	Cost
Chemical and physical properties of drug	Availability of raw materials
Drug product considerations	Stability
Pharmacokinetics of drug	Quality control
Bioavailability of drug	Method of manufacturing
Route of drug administration	
Desired drug dosage form	
Desired dose of drug	

The finished drug product is a compromise of various factors, including therapeutic objectives, pharmacokinetics, physical and chemical properties, manufacturing, cost, and patient acceptance. Most important, the finished drug product should meet the therapeutic objective by delivering the drug with maximum bioavailability and minimum adverse effects.

PHARMACODYNAMIC CONSIDERATIONS

Therapeutic considerations concern the pharmacodynamic and pharmacologic properties of the drug, including the desired therapeutic response as well as the type and frequency of toxic and/or adverse reactions of the drug. The therapeutic objective will influence the type of drug product to be manufactured. A drug used to treat an acute illness should be formulated to release the drug rapidly, allowing for quick absorption and rapid onset. For example, nitroglycerin is formulated in a sublingual tablet for the treatment of angina pectoris. For prophylactic use in the treatment of certain chronic diseases such as asthma, an extended- or controlled-release dosage form is preferred. The extended-release dosage form releases the drug slowly, thereby controlling the rate of drug absorption and allowing for more constant plasma drug concentrations. In some cases, an immediate-drug-release component is included in the extended-release dosage form, to allow for both rapid onset followed by a slower sustained release of the drug. Controlled release and modified release dosage forms are discussed in Chapter 17.

DRUG CONSIDERATIONS

As discussed earlier, the physicochemical properties of the drug (Table 14.1) are major factors that are controlled or modified by the formulator. These physicochemical properties influence the type of dosage form and the process for the manufacture of the dosage form. Physical properties of the drug—such as dissolution, particle size, and crystalline form—are influenced by methods of processing and manufacturing. If the drug has low aqueous solubility and an intravenous injection is desired, a soluble salt of the drug may be prepared. Chemical instability or chemical interactions with certain excipients will also affect the type of drug product and its method of fabrication. There are many creative approaches to improve the product; only a few are discussed in this chapter.

DRUG PRODUCT CONSIDERATIONS

Pharmacokinetics of the Drug

Knowledge of the pharmacokinetic profile of the drug is important to estimate the appropriate amount (dose) of drug in the drug product and a release rate that will maintain a desired drug level in the body. The therapeutic window determines the desired or target plasma drug concentration that will be effective with minimal adverse effects. Drug concentrations higher than the therapeutic window (eg, minimum toxic concentration) may cause more intense pharmacodynamic and/or toxic response; drug concentrations below the therapeutic window (eg, minimum effective concentration) may be subtherapeutic. For drugs with a narrow therapeutic window, knowledge of the pharmacokinetic profile enhances drug therapy for many products through the development of an appropriate dosage regimen, including the size of the dose and the dosing frequency, to achieve and maintain the target drug concentration.

Bioavailability of the Drug

The stability of the drug in the gastrointestinal tract, including the stomach and intestine, is another consideration. Some drugs, such as penicillin G, are unstable in the acidic medium of the stomach. The addition of buffering in the formulation or the use of an enteric coating on the dosage form will protect the drug from degradation at a low pH. Some drugs have poor bioavailability because of first-pass effects (presystemic elimination). If oral drug bioavailability is poor due to metabolism by enzymes in the gastrointestinal tract or in the liver, then a higher dose may be needed, as in the case of propranolol, or an alternative route of drug administration, as in the case of insulin. Drugs that are only partially absorbed after oral administration usually leave residual drug in the gastrointestinal tract, which may cause local bowel irritation or alter the normal gastrointestinal flora. Designing dosage forms to contain unabsorbed drug contains risk that under unusual conditions (eg, change in diet or disease condition), complete drug absorption can occur leading to excessive drug bioavailability and toxicity. If the drug is not absorbed after the oral route or a higher dose causes toxicity, then the drug must be given by an alternative route of administration, and a different dosage form such as a parenteral drug product might be needed.

Dose Considerations

The size of the dose in the drug product is based on the inherent potency of the drug and its apparent volume of distribution, which determines the target plasma drug concentration needed for the desired therapeutic effect. For some drugs, wide variation in the size of the dose is needed for different patients because of large intersubject differences in the pharmacokinetics and bioavailability of the drug. Therefore, the drug product must be available in several dose strengths to allow for individualized dosing. Some tablets are also scored for breaking, to allow the administration of fractional doses.

The size and shape of a solid oral drug product are designed for easy swallowing. The total size of a drug product is determined by the dose of the drug and any additional excipients needed to manufacture the desired dosage form. For oral dosage forms, if the required dose is large (1 g or more), then the patient may have difficulty in swallowing the drug product. For example, many patients may find a capsule-shaped tablet (caplet) easier to swallow than a large round tablet. Large or oddly shaped tablets, which may become lodged in the esophageal sphincter during swallowing, are generally not manufactured. Some esophageal injuries due to irritating drug lodged in the esophagus have been reported with potassium chloride tablets and other drugs. Older patients may have more difficulties in swallowing large tablets and capsules. Most of these swallowing difficulties may be overcome by taking the product with a large amount of fluid.

Dosing Frequency

The dosing frequency is related to the clearance of the drug and the target plasma drug concentration. If the pharmacokinetics show that the drug has a short duration of action due to a short elimination half-life or rapid clearance from the body, the drug must be given more frequently. To minimize fluctuating plasma drug concentrations and improve patient compliance, an extended-release drug product may be preferred. An extended-release product contains two or more doses of the drug that are released over a prolonged period (Chapter 17).

PATIENT CONSIDERATIONS

The drug product must be acceptable to the patient. Poor patient compliance may result from poor product attributes, such as difficulty in swallowing, disagreeable odor, bitter medicine taste, or two frequent and/or unusual dosage requirements. In recent years, creative packaging has allowed the patient to remove one tablet each day from a specially designed package so that the daily doses are not missed. This innovation improves compliance. Of course, pharmacodynamic factors, such as side effects of the drug or an allergic reaction, also influence patient compliance.

ROUTE OF DRUG ADMINISTRATION

The route of drug administration (Chapter 13) affects the bioavailability of the drug, thereby affecting the onset and duration of the pharmacologic effect. In the design of a drug dosage form, the pharmaceutical manufacturer must consider (1) the intended route of administration; (2) the size of the dose; (3) the anatomic and physiologic characteristics of the administration site, such as membrane permeability and blood flow; (4) the physicochemical properties of the site, such as pH, osmotic pressure, and presence of physiologic fluids; and (5) the interaction

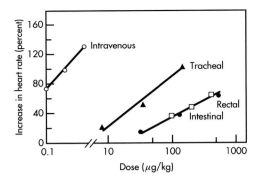

Figure 14-16. Dose–response curve to isoproterenol by various routes in dogs.
(From Gillette and Mitchell, 1975, with permission.)

of the drug and dosage form at the administration site, including alteration of the administration site due to the drug and/or dosage form.

Although drug responses are quite similar with different routes of administration, there are examples in which severe differences in response may occur. For example, with the drug isoproterenol, a difference in activity of a thousandfold has been found, attributed to different routes of administration. Figure 14-16 shows the change in heart rate due to isoproterenol with different routes of administration. Studies have shown that isoproterenol is metabolized in the gut and during passage through the liver. The rate and types of metabolite formed are found to be different depending on the routes of administration.

Oral Drug Products

The major advantages of oral drug products are the convenience of administration, safety, and the elimination of discomforts involved with injections. The hazard of rapid intravenous administration causing toxic high concentration of drug in the blood is avoided. The main disadvantages of oral drug products are the potential problems of reduced, erratic, or incomplete bioavailability. Unabsorbed drug may also alter the contents and microbiologic flora of the gastrointestinal tract. In addition, nausea or gastrointestinal discomfort may occur with drugs that cause local irritation. Bioavailability may be altered by drug and food interactions (see Chapter 13).

Highly ionized drug molecules are not absorbed easily. The ganglion-blocking drugs hexamethonium, pentolinium, and bretylium are ionized at intestinal pH. Therefore, they are not sufficiently absorbed orally to be effective. Neomycin, gentamicin, and cefamandole are not well absorbed orally. In the case of neomycin, after oral administration the drug will concentrate in the gastrointestinal tract to exert its local antibacterial effect. Drugs with large molecular weights may not be well absorbed when given orally. There is some evidence that large drug molecules may be absorbed through the lymphatic system when formulated with a "carrier." The mechanism is not known. Some large molecules are absorbed when administered in solution with a surface-active agent. For example, cyclosporine has been given orally with good absorption when formulated with a surfactant in oil. A possible role of the oil is to stimulate the flow of lymph as well as to delay retention of the drug. Oily vehicles have been used to lengthen the gastrointestinal transit time of oral preparations.

Absorption of Lipid-Soluble Drugs

Most hydrophobic drugs are poorly soluble in water and generally are not well absorbed orally because of failure of the drug to dissolve in the fluids of the gastrointestinal tract. These lipophilic drugs are more soluble in lipids or oily vehicles. Lipid-soluble drugs given with fatty excipients mix with digested fatty acids, which are emulsified by bile in the small intestine. The emulsified drug is then absorbed through the GI mucosa or through the lymphatic system. A normal digestive function of the small intestine is the digestion and absorption of fats such as triglycerides. These fats are first hydrolyzed into monoglycerides and fatty acids by pancreatic lipase. The fatty acids then react with carrier lipoproteins to form chylomicrons, which are absorbed through the lymph. The chylomicrons eventually release the fatty acids, and any lipophilic drugs incorporated in the oil phase. Fat substances trigger receptors in the stomach to delay stomach emptying and reduce GI transit rates. Prolonged transit time allows more contact time for increased drug absorption.

When griseofulvin or phenytoin was given orally in corn oil suspensions, an increase in drug absorption was demonstrated (Bates and Equeira, 1975). The increase in absorption was attributed to the formation of mixed micelles with bile secretions, which aid drug dissolution.

The bioavailability of metaxalone (Skelaxin), a hydrophobic drug, is greatly increased when it is given with a high-fat meal. In addition, stomach emptying may be delayed depending on the volume and nature of the oil. Long-chain fatty acids (above C-10) are more effective than short-chain acids in delaying stomach emptying. Unsaturated fatty acids are more effective than saturated straight-chain fatty acids; triglycerides are not as effective as fatty acids. Oleic acid, arachis oil, and myristic acid also delay stomach emptying. For example, the bioavailability of a water-insoluble antimalarial drug was increased in dogs when oleic acid was incorporated as part of a vehicle into a soft gelatin capsule (Stella et al, 1978).

Calcium carbonate, a source of calcium for the body, was only about 30% available in a solid dosage form, but was almost 60% bioavailable when dispersed in a special vehicle as a soft gelatin capsule (Fordtran et al, 1986). Bleomycin, an anticancer drug (MW 1500), is poorly absorbed orally and therefore was formulated for absorption through the lymphatic system. The lymphotropic carrier was dextran sulfate. Bleomycin was linked ionically to the carrier to form a complex. The carrier dextran (MW 500,000) was too large to be absorbed through the membrane and pass into the lymphatic vessels (Yoshikawa et al, 1989).

Gastrointestinal Side Effects

Many orally administered drugs are irritating to the stomach. These drugs may cause nausea or stomach pain when taken on an empty stomach. In some cases, food or antacids may be given together with the drug to reduce stomach irritation. Alternatively, the drug may be enteric coated to reduce gastric irritation. A common drug that causes irritation is aspirin. Buffered aspirin tablets, enteric-coated tablets, and granules are available. However, enteric coating may sometimes delay or reduce the amount of drug absorbed. Furthermore, enteric coating may not abolish gastric irritation completely, because the drug may occasionally be regurgitated back to the stomach after the coating dissolves in the intestine. Enteric-coated tablets may be greatly affected by the presence of food in the stomach. The drug may not be released from the stomach for several hours when stomach emptying is delayed by food.

Buffering material or antacid ingredients have also been used with aspirin to reduce stomach irritation. When a large amount of antacid or buffering material is included in the formulation, dissolution of aspirin may occur quickly, leading to reduced irritation to the stomach. However, many buffered aspirin formulations do not contain sufficient buffering material to make a difference in dissolution in the stomach.

Certain drugs have been formulated into soft gelatin capsules to improve drug bioavailability and reduce gastrointestinal side effects. If the drug is formulated in the soft gelatin capsule as a solution, the drug may disperse and dissolve more rapidly, leaving less residual drug in the gut and causing less irritation. This approach may be useful for a drug that causes local irritation but will be ineffective if the drug is inherently ulcerogenic. Indomethacin, for example, may cause ulceration in animals even when administered parenterally.

There are many options available to the formulator to improve the tolerance of the drug and minimize gastric irritation. The nature of excipients and the physical state of the drugs are important and must be carefully assessed before a drug product is formulated. Some excipients may improve the solubility of the drug and facilitate absorption, whereas others may physically adsorb the drug to reduce irritation. Often, a great number of formulations must be tested before an acceptable one is chosen.

Buccal and Sublingual Tablets

A drug that diffuses and penetrates rapidly across mucosal membranes may be placed under the tongue and be rapidly absorbed. A tablet designed for release under the tongue is called a *sublingual tablet*. Nitroglycerin, isoproterenol, erythrityl tetranitrate, and isosorbide dinitrate are common examples. Sublingual tablets usually dissolve rapidly.

A tablet designed for release and absorption of the drug in the buccal (cheek) pouch is called a *buccal tablet*. The buccal cavity is the space between the mandibular arch and the oral mucosa, an area well supplied with blood vessels for efficient drug absorption. A buccal tablet may release drug rapidly or may be designed to release drug slowly for a prolonged effect. For example, Sorbitrate sublingual tablet, Sorbitrate chewable tablet, and Sorbitrate oral tablet (Zeneca) are three different dosage forms of isosorbide dinitrate for the relief and prevention of angina pectoris. The sublingual tablet is a lactose formulation that dissolves rapidly under the tongue and is then absorbed. The chewable tablet is chewed, and some drug is absorbed in the buccal cavity; the oral tablet is simply a conventional product for GI absorption. The chewable tablet contains flavor, confectioner's sugar, and mannitol, which are absent in both the oral and sublingual tablets. The sublingual tablet contains lactose and starch for rapid dissolution. The onset of sublingual nitroglycerin is rapid, much faster than when nitroglycerin is taken orally or absorbed through the skin. The duration of action, however, is shorter than with the other two routes. Drug absorbed through the buccal mucosa will not pass through the liver before general distribution. Consequently, for a drug with significant first-pass effect, buccal absorption may provide better bioavailability than oral administration. Some peptide drugs have been reported to be absorbed by the buccal route, which provides a route of administration without the drug being destroyed by enzymes in the GI tract.

A newer approach to drug absorption from the oral cavity has been the development of a translingual nitroglycerin spray (Nitrolinqual Pumpspray). The spray, containing 0.4 mg per metered dose, is given by spraying one or two metered doses onto the oral mucosa at the onset of an acute angina attack.

Fentanyl citrate is a potent, lipid-soluble opioid agonist that crosses mucosal membranes rapidly. Fentanyl has been formulated as a transdermal drug product (Durapress) and as an oral lozenge on a handle (Actiq) containing fentanyl citrate for oral transmucosal delivery. According to the manufacturer, fentanyl bioavailability from Actiq is about 50%, representing a combination of rapid absorption across the oral mucosa and slower absorption through swallowing and transport across the gastrointestinal mucosa.

Nasal Drug Products

Nasal products provide a simple means of local and/or systemic drug delivery. The nasal mucosa are highly vascularized and easily accessible. The vehicle used for nasal administration must be nonirritating and well tolerated. The most common drug products for local activity are the nasal vasoconstrictors phenylephrine and naphazoline. An example of a new nasal delivery for both local and systemic effect is ipratropium bromide, a drug used for rhinitis and the common cold. In patients with perennial rhinitis, about 10% of the drug was absorbed intranasally (Wood et al, 1995).

Nasacort AQ nasal spray (Rhone-Poulenc-Rorer) is triamcinolone acetonide delivered to the nasal area by spray. Each puff delivers about 50 μg of the drug. It is useful for allergic rhinitis. The action is partially systemic and local. Another example is levocabastine, a histamine H1-receptor antagonist developed as levocabastine nasal spray. Peak plasma concentrations (C_{max}) occur within 1 to 2 hours, with systemic availability ranging from 60% to 80% (Heykants et al, 1995). Benefits of levocabastine are predominantly mediated through local antihistaminic effects, with some systemic contribution. Butorphanol tartrate nasal spray (Stadol NS) is an opioid analgesic available as a nasal spray for the treatment of pain as a preoperative or preanesthetic medication, as well as for pain relief during labor and for migraine headache. The nasal route offers an alternative to injection. Some biological products such as peptides and proteins have been suggested for nasal delivery, because they are then not digested by enzymes as they are in the GI tract. The luteinizing hormone-releasing hormone agonist buserelin acetate (Suprefact[R] nasal spray—Aventis Pharma) has been formulated with oleic acid for systemic nasal delivery in an experimental formulation. Therapeutic proteins, such as recombinant interferon-alpha/D, have also been investigated for nasal delivery. Detectable levels of interferon-alpha β/D in serum were achieved via the nasal route and in the lung. Drug bioavailability was 6.8% from the lung in the rat, and 2.9% from the nasal cavity in the rabbit (Bayley et al, 1995). Other examples of nasal delivery drug products for systemic drug absorption are Nicotrol for the delivery of nicotine to aid smokers in quitting smoking, and Miacalcin for the delivery of calcitonin salmon, a parathyroid agent for the treatment of postmenopausal osteoporosis.

An *in-vitro* human nasal model was developed as a tool to study the local tolerability of nasal powder forms using excised nasal mucosa in a diffusion chamber (De Fraissinettea et al, 1995). The suitability of this model was tested using Sandostatin, an octapeptide analog of somatostatin. The drug is also used for ocular treatment of allergic rhinoconjunctivitis as eye drops; it was about 30–60% available systemically by that route.

Recently, a live influenza virus vaccine, FluMist[R] (influenza virus vaccine live, intranasal—Wyeth), has been marketed for intranasal delivery. FluMist is indicated for active immunization for the prevention of disease caused by influenza A and B viruses.

Colonic Drug Delivery

There has been considerable research into the delivery of drugs specifically to the colon after oral administration (Shareef et al, 2003). Crohn's disease or chronic inflammatory colitis may be more effectively treated by direct drug delivery to the colon. One such drug, mesalamine (5-aminosalicylic acid, Asacol) is available in a delayed-release tablet coated with an acrylic-based resin that delays the release of the drug until it reaches the distal ileum and beyond. Protein drugs are generally unstable in the acidic environment of the stomach and are also degraded by proteolytic enzymes present in the stomach and small intestine. Researchers are investigating the oral delivery of protein and peptide drugs by protecting them against enzymatic degradation for later release in the colon.

Over 500 different bacterial species inhabit the colon, although five frequent species dominate the microflora. Within the cecum and colon, anaerobic species dominate and bacterial counts of 10^{12}/mL have been reported. Drugs such as the β-blockers, oxprenolol and metoprolol, and isosorbide-5-mononitrate are well absorbed in the colon, similar to absorption in the small intestine. Thus, these drugs are suitable candidates for colonic delivery. The nonsteroidal anti-inflammatory drug naproxen has been formed into a prodrug naproxen-dextran that survives intestinal enzyme and intestinal absorption. The prodrug reaches the colon, where it is enzymatically decomposed into naproxen and dextran (Harboe et al, 1989).

Rectal and Vaginal Drug Delivery

Products for rectal or vaginal drug delivery may be administered in either solid or liquid dosage forms. Rectal drug administration can be used for either local or systemic drug delivery. Rectal drug delivery for systemic absorption is preferred for drugs that cannot be tolerated orally (eg, when a drug causes nausea) or in situations where the drug cannot be given orally. A sustained-release preparation may be prepared for rectal administration. The rate of release of the drug from this preparation is dependent on the nature of the base composition and on the solubility of the drug involved. Rectal drug absorption may partially bypass the first-pass effects due to enzymes in the liver. Drug absorbed in the lower rectal region does not pass through the liver, whereas drug absorbed in the upper rectal region passes through the hepatic portal vein. Release of drug from a suppository depends on the composition of the suppository base. A water-soluble base, such as polyethylene glycol and glycerin, generally dissolves and releases the drug; on the other hand, an oleaginous base with a low melting point may melt at body temperature and release the drug. Some suppositories contain an emulsifying agent that keeps the fatty oil emulsified and the drug dissolved in it.

Vaginal drug delivery is generally for local drug delivery, but some systemic drug absorption can occur. Progesterone vaginal suppositories have been evaluated for the treatment of premenstrual symptoms of anxiety and irritability. Antifungal agents are often formulated into suppositories for treating vaginal infections. Fluconazole, a triazole antifungal agent, has been formulated to treat vulvovaginal candidiasis. The result of oral doses is comparable with that of a clotrimazole vaginal suppository. Many vaginal preparations are used for the delivery of antifungal agents.

Parenteral Drug Products

In general, intravenous (IV) bolus administration of a drug provides the most rapid onset of drug action. After IV bolus injection, the drug is distributed via the circulation to all parts of the body within a few minutes. After intramuscular (IM) injection, drug is absorbed from the injection site into the bloodstream (Fig. 14-17). Plasma drug input after oral and IM administration involves an absorption phase in which the drug concentration rises slowly to a peak and then declines according to the elimination half-life of the drug. (Note that the systemic elimination of all products is essentially similar; only the rate and extent of absorption may be modified by formulation.) The plasma drug level peaks instantaneously after an IV bolus injection, so a peak is usually not visible. After 3 hours, however, the plasma level of the drug after intravenous administration has declined to a lower level than after the oral and intramuscular administration. In this example (Fig. 14-17), the areas under the plasma curves are all approximately equal, indicating that the oral and intramuscular preparations are both well formulated and are 100% available.

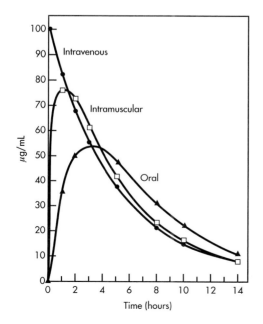

Figure 14-17.   Plasma concentration of a drug after the same dose is administered by three different routes.

Frequently, because of incomplete absorption or metabolism, oral preparations may have a lower area under the curve.

Drug absorption after an intramuscular injection may be faster or slower absorption than after oral drug administration. Intramuscular preparations are generally injected into a muscle mass such as in the buttocks (gluteus muscle) or in the deltoid muscle. Drug absorption occurs as the drug diffuses from the muscle into the surrounding tissue fluid and then into the blood. Different muscle tissues have different blood flow. For example, blood flow to the deltoid muscle is higher than blood flow to the gluteus muscle. Intramuscular injections may be formulated to have a faster or slower drug release by changing the vehicle of the injection preparation. Aqueous solutions release drug more rapidly, and the drug is more rapidly absorbed from the injection site, whereas a viscous, oily, or suspension vehicle may result in a slow drug release and consequently slow and sustained drug absorption. Viscous vehicles generally slow down drug diffusion and distribution. A drug in an oily vehicle must partition into an aqueous phase before systemic absorption. A drug that is very soluble in oil and relatively insoluble in water may have a relatively long and sustained release from the absorption site because of slow partitioning. Drugs, including peptides and proteins, have also been formulated as emulsions, suspensions, liposomes, and nanoparticles for parenteral injection. A change in a parenteral drug product from a solution to an emulsion, liposome, etc, will alter the drug's distribution and pharmacokinetic profile.

CLINICAL EXAMPLE

Haloperidol (Haldol) is a butyrophenone antipsychotic agent with pharmacologic effects similar to the piperazine phenothiazines. Haloperidol is available for oral and IM administration. Two IM preparations of haloperidol are available, including haloperidol lactate in an aqueous vehicle and haloperidol deconate in a nonaqueous sesame oil vehicle. Table 14.10 shows the t_{max} and elimination half-life of haloperidol after the oral, IM, or IV administration.

Haloperidol lactate is given in an aqueous solution and after intramuscular injection has a time for peak drug concentration of 20 minutes and an elimination

TABLE 14.10 Pharmacokinetic Parameters for Haloperidol after Oral and Parenteral Administration

ROUTE	PERCENT ABSORPTION	TIME FOR PEAK CONCENTRATION, t_{max}	ELIMINATION HALF-LIFE
Oral	60	3–5 hr	24 (12–38) hr
IM	75	0.33 hr	21 (13–36) hr
Deconate		6th day (4–11 days)	3 wk
IV	100	Immediate	14 (10–19) hr

Adapted from *Facts and Comparisons* (1997).

half-life of 21 days. In contrast, haloperidol deconate, the deconate ester of the butyrophenone, is lipid soluble and is formulated in sesame oil. Due to the slow drug release from the oil after IM administration, the time for peak drug concentration is 4–11 days and the elimination half-life is about 3 weeks. Thus, the suggested dosage interval between intramuscular injections for haloperidol deconate is 4 weeks.

A major advantage of intramuscular injections compared to intravenous bolus injections is the flexibility of formulation. A drug that is not water soluble cannot be easily administered by the intravenous route. A nonaqueous injection for intravenous administration must be given very slowly to avoid any drug precipitation in the vein. Propylene glycol and PEG 400 in combination with other solvents have been used in intravenous preparations.

Parenteral dosage forms for intravenous administration containing suspensions, liposomes, or nanoparticles have been developed for the administration of antineoplastic drugs. In this case, the dosage form may alter the distribution of the drug, because small particles are engulfed by macrophages of the reticuloendothelial system, resulting in drug concentration in the liver and spleen.

Inhalation Drug Products

Drugs administered into the respiratory system, such as bronchodilators and corticosteroids, may be formulated as aerosols or inhalation solutions. An aerosol preparation with suitable propellant can administer drug rapidly into the bronchial region. The advantages of drugs given by inhalation include (1) rapid absorption and rapid onset of activity (eg, bronchodilators), (2) avoidance of first-pass effects or metabolism prior to systemic absorption (eg, isoproterenol, bitolterol), and (3) localization of drug activity to the lung and minimum systemic toxicity (eg, dexamethasone).

The particle size of the suspension (or, in the case of a solution, the size of the mist particles) is important in determining the extent of penetration into the bronchioles. For coarse particles, inertia carries the drug for a short distance up the nasal cavity. Drugs with small particles move by sedimentation or brownian movement deeper into the bronchioles.

Many aerosol products are designed for drug therapy of chronic obstructive pulmonary disease (COPD), particularly asthma. For example, Intal (Rhone-Poulenc-Rorer) delivers sodium cromolyn to a patient through inhalation. The propellants for aerosols have been the chlorinated fluorocarbons (CFCs, such as Freons, DuPont). Freons commonly used include dichlorodifluoromethane (Freon-12) and dichlortetrafluoroethane (Freon-114). However, these compounds deplete the ozone layer of the stratosphere, and other propellants are now being investigated to replace CFCs. The new propellants include classes of hydrofluoroalkanes (HFAs), which do not contain chlorines. HFA-227 and HFA-134a show promise as new propellents for medical inhalers because they are nonflammable, not chemically reactive, and do not have ozone-depleting potential. Some examples of inhalation and intranasal products are shown in Table 14.11.

TABLE 14.11   Examples of Inhalation and Intranasal Drug Products

	DRUG PRODUCT	GENERIC NAME	INDICATION
Inhalation	Proventil	Albuterol	Bronchodilator
	Beconase	Beclomethasone diproprionate	Anti-inflammatory steroid
	Foradil Aerolizer	Formoterol fumarate inhalation powder	Bronchodilator
	Pulmicort Turbuhaler	Budesonide inhalation powder	Anti-inflammatory steroid
	Virazole	Ribavirin for inhalation solution	Antiviral nucleoside
	Mucomyst	Acetylcysteine	Mucolytic
Intranasal	Flonase	Fluticasone proprionate	Anti-inflammatory steroid
	FluMist	Influenza virus intranasal vaccine	Live (attenuated) influenza virus
	Nasalcrom	Cromolyn sodium	Mast cell stabilizer
	Nasalcort	Triamcinolone actonide	Anti-inflammatory steroid

Transdermal Drug Products

Transdermal administration delivers a drug into the patient's systemic circulation through the skin for systemic activity. For example, scopolamine has been delivered through the skin of the ear for relief of motion sickness. Transdermal administration may release the drug over an extended period of several hours or days without the discomforts of gastrointestinal side effects or first-pass effects. For example, Estraderm delivers estradiol for estrogen replacement therapy in post-menopausal women and is applied twice a week. Many transdermal products deliver drug at a constant rate to the body, similar to a zero-order infusion process. As a result, a stable, plateau level of the drug may be maintained. Many therapeutic categories of drugs are now available as transdermal products (Table 14.12).

Transdermal products vary in design. In general, the patch contains several parts: (1) a backing or support layer; (2) a drug layer (reservoir containing the dose); (3) a release-controlling layer (usually a semipermeable film), (4) a pressure-sensitive

TABLE 14.12 Transdermal Products

DRUG	PRODUCT	DRUG CLASS
Estradiol	Vivelle	Estrogen
Fentanyl	Duragesic	Opiate agonist
Nicotine	Habitrol Tran	Smoking control
	Nicoderm	Smoking control
	Nicotrol	Smoking control
	Prostep patch	Smoking control
Naftifine HCl	Naftin	Antifungal
Nifedipine	Adalat	Calcium channel blocker
Nitroglycerin	Nitrodisc	Antiangina
	Nitro-Dur	Antiangina
Clonidine	Catopress	Antihypertensive
Ethinylestradiol and norelgestromin	Evra	Contraception

adhesive (PSA); and (5) a protective strip, which must be removed prior to application. (See Chapter 17, Fig. 17-14). The release-controlling membrane may be a polymeric film such as ethylvinyl copolymer, which controls the release rate of the dose and its duration of action. The PSA layer is important for maintaining uninterrupted skin contact for drug diffusion through the skin. In some cases, the drug is blended directly into an adhesive, such as acrylate or silicone; performing the dual functions of release control and adhesion, this product is known as "drug in adhesive." In other products, the drug dose may be placed in a separate insoluble matrix layer, which helps control the release rate. This is generally known as a "matrix patch," and provides a little more control of the release rate as compared to the simple "reservoir" type of patch. Multilayers of drugs may be involved in other transdermal products using a "laminate" design. In many cases, drug permeation through the skin is the slowest step in the transdermal delivery of drug into the body. See Chapter 17 for discussion of modified-release patches.

Scale-up and Postapproval Changes (SUPAC)

Any changes in a drug product after it has been approved for marketing by the FDA is known as a *postapproval change.* Postapproval changes may include analytical, manufacturing, and packaging changes in a drug product after it has been approved for marketing by the FDA (FDA Guidance November, 1999). A major concern of industry and the FDA is that if a pharmaceutical manufacturer makes any change in the formulation, scales up the formulation to a larger batch size, changes the process, equipment, or manufacturing site, whether these changes will affect the identity, strength, purity, quality, safety, or efficacy of the approved drug product. In addition any changes in raw material (ie, material used for preparing active pharmaceutical ingredient), excipients, or packaging (including container closure system) should also be shown not to affect the quality of the drug product. SUPAC is discussed in more detail in Chapter 16.

FREQUENTLY ASKED QUESTIONS

1. What physical or chemical properties of a drug substance are important in designing a drug for (a) oral administration or (b) parenteral administration?

2. For a lipid-soluble drug that has very poor aqueous solubility, what strategies could be used to make this drug more bioavailable after oral administration?

3. For a weak ester drug that is unstable in highly acid or alkaline solutions, what strategies could be used to make this drug more bioavailable after oral administration?

4. How do excipients in a drug product that are physically inert, chemically inert, and nontoxic change the bioavailability of the active drug substance?

LEARNING QUESTIONS

1. What are the two rate-limiting steps possible in the oral absorption of a solid drug product? Which one would apply to a soluble drug? Which one could be altered by the pharmacist? Give examples.

2. What is the physiologic transport mechanism for the absorption of most drugs from the gastrointestinal tract? What area of the gastrointestinal tract is most favorable for the absorption of drugs? Why?

3. Explain why the absorption rate of a soluble drug tends to be greater than the elimination rate of the drug.

4. What type of oral dosage form generally yields the greatest amount of systemically available drug in the least amount of time? (Assume that the drug can be prepared in any form.) Why?

5. What effect does the oral administration of an anticholinergic drug, such as atropine sulfate, have on the bioavailability of aspirin from an enteric-coated tablet? (*Hint:* Atropine sulfate decreases gastrointestinal absorption.)

6. Drug formulations of erythromycin, including its esters and salts, have significant differences in bioavailability. Erythromycin is unstable in an acidic medium. Suggest a method for preventing a potential bioavailability problem for this drug.

REFERENCES

Aguiar AJ, Krc J, Kinkel AW, Samyn JC: Effect of polymorphism on the absorption of chloramphenical from chloramphenical palmitate. *J Pharm Sci* **56**:847–853, 1967

Allen PV, Rahn PD, Sarapu AC, Vandewielen AJ: Physical characteristic of erythromycin anhydrate, and dihydrate crystalline solids. *J Pharm Sci* **67**:1087–1093, 1978

Bates TR, Equeira JA: Bioavailability of micronized grieseofulvin from corn oil in water emulsion, aqueous suspension and commercial dosage form in humans. *J Pharm Sci* **64**:793–797, 1975

Bayley D, Temple C, Clay V, Steward A, Lowther N: The transmucosal absorption of recombinant human interferon-alpha B/D hybrid in the rat and rabbit. *J Pharm Pharmacol* **47**(9):721–724, 1995

Cameron CG, Cuff GW, McGinity J: Development and evaluation of controlled release theophylline tablet formulations containing acrylic resins: Comparison of dissolution test methodologies (abstr). American Pharmaceutical Association Meeting, New Orleans, LA, April 1983

De Fraissinette A, Kolopp M, Schiller I, Fricker G, Gammert C, Pospischil A, Vonderscher J, Richter F: *In vitro* tolerability of human nasal mucosa: Histopathological and scanning electron-microscopic evaluation of nasal forms containing Sandostatin. *Cell Biol Toxicol* **11**(5):295–301, 1995

Facts and Comparisons, Walter Kluwer Health, St. Louis, MO, 1977

FDA Guidance for Industry: *Changes to an Approved NDA or ANDA*, November 1999

FDA Guidance for Industry: *Waiver of In Vivo Bioavailability and Bioequivalence Studies for Immediate-Release Solid Oral Dosage Forms Based on a Biopharmaceutics Classification System*, August 2000

Fordtran J, Patrawala M, Chakrabarti S: Influence of vehicle composition on *in vivo* absorption of calcium from soft elastic gelatin capsule. *Pharm Res* **3**(suppl):645, 1986

Gillette JR, Mitchell JR: Routes of drug administration and response. In *Concepts in Biochemical Pharmacology*. Berlin, Springer-Verlag, 1975, chap 64

Gray VA, Brown CK, Dressman JB, Leeson J: A new general chapter on dissolution. *Pharm Forum* **27**:3432–3439, 2001

Harboe E, Larsen C, Johansen A, Olesen HP: Macromolecular prodrugs. XV. Colon-targeted delivery—bioavailability of naproxen from orally administered dextran-naproxen ester prodrugs varying in molecular size in the pig. *Pharm Res* **6**(11):919–23, 1989

Heykants J, Van Peer A, Van de Velde V, Snoeck E, Meuldermans W, Woestenborghs R: The pharmacokinetic properties of topical levocabastine. A review. *Clin Pharmacokinet* **29**(4):221–230, 1995

Hofer JD, Gray VA: Examination of selection of immediate release dissolution acceptance criteria. *Pharm Forum* **29**:334–340, 2003

Leeson LJ: *In vivo–in-vitro* correlations. *Pharm Forum* **28**:1315–1319, 2002

Levy G, Leonards J, Procknal JA: Development of *in vitro* tests which correlate quantitatively with dissolution rate-limited drug absorption in man. *J Pharm Sci* **54**:1719, 1965

Masih SZ, Jacob KC, Majuh M, Fatmi A: Comparison of USP basket and paddle method for evaluation of sustained release formulation containing pseudoephedrine and guaifenesin (abstr). American Pharmaceutical Association Meeting, New Orleans, LA, April 1983

Philip J, Daly RE: Test for selection of erythromycin stearate bulk drug for tablet preparation. *J Pharm Sci* **72**:979–980, 1983

Prasad V, Shah V, Knight P, et al: Importance of media selection in establishment of *in vitro–in vivo* relationship for quinidine gluconate. *Int J Pharm* **13**:1–7, 1983

Shah VP, Prasad VK, Alston T, et al: Phenytoin I: *In vitro* correlation for 100 mg phenytoin sodium capsules. *J Pharm Sci* **72**:306–308, 1983

Shareef MA, Ahuja A, Ahmad FJ, Raghava S: Colonic drug delivery: An updated review, *AAPS PharmSci* **5**:161–186, 2003.

Stella V, Haslam J, Yata N, et al: Enhancement of bioavailability of a hydrophobic amine antimalarial by formulation with oleic acid in a soft gelatin capsule. *J Pharm Sci* **67**:1375–1377, 1978

United States Pharmacopeial Convention: *The United States Pharmacopeia*, 23rd ed. Easton, PA, Mark, 1995. Published by United States Pharmacopeia Convention, Inc. Rockville, MD, now published annually 24th Ed. 2004

Wood CC, Fireman P, Grossman J, Wecker M, MacGregor T: Product characteristics and pharmacokinetics of intranasal ipratropium bromide. *J Allergy Clin Immunol* **95**(5 pt 2):1111–1116, 1995

Wood JH: *In vitro* evaluation of physiological availability of compressed tablets. *Pharm Acta Helv* **42**:129, 1966

Yoshikawa H, Nakao Y, Takada K, et al: Targeted and sustained delivery of aclarubicin to lymphatics by lactic acid oligomer microsphere in rat. *Chem Pharm Bull* **37**:802–804, 1989

BIBLIOGRAPHY

Aguiar AJ: Physical properties and pharmaceutical manipulations influencing drug absorption. In Forth IW, Rummel W (eds), *Pharmacology of Intestinal Absorption: Gastrointestinal Absorption of Drugs*. New York, Pergamon, 1975, vol 1, chap 6

Amidon GL, Lennernas H, Shah VP, Crison JR: A theoretical basis for a biopharmaceutic drug classification: The correlation of *in vitro* drug product dissolution and *in vivo* bioavailability, *Pharm Res* **12**:413–420, 1995

Barr WH: The use of physical and animal models to assess bioavailability. *Pharmacology* **8**:88–101, 1972

Berge S, Bighley L, Monkhouse D: Pharmaceutical salts. *J Pharm Sci* **66**:1–19, 1977

Blanchard J: Gastrointestinal absorption, II. Formulation factors affecting bioavailability. *Am J Pharm* **150**:132–151, 1978

Blanchard J, Sawchuk RJ, Brodie BB: *Principles and Perspectives in Drug Bioavailability*. New York, Karger, 1979

Burks TF, Galligan JJ, Porreca F, Barber WD: Regulation of gastric emptying. *Fed Proc* **44**:2897–2901, 1985

Cabana BE, O'Neil R: FDA's report on drug dissolution. *Pharm Forum* **6**:71–75, 1980

Cadwalder DE: *Biopharmaceutics and Drug Interactions*. Nutley, NJ, Roche Laboratories, 1971

Christensen J: The physiology of gastrointestinal transit. *Med Clin N Am* **58**:1165–1180, 1974

Dakkuri A, Shah AC: Dissolution methodology: An overview. *Pharm Technol* **6**:28–32, 1982

Dressman JB, Amidon GL, Reppas C, Shah VP: Dissolution testing as a prognostic tool for oral drug absorption: Immediate release dosage forms. *Pharm Res* **15**:11–22, 1998

Eye IS: A review of the physiology of the gastrointestinal tract in relation to radiation doses from radioactive materials. *Health Phys* **12:**131–161, 1966

Gilbaldi M: *Biopharmaceutics and Clinical Pharmacokinetics.* Philadelphia, Lea & Febiger, 1977

Hansen WA: *Handbook of Dissolution Testing.* Springfield, OR, Pharmaceutical Technology Publications, 1982

Hardwidge E, Sarapu A, Laughlin W: Comparison of operating characteristics of different dissolution test systems. *J Pharm Sci* **6:**1732–1735, 1978

Houston JB, Wood SG: Gastrointestinal absorption of drugs and other xenobiotics. In Bridges JW, Chasseaud LF (eds), *Progress in Drug Metabolism.* London, Wiley, 1980, vol 4, chap 2

Jollow DJ, Brodie BB: Mechanisms of drug absorption and drug solution. *Pharmacology* **8:**21–32, 1972

LaDu BN, Mandel HG, Way EL: *Fundamentals of Drug Metabolism and Drug Disposition.* Baltimore, Williams & Wilkins, 1971

Leesman GD, Sinko PJ, Amidon GL: Simulation of oral drug absorption: Gastric emptying and gastrointestinal motility. In Welling PW, Tse FLS (eds), *Pharmacokinetics: Regulatory, Industry, Academic Perspectives.* New York, Marcel Dekker, 1988, chap 6

Leeson LJ, Carstensen JT: Industrial pharmaceutical technology. In Leeson L, Carstensen JT (eds), *Dissolution Technology.* Washington, DC, Academy of Pharmaceutical Sciences, 1974

Levine RR: Factors affecting gastrointestinal absorption of drugs. *Dig Dis* **15:**171–188, 1970

McElnay JC: Buccal absorption of drugs. In Swarbrick J, Boylan JC (eds), *Encyclopedia of Pharmaceutical Technology.* New York, Marcel Dekker, 1990, vol 2, pp 189–211

Mojaverian P, Vlasses PH, Kellner PE, Rocci ML Jr: Effects of gender, posture and age on gastric residence of an indigestible solid: Pharmaceutical considerations. *Pharm Res* **5:**639–644, 1988

Neinbert R: Ion pair transport across membranes. *Pharm Res* **6:**743–747, 1989

Niazi S: *Textbook of Biopharmaceutics and Clinical Pharmacokinetics.* New York, Appleton, 1979

Notari RE: *Biopharmaceutics and Pharmacokinetics: An Introduction.* New York, Marcel Dekker, 1975

Palin K: Lipids and oral drug delivery. *Pharm Int* **Nov:**272–275, 1985

Palin K, Whalley D, Wilson C, et al: Determination of gastric-emptying profiles in the rat: Influence of oil structure and volume. *Int J Pharm* **12:**315–322, 1982

Parrott EL: *Pharmaceutical Technology.* Minneapolis, Burgess, 1970

Pernarowski M: Dissolution methodology. In Leeson L, Carstensen JT (eds), *Dissolution Technology.* Washington, DC, Academy of Pharmaceutical Sciences, 1975, p 58

Pharmacopeial Forum: FDA report on drug dissolution. *Pharm Forum* **6:**71–75, 1980

Prasad VK, Shah VP, Hunt J, et al: Evaluation of basket and paddle dissolution methods using different performance standards. *J Pharm Sci* **72:**42–44, 1983

Robinson JR: *Sustained and Controlled Release Drug Delivery Systems.* New York, Marcel Dekker, 1978

Robinson JR, Eriken SP: Theoretical formulation of sustained release dosage forms. *J Pharm Sci* **55:**1254, 1966

Rubinstein A, Li VHK, Robinson JR: Gastrointestinal–physiological variables affecting performance of oral sustained release dosage forms. In Yacobi A, Halperin-Walega E (eds), *Oral Sustained Release Formulations: Design and Evaluation.* New York, Pergamon, 1988, chap 6

Schwarz-Mann WH, Bonn R: Principles of transdermal nitroglycerin administration. *Eur Heart J* **10**(suppl A):26–29, 1989

Shaw JE, Chandrasekaran K: Controlled topical delivery of drugs for system in action. *Drug Metab Rev* **8:**223–233, 1978

Swarbrick J: *In vitro* models of drug dissolution. In Swarbrick J (ed), *Current Concepts in the Pharmaceutical Sciences: Biopharmaceutics.* Philadelphia, Lea & Febiger, 1970

Wagner JG: *Biopharmaceutics and Relevant Pharmacokinetics.* Hamilton, IL, Drug Intelligence Publications, 1971

Welling PG: Dosage route, bioavailability and clinical efficacy. In Welling PW, Tse FLS (eds), *Pharmacokinetics: Regulatory, Industry, Academic Perspectives.* New York, Marcel Dekker, 1988, chap 3

Wurster DE, Taylor PW: Dissolution rates. *J Pharm Sci* **54:**169–175, 1965

Yoshikawa H, Muranishi S, Sugihira N, Seaki H: Mechanism of transfer of bleomycin into lymphatics by bifunctional delivery system via lumen of small intestine. *Chem Pharm Bull* **31:**1726–1732, 1983

York P: Solid state properties of powders in the formulation and processing of solid dosage form. *Int J Pharm* **14:**1–28, 1983

Zaffaroni A: Therapeutic systems: The key to rational drug therapy. *Drug Metab Rev* **8:**191–222, 1978

15

BIOAVAILABILITY AND BIOEQUIVALENCE

A *multisource drug product* is a drug product that contains the same active drug substance in the same dosage form and is marketed by more than one pharmaceutical manufacturer. *Single-source drug products* are drug products for which the patent has not yet expired or has certain exclusivities so that only one manufacturer can make it. Single-source drug products are usually brand-name (innovator) drug products. After the patent and other exclusivities for the brand-name drug expires, a pharmaceutical firm may manufacture a generic drug product that can be substituted for the branded drug product. Since the formulation and method of manufacture of the drug product can affect the bioavailability and stability of the drug, the generic drug manufacturer must demonstrate that the generic drug product is bioequivalent and therapeutically equivalent to the brand-name drug product.

Drug product selection and generic drug product substitution are major responsibilities for physicians, pharmacists, and others who prescribe, dispense, or purchase drugs. To facilitate such decisions, the U.S. Food and Drug Administration (FDA) publishes annually, in print and on the Internet, *Approved Drug Products with Therapeutic Equivalence Evaluations*, also known as the *Orange Book* (www.fda.gov/cder/ob/default.htm). The *Orange Book* identifies drug products approved on the basis of safety and effectiveness by the FDA and contains therapeutic equivalence evaluations for approved multisource prescription drug products. These evaluations serve as public information and advice to state health agencies, prescribers, and pharmacists to promote public education in the area of drug product selection and to foster containment of health care costs. The following definitions are from the *2003 Orange Book, Code of Federal Regulations*, 21 CFR 320, and other sources.

DEFINITIONS

- *Bioavailability.* Bioavailability means the rate and extent to which the active ingredient or active moiety is absorbed from a drug product and becomes available at

453

the site of action. For drug products that are not intended to be absorbed into the bloodstream, bioavailability may be assessed by measurements intended to reflect the rate and extent to which the active ingredient or active moiety becomes available at the site of action.

- *Bioequivalence requirement.* A requirement imposed by the FDA for *in-vitro* and/or *in-vivo* testing of specified drug products, which must be satisfied as a condition for marketing.

- *Bioequivalent drug products.* This term describes pharmaceutical equivalent or pharmaceutical alternative products that display comparable bioavailability when studied under similar experimental conditions. For systemically absorbed drugs, the test (generic) and reference listed drug (brand-name) shall be considered bioequivalent if: (1) the rate and extent of absorption of the test drug do not show a significant difference from the rate and extent of absorption of the reference drug when administered at the same molar dose of the therapeutic ingredient under similar experimental conditions in either a single dose or multiple doses; or (2) the extent of absorption of the test drug does not show a significant difference from the extent of absorption of the reference drug when administered at the same molar dose of the therapeutic ingredient under similar experimental conditions in either a single dose or multiple doses and the difference from the reference drug in the rate of absorption of the drug is intentional, is reflected in its proposed labeling, is not essential to the attainment of effective body drug concentrations on chronic use, and is considered medically insignificant for the drug.

  When the above methods are not applicable (eg, for drug products that are not intended to be absorbed into the bloodstream), other *in-vivo* or *in-vitro* test methods to demonstrate bioequivalence may be appropriate. Bioequivalence may sometimes be demonstrated using an *in-vitro* bioequivalence standard, especially when such an *in-vitro* test has been correlated with human *in-vivo* bioavailability data. In other situations, bioequivalence may sometimes be demonstrated through comparative clinical trials or pharmacodynamic studies.

  Bioequivalent drug products may contain different inactive ingredients, provided the manufacturer identifies the differences and provides information that the differences do not affect the safety or efficacy of the product.

- *Brand name.* The trade name of the drug. This name is privately owned by the manufacturer or distributor and is used to distinguish the specific drug product from competitor's products (eg, Tylenol, McNeil Laboratories).

- *Chemical name.* The name used by organic chemists to indicate the chemical structure of the drug (eg, N-acetyl-*p*-aminophenol).

- *Abbreviated New Drug Application* (ANDA). Drug manufacturers must file an ANDA for approval to market a generic drug product. The generic manufacturer is not required to perform clinical efficacy studies or nonclinical toxicology studies for the ANDA.

- *Drug product.* The finished dosage form (eg, tablet, capsule, or solution) that contains the active drug ingredient, generally, but not necessarily, in association with inactive ingredients.

- *Drug product selection.* The process of choosing or selecting the drug product in a specified dosage form.

- *Drug substance.* A drug substance is the active pharmaceutical ingredient (API) or component in the drug product that furnishes the pharmacodynamic activity.

- *Equivalence.* Relationship in terms of bioavailability, therapeutic response, or a set of established standards of one drug product to another.

- *Generic name.* The established, nonproprietary, or common name of the active drug in a drug product (eg, acetaminophen).

- *Generic substitution.* The process of dispensing a different brand or an un-branded drug product in place of the prescribed drug product. The substituted drug product contains the same active ingredient or therapeutic moiety as the same salt or ester in the same dosage form but is made by a different manufacturer. For example, a prescription for Motrin brand of ibuprofen might be dispensed by the pharmacist as Advil brand of ibuprofen or as a non-branded generic ibuprofen if generic substitution is permitted and desired by the physician.

- *Pharmaceutical alternatives.* Drug products that contain the same therapeutic moiety but as different salts, esters, or complexes. For example, tetracycline phosphate or tetracycline hydrochloride equivalent to 250 mg tetracycline base are considered pharmaceutical alternatives. Different dosage forms and strengths within a product line by a single manufacturer are pharmaceutical alternatives (eg, an extended-release dosage form and a standard immediate-release dosage form of the same active ingredient). The FDA currently considers a tablet and capsule containing the same active ingredient in the same dosage strength as pharmaceutical alternatives.

- *Pharmaceutical equivalents.* Drug products in identical dosage forms that contain the same active ingredient(s), ie, the same salt or ester, are of the same dosage form, use the same route of administration, and are identical in strength or concentration (eg, chlordiazepoxide hydrochloride, 5-mg capsules). Pharmaceutically equivalent drug products are formulated to contain the same amount of active ingredient in the same dosage form and to meet the same or compendial or other applicable standards (ie, strength, quality, purity, and identity), but they may differ in characteristics such as shape, scoring configuration, release mechanisms, packaging, excipients (including colors, flavors, preservatives), expiration time, and, within certain limits, labeling. When applicable, pharmaceutical equivalents must meet the same content uniformity, disintegration times, and/or dissolution rates. Modified-release dosage forms that require a reservoir or overage or certain dosage forms such as prefilled syringes in which residual volume may vary must deliver identical amounts of active drug ingredient over an identical dosing period.

- *Pharmaceutical substitution.* The process of dispensing a pharmaceutical alternative for the prescribed drug product. For example, ampicillin suspension is dispensed in place of ampicillin capsules, or tetracycline hydrochloride is dispensed in place of tetracycline phosphate. Pharmaceutical substitution generally requires the physician's approval.

- *Reference listed drug.* The reference listed drug (RLD) is identified by the FDA as the drug product on which an applicant relies when seeking approval of an Abbreviated New Drug Application (ANDA). The RLD is generally the brand-name drug that has a full New Drug Application (NDA). The FDA designates a single reference listed drug as the standard to which all generic versions must be shown to be bioequivalent. The FDA hopes to avoid possible significant variations among generic drugs and their brand-name counterparts. Such variations could result if generic drugs were compared to different reference listed drugs.

- *Therapeutic alternatives.* Drug products containing different active ingredients that are indicated for the same therapeutic or clinical objectives. Active ingredients in therapeutic alternatives are from the same pharmacologic class and are expected to have the same therapeutic effect when administered to patients for such condition of use. For example, ibuprofen is given instead of aspirin; cimetidine may be given instead of ranitidine.

- *Therapeutic equivalents.* Drug products are considered to be therapeutic equivalents only if they are pharmaceutical equivalents and if they can be expected to have the same clinical effect and safety profile when administered to patients under the conditions specified in the labeling. The FDA classifies as therapeutically equivalent those products that meet the following general criteria: (1) they are approved as safe and effective; (2) they are pharmaceutical equivalents in that they (a) contain identical amounts of the same active drug ingredient in the same dosage form and route of administration, and (b) meet compendial or other applicable standards of strength, quality, purity, and identity; (3) they are bioequivalent in that (a) they do not present a known or potential bioequivalence problem, and they meet an acceptable *in-vitro* standard, or (b) if they do present such a known or potential problem, they are shown to meet an appropriate bioequivalence standard; (4) they are adequately labeled; and (5) they are manufactured in compliance with Current Good Manufacturing Practice regulations. The FDA believes that products classified as therapeutically equivalent can be substituted with the full expectation that the substituted product will produce the same clinical effect and safety profile as the prescribed product.

- *Therapeutic substitution.* The process of dispensing a therapeutic alternative in place of the prescribed drug product. For example, amoxicillin is dispensed instead of ampicillin or ibuprofen is dispensed instead of naproxen. Therapeutic substitution can also occur when one NDA-approved drug is substituted for the same drug which has been approved by a different NDA, eg, the substitution of Nicoderm (nicotine transdermal system) for Nicotrol (nicotine transdermal system).

PURPOSE OF BIOAVAILABILITY STUDIES

Bioavailability studies are performed for both approved active drug ingredients and therapeutic moieties not yet approved for marketing by the FDA. New formulations of active drug ingredients must be approved by the FDA before marketing. In approving a drug product for marketing, the FDA ensures that the drug product is safe and effective for its labeled indications for use. Moreover, the drug product must meet all applicable standards of identity, strength, quality, and purity. To ensure that these standards are met, the FDA requires bioavailability/pharmacokinetic studies and, where necessary, bioequivalence studies for all drug products (*FDA Guidance for Industry,* 2003). Bioavailability may be considered as one aspect of drug product quality that links *in-vivo* performance of the drug product used in clinical trials to studies demonstrating evidence of safety and efficacy.

For unmarketed drugs that do not have full NDA approval by the FDA, *in-vitro* and/or *in-vivo* bioequivalence studies must be performed on the drug formulation proposed for marketing as a generic drug product. Furthermore, the essential pharmacokinetics of the active drug ingredient or therapeutic moiety must be characterized. Essential pharmacokinetic parameters, including the rate and extent of systemic absorption, elimination half-life, and rates of excretion and metabolism, should be established after single- and multiple-dose administration. Data from these *in-vivo* bioavailability studies are important to establish recommended dosage regimens and to support drug labeling.

In-vivo bioavailability studies are also performed for new formulations of active drug ingredients or therapeutic moieties that have full NDA approval and are approved for marketing. The purpose of these studies is to determine the bioavailability and to characterize the pharmacokinetics of the new formulation, new dosage form, or new salt or ester relative to a reference formulation.

In summary, clinical studies are useful in determining the safety and efficacy of drug products. *Bioavailability* studies are used to define the effect of changes in the physicochemical properties of the drug substance and the effect of the drug product (dosage form) on the pharmacokinetics of the drug. *Bioequivalence* studies are used to compare the bioavailability of the same drug (same salt or ester) from various drug products. Bioavailability and bioequivalence can also be considered as performance measures of the drug product *in-vivo*. If the drug products are bioequivalent and therapeutically equivalent (as defined above), then the clinical efficacy and the safety profile of these drug products are assumed to be similar and may be substituted for each other.

RELATIVE AND ABSOLUTE AVAILABILITY

The area under the drug concentration–time curve (AUC) is used as a measure of the total amount of unaltered drug that reaches the systemic circulation. The AUC is dependent on the total quantity of available drug, FD_0, divided by the elimination rate constant, k, and the apparent volume of distribution, V_D. F is the fraction of the dose absorbed. After IV administration, F is equal to unity, because the entire dose enters the systemic circulation. Therefore, the drug is considered to be completely available after IV administration. After oral administration of a drug, F may vary from a value of 0 (no drug absorption) to 1 (complete drug absorption).

Relative Availability

Relative (apparent) availability is the availability of the drug from a drug product as compared to a recognized standard. The fraction of dose systemically available from an oral drug product is difficult to ascertain. The availability of drug in the formulation is compared to the availability of drug in a standard dosage formulation, usually a solution of the pure drug evaluated in a crossover study. The relative availability of two drug products given at the same dosage level and by the same route of administration can be obtained using the following equation:

$$\text{Relative availability} = \frac{[\text{AUC}]_A}{[\text{AUC}]_B} \tag{15.1}$$

where drug product B is the recognized reference standard. This fraction may be multiplied by 100 to give percent relative availability.

When different doses are administered, a correction for the size of the dose is made, as in the following equation:

$$\text{Relative availability} = \frac{[\text{AUC}]_A / \text{dose A}}{[\text{AUC}]_B / \text{dose B}} \tag{15.2}$$

Urinary drug excretion data may also be used to measure relative availability, as long as the total amount of intact drug excreted in the urine is collected. The percent relative availability using urinary excretion data can be determined as follows:

$$\text{Percent relative availability} = \frac{[D_u]_A^\infty}{[D_u]_B^\infty} \times 100 \tag{15.3}$$

where $[D_u]^\infty$ is the total amount of drug excreted in the urine.

Absolute Availability

The absolute availability of drug is the systemic availability of a drug after extravascular administration (eg, oral, rectal, transdermal, subcutaneous) compared to IV dosing. The absolute availability of a drug is generally measured by comparing the respective AUCs after extravascular and IV administration. This measurement may be performed as long as V_D and k are independent of the route of administration. Absolute availability after oral drug administration using plasma data can be determined as follows:

$$\text{Absolute availability} = F = \frac{[\text{AUC}]_{PO} / \text{dose}_{PO}}{[\text{AUC}]_{IV} / \text{dose}_{IV}} \tag{15.4}$$

Absolute availability, F, may be expressed as a fraction or as a percent by multiplying $F \times 100$. Absolute availability using urinary drug excretion data can be determined by the following:

$$\text{Absolute availability} = \frac{[D_u]_{PO}^\infty / \text{dose}_{PO}}{[D_u]_{IV}^\infty / \text{dose}_{IV}} \tag{15.5}$$

The absolute bioavailability is also equal to F, the fraction of the dose that is bioavailable. Absolute availability is sometimes expressed as a percent, ie, $F = 1$, or 100%. For drugs given intravascularly, such as by IV bolus injection, $F = 1$ because all of the drug is completely absorbed. For all extravascular routes of administration, such as the oral route (PO), the absolute bioavailability F may not exceed 100% ($F > 1$). F is usually determined by Equation 15.4 or 15.5, where PO is the oral route or any other extravascular route of drug administration.

PRACTICE PROBLEM

The bioavailability of a new investigational drug was studied in 12 volunteers. Each volunteer received either a single oral tablet containing 200 mg of the drug, 5 mL of a pure aqueous solution containing 200 mg of the drug, or a single IV bolus injection containing 50 mg of the drug. Plasma samples were obtained periodically up to 48 hours after the dose and assayed for drug concentration. The average AUC values (0–48 hours) are given in the table below. From these data, calculate (a) the relative bioavailability of the drug from the tablet compared to the oral solution and (b) the absolute bioavailability of the drug from the tablet.

Drug Product	Dose (mg)	AUC (μg hr/mL)	Standard Deviation
Oral tablet	200	89.5	19.7
Oral solution	200	86.1	18.1
IV bolus injection	50	37.8	5.7

Solution

The relative bioavailability of the drug from the tablet is estimated using Equation 15.1. No adjustment for dose is necessary.

$$\text{Relative bioavailability} = \frac{89.5}{86.1} = 1.04 \quad \text{or} \quad 104\%$$

The relative bioavailability of the drug from the tablet is 1.04, or 104%, compared to the solution. In this study, the difference in drug bioavailability between tablet and solution was not statistically significant. It is possible for the relative bioavailability to be greater than 100%.

The absolute drug bioavailability from the tablet is calculated using Equation 15.4 and adjusting for the dose.

$$F = \text{absolute bioavailability} = \frac{89.5/200}{37.8/50} = 0.592 \quad \text{or} \quad 59.2\%$$

Because F, the fraction of dose absorbed from the tablet, is less than 1, the drug is not completely absorbed systemically, as a result of either poor absorption or metabolism by first-pass effect. The relative bioavailability of the drug from the tablet is approximately 100% when compared to the oral solution.

Results from bioequivalence studies may show that the relative bioavailability of the test oral product is greater than, equal to, or less than 100% compared to the reference oral drug product. However, the results from these bioequivalence studies should not be misinterpreted to imply that the absolute bioavailability of the drug from the oral drug products is also 100% unless the oral formulation was compared to an intravenous injection of the drug.

METHODS FOR ASSESSING BIOAVAILABILITY

Direct and indirect methods may be used to assess drug bioavailability. The *in-vivo* bioavailability of a drug product is demonstrated by the rate and extent of drug absorption, as determined by comparison of measured parameters, eg, concentration of the active drug ingredient in the blood, cumulative urinary excretion rates, or pharmacological effects. For drug products that are not intended to be absorbed into the bloodstream, bioavailability may be assessed by measurements intended to reflect the rate and extent to which the active ingredient or active moiety becomes available at the site of action. The design of the bioavailability study depends on the objectives of the study, the ability to analyze the drug (and metabolites) in biological fluids, the pharmacodynamics of the drug substance, the route of drug administration, and the nature of the drug product. Pharmacokinetic and/or pharmacodynamic parameters as well as clinical observations and *in-vitro* studies may be used to determine drug bioavailability from a drug product (Table 15.1).

Plasma Drug Concentration

Measurement of drug concentrations in blood, plasma, or serum after drug administration is the most direct and objective way to determine systemic drug bioavailability. By appropriate blood sampling, an accurate description of the plasma drug concentration–time profile of the therapeutically active drug substance(s) can be obtained using a validated drug assay.

> **t_{max}.** The *time of peak plasma concentration*, t_{max}, corresponds to the time required to reach maximum drug concentration after drug administration. At t_{max}, peak drug absorption occurs and the rate of drug absorption exactly equals the rate of drug elimination (Fig. 15-1). Drug absorption still continues after t_{max} is reached, but at a slower rate. When comparing drug products, t_{max} can be used as an approximate indication of drug absorption rate. The value for t_{max} will become smaller (indicating less time required to reach peak

TABLE 15.1   *Methods for Assessing Bioavailability and Bioequivalence*

Plasma drug concentration
Time for peak plasma (blood) concentration (t_{max})
Peak plasma drug concentration (C_{max})
Area under the plasma drug concentration–time curve (AUC)
Urinary drug excretion
Cumulative amount of drug excreted in the urine (D_u)
Rate of drug excretion in the urine (dD_u/dt)
Time for maximum urinary excretion (t)
Acute pharmacodynamic effect
Maximum pharmacodynamic effect (E_{max})
Time for maximum pharmacodynamic effect
Area under the pharmacodynamic effect–time curve
Onset time for pharmacodynamic effect
Clinical observations
Well-controlled clinical trials
***In-vitro* studies**
Drug dissolution

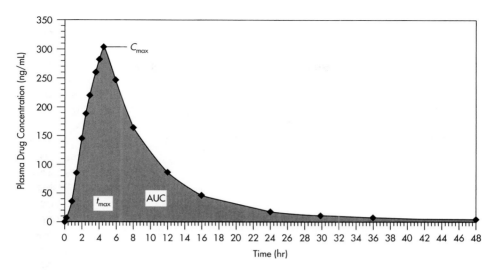

Figure 15-1. *Plasma drug concentration–time curve.*

plasma concentration) as the absorption rate for the drug becomes more rapid. Units for t_{max} are units of time (eg, hours, minutes).

***C*max.** The *peak plasma drug concentration*, C_{max}, represents the maximum plasma drug concentration obtained after oral administration of drug. For many drugs, a relationship is found between the pharmacodynamic drug effect and the plasma drug concentration. C_{max} provides indications that the drug is sufficiently systemically absorbed to provide a therapeutic response. In addition, C_{max} provides warning of possibly toxic levels of drug. The units of C_{max} are concentration units (eg, mg/mL, ng/mL). Although not a unit for rate, C_{max} is often used in bioequivalence studies as a surrogate measure for the rate of drug bioavailability.

AUC. The *area under the plasma level–time curve*, AUC, is a measurement of the *extent* of drug bioavailability (Fig. 15-1). The AUC reflects the total amount of active drug that reaches the systemic circulation. The AUC is the area under the drug plasma level–time curve from $t = 0$ to $t = \infty$, and is equal to the amount of unchanged drug reaching the general circulation divided by the clearance.

$$[\mathrm{AUC}]_0^\infty = \int_0^\infty C_p\, dt \tag{15.6}$$

$$[\mathrm{AUC}]_0^\infty = \frac{FD_0}{\mathrm{clearance}} = \frac{FD_0}{kV_D} \tag{15.7}$$

where F = fraction of dose absorbed, D_0 = dose, k = elimination rate constant, and V_D = volume of distribution. The AUC is independent of the route of administration and processes of drug elimination as long as the elimination processes do not change. The AUC can be determined by a numerical integration procedure, such as the trapezoidal rule method. The units for AUC are concentration time (eg, μg hr/mL).

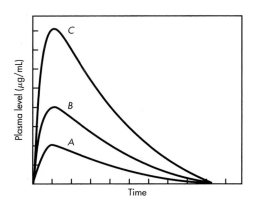

Figure 15-2. Plasma level–time curve following administration of single doses of **(A)** 250 mg, **(B)** 500 mg, and **(C)** 1000 mg of drug.

For many drugs, the AUC is directly proportional to dose. For example, if a single dose of a drug is increased from 250 to 1000 mg, the AUC will also show a fourfold increase (Figs. 15-2 and 15-3).

In some cases, the AUC is not directly proportional to the administered dose for all dosage levels. For example, as the dosage of drug is increased, one of the pathways for drug elimination may become saturated (Fig. 15-4). Drug elimination includes the processes of metabolism and excretion. Drug metabolism is an enzyme-dependent process. For drugs such as salicylate and phenytoin, continued increase of the dose causes saturation of one of the enzyme pathways for drug metabolism and consequent prolongation of the elimination half-life. The AUC thus increases disproportionally to the increase in dose, because a smaller amount of drug is being eliminated (ie, more drug is retained). When the AUC is not directly proportional to the dose, bioavailability of the drug is difficult to evaluate because drug kinetics may be dose dependent.

Urinary Drug Excretion Data

Urinary drug excretion data is an indirect method for estimating bioavailability. The drug must be excreted in significant quantities as unchanged drug in the urine. In addition, timely urine samples must be collected and the total amount of urinary drug excretion must be obtained (see Chapter 3).

Figure 15-3. Linear relationship between AUC and dose (data from Fig. 15-2).

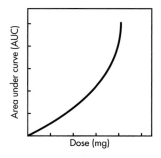

Figure 15-4. Relationship between AUC and dose when metabolism is saturable.

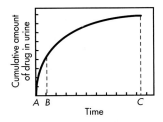

Figure 15-5. Corresponding plots relating the plasma level–time curve and the cumulative urinary drug excretion.

D_u^∞. The *cumulative amount of drug excreted in the urine*, D_u^∞, is related directly to the total amount of drug absorbed. Experimentally, urine samples are collected periodically after administration of a drug product. Each urine specimen is analyzed for free drug using a specific assay. A graph is constructed that relates the cumulative drug excreted to the collection-time interval (Fig. 15-5).

The relationship between the cumulative amount of drug excreted in the urine and the plasma level–time curve is shown in Figure 15-6. When the drug is almost completely eliminated (point C), the plasma concentration approaches zero and the maximum amount of drug excreted in the urine, D_u^∞, is obtained.

dD_u/dt. The *rate of drug excretion*. Because most drugs are eliminated by a first-order rate process, the rate of drug excretion is dependent on the first-order elimination rate constant k and the concentration of drug in the plasma C_p. In Figure 15-6, the *maximum rate of drug excretion*, $(dD_u/dt)_{max}$, is at point B, whereas the minimum rate of drug excretion is at points A and C. Thus, a graph comparing the rate of drug excretion with respect to time should be similar in shape as the plasma level–time curve for that drug (Fig. 15-7).

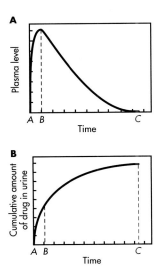

Figure 15-6. Corresponding plots relating the plasma level–time curve and the cumulative urinary drug excretion.

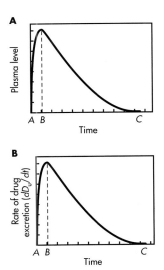

Figure 15-7. Corresponding plots relating the plasma level–time curve and the rate of urinary drug excretion.

t^{∞}. The *total time for the drug to be excreted*. In Figures 15-6 and 15-7, the slope of the curve segment A–B is related to the rate of drug absorption, whereas point C is related to the total time required after drug administration for the drug to be absorbed and completely excreted $t = \infty$. The t^{∞} is a useful parameter in bioequivalence studies that compare several drug products, as will be described later in this chapter.

Acute Pharmacodynamic Effect

In some cases, the quantitative measurement of a drug in plasma or urine lacks an assay with sufficient accuracy and/or reproducibility. For locally acting, non-systemically absorbed drug products, such as topical corticosteroids, plasma drug concentrations may not reflect the bioavailability of the drug at the site of action. An acute pharmacodynamic effect, such as an effect on forced expiratory volume, FEV_1 (inhaled bronchodilators) or skin blanching (topical corticosteroids) can be used as an index of drug bioavailability. In this case, the acute pharmacodynamic effect is measured over a period of time after administration of the drug product. Measurements of the pharmacodynamic effect should be made with sufficient frequency to permit a reasonable estimate for a time period at least three times the half-life of the drug (Gardner, 1977). This approach may be particularly applicable to dosage forms that are not intended to deliver the active moiety to the bloodstream for systemic distribution.

The use of an acute pharmacodynamic effect to determine bioavailability generally requires demonstration of a dose–response curve (see Chapter 19). Bioavailability is determined by characterization of the dose–response curve. For bioequivalence determination, pharmacodynamic parameters including the total area under the acute pharmacodynamic effect–time curve, peak pharmacodynamic effect, and time for peak pharmacodynamic effect are obtained from the pharmacodynamic effect–time curve. The onset time and duration of the pharmacokinetic effect may also be included in the analysis of the data. The use of pharmacodynamic endpoints for the determination of bioavailability and bioequivalence is much more variable than the measurement of plasma or urine drug concentrations.

Clinical Observations

Well-controlled clinical trials in humans establish the safety and effectiveness of drug products and may be used to determine bioavailability. However, the clinical trials approach is the least accurate, least sensitive, and least reproducible of the general approaches for determining *in-vivo* bioavailability. The FDA considers this approach only when analytical methods and pharmacodynamic methods are not available to permit use of one of the approaches described above. Comparative clinical studies have been used to establish bioequivalence for topical antifungal drug products (eg, ketoconazole) and for topical acne preparations. For dosage forms intended to deliver the active moiety to the bloodstream for systemic distribution, this approach may be considered acceptable only when analytical methods cannot be developed to permit use of one of the other approaches

In-Vitro Studies

Drug dissolution studies may under certain conditions give an indication of drug bioavailability. Ideally, the *in-vitro* drug dissolution rate should correlate with *in-vivo* drug bioavailability (see Chapters 7 and 14 on *in-vivo–in-vitro* correlation, IVIVC). Dissolution studies are often performed on several test formulations of the same drug. The test formulation that demonstrates the most rapid rate of drug dissolution *in vitro* will generally have the most rapid rate of drug bioavailability *in vivo*.

The FDA may also use other *in-vitro* approaches for establishing bioequivalence. For example, cholestyramine resin is a basic quaternary ammonium anion-exchange resin that is hydrophilic, insoluble in water, and not absorbed in the gastrointestinal tract. The bioequivalence of cholestyramine resin is performed by equilibrium and kinetic binding studies of the resin to bile acid salts (www.fda.gov/cder/guidance/cholesty.pdf).

BIOEQUIVALENCE STUDIES

Differences in the predicted clinical response or an adverse event may be due to differences in the pharmacokinetic and/or pharmacodynamic behavior of the drug among individuals or to differences in the bioavailability of the drug from the drug product. Bioequivalent drug products that have the same systemic drug bioavailability will have the same predictable drug response. However, variable clinical responses among individuals that are unrelated to bioavailability may be due to differences in the pharmacodynamics of the drug. Differences in pharmacodynamics, ie, the relationship between the drug and the receptor site, may be due to differences in receptor sensitivity to the drug. Various factors affecting pharmacodynamic drug behavior may include age, drug tolerance, drug interactions, and unknown pathophysiologic factors.

The bioavailability of a drug may be more reproducible among fasted individuals in controlled studies who take the drug on an empty stomach. When the drug is used on a daily basis, however, the nature of an individual's diet and lifestyle may affect the plasma drug levels because of variable absorption in the presence of food or even a change in the metabolic clearance of the drug. Feldman and associates (1982) reported that patients on a high-carbohydrate diet have a much longer elimination half-life of theophylline, due to the reduced metabolic clearance of the drug ($t_{1/2}$, 18.1 hours), compared to patients on normal diets ($t_{1/2} = 6.76$ hours). Previous studies demonstrated that the theophylline drug product was completely bioavailable. The higher plasma drug concentration resulting from a carbohydrate diet may subject the patient to a higher risk of drug intoxication with theophylline. The effect of food on the availability of theophylline has been reported by the FDA concerning the risk of higher theophylline plasma concentrations from a 24-hour sustained-release drug product taken with food. Although most bioavailability drug studies use fasted volunteers, the diet of patients actually using the drug product may increase, decrease, or have no affect on the bioavailability of the drug (Hendles et al, 1984).

Bases for Determining Bioequivalence

Bioequivalence is established if the *in-vivo* bioavailability of a test drug product (usually the generic product) does not differ significantly (ie, statistically insignificant) in the product's rate and extent of drug absorption, as determined by comparison of measured parameters (eg, concentration of the active drug ingredient in the blood, urinary excretion rates, or pharmacodynamic effects), from that of the *reference listed drug* (usually the brand-name product) when administered at the same molar dose of the active moiety under similar experimental conditions, either single dose or multiple dose.

In a few cases, a drug product that differs from the reference listed drug in its rate of absorption, but not in its extent of absorption, may be considered bioequivalent if the difference in the rate of absorption is intentional and appropriately reflected in the labeling and/or the rate of absorption is not detrimental to the safety and effectiveness of the drug product.

Drug Products with Possible Bioavailability and Bioequivalence Problems

Lack of bioavailability or bioequivalence may be suspected when evidence from well-controlled clinical trials or controlled observations in patients of various marketed drug products do not give comparable therapeutic effects. These drug products need to be evaluated either *in vitro* (eg, drug dissolution/release test) or *in vivo* (eg, bioequivalence study) to determine if the drug product has a bioavailability problem (see also U.S. Code of Federal Regulations, 21 CFR 320.33).

In addition, during the development of a drug product, certain biopharmaceutical properties of the active drug substance or the formulation of the drug product may indicate that the drug may have variable bioavailability and/or a bioequivalence problem. Some of these biopharmaceutic properties include:

- The active drug ingredient has low solubility in water (eg, less than 5 mg/mL).
- The dissolution rate of one or more such products is slow (eg, less than 50% in 30 minutes when tested with a general method specified by the FDA).
- The particle size and/or surface area of the active drug ingredient is critical in determining its bioavailability.
- Certain structural forms of the active drug ingredient (eg, polymorphic forms, solvates, complexes, and crystal modifications) dissolve poorly, thus affecting absorption.
- Drug products that have a high ratio of excipients to active ingredients (eg, greater than 5:1).
- Specific inactive ingredients (eg, hydrophilic or hydrophobic excipients and lubricants) either may be required for absorption of the active drug ingredient or therapeutic moiety or may interfere with such absorption.
- The active drug ingredient, therapeutic moiety, or its precursor is absorbed in large part in a particular segment of the GI tract or is absorbed from a localized site.

- The degree of absorption of the active drug ingredient, therapeutic moiety, or its precursor is poor (eg, less than 50%, ordinarily in comparison to an intravenous dose), even when it is administered in pure form (eg, in solution).
- There is rapid metabolism of the therapeutic moiety in the intestinal wall or liver during the absorption process (first-order metabolism), so that the rate of absorption is unusually important in the therapeutic effect and/or toxicity of the drug product.
- The therapeutic moiety is rapidly metabolized or excreted, so that rapid dissolution and absorption are required for effectiveness.
- The active drug ingredient or therapeutic moiety is unstable in specific portions of the GI tract and requires special coatings or formulations (eg, buffers, enteric coatings, and film coatings) to ensure adequate absorption.
- The drug product is subject to dose-dependent kinetics in or near the therapeutic range, and the rate and extent of absorption are important to bioequivalence.

DESIGN AND EVALUATION OF BIOEQUIVALENCE STUDIES

Bioequivalence studies are performed to compare the bioavailability of the generic drug product to the brand-name product. Statistical techniques should be of sufficient sensitivity to detect differences in rate and extent of absorption that are not attributable to subject variability. Once bioequivalence is established, it is likely that both the generic and brand-name dosage forms will produce the same therapeutic effect. The FDA publishes guidances for bioequivalence studies (www.fda.gov/cder/guidance; see also 21 CFR 320.25). Sponsors may also request a meeting with the FDA to review the study design for a specific drug product.

Design

The design and evaluation of well-controlled bioequivalence studies require cooperative input from pharmacokineticists, statisticians, clinicians, bioanalytical chemists, and others. The basic design for a bioequivalence study is determined by (1) the scientific questions to be answered, (2) the nature of the reference material and the dosage form to be tested, (3) the availability of analytical methods, and (4) benefit–risk and ethical considerations with regard to testing in humans. For some generic drugs, the FDA offers general guidelines for conducting these studies. For example, *Statistical Procedures for Bioequivalence Studies Using a Standard Two-Treatment Crossover Design* is available from the FDA; the publication addresses three specific aspects, including (1) logarithmic transformation of pharmacokinetic data, (2) sequence effect, and (3) outlier consideration. However, even with the availability of such guidelines, the principal investigator should prepare a detailed protocol for the study. Some of the elements of a protocol for an *in-vivo* bioavailability study are listed in Table 15.2. Bioavailability studies for controlled-release dosage forms are discussed in Chapter 17.

TABLE 15.2   Elements of a Bioavailability Study Protocol

I. Title	C. Inclusion/exclusion criteria
A. Principal investigator (study director)	1. Inclusion criteria
B. Project/protocol number and date	2. Exclusion criteria
II. Study objective	D. Restrictions/prohibitions
III. Study design	V. Clinical procedures
A. Design	A. Dosage and drug administration
B. Drug products	B. Biological sampling schedule and handling procedures
1. Test product(s)	C. Activity of subjects
2. Reference product	VI. Ethical considerations
C. Dosage regimen	A. Basic principles
D. Sample collection schedule	B. Institutional review board
E. Housing/confinement	C. Informed consent
F. Fasting/meals schedule	D. Indications for subject withdrawal
G. Analytical methods	E. Adverse reactions and emergency procedures
IV. Study population	VII. Facilities
A. Subjects	VIII. Data analysis
B. Subject selection	A. Analytical validation procedure
1. Medical history	B. Statistical treatment of data
2. Physical examination	IX. Drug accountability
3. Laboratory tests	X. Appendix

For bioequivalence studies, the test and reference drug formulations must contain the pharmaceutical equivalent drug in the same dose strength, in similar dosage forms (eg, immediate release or controlled release), and be given by the same route of administration. Both a single-dose and/or a multiple-dose (steady-state) study may be required. Before beginning the study, the *Institutional Review Board* (IRB) of the clinical facility in which the study is to be performed must approve the study. The IRB is composed of both professional and lay persons with diverse backgrounds, who have clinical experience and expertise as well as sensitivity to ethical issues and community attitudes. The IRB is responsible for safeguarding the rights and welfare of human subjects.

The basic guiding principle in performing studies is *do not do unnecessary human research.* Generally, the study is performed in normal, healthy male and female volunteers who have given informed consent to be in the study. Critically ill patients are not included in an *in-vivo* bioavailability study unless the attending physician determines that there is a potential benefit to the patient. The number of subjects in the study will depend on the expected intersubject and intrasubject variability. Patient selection is made according to certain established criteria for inclusion into, or exclusion from, the study. For example, the study might exclude any volunteers who have known allergies to the drug, are overweight, or have taken any medication within a specified period (often 1 week) prior to the study. Smokers are often included in these studies. The subjects are generally fasted for 10 to 12 hours (overnight) prior to drug administration and may continue to fast for a 2- to 4-hour period after dosing.

Analytical Methods

The analytical method used in an *in-vivo* bioavailability or bioequivalence study to measure the concentration of the active drug ingredient or therapeutic moiety, or its active metabolite(s), in body fluids or excretory products, or the method used to measure an acute pharmacological effect, must be demonstrated to be accurate and of sufficient sensitivity to measure, with appropriate precision, the actual concentration of the active drug ingredient or therapeutic moiety, or its active metabolite(s), achieved in the body. For bioavailability studies, both the parent drug and its major active metabolites are generally measured. For bioequivalence studies, the parent drug is measured. The active metabolite might be measured for some very high hepatic clearance (first-pass metabolism) drugs when the parent drug concentrations are too low to be reliable.

Reference Standard

For bioequivalence studies, one formulation of the drug is chosen as a reference standard against which all other formulations of the drug are compared. The reference drug product should be administered by the same route as the comparison formulations unless an alternative route or additional route is needed to answer specific pharmacokinetic questions. For example, if an active drug is poorly bioavailable after oral administration, the drug may be compared to an oral solution or an intravenous injection. For bioequivalence studies on a proposed generic drug product the reference standard is the *reference listed drug* (RLD), which is listed in *Approved Drug Products with Therapeutic Equivalence Evaluations*—the *Orange Book* (www.fda.gov/cder/ob/default.htm), and the proposed generic drug product is often referred to as the "Test" drug product. The RLD is generally a formulation currently marketed with a fully approved NDA for which there are valid scientific safety and efficacy data. The RLD is usually the innovator's or original manufacturer's brand-name product and is administered according to the dosage recommendations in the labeling.

Before beginning an *in-vivo* bioequivalence study, the total content of the active drug substance in the test product (generally the generic product) must be within 5% of that of the reference product. Moreover, *in-vitro* comparative dissolution or drug-release studies under various specified conditions are usually performed for both test and reference products before performing the *in-vivo* bioequivalence study.

Extended-Release Formulations

The purpose of an *in-vivo* bioavailability study involving an extended-release drug product is to determine if (1) the drug product meets the controlled-release claims made for it, (2) the bioavailability profile established for the drug product rules out the occurrence of any *dose dumping*, (3) the drug product's steady-state performance is equivalent to that of a currently marketed non-extended-release formulation, and (4) the drug product's formulation provides consistent pharmacokinetic performance between individual dosage units. A comparison bioavailability study is used for the development of a new extended release drug product in which the reference drug product may be either a solution or suspension of the active ingredient or a currently marketed non-controlled release drug product such as a tablet or capsule. For example, the bioavailability of a non-controlled-release (immediate-release) drug product given at a dose of 25 mg every 8 hours is compared to an extended-release product containing 75 mg of the same drug given once daily. For a bioequivalence study of a new generic extended release drug product, the reference drug product is the currently marketed extended release drug product listed as the RLD in the Orange Book and is administered according to the dosage recommendations in the approved labeling.

Combination Drug Products

Generally, the purpose of an *in-vivo* bioavailability study involving a combination drug product containing more than one active drug substance is to determine if the rate and extent of absorption of each active drug ingredient or therapeutic moiety in the combination drug product is equivalent to the rate and extent of absorption of each active drug ingredient or therapeutic moiety administered concurrently in separate single-ingredient preparations. The reference material in such a bioavailability study should be two or more currently marketed, single-ingredient drug products, each of which contains one of the active drug ingredients in the combination drug product. The FDA may, for valid scientific reasons, specify that the reference material be a combination drug product that is the subject of an approved NDA.

STUDY DESIGNS

For many drug products, the FDA, Division of Bioequivalence, Office of Generic Drugs, provides guidance for the performance of *in-vitro* dissolution and *in-vivo* bioequivalence studies. Similar guidelines appear in the United States Pharmacopeia NF. Currently, three different studies may be required for solid oral dosage forms, including (1) a fasting study, (2) a food intervention study, and/or (3) a multiple-dose (steady-state) study. Other study designs have been proposed by the FDA. For example, the FDA published two draft guidelines in October and December 1997 to consider the performance of individual bioequivalence studies using a replicate design and a two-way crossover food intervention study. Proper study design and statistical evolution are important considerations for the determination of bioequivalence. Some of the designs listed above are summarized here.

Fasting Study

Bioequivalence studies are usually evaluated by a single-dose, two-period, two-treatment, two-sequence, open-label, randomized crossover design comparing equal doses of the test and reference products in fasted, adult, healthy subjects. This study is required for all immediate-release and modified-release oral dosage forms. Both male and female subjects may be used in the study. Blood sampling is performed just before (zero time) the dose and at appropriate intervals after the dose to obtain an adequate description of the plasma drug concentration–time profile. The subjects should be in the fasting state (overnight fast of at least 10 hours) before drug administration and should continue to fast for up to 4 hours after dosing. No other medication is normally given to the subject for at least 1 week prior to the study. In some cases, a parallel design may be more appropriate for certain drug products, containing a drug with a very long elimination half-life. A replicate design may be used for a drug product containing a drug that has high intrasubject variability.

Food Intervention Study

Co-administration of food with an oral drug product may affect the bioavailability of the drug. Food intervention or food effect studies are generally conducted using meal conditions that are expected to provide the greatest effects on GI physiology so that systemic drug availability is maximally affected. The test meal is a high-fat (approximately 50% of total caloric content of the meal) and high-calorie (approximately 800–1000 calories) meal. A typical test meal is two eggs fried in butter, two strips of bacon, two slices of toast with butter, 4 ounces of brown potatoes, and 8 ounces of milk. This test meal derives approximately 150, 250, and 500–600 calories from protein, carbohydrate, and fat, respectively (www.fda.gov/cder/guidance/4613dft.pdf).

For bioequivalence studies, drug bioavailability from both the test and reference products should be affected similarly by food. The study design uses a single-dose, randomized, two-treatment, two-period, crossover study comparing equal doses of the test and reference products. Following an overnight fast of at least 10 hours, subjects are given the recommended meal 30 minutes before dosing. The meal is consumed over 30 minutes, with administration of the drug product immediately after the meal. The drug product is given with 240 mL (8 fluid ounces) of water. No food is allowed for at least 4 hours postdose. This study is required for all modified-release dosage forms and may be required for immediate-release dosage forms if the bioavailability of the active drug ingredient is known to be affected by food (eg, ibuprofen, naproxen). For certain extended-release capsules that contain coated beads, the capsule contents are sprinkled over soft foods such as apple sauce, which is taken by the fasted subject and the bioavailability of the drug is then measured. Bioavailability studies might also examine the affects of other foods and special vehicles such as apple juice.

Multiple-Dose (Steady-State) Study

In a few cases, a multiple-dose, steady-state, randomized, two-treatment, two-way crossover study comparing equal doses of the test and reference products may be performed in adult, healthy subjects. For these studies, three consecutive trough concentrations (C_{min}) on three consecutive days should be determined to ascertain that the subjects are at steady state. The last morning dose is given to the subject after an overnight fast, with continual fasting for at least 2 hours following dose administration. Blood sampling is performed similarly to the single-dose study.

Crossover Designs

Subjects who meet the inclusion and exclusion study criteria and have given informed consent are selected at random. A complete crossover design is usually employed, in which each subject receives the test drug product and the reference product. Examples of *Latin-square crossover designs* for a bioequivalence study in human

TABLE 15.3   Latin-Square Crossover Design for a Bioequivalence Study of Three Drug Products in Six Human Volunteers

SUBJECT	DRUG PRODUCT		
	Study Period 1	Study Period 2	Study Period 3
1	A	B	C
2	B	C	A
3	C	A	B
4	A	C	B
5	C	B	A
6	B	A	C

volunteers, comparing three different drug formulations (A, B, C) or four different drug formulations (A, B, C, D), are described in Tables 10.3 and 10.4. The Latin-square design plans the clinical trial so that each subject receives each drug product only once, with adequate time between medications for the elimination of the drug from the body (Table 15.3). In this design, each subject is his own control, and subject-to-subject variation is reduced. Moreover, variation due to sequence, period, and treatment (formulation) are reduced, so that all patients do not receive the same drug product on the same day and in the same order. Possible carryover effects from any particular drug product are minimized by changing the sequence or order in which the drug products are given to the subject. Thus, drug product B may be followed by drug product A, D, or C (Table 15.4). After each subject receives a drug product, blood samples are collected at appropriate time intervals so that a valid blood drug level–time curve is obtained. The time intervals should be spaced so that the peak blood concentration, the total area under the curve, and the absorption and elimination phases of the curve may be well described.

TABLE 15.4   Latin-Square Crossover Design for a Bioequivalency Study of Four Drug Products in 16 Human Volunteers

SUBJECT	DRUG PRODUCT			
	Study Period 1	Study Period 2	Study Period 3	Study Period 4
1	A	B	C	D
2	B	C	D	A
3	C	D	A	B
4	D	A	B	C
5	A	B	D	C
6	B	D	C	A
7	D	C	A	B
8	C	A	B	D
9	A	C	B	D
10	C	B	D	A
11	B	D	A	C
12	D	A	C	B
13	A	C	D	B
14	C	D	B	A
15	D	B	A	C
16	B	A	C	D

Period refers to the time period in which a study is performed. A two-period study is a study that is performed on two different days (time periods) separated by a *washout period* during which most of the drug is eliminated from the body—generally about 10 elimination half-lives. A *sequence* refers to the number of different orders in the treatment groups in a study. For example, a two-sequence, two-period study would be designed as follows:

	Period 1	**Period 2**
Sequence 1	T	R
Sequence 2	R	T

where R = reference and T = treatment.

Table 15.4 shows a design for three different drug treatment groups given in a three-period study with six different sequences. The order in which the drug treatments are given should not stay the same in order to prevent any bias in the data due to a residual effect from the previous treatment.

Replicated Crossover Design

Replicated crossover designs are used for the determination of individual bioequivalence, to estimate within-subject variance for both the Test and Reference drug products, and to provide an estimate of the subject-by-formulation interaction variance. Generally, a four-period, two-sequence, two-formulation design is recommended by the FDA.

	Period 1	**Period 2**	**Period 3**	**Period 4**
Sequence 1	T	R	T	R
Sequence 2	R	T	R	T

where R = reference and T = treatment.

The same reference and the same test are each given twice to the same subject. Other sequences are possible. In this design, Reference-to-Reference and Test-to-Test comparisons may also be made.

EVALUATION OF THE DATA

Analytical Method

The analytical method for measurement of the drug must be validated for accuracy, precision, sensitivity, and specificity. The use of more than one analytical method during a bioequivalence study may not be valid, because different methods may yield different values. Data should be presented in both tabulated and graphic form for evaluation. The plasma drug concentration–time curve for each drug product and each subject should be available.

Pharmacokinetic Evaluation of the Data

For single-dose studies, including a fasting study or a food intervention study, the pharmacokinetic analyses include calculation for each subject of the area under the curve to the last quantifiable concentration (AUC_{0-t}) and to infinity ($AUC_{0-\infty}$), T_{max}, and C_{max}. Additionally, the elimination rate constant, k, the elimination half-life, $t_{1/2}$, and other parameters may be estimated. For multiple-dose studies, pharmacokinetic analysis includes calculation for each subject of the steady-state area under the curve, (AUC_{0-t}), T_{max}, C_{min}, C_{max}, and the percent fluctuation [$100 \times (C_{max} - C_{min})/C_{min}$]. Proper statistical evaluation should be performed on the estimated pharmacokinetic parameters.

Statistical Evaluation of the Data

Bioequivalence is generally determined using a comparison of population averages of a bioequivalence metric, such as AUC and C_{max}. This approach, termed *average bioequivalence*, involves the calculation of a 90% confidence interval for the ratio of averages (population geometric means) of the bioequivalence metrics for the Test and Reference drug products. To establish bioequivalence, the calculated confidence interval should fall within a prescribed bioequivalence limit, usually, 80–125% for the ratio of the product averages. Standard crossover design studies are used to obtain the data. Another approach proposed by the FDA and others is termed *individual bioequivalence*. Individual bioequivalence requires a replicate crossover design, and estimates within-subject variability for the Test and Reference drug products, as well as subject-by-formulation interaction. Presently, only average bioequivalence estimates are used to establish bioequivalence of generic drug products.

To prove bioequivalence, there must be no statistical difference between the bioavailability of the Test product and the Reference product. Several statistical approaches are used to compare the bioavailability of drug from the test dosage form to the bioavailability of the drug from the reference dosage form. Many statistical approaches (parametric tests) assume that the data are distributed according to a normal distribution or "bell-shaped curve" (see Appendix A). The distribution of many biological parameters such as C_{max} and AUC have a longer right tail than would be observed in a normal distribution (Midha et al, 1993). Moreover, the true distribution of these biological parameters may be difficult to ascertain because of the small number of subjects used in a bioequivalence study. The distribution of data that has been transformed to log values resembles more closely a normal distribution compared to the distribution of non-log-transformed data. Therefore, log transformation of the bioavailability data (eg, C_{max}, AUC) is performed before statistical data evaluation for bioequivalence determination.

Analysis of Variance (ANOVA)

An analysis of variance (ANOVA) is a statistical procedure (Appendix A) used to test the data for differences within and between treatment and control groups. A bioequivalent product should produce no significant difference in all pharmacokinetic parameters tested. The parameters tested usually include AUC_{0-t}, $AUC_{0-\infty}$, t_{max}, and C_{max} obtained for each treatment or dosage form. Other metrics of bioavailability have also been used to compare the bioequivalence of two or more formulations. The ANOVA may evaluate variability in subjects, treatment groups, study period, formulation, and other variables, depending on the study design. If the variability in the data is large, the difference in means for each pharmacokinetic parameter, such as AUC, may be masked, and the investigator might erroneously conclude that the two drug products are bioequivalent.

A statistical difference between the pharmacokinetic parameters obtained from two or more drug products is considered statistically significant if there is a probability of less than 1 in 20 times or 0.05 probability ($p \leq 0.05$) that these results would have happened on the basis of chance alone. The probability, p, is used to indicate the level of statistical significance. If $p < 0.05$, the differences between the two drug products are not considered statistically significant.

To reduce the possibility of failing to detect small differences between the test products, a *power test* is performed to calculate the probability that the conclusion of the ANOVA is valid. The power of the test will depend on the sample size, variability of the data, and desired level of significance. Usually the power is set at 0.80 with a $\beta = 0.2$ and a level of significance of 0.05. The higher the power, the more sensitive the test and the greater the probability that the conclusion of the ANOVA is valid.

Two One-Sided Tests Procedure

The two one-sided tests procedure is also referred to as the *confidence interval approach* (Schuirmann, 1987). This statistical method is used to demonstrate if the bioavailability of the drug from the Test formulation is too low or high in comparison to that of the Reference product. The objective of the approach is to determine if there are large differences (ie, greater than 20%) between the mean parameters.

The 90% confidence limits are estimated for the sample means. The interval estimate is based on a Student's t distribution of the data. In this test, presently required by the FDA, a 90% confidence interval about the ratio of means of the two drug products must be within ±20% for measurement of the rate and extent of drug bioavailability. For most drugs, up to a 20% difference in AUC or C_{max} between two formulations would have no clinical significance. The lower 90% confidence interval for the ratio of means cannot be less than 0.80, and the upper 90% confidence interval for the ratio of the means cannot be greater than 1.20. When log-transformed data are used, the 90% confidence interval is set at 80–125%. These confidence limits have also been termed the *bioequivalence interval* (Midha et al, 1993). The 90% confidence interval is a function of sample size and study variability, including inter- and intrasubject variability.

For a single-dose, fasting study, an analysis of variance (ANOVA) is usually performed on the log-transformed AUC and C_{max} values. There should be no statistical differences between the mean AUC and C_{max} parameters for the Test (generic) and Reference drug products. In addition, the 90% confidence intervals about the ratio of the means for AUC and C_{max} values of the Test drug product should not be less than 0.80 (80%) nor greater than 1.25 (125%) of that of the Reference product based on log-transformed data.

BIOEQUIVALENCE EXAMPLE

A simulated example of the results for a single-dose, fasting study is shown in Table 15.5 and in Figure 15-8. As shown by the ANOVA, no statistical differences

TABLE 15.5 Bioavailability Comparison of a Generic (Test) and Brand-Name (Reference) Drug Products (Log-Normal Transformed Data)

VARIABLE	UNITS	GEOMETRIC MEAN		% RATIO	90% CONFIDENCE INTERVAL (LOWER LIMIT, UPPER LIMIT)	p VALUES FOR PRODUCT EFFECTS	POWER OF ANOVA	ANOVA % CV
		Test	Reference					
C_{max}	ng/mL	344.79	356.81	96.6	(89.5,112)	0.3586	0.8791	17.90%
AUC_{0-t}	ng hr/mL	2659.12	2674.92	99.4	(95.1,104)	0.8172	1.0000	12.60%
AUC_∞		2708.63	2718.52	99.6	(95.4,103)	0.8865	1.0000	12.20%
T_{max}	hr	4.29	4.24	101				
K_{elim}	1/hr	0.0961	0.0980	98.1				
$t_{1/2}$	hr	8.47	8.33	101.7				

The results were obtained from a two-way, crossover, single-dose study in 36 fasted, healthy, adult male and female volunteers. No statistical differences were observed for the mean values between Test and Reference products.

for the pharmacokinetic parameters AUC_{0-t}, $AUC_{0-\infty}$, and C_{max} were observed between the Test product and the brand-name product. The 90% confidence limits for the mean pharmacokinetic parameters of the Test product were within 0.80–1.25 (80–125%) of the reference product means based on log transformation of the data. The power test for the AUC measures were above 99%, showing good precision of the data. The power test for the C_{max} values was 87.9%, showing that this parameter was more variable.

Table 15.6 shows the results for a hypothetical bioavailability study in which three different tablet formulations were compared to a solution of the drug given in the same dose. As shown in the table, the bioavailability from all three tablet formulations was greater than 80% of that of the solution. According to the ANOVA, the

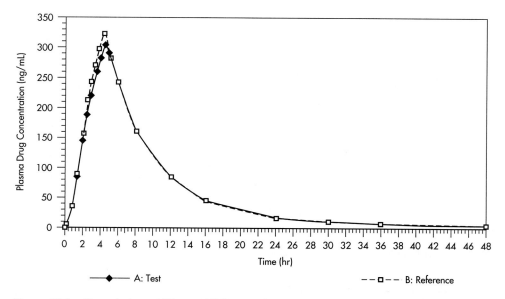

Figure 15-8. Bioequivalence of Test and Reference drug products: mean plasma drug concentrations.

TABLE 15.6   Summary of the Results of a Bioavailability Study[a]

DOSAGE FORM	C_{max} (μg/mL)	t_{max} (hr)	AUC_{0-24} (μg hr/mL)	F^b	90% CONFIDENCE INTERVAL FOR AUC
Solution	16.1 ± 2.5	1.5 ± 0.85	1835 ± 235		
Tablet A	10.5 ± 3.2[c]	2.5 ± 1.0[c]	1523 ± 381	81	74–90%
Tablet B	13.7 ± 4.1	2.1 ± 0.98	1707 ± 317	93	88–98%
Tablet C	14.8 ± 3.6	1.8 ± 0.95	1762 ± 295	96	91–103%

[a] The bioavailability of a drug from four different formulations was studied in 24 healthy, adult male subjects using a four-way Latin-square crossover design. The results represent the mean ± standard deviation.
[b] Oral bioavailability relative to the solution.
[c] $p \leq 0.05$.

mean AUC values were not statistically different from each other nor different from that of the solution. However, the 90% confidence interval for the AUC showed that for tablet A, the bioavailability was less than 80% (ie, 74%), compared to the solution at the low-range estimate and would not be considered bioequivalent based on AUC.

For illustrative purposes, consider a drug that has been prepared at the same dosage level in three formulations, A, B, and C. These formulations are given to a group of volunteers using a three-way, randomized crossover design. In this experimental design, all subjects receive each formulation once. From each subject, plasma drug level and urinary drug excretion data are obtained. With these data we can observe the relationship between plasma and urinary excretion parameters and drug bioavailability (Fig. 15-9). The rate of drug absorption from formulation A is more rapid than that from formulation B, because the t_{max} for formulation A is shorter. Because the AUC for formulation A is identical to the AUC for formulation B, the extent of bioavailability from both of these formulations is the same. Note, however,

Figure 15-9. Corresponding plots relating plasma concentration and urinary excretion data.

TABLE 15.7   Relationship of Plasma Level and Urinary Excretion Parameters to Drug Bioavailability

EXTENT OF DRUG BIOAVAILABILITY DECREASES		RATE OF DRUG BIOAVAILABILITY DECREASES	
Parameter	**Change**	**Parameter**	**Change**
Plasma data			
t_{max}	Same	t_{max}	Increase
C_{max}	Decrease	C_{max}	Decrease
AUC	Decrease	AUC	Same
Urine data			
t^{∞}	Same	t^{∞}	Increase
$[dD_u/dt]_{max}{}^a$	Decrease	$[dD_u/dt]_{max}{}^a$	Decrease
D_u^{∞}	Decrease	D_u^{∞}	Same

[a] Maximum rate of urinary drug excretion.

the C_{max} for A is higher than that for B, because the rate of drug absorption is more rapid.

The C_{max} is generally higher when the extent of drug bioavailability is greater. The rate of drug absorption from formulation C is the same as that from formulation A, but the extent of drug available is less. The C_{max} for formulation C is less than that for formulation A. The decrease in C_{max} for formulation C is proportional to the decrease in AUC in comparison to the drug plasma level data for formulation A. The corresponding urinary excretion data confirm these observations. These relationships are summarized in Table 15.7. The table illustrates how bioavailability parameters for plasma and urine change when only the extent and rate of bioavailability are changed, respectively. Formulation changes in a drug product may affect both the rate and extent of drug bioavailability.

STUDY SUBMISSION AND DRUG REVIEW PROCESS

The contents of New Drug Applications (NDAs) and Abbreviated New Drug Applications (ANDAs) are similar in terms of the quality of manufacture (Table 15.8).

TABLE 15.8   NDA Versus ANDA Review Process

BRAND–NAME DRUG NDA REQUIREMENTS	GENERIC DRUG ANDA REQUIREMENTS
1. Chemistry	1. Chemistry
2. Manufacturing	2. Manufacturing
3. Controls	3. Controls
4. Labeling	4. Labeling
5. Testing	5. Testing
6. Animal studies	6. Bioequivalence
7. Clinical studies	
8. Bioavailability	

Source: Center for Drug Evaluation & Research, U.S. Food & Drug Administration.

The submission for a NDA must contain safety and efficacy study as provided by animal toxicology studies, clinical efficacy studies, and pharmacokinetic/bioavailability studies. For the generic drug manufacturer, the bioequivalence study is the pivotal study in the ANDA that replaces the animal, clinical, and pharmacokinetic studies.

An outline for the submission of a completed bioavailability study for submission to the FDA is shown in Table 15.9. The investigator should be sure that the study has been properly designed, the objectives are clearly defined, and the method of analysis has been validated (ie, shown to measure precisely and accurately the plasma drug concentration). The results are analyzed both statistically and pharmacokinetically. These results, along with case reports and various data supporting the validity of the analytical method, are included in the submission. The FDA reviews the study in detail according to the outline presented in Table 15.10. If necessary, an FDA investigator may inspect both the clinical and analytical facilities used in the study and audit the raw data used in support of the bioavailability study. For ANDA applications, the FDA Office of Generic Drugs reviews the entire ANDA as shown in Figure 15-10. If the application is incomplete, the FDA will not review the submission and the sponsor will receive a Refusal to File letter.

Waivers of *In-Vivo* Bioequivalence Studies (Biowaivers)

In some cases, *in-vitro* dissolution testing may be used in lieu of *in-vivo* bioequivalence studies. When the drug product is in the same dosage form but in different strengths, and is proportionally similar in active and inactive ingredients, an *in-vivo* bioequivalence study of one or more lower strengths can be waived based on the dissolution tests and an *in-vivo* bioequivalence study on the highest strength. Ideally, if there is a strong correlation between dissolution of the drug and the bioavailability of the drug, then the comparative dissolution tests comparing the test product to the reference product should be sufficient to demonstrate bioequivalence. For most drug products, especially immediate-release tablets and capsules, no strong correlation exists, and the FDA requires an *in-vivo* bioequivalence study. For oral solid dosage forms, an *in-vivo* bioequivalence study may be required to support at least one dose strength of the product. Usually, an *in-vivo* bioequivalence study is required for the highest dose strength. If the lower-dose-strength test product is substantially similar in active and inactive ingredients, then only a comparison *in-vitro* dissolution between the test and brand-name formulations may be used.

For example, an immediate-release tablet is available in 200-mg, 100-mg, and 50-mg strengths. The 100- and 50-mg-strength tablets are made the same way as the highest-strength tablet. A human bioequivalence study is performed on the highest or 200-mg strength. Comparative *in-vitro* dissolution studies are performed on the 100-mg and 50-mg dose strengths. If these drug products have no known bioavailability problems, are well absorbed systemically, are well correlated with *in-vitro* dissolution, and have a large margin of safety, then arguments for not performing an *in-vivo* bioavailability study may be valid. Methods for correlation of *in-vitro* dissolution of the drug with *in-vivo* drug bioavailability are discussed in Chapters 14 and 17. The manufacturer does not need to perform additional *in-vivo* bioequivalence studies on the lower-strength products if the products meet all *in-vitro* criteria.

TABLE 15.9   Proposed Format and Contents of an *in-Vivo* Bioequivalence Study Submission and Accompanying *in-Vitro* Data

Title page
  Study title
  Name of sponsor
  Name and address of clinical laboratory
  Name of principal investigator(s)
  Name of clinical investigator
  Name of analytical laboratory
  Dates of clinical study (start, completion)
  Signature of principal investigator (and date)
  Signature of clinical investigator (and date)

Table of contents
  I. Study Résumé
    Product information
    Summary of bioequivalence study
    Summary of bioequivalence data
      Plasma
      Urinary excretion
    Figure of mean plasma concentration–time profile
    Figure of mean cumulative urinary excretion
    Figure of mean urinary excretion rates
  II. Protocol and Approvals
    Protocol
    Letter of acceptance of protocol from FDA
    Informed consent form
    Letter of approval of Institutional Review Board
    List of members of Institutional Review Board
  III. Clinical Study
    Summary of the study
    Details of the study
    Demographic characteristics of the subjects
    Subject assignment in the study
    Mean physical characteristics of subjects arranged by sequence
    Details of clinical activity
    Deviations from protocol
    Vital signs of subjects
    Adverse reactions report
  IV. Assay Methodology and Validation
    Assay method description
    Validation procedure
    Summary of validation
    Data on linearity of standard samples
    Data on interday precision and accuracy
    Data on intraday precision and accuracy
    Figure for standard curve(s) for low/high ranges
    Chromatograms of standard and quality control samples
    Sample calculation

  V. Pharmacokinetic Parameters and Tests
    Definition and calculations
    Statistical tests
    Drug levels at each sampling time and pharmacokinetic parameters
    Figure of mean plasma concentration–time profile
    Figures of individual subject plasma concentration–time profiles
    Figure of mean cumulative urinary excretion
    Figures of individual subject cumulative urinary excretion
    Figure of mean urinary excretion rates
    Figures of individual subject urinary excretion rates
    Tables of individual subject data arranged by drug, drug/period, drug/sequence
  VI. Statistical Analyses
    Statistical considerations
    Summary of statistical significance
    Summary of statistical parameters
    Analysis of variance, least squares estimates and least-squares means
    Assessment of sequence, period, and treatment effects
    90% Confidence intervals for the difference between Test and Reference products for the log-normal-transformed parameters of AUC_{0-t}, $AUC_{0-\infty}$, and C_{max} should be within 80% and 125%
  VII. Appendices
    Randomization schedule
    Sample identification codes
    Analytical raw data
    Chromatograms of at least 20% of subjects
    Medical record and clinical reports
    Clinical facilities description
    Analytical facilities description
    Curricula vitae of the investigators
  VIII. *In-Vitro* Testing
    Dissolution testing
    Dissolution assay methodology
    Content uniformity testing
    Potency determination
  IX. Batch Size and Formulation
    Batch record
    Quantitative formulation

Modified from Dighe and Adams (1991), with permission.

TABLE 15.10   *General Elements of a Biopharmaceutics Review*

Introduction	Summary and analysis of data
Study design	Comments
Study objective(s)	Deficiencies
Assay description and validation	Recommendation
Assay for individual samples checked	

Dissolution Profile Comparison

Comparative dissolution profiles are used as (1) the basis for formulation development of bioequivalent drug products and proceeding to the pivotal *in-vivo* bioequivalence study; (2) comparative dissolution profiles are used for demonstrating the equivalence of a change in the formulation of a drug product after the drug product has been approved for marketing (see SUPAC in Chapter 16); and (3) the basis of a biowaiver of a lower-strength drug product that is dose proportional in active and inactive ingredients to the higher-strength drug product.

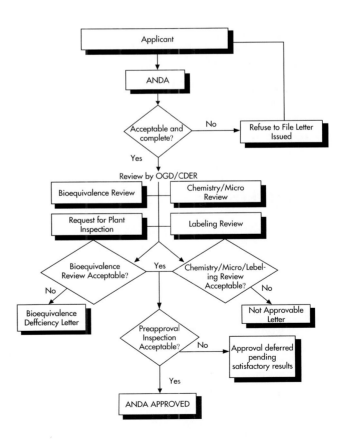

Figure 15-10.   Generic drug review process.
Source: Office of Generic Drugs, Center for Drug Evaluation & Research, U.S. Food & Drug Administration.

A model-independent mathematical method was developed by Moore and Flanner (1996) to compare dissolution profiles using two factors, f_1 and f_2. The factor f_2, known as the *similarity factor*, measures the closeness between the two profiles:

$$f_2 = 50 \times \log \left\{ \left[1 + \frac{1}{n} \sum_{t=1}^{n} (R_1 - T_1)^2 \right]^{-5} \times 100 \right\}$$

where n is the number of time points, R_1 is the dissolution value of the Reference product at time t, and T_1 is the dissolution value of the Test product batch at time t.

The Reference may be the original drug product before a formulation change (prechange) and the Test may be the drug product after the formulation was changed (postchange). Alternatively, the Reference may be the higher-strength drug product and the Test may be the lower-strength drug product. The f_2 comparison is the focus of several FDA guidances and is of regulatory interest in knowing the similarity of the two dissolution curves. When the two profiles are identical, $f_2 = 100$. An average difference of 10% at all measured time points results in a f_2 value of 50. The FDA has set a public standard for f_2 value between 50 and 100 to indicate similarity between two dissolution profiles.

In some cases, two generic drug products may have dissimilar dissolution profiles and still be bioequivalent *in-vivo*. For example, Polli et al (1997) have shown that slow-, medium-, and fast-dissolving formulations of metoprolol tartrate tablets were bioequivalent. Furthermore, bioequivalent modified-release drug products may have different drug release mechanisms and therefore different dissolution profiles. For example, for theophylline extended-release capsules, the *United States Pharmacopeia* (USP) lists 10 individual drug release tests for products labeled for dosing every 12 hours. However, only generic drug products that are FDA approved as bioequivalent drug products and listed in the current edition of the *Orange Book* may be substituted for each other.

THE BIOPHARMACEUTICS CLASSIFICATION SYSTEM (BCS)

A theoretical basis for correlating *in-vitro* drug dissolution with *in-vivo* bioavailability was developed by Amidon et al (1995). This approach is based on the aqueous solubility of the drug and the permeation of the drug through the gastrointestinal tract. The classification system is based on Fick's first law applied to a membrane:

$$J_w = P_w C_w$$

where J_w is the drug flux (mass/area/time) through the intestinal wall at any position and time, P_w is the permeability of the membrane, and C_w is the drug concentration at the intestinal membrane surface.

This approach assumes that no other components in the formulation affect the membrane permeability and/or intestinal transport. Using this approach, Amidon et al (1995) studied the solubility and permeability characteristics of various representative drugs and obtained a biopharmaceutic drug classification (Table 15.11) for predicting the *in-vitro* drug dissolution of immediate-release solid oral drug products with *in-vivo* absorption.

TABLE 15.11   Biopharmaceutics Classification System

CLASS	SOLUBILITY	PERMEABILITY	COMMENTS
Class 1	High	High	Drug dissolves rapidly and is well absorbed. Bioavailability problem is not expected for immediate release drug products.
Class 2	Low	High	Drug is dissolution limited and well absorbed. Bioavailability is controlled by the dosage form and rate of release of the drug substance.
Class 3	High	Low	Drug is permeability limited. Bioavailability may be incomplete if drug is not released and dissolved within absorption window.
Class 4	Low	Low	Difficulty in formulating a drug product that will deliver consistent drug bioavailability. An alternate route of administration may be needed.

From *FDA Guidance for Industry: Waiver of In Vivo Bioavailability and Bioequivalence Studies for Immediate Release Solid Oral Dosage Forms Containing Certain Active Moieties/Active Ingredients Based on a Biopharmaceutics Classification System* (2000), and Amidon et al (1995).

The FDA may waive the requirement for performing an *in-vivo* bioavailability or bioequivalence study for certain immediate-release solid oral drug products that meet very specific criteria, namely, the permeability, solubility, and dissolution of the drug. These characteristics include the *in-vitro* dissolution, of the drug product in various media, drug permeability information, and assuming ideal behavior of the drug product, drug dissolution, and absorption in the GI tract. For regulatory purpose, drugs are classified according to the Biopharmaceutics Classification System (BCS) in accordance the solubility, permeability, and dissolution characteristics of the drug (*FDA Guidance for Industry*, 2000; Amidon et al, 1995).

Solubility

An objective of the BCS approach is to determine the equilibrium solubility of a drug under approximate physiologic conditions. For this purpose, determination of pH–solubility profiles over a pH range of 1–8 is suggested. The solubility class is determined by calculating what volume of an aqueous medium is sufficient to dissolve the highest anticipated dose strength. A drug substance is considered highly soluble when the highest dose strength is soluble in 250 mL or less of aqueous medium over the pH range 1–8. The volume estimate of 250 mL is derived from typical bioequivalence study protocols that prescribe administration of a drug product to fasting human volunteers with a glass (8 ounces) of water.

Permeability

Studies of the extent of absorption in humans, or intestinal permeability methods, can be used to determine the permeability class membership of a drug. To be classified as highly permeable, a test drug should have an extent of absorption > 90% in humans. Supportive information on permeability characteristics of the drug substance should also be derived from its physical-chemical properties (eg, octanol: water partition coefficient).

Some methods to determine the permeability of a drug from the gastrointestinal tract include: (1) *in-vivo* intestinal perfusion studies in humans; (2) *in-vivo* or *in-situ* intestinal perfusion studies in animals; (3) *in-vitro* permeation experiments using excised human or animal intestinal tissues; and (4) *in-vitro* permeation experiments across a monolayer of cultured human intestinal cells. When using these methods, the experimental permeability data should correlate with the known extent-of-absorption data in humans.

Dissolution

The dissolution class is based on the *in-vitro* dissolution rate of an immediate-release drug product under specified test conditions and is intended to indicate rapid *in-vivo* dissolution in relation to the average rate of gastric emptying in humans under fasting conditions. An immediate-release drug product is considered rapidly dissolving when not less than 85% of the label amount of drug substance dissolves within 30 minutes using USP Apparatus I (see Chapter 14) at 100 rpm or Apparatus II at 50 rpm in a volume of 900 mL or less in each of the following media: (1) acidic media such as 0.1 N HCl or Simulated Gastric Fluid USP without enzymes, (2) a pH 4.5 buffer, and (3) a pH 6.8 buffer or Simulated Intestinal Fluid USP without enzymes.

Drug Products for Which Bioavailability or Bioequivalence May Be Self-Evident

The best measure of a drug product's performance is to determine the *in-vivo* bioavailability of the drug. For some well-characterized drug products and for certain drug products in which bioavailability is self-evident (eg, sterile solutions for injection), *in-vivo* bioavailability studies may be unnecessary or unimportant to the achievement of the product's intended purposes. The FDA will waive the requirement for submission of *in-vivo* evidence demonstrating the bioavailability of the drug product if the product meets one of the following criteria (U.S. Code of Federal Regulations, 21 CFR 320.22). However, there may be specific requirements for certain drug products, and the appropriate FDA division should be consulted.

1. The drug product (a) is a solution intended solely for intravenous administration and (b) contains an active drug ingredient or therapeutic moiety combined with the same solvent and in the same concentration as in an intravenous solution that is the subject of an approved, full, New Drug Application.
2. The drug product is a topically applied preparation (eg, a cream, ointment, or gel intended for local therapeutic effect). The FDA has released guidances for the performance of bioequivalence studies on topical corticosteroids and antifungal agents. The FDA is also considering performing dermatopharmacokinetic (DPK) studies on other topical drug products. In addition, *in-vitro* drug release and diffusion studies may be required.
3. The drug product is in an oral dosage form that is not intended to be absorbed (eg, an antacid or a radiopaque medium). Specific *in-vitro* bioequivalence studies may be required by the FDA. For example, the bioequivalence of cholestyramine resin is demonstrated *in-vitro* by the binding of bile acids to the resin.

4. The drug product meets both of the following conditions:

    a. It is administered by inhalation as a gas or vapor (eg, as a medicinal or as an inhalation anesthetic).

    b. It contains an active drug ingredient or therapeutic moiety in the same dosage form as a drug product that is the subject of an approved, full, New Drug Application(NDA).

5. The drug product meets all of the following conditions:

    a. It is an oral solution, elixir, syrup, tincture, or similar other solubilized form.

    b. It contains an active drug ingredient or therapeutic moiety in the same concentration as a drug product that is the subject of an approved, full, New Drug Application.

    c. It contains no inactive ingredient that is known to significantly affect absorption of the active drug ingredient or therapeutic moiety.

GENERIC BIOLOGICS

Biologics, in contrast to drugs that are chemically synthesized, are derived from living sources such as human, animal, or microorganisms. Many biologics are complex mixtures that are not easily identified or characterized and are manufactured by biotechnology. Other biological drugs, such as insulin and growth hormone, are proteins derived by biotechnology and have been well characterized.

Presently, there is no FDA regulatory pathway to establish the bioequivalence of a biotechnology-derived drug product. Scientifically, there are advocates for and against the feasibility for the manufacture of generic biotechnology-derived drug products (generic biologics) that are bioequivalent to the innovator or brand-drug product.

Those opposed to the development of generic biologics have claimed that generic manufacturers do not have the ability to fully characterize the active ingredient(s), that immunogenicity-related impurities may be present in the product, and that the manufacture of a biologic drug product is process dependent.

Many biologic drug products are given parenterally. The efficacy of the biologic may be affected by the development of antibodies to the active ingredient or to product-related impurities. The degree of immunogenicity and subsequent antibody formation to a foreign peptide or protein will alter the efficacy of the drug. Antibodies can increase bioavailability if they are not neutralizing, which would result in higher drug levels in the body. In contrast, antibodies can decrease bioavailability of the biologic drug by forming an antibody–protein complex that results in a change in drug distribution and a change in clearance.

Advocates for the manufacture of generic biologics argue that bioequivalent biotechnology-derived drug products can be made on a case-by-case basis. Currently, manufacturers of marketed biotechnology drugs may seek to make changes in the manufacturing process used to make a particular product for a variety of reasons, including improvement of product quality, yield, and manufacturing efficiency. These manufacturers have developed improvements in production methods, process and control test methods, and test methods for product characterization.

For example, a biologics manufacturer institutes a change in its manufacturing process, before FDA approval of its product but after completion of a pivotal clinical study. The FDA may not require the manufacturer to perform additional clinical studies to demonstrate that the resulting product is still safe, pure, and potent. Such manufacturing process changes, implemented before or after product approval, have included changes implemented during expansion from pilot-scale to full-scale production, the move of production facilities from one legal entity to another legal entity, and the implementation of changes in different stages of the manufacturing process such as fermentation, purification, and formulation. The manufacturer may be able to demonstrate product comparability between a biological product made after a manufacturing change ("new" product) and a product made before implementation of the change ("old" product) through different types of analytical and functional testing, with or without preclinical animal testing. The FDA may determine that two products are comparable if the results of the comparability testing demonstrate that the manufacturing change does not affect safety, identity, purity, or potency (*FDA Guidance Concerning Demonstration of Comparability of Human Biological Products, Including Therapeutic Biotechnology-Derived Products*, 1996). The FDA currently requires that manufacturers should carefully assess manufacturing changes and evaluate the product resulting from these changes for comparability to the preexisting product. Determinations of product comparability may be based on chemical, physical, and biological assays and, in some cases, other nonclinical data.

It is important to note that the FDA uses such terms as *comparable* and *similar* for approval of manufacturing changes of biologic drug products (*FDA Guidance*, 1996). In contrast, the FDA uses the term *bioequivalence* for approval of manufacturing changes of drug products that contain chemically derived active ingredients. Advocates for the manufacturer of generic biologics feel that the science and technology for the manufacture of certain bioequivalent biologic drug products are already available. Moreover, if the innovator manufacturer of a marketed biologic drug product can perform a manufacturing change and demonstrate the comparability of the "new" to the "old" marketed biologic drug product, then a generic manufacturer should be able to use similar techniques to demonstrate bioequivalence of the generic drug product.

CLINICAL SIGNIFICANCE OF BIOEQUIVALENCE STUDIES

Bioequivalence of different formulations of the same drug substance involves equivalence with respect to rate and extent of systemic drug absorption. Clinical interpretation is important in evaluating the results of a bioequivalence study. A small difference between drug products, even if statistically significant, may produce very little difference in therapeutic response. Generally, two formulations whose rate and extent of absorption differ by 20% or less are considered bioequivalent. The Report by the Bioequivalence Task Force (1988) considered that differences of less than 20% in AUC and C_{max} between drug products are "unlikely to be clinically significant in patients." The Task Force further stated that "clinical studies of effectiveness have difficulty detecting differences in doses of even 50–100%."

Therefore, normal variation is observed in medical practice and plasma drug levels may vary among individuals greater than 20%.

According to Westlake (1972), a small, statistically significant difference in drug bioavailability from two or more dosage forms may be detected if the study is well controlled and the number of subjects is sufficiently large. When the therapeutic objectives of the drug are considered, an equivalent clinical response should be obtained from the comparison dosage forms if the plasma drug concentrations remain above the minimum effective concentration (MEC) for an appropriate interval and do not reach the minimum toxic concentration (MTC). Therefore, the investigator must consider whether any statistical difference in bioavailability would alter clinical efficiency.

Special populations, such as the elderly or patients on drug therapy, are generally not used for bioequivalence studies. Normal, healthy volunteers are preferred for bioequivalence studies, because these subjects are less at risk and may more easily endure the discomforts of the study, such as blood sampling. Furthermore, the objective of these studies is to evaluate the bioavailability of the drug from the dosage form, and use of healthy subjects should minimize both inter- and intrasubject variability. It is theoretically possible that the excipients in one of the dosage forms tested may pose a problem in a patient who uses the generic dosage form.

For the manufacture of a dosage form, specifications are set to provide uniformity of dosage forms. With proper specifications, quality control procedures should minimize product-to-product variability by different manufacturers and lot-to-lot variability with a single manufacturer (see Chapter 16).

SPECIAL CONCERNS IN BIOAVAILABILITY AND BIOEQUIVALENCE STUDIES

The general bioequivalence study designs and evaluation, such as the comparison of AUC, C_{max}, and t_{max}, may be used for systemically absorbed drugs and conventional oral dosage forms. However, for certain drugs and dosage forms, systemic bioavailability and bioequivalence are difficult to ascertain (Table 15.12).

TABLE 15.12   Problems in Bioavailability and Bioequivalence

Drugs with high intrasubject variability	Inhalation
Drugs with long elimination half-life	Ophthalmic
Biotransformation of drugs	Intranasal
Stereoselective drug metabolism	Bioavailable drugs that should not produce peak drug
Drugs with active metabolites	levels
Drugs with polymorphic metabolism	Potassium supplements
Nonbioavailable drugs (drugs intended for local effect)	Endogeneous drug levels
Antacids	Hormone replacement therapy
Local anesthetics	Biotechnology-derived drugs
Anti-infectives	Erythropoietin interferon
Anti-inflammatory steroids	Protease inhibitors
Dosage forms for nonoral administration	Complex drug substances
Transdermal	Conjugated estrogens

Drugs and drug products (eg, cyclosporine, chlorpromazine, verapamil, isosorbide dinitrate, sulindac) are considered to be highly variable if the intrasubject variability in bioavailability parameters is greater than 30% by analysis of variance coefficient of variation (Shah et al, 1996). The number of subjects required to demonstrate bioequivalence for these drug products may be excessive, requiring more than 60 subjects to meet current FDA bioequivalence criteria. The intrasubject variability may be due to the drug itself or to the drug formulation or to both. The FDA has held public forums to determine whether the current bioequivalence guidelines need to be changed for these highly variable drugs (Shah et al, 1996).

For drugs with very long elimination half-lives or a complex elimination phase, a complete plasma drug concentration–time curve (ie, three elimination half-lives or an AUC representing 90% of the total AUC) may be difficult to obtain for a bioequivalence study using a crossover design. For these drugs, a truncated (shortened) plasma drug concentration–time curve (0–72 hr) may be more practical. The use of a truncated plasma drug concentration-time curve allows for the measurement of peak absorption and decreases the time and cost for performing the bioequivalence study.

Many drugs are stereoisomers, and each isomer may give a different pharmacodynamic response and may have a different rate of biotransformation. The bioavailability of the individual isomers may be difficult to measure because of problems in analysis. Some drugs have active metabolites, which should be quantitated as well as the parent drug. Drugs such as thioridazine and selegilene have two active metabolites. The question for such drugs is whether bioequivalence should be proven by matching the bioavailability of both metabolites and the parent drug. Assuming both biotransformation pathways follow first-order reaction kinetics, then the metabolites should be in constant ratio to the parent drug. Genetic variation in metabolism may present a bioequivalence problem. For example, the acetylation of procainamide to N-acetylprocainamide demonstrates genetic polymorphism, with two groups of subjects consisting of rapid acetylators and slow acetylators. To decrease intersubject variability, a bioequivalence study may be performed on only one phenotype, such as the rapid acetylators.

Some drugs (eg, benzocaine, hydrocortisone, anti-infectives, antacids) are intended for local effect and formulated as topical ointments, oral suspensions, or rectal suppositories. These drugs should not have significant systemic bioavailability from the site of administration. The bioequivalence determination for drugs that are not absorbed systemically from the site of application can be difficult to assess. For these nonsystemic-absorbable drugs, a "surrogate" marker is needed for bioequivalence determination (Table 15.13). For example, the acid-neutralizing capacity of an oral antacid and the binding of bile acids to cholestyramine resin have been used as surrogate markers in lieu of *in-vivo* bioequivalence studies.

Various drug delivery systems and newer dosage forms are designed to deliver the drug by a nonoral route, which may produce only partial systemic bioavailability. For the treatment of asthma, inhalation of the drug (eg, albuterol, beclomethasone dipropionate) has been used to maximize drug in the respiratory passages and to decrease systemic side effects. Drugs such as nitroglycerin given transdermally may differ in release rates, in the amount of drug in the transdermal delivery system,

TABLE 15.13 *Possible Surrogate Markers for Bioequivalence Studies*

DRUG PRODUCT	DRUG	POSSIBLE SURROGATE MARKER FOR BIOEQUIVALENCE
Metered-dose inhaler	Albuterol	Forced expiratory volume (FEV_1)
Topical steroid	Hydrocortisone	Skin blanching
Anion-exchange resin	Cholestyramine	Binding to bile acids
Antacid	Magnesium and aluminum hydroxide gel	Neutralization of acid
Topical antifungal	Ketoconazole	Drug uptake into stratum corneum

and in the surface area of the skin to which the transdermal delivery system is applied. Thus, the determination of bioequivalence among different manufacturers of transdermal delivery systems for the same active drug is difficult. Dermatokinetics are pharmacokinetic studies that investigate drug uptake into skin layers after topical drug administration. The drug is applied topically, the skin is peeled at various time periods after the dose, using transparent tape, and the drug concentrations are measured in the skin.

Drugs such as potassium supplements are given orally and may not produce the usual bioavailability parameters of AUC, C_{max}, and t_{max}. For these drugs, more indirect methods must be used to ascertain bioequivalence. For example, urinary potassium excretion parameters are more appropriate for the measurement of bioavailability of potassium supplements. However, for certain hormonal replacement drugs (eg, levothyroxine), the steady-state hormone concentration in hypothyroid individuals, the thyroidal-stimulating hormone level, and pharmacodynamic endpoints may also be appropriate to measure.

GENERIC SUBSTITUTION

To contain drug costs, most states have adopted generic substitution laws to allow pharmacists to dispense a generic drug product for a brand-name drug product that has been prescribed. Some states have adopted a *positive formulary*, which lists therapeutically equivalent or interchangeable drug products that pharmacists may dispense. Other states use a *negative formulary*, which lists drug products that are not therapeutically equivalent, and/or the interchange of which is prohibited. If the drug is not in the negative formulary, the unlisted generic drug products are assumed to be therapeutically equivalent and may be interchanged.

Approved Drug Products with Therapeutic Equivalence Evaluations (*Orange Book*)

Due to public demand, the FDA Center for Drug Evaluation and Research publishes annually a listing of approved drug products, *Approved Drug Products with Therapeutic Equivalence Evaluations* (commonly known as the *Orange Book*). The Orange Book is available on the Internet at www.fda.gov/cder/ob/default.htm.

TABLE 15.14   Therapeutic Equivalence Evaluation Codes

A Codes

Drug products considered to be therapeutically equivalent to other pharmaceutically equivalent products

AA	Products in conventional dosage forms not presenting bioequivalence problems
AB	Products meeting bioequivalence requirements
AN	Solutions and powders for aerosolization
AO	Injectable oil solutions
AP	Injectable aqueous solutions
AT	Topical products

B Codes

Drug products that the FDA does not consider to be therapeutically equivalent to other pharmaceutically equivalent products

B*	Drug products requiring further FDA investigation and review to determine therapeutic equivalence
BC	Extended-release tablets, extended-release capsules, and extended-release injectables
BD	Active ingredients and dosage forms with documented bioequivalence problems
BE	Delayed-release oral dosage forms
BN	Products in aerosol–nebulizer drug delivery systems
BP	Active ingredients and dosage forms with potential bioequivalence problems
BR	Suppositories or enemas for systemic use
BS	Products having drug standard deficiencies
BT	Topical products with bioequivalence issues
BX	Insufficient data

Adopted from: *Approved Drug Products with Therapeutic Equivalence Evaluations* (Orange Book) (www.fda.cder/ob/default.htm) 2003.

The Orange Book contains therapeutic equivalence evaluations for approved drug products made by various manufacturers. These marketed drug products are evaluated according to specific criteria. The evaluation codes used for these drugs are listed in Table 15.14. The drug products are divided into two major categories: "A" codes apply to drug products considered to be therapeutically equivalent to other pharmaceutically equivalent products, and "B" codes apply to drug products that the FDA does not at this time consider to be therapeutically equivalent to other pharmaceutically equivalent products. A list of therapeutic-equivalence-related terms and their definitions is also given in the monograph. According to the FDA, evaluations do not mandate that drugs be purchased, prescribed, or dispensed, but provide public information and advice. The FDA evaluation of the drug products should be used as a guide only, with the practitioner exercising professional care and judgment.

The concept of therapeutic equivalence as used to develop the Orange Book applies only to drug products containing the same active ingredient(s) and does not encompass a comparison of different therapeutic agents used for the same condition (eg, propoxyphene hydrochloride versus pentazocine hydrochloride for the treatment of pain). Any drug product in the Orange Book that is repackaged and/or distributed by other than the application holder is considered to be therapeutically equivalent to the application holder's drug product even if the application holder's drug product is single source or coded as nonequivalent (eg, BN). Also, distributors or repackagers of an application holder's drug product are considered to have the same code as the application holder. Therapeutic equivalence determinations are not made for unapproved, off-label indications. With this limitation, however, the FDA believes that products classified as therapeutically equivalent can be substituted with the full expectation that the substituted product will produce the same clinical effect and safety profile as the prescribed product (www.fda.gov/cder/ob/default.htm).

Professional care and judgment should be exercised in using the Orange Book. Evaluations of therapeutic equivalence for prescription drugs are based on scientific and medical evaluations by the FDA. Products evaluated as therapeutically equivalent can be expected, in the judgment of the FDA, to have equivalent clinical effect and no difference in their potential for adverse effects when used under the conditions of their labeling. However, these products may differ in other characteristics such as shape, scoring configuration, release mechanisms, packaging, excipients (including colors, flavors, preservatives), expiration date/time, and, in some instances, labeling. If products with such differences are substituted for each other, there is a potential for patient confusion due to differences in color or shape of tablets, inability to provide a given dose using a partial tablet if the proper scoring configuration is not available, or decreased patient acceptance of certain products because of flavor. There may also be better stability of one product over another under adverse storage conditions, or allergic reactions in rare cases due to a coloring or a preservative ingredient, as well as differences in cost to the patient.

FDA evaluation of therapeutic equivalence in no way relieves practitioners of their professional responsibilities in prescribing and dispensing such products with due care and with appropriate information to individual patients. In those circumstances where the characteristics of a specific product, other than its active ingredient, are important in the therapy of a particular patient, the physician's specification of that product is appropriate. Pharmacists must also be familiar with the expiration dates/times and labeling directions for storage of the different products, particularly for reconstituted products, to assure that patients are properly advised when one product is substituted for another.

 # FREQUENTLY ASKED QUESTIONS

1. Why are preclinical animal toxicology studies and clinical efficacy drug studies in human subjects not required by the FDA to approve a generic drug product as a therapeutic equivalent to the brand-name drug product?

2. What do sequence, washout period, and period mean in a crossover bioavailability study?

3. Why does the FDA require a food intervention (food effect) study for some generic drug products before granting approval? For which drug products are food effect studies required?

4. What type of bioequivalence studies are required for drugs that are not systemically absorbed or for those drugs in which the C_{max} and AUC cannot be measured in the plasma?

5. How does inter- and intrasubject variability affect the statistical demonstration of bioequivalence for a drug product?

6. Can chemically equivalent drug products that are not bioequivalent (ie, bioinequivalent) to each other have similar clinical efficacy?

LEARNING QUESTIONS

1. An antibiotic was formulated into two different oral dosage forms, A and B. Biopharmaceutic studies revealed different antibiotic blood level curves for each drug product (Fig. 15-11). Each drug product was given in the same dose as the other. Explain how the various possible formulation factors could have caused the differences in blood levels. Give examples where possible. How would the corresponding urinary drug excretion curves relate to the plasma level–time curves?

2. Assume that you have just made a new formulation of acetaminophen. Design a protocol to compare your drug product against the acetaminophen drug products on the market. What criteria would you use for proof of bioequivalence for your new formulation? How would you determine if the acetaminophen was completely (100%) systemically absorbed?

3. The data in Table 15.15 represent the average findings in antibiotic plasma samples taken from 10 humans (average weight 70 kg), tabulated in a four-way crossover design.

   a. Which of the four drug products in Table 15.15 would be preferred as a reference standard for the determination of relative bioavailability? Why?

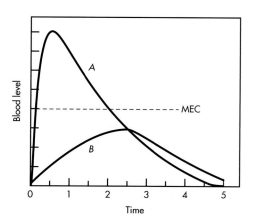

Figure 15-11. Blood-level curves for two different oral dosage forms of a hypothetical antibiotic.

TABLE 15.15 Comparison of Plasma Concentrations of Antibiotic, as Related to Dosage Form and Time

TIME AFTER DOSE (hr)	PLASMA CONCENTRATION (μg/ml)			
	IV Solution (2 mg/kg)	Oral Solution (10 mg/kg)	Oral Tablet (10 mg/kg)	Oral Capsule (10 mg/kg)
0.5	5.94	23.4	13.2	18.7
1.0	5.30	26.6	18.0	21.3
1.5	4.72	25.2	19.0	20.1
2.0	4.21	22.8	18.3	18.2
3.0	3.34	18.2	15.4	14.6
4.0	2.66	14.5	12.5	11.6
6.0	1.68	9.14	7.92	7.31
8.0	1.06	5.77	5.00	4.61
10.0	0.67	3.64	3.16	2.91
12.0	0.42	2.30	1.99	1.83
AUC $\left(\dfrac{\mu g}{mL} \times hr\right)$	29.0	145.0	116.0	116.0

b. From which oral drug product is the drug absorbed more rapidly?

c. What is the absolute bioavailability of the drug from the oral solution?

d. What is the relative bioavailability of the drug from the oral tablet compared to the reference standard?

e. From the data in Table 15.15, determine:

(1) Apparent V_D

(2) Elimination $t_{1/2}$

(3) First-order elimination rate constant k

(4) Total body clearance

f. From the data above, graph the cumulative urinary excretion curves that would correspond to the plasma concentration time curves.

4. Aphrodisia is a new drug manufactured by the Venus Drug Company. When tested in humans, the pharmacokinetics of the drug assume a one-compartment open model with first-order absorption and first-order elimination:

$$D_{GI} \xrightarrow{k_a} D_B V_D \xrightarrow{k}$$

The drug was given in a single oral dose of 250 mg to a group of college students 21–29 years of age. Mean body weight was 60 kg. Samples of blood were obtained at various time intervals after the administration of the drug, and the plasma fractions were analyzed for active drug. The data are summarized in Table 15.16.

a. The minimum effective concentration of Aphrodisia in plasma is 2.3 μg/mL. What is the onset time of this drug?

b. The minimum effective concentration of Aphrodisia in plasma is 2.3 μg/mL. What is the duration of activity of this drug?

TABLE 15.16   Data Summary of Active Drug Concentration in Plasma Fractions

TIME (hr)	C_p (μg/mL)	TIME (hr)	C_p (μg/mL)
0	0	12	3.02
1	1.88	18	1.86
2	3.05	24	1.12
3	3.74	36	0.40
5	4.21	48	0.14
7	4.08	60	0.05
9	3.70	72	0.02

   c. What is the elimination half-life of Aphrodisia in college students?

   d. What is the time for peak drug concentration (t_{max}) of Aphrodisia?

   e. What is the peak drug concentration (C_{max})?

   f. Assuming that the drug is 100% systemically available (ie, fraction of drug absorbed equals unity), what is the AUC for Aphrodisia?

5. You wish to do a bioequivalence study on three different formulations of the same active drug. Lay out a Latin-square design for the proper sequencing of these drug products in six normal, healthy volunteers. What is the main reason for using a crossover design in a bioequivalence study? What is meant by a "random" population?

6. Four different drug products containing the same antibiotic were given to 12 volunteer adult males (age 19–28 years, average weight 73 kg) in a four-way crossover design. The volunteers were fasted for 12 hours prior to taking the drug product. Urine samples were collected up to 72 hours after the administration of the drug to obtain the maximum urinary drug excretion, D_u^∞. The data are presented in Table 15.17.

   a. What is the absolute bioavailability of the drug from the tablet?

   b. What is the relative bioavailability of the capsule compared to the oral solution?

7. According to the prescribing information for cimetidine (Tagamet), following IV or IM administration, 75% of the drug is recovered from the urine after 24 hours as the parent compound. Following a single oral dose, 48% of the drug is recovered from the urine after 24 hours as the parent compound. From this information, determine what fraction of the drug is absorbed systemically from an oral dose after 24 hours.

TABLE 15.17   Urinary Drug Excretion Data Summary

DRUG PRODUCT	DOSE (mg/kg)	CUMULATIVE URINARY DRUG EXCRETION (D_u^∞), 0–72 hr (mg)
IV solution	0.2	20
Oral solution	4	380
Oral tablet	4	340
Oral capsule	4	360

TABLE 15.18   Blood Level Data Summary for Two Drug Products

KINETIC VARIABLE	UNIT	DRUG PRODUCT A 4 × 250-mg Tablet	DRUG PRODUCT B 1000-mg Tablet	STATISTIC
Time for peak drug concentration (range)	hr	1.3 (0.7–1.5)	1.8 (1.5–2.2)	$p < 0.05$
Peak concentration (range)	$\mu g/mL$	53 (46–58)	47 (42–51)	$p < 0.05$
AUC (range)	$\mu g\ hr/mL$	118 (98–125)	103 (90–120)	NS
$t_{1/2}$	hr	3.2 (2.5–3.8)	3.8 (2.9–4.3)	NS

8. Define *bioequivalence requirement*. Why does the FDA require a bioequivalence requirement for the manufacture of a generic drug product?

9. Why can we use the time for peak drug concentration (t_{max}) in a bioequivalence study for an estimate of the rate of drug absorption, rather than calculating the k_a?

10. Ten male volunteers (18–26 years of age) weighing an average of 73 kg were given either 4 tablets each containing 250 mg of drug (drug product A) or 1 tablet containing 1000 mg of drug (drug product B). Blood levels of the drug were obtained and the data are summarized in Table 15.18.

   a. State a possible reason for the difference in the time for peak drug concentration ($t_{max,A}$) after drug product A compared to the $t_{max,B}$ after drug product B. (Assume that all the tablets were made from the same formulation—that is, the drug is in the same particle size, same salt form, same excipients, and same ratio of excipients to active drug.)

   b. Draw a graph relating the cumulative amount of drug excreted in urine of patients given drug product A compared to the cumulative drug excreted in urine after drug product B. Label axes!

   c. In a second study using the same 10 male volunteers, a 125-mg dose of the drug was given by IV bolus and the AUC was computed as 20 µg hr/mL. Calculate the fraction of drug systemically absorbed from drug product B (1 × 1000 mg) tablet using the data in Table 15.19.

11. After performing a bioequivalence test comparing a generic drug product to a brand-name drug product, it was observed that the generic drug product had greater bioavailability than the brand-name drug product.

   a. Would you approve marketing the generic drug product, claiming it was superior to the brand-name drug product?

   b. Would you expect identical pharmacodynamic responses to both drug products?

   c. What therapeutic problem might arise in using the generic drug product that might not occur when using the brand-name drug product?

TABLE 15.19   Disintegration Times and Dissolution Rates of Tolazamide Tablets[a]

TABLET	MEAN DISINTEGRATION TIME[b] MIN (RANGE)	PERCENT DISSOLVED IN 30 MIN[c] (RANGE)
A	3.8 (3.0–4.0)	103.9 (100.5–106.3)
B	2.2 (1.8–2.5)	10.9 (9.3–13.5)
C	2.3 (2.0–2.5)	31.6 (26.4–37.2)
D	26.5 (22.5–30.5)	29.7 (20.8–38.4)

[a] $N = 6$.
[b] By the method of USP-23.
[c] Dissolution rates in pH 7.6 buffer.

From Welling et al (1982), with permission.

12. The following study is from Welling and associates (1982):

Tolazamide Formulations. Four tolazamide tablet formulations were selected for this study. The tablet formulations were labeled A, B, C, and D. Disintegration and dissolution tests were performed by standard USP-23 procedures.

Subjects. Twenty healthy adult male volunteers between the ages of 18 and 38 (mean, 26 years) and weighing between 61.4 and 95.5 kg (mean, 74.5 kg) were selected for the study. The subjects were randomly assigned to 4 groups of 5 each. The four treatments were administered according to 4×4 Latin-square design. Each treatment was separated by 1-week intervals. All subjects fasted overnight before receiving the tolazamide tablet the following morning. The tablet was given with 180 mL of water. Food intake was allowed at 5 hours postdose. Blood samples (10 mL) were taken just before the dose and periodically after dosing. The serum fraction was separated from the blood and analyzed for tolazamide by high-pressure liquid chromatography.

Data Analysis. Serum data were analyzed by a digital computer program using a regression analysis and by the percent of drug unabsorbed by the method of Wagner and Nelson, 1963 (see Chapter 7). AUC was determined by the trapezoidal rule and an analysis of variance was determined by Tukey's method.

a. Why was a Latin-square crossover design used in this study?

b. Why were the subjects fasted before being given the tolazamide tablets?

c. Why did the authors use the Wagner–Nelson method rather than the Loo–Riegelman method for measuring the amount of drug absorbed?

d. From the data in Table 15.20 only, from which tablet formulation would you expect the highest bioavailability? Why?

e. From the data in Table 15.20, did the disintegration times correlate with the dissolution times? Why?

f. Do the data in Table 15.20 appear to correlate with the data in Table 15.19? Why?

g. Draw the expected cumulative urinary excretion–time curve for formulations A and B. Label axes and identify each curve.

h. Assuming formulation A is the reference formulation, what is the relative bioavailability of formulation D?

TABLE 15.20   Mean Tolazamide Concentrations[a] in Serum

TIME (hr)	TREATMENT (μg/mL) A	B	C	D	STATISTIC[b]
0	10.8 ± 7.4	1.3 ± 1.4	1.8 ± 1.9	3.5 ± 2.6	A̅D̅C̅B̅
1	20.5 ± 7.3	2.8 ± 2.8	5.4 ± 4.8	13.5 ± 6.6	A̅D̅C̅B̅
3	23.9 ± 5.3	4.4 ± 4.3	9.8 ± 5.6	20.0 ± 6.4	A̅D̅C̅B̅
4	25.4 ± 5.2	5.7 ± 4.1	13.6 ± 5.3	22.0 ± 5.4	A̅D̅C̅B̅
5	24.1 ± 6.3	6.6 ± 4.0	15.1 ± 4.7	22.6 ± 5.0	A̅D̅C̅B̅
6	19.9 ± 5.9	6.8 ± 3.4	14.3 ± 3.9	19.7 ± 4.7	A̅D̅C̅B̅
8	15.2 ± 5.5	6.6 ± 3.2	12.8 ± 4.1	14.6 ± 4.2	A̅D̅C̅B̅
12	8.8 ± 4.8	5.5 ± 3.2	9.1 ± 4.0	8.5 ± 4.1	C̅A̅D̅B̅
16	5.6 ± 3.8	4.6 ± 3.3	6.4 ± 3.9	5.4 ± 3.1	C̅A̅D̅B̅
24	2.7 ± 2.4	3.1 ± 2.6	3.1 ± 3.3	2.4 ± 1.8	C̅B̅A̅D̅
C_{max}, μg/mL[c]	27.8 ± 5.3	7.7 ± 4.1	16.4 ± 4.4	24.0 ± 4.5	A̅D̅C̅B̅
t_{max}, hr[d]	3.3 ± 0.9	7.0 ± 2.2	5.4 ± 2.0	4.0 ± 0.9	B̅C̅D̅A̅
AUC_{0-24}, μg hr/mL[e]	260 ± 81	112 ± 63	193 ± 70	231 ± 67	A̅D̅C̅B̅

[a]Concentrations $\pm$ 1 SD, $n = 20$.
[b]For explanation see text.
[c]Maximum concentration of tolazamide in serum.
[d]Time of maximum concentration.
[e]Area under the 0–24-hr serum tolazamide concentration curve calculated by trapezoidal rule.

From Welling et al (1982), with permission.

> **i.** Using the data in Table 15.20 for formulation A, calculate the elimination half-life ($t_{1/2}$) for tolazamide.

13. If *in-vitro* drug dissolution and/or release studies for an oral solid dosage form (eg, tablet) does not correlate with the bioavailability of the drug *in-vivo*, why should the pharmaceutical manufacturer continue to perform *in-vitro* release studies for each production batch of the solid dosage form?

14. Is it possible for two pharmaceutically equivalent solid dosage forms containing different inactive ingredients (ie, excipients) to demonstrate bioequivalence *in-vivo* even though these drug products demonstrate differences in drug dissolution tests *in-vitro*?

15. For bioequivalence studies, t_{max}, C_{max}, and AUC, along with an appropriate statistical analyses, are the parameters generally used to demonstrate the bioequivalence of two similar drug products containing the same active drug.

> **a.** Why are the parameters t_{max}, C_{max}, and AUC acceptable for proving that two drug products are bioequivalent?
>
> **b.** Are pharmacokinetic models needed in the evaluation of bioequivalence?
>
> **c.** Is it necessary to use a pharmacokinetic model to completely describe the plasma drug concentration–time curve for the determination of t_{max}, C_{max}, and AUC?
>
> **d.** Why are log-transformed data used for the statistical evaluation of bioequivalence?
>
> **e.** What is an add-on study?

REFERENCES

Amidon, GL, Lennernas H, Shah VP, Crison JR: A theoretical basis for a biopharmaceutic drug classification: The correlation of *in-vitro* drug product dissolution and *in vivo* bioavailability. *Pharm Res* **12:**413–420, 1995

Dighe SV, Adams WP: Bioequivalence: A United States regulatory perspective. In Welling PG, Tse FLS, Dighe SV (eds), *Pharmaceutical Bioequivalence*. New York, Marcel Dekker, 1991, chap 12

FDA Guidance Concerning Demonstration of Comparability of Human Biological Products, Including Therapeutic Biotechnology-Derived Products, April 1996

FDA Guidance for Industry: Bioavailability and Bioequivalence Studies for Orally Administered Drug Products—General Considerations, March 2003

FDA Guidance for Industry: Dissolution Testing of Immediate Release Solid Oral Dosage Forms, August 1997

FDA Guidance for Industry: Statistical Approaches to Establishing Bioequivalence, January 2001

FDA Guidance for Industry: Waiver of In Vivo Bioavailability and Bioequivalence Studies for Immediate Release Solid Oral Dosage Forms Containing Certain Active Moieties/Active Ingredients Based on a Biopharmaceutics Classification System, August 2000

Feldman CH, Hutchinson VE, Sher TH, et al: Interaction between nutrition and theophylline metabolism in children. *Ther Drug Monit* **4:**69–76, 1982

Gardner S: Bioequivalence requirements and *in vivo* bioavailability procedures. *Fed Reg* **42:**1651, 1977

Hendles L, Iafrate RP, Weinberger M: A clinical and pharmacokinetic basis for the selection and use of slow release theophylline products. *Clin Pharmacokinet* **9:**95–135, 1984

Midha KA, Ormsby ED, Hubbard JW, McKay G, Hawes EM, Gavalas, McGilvery IJ: Logarithmic transformation in bioequivalence: Application with two formulations of perphenazine. *J Pharm Sci* **82:**138–144, 1993

Moore JW, Flanner HH: Mathematical comparison of curves with an emphasis on *in vitro* dissolution profiles. *Pharm Tech* **20**(6):64–74, 1996

Mordenti J, Cavagnaro JA, Green JD: Design of biological equivalence programs for therapeutic biotechnology products in clinical development: A perspective. *Pharm Res* **13:**1427–1437, 1996

Polli JE, Rekhi GS, Augsburger LL, Shah VP: Methods to compare dissolution profiles and a rationale for wide dissolution specifications for metoprolol tartrate tablets. *J Pharm Sci* **86**(6):690–700, 1997

Purich E: Bioavailability/bioequivalence regulations: An FDA perspective. In Albert KS (ed), *Drug Absorption and Disposition, Statistical Considerations*. Washington, DC, American Pharmaceutical Association, 1980

Report by the Bioequivalence Task Force 1988 on Recommendations from the Bioequivalence Hearings Conducted by the Food and Drug Administration, Sept 29–Oct 1, 1986. Rockville, MD, FDA, 1988

Schuirmann DJ: A comparison of the two one-sided tests procedure and the power approach for assessing the equivalence of average bioavailability. *J Pharmacokinet Biopharmaceut* **15:**657–680, 1987

Shah P, Yacobi A, Barr WH, Benet LZ, Breimer D, et al: Evaluation of orally administered highly variable drugs and drug formulations. *Pharm Res* **13:**1590–1595, 1996

Wagner JG, Nelson E: Percent absorbed time plots from blood level and for urinary excretion data. *J Pharm Sci* **52:**610–61, 1963

Welling PG, Patel RB, Patel UR, et al: Bioavailability of tolazamide from tablets: Comparison of *in vitro* and *in vivo* results. *J Pharm Sci* **71:**1259–1263, 1982

Westlake WJ: Use of confidence intervals in analysis of comparative bioavailability trials. *J Pharm Sci* **61:**1340–1341, 1972

Yu LX, Amidon GL, Polli JE, Zhao H, Mehta MU, Conner DP, Shah VP, Lesko LJ, Chen ML, Lee VH, Hussain AS: Biopharmaceutics classification system: The scientific basis for biowaiver extensions. *Pharm Res* **19**(7):921–925, 2002

BIBLIOGRAPHY

Abdou HM: *Dissolution, Bioavailability and Bioequivalence*. Easton, PA, Mack, 1989

Bennett RW, Popovitch NG: Statistical inferences as applied to bioavailability data: A guide for the practicing pharmacist. *Am J Hosp Pharm* **34:**712–723, 1977

Chodes DJ, DiSanto AR: *Basics of Bioavailability.* Kalamazoo, MI, Upjohn, 1974

Dighe SV: Biopharmaceutics program. *Clin Res Pract Drug Res Aff* **1:**61–76, 1983

DiSanto AR, Desante KA: Bioavailability and pharmacokinetics of prednisone in humans. *J Pharm Sci* **64:**109–112, 1975

Hendeles L, Wienberger M, Bighley L: Absolute bioavailability of oral theophylline. *Am J Hosp Pharm* **34:**525–527, 1977

Kennedy D: Therapeutically equivalent drugs. *Fed Reg* **44:**2932–2952, 1979

Martin A, Dolusio JT (eds): *Industrial Bioavailability and Pharmacokinetics: Guidelines, Regulations and Controls.* Austin, TX, Austin Drug Dynamics Institute, University of Texas, 1977

Metzler CM: Bioavailability: A problem in equivalence. *Biometrics* **30:**309–317, 1974

Report of the Blue Ribbon Committee on Generic Medicines. Generic Medicines: Restoring Public Confidence. Rockville, MD, FDA, 1990

Schumacher GE: Use of bioavailability data by practitioners, I. Pitfalls in interpreting the data. *Am J Hosp Pharm* **32:**839–842, 1975

Schumacher GE: Interpretation of bioavailability data by practitioners. *J Clin Pharmacol* **16:**554–559, 1976

Wagner JG: An overview of the analysis and interpretation of bioavailability studies in man. *Pharmacology* **8:**102–117, 1972

Welling PG, Tse FLS, Dighe SV (eds): *Pharmaceutical Bioequivalence.* New York, Marcel Dekker, 1991

Westlake WJ: The design and analysis of comparative blood level trials. In Swarbrick J (ed), *Current Concepts in Pharmaceutical Sciences: Dosage Form Design and Bioavailability.* Philadelphia, Lea & Febiger, 1973, chap 5

Westlake WJ: Use of statistical methods in evaluation of *in vivo* performance of dosage forms. *J Pharm Sci* **62:**1579–1589, 1973

16

IMPACT OF DRUG PRODUCT QUALITY AND BIOPHARMACEUTICS ON CLINICAL EFFICACY

RISKS FROM MEDICINES

The U.S. Food and Drug Administration (FDA) Center for Drug Evaluation and Research (CDER) has summarized various types of safety and efficacy risks from medicines (Fig. 16-1). Known side effects are observed adverse events that are identified in the drug's labeling. Side effects from the use of drugs are the major cause of drug related injuries, adverse events, and deaths. Some side effects are avoidable, and others are unavoidable. Avoidable side effects may include known drug–drug or drug–food interactions, contraindications, improper compliance, etc. In many cases, drug therapy requires an individualized drug treatment plan and careful patient monitoring. Some known side effects occur with the best medical practice and even when the drug is used appropriately. Examples include nausea from antibiotics or bone marrow suppression from chemotherapy. Medication errors include wrong drug, wrong dose, or incorrect administration. Some side effects are unavoidable. These uncertainties include unexpected adverse events, side effects due to long-term therapy, and unstudied uses and unstudied populations. For example, a rare adverse event occurring in fewer than 1 in 10,000 persons would not be identified in normal premarket testing.

Product quality defects are an important source of risk that may affect safety and efficacy. Product quality includes strength and purity of the drug substance

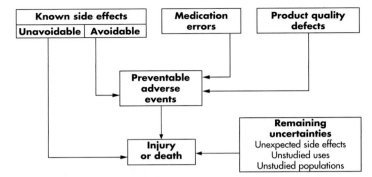

Figure 16-1   Sources of risk from drug products.
(*Source:* FDA, CDER Report to the Nation: 2001.)

and drug product and is also controlled through Good Manufacturing Practices and monitoring of the manufacturing operations. This chapter will focus on drug product quality and risks of product quality defects. Individualization of drug therapy and drug–drug interactions are discussed in later chapters.

Drug Product Quality

Drug product quality relates to the biopharmaceutic and physicochemical properties of the drug substance and the drug product, as discussed in previous chapters. The performance of each drug product must be consistent and predictable to assure both clinical efficacy and safety. Product attributes and performance are critical factors that influence product quality (Table 16.1). Each component of the drug product and the method of manufacture contribute to quality. Quality must be built into the product during research, development, and production. Quality is maintained by implementing systems and procedures that are followed during the development and manufacture of the drug product.

An independent *quality assurance* (QA) unit is a vital part of drug development and manufacture. QA is responsible for ensuring that all the appropriate procedures have been followed and documented. QA provides a high probability that each dose or package of a drug product will have predictable characteristics and perform according to its labeled use. The *quality control* (QC) unit is responsible for the in-process tests beginning from receipt of raw materials, throughout production, finished product, packaging, and distribution.

Principles of quality assurance include: (1) quality, safety, and effectiveness must be designed and built into the product; (2) quality cannot be inspected or tested into the finished product; and (3) each step of the manufacturing process must be

TABLE 16.1   Product Quality and Performance Attributes

Product quality	Chemistry, manufacturing and controls (CMC)
	Microbiology
	Information that pertains to the identity, strength, quality, purity and potency of the drug product
Product performance	Bioavailability and bioequivalence information
	Drug release/dissolution

controlled to maximize the probability that the finished product meets all quality and design specifications.

QA/QC has the responsibility and authority to approve or reject all components, drug product containers, closures, in-process materials, packaging material, labeling, and drug products, and the authority to review production records to assure that no errors have occurred or, if errors have occurred, that they have been fully investigated. QA/QC is responsible for approving or rejecting drug products manufactured, processed, packed, or held under contract by another company.

Good Manufacturing Practices

Good Manufacturing Practices (GMPs) are FDA regulations that describe the methods, equipment, facilities, and controls required for producing human and veterinary products. GMPs define a quality system that manufacturers use to build quality into their products. For example, approved drug products developed and produced according to GMPs are considered safe, properly identified, of the correct strength, pure, and of high quality. The U.S. regulations are called *current* Good Manufacturing Practices (cGMPs), to emphasize that the expectations are dynamic. These regulations are minimum requirements that may be exceeded by the manufacturer. GMPs help prevent inadvertent use or release of unacceptable drug products into manufacturing and distribution. GMP requirements include well-trained personnel and management, buildings and facilities, and written and approved Standard Operating Procedures (SOPs), as listed in Table 16.2.

Guidances for Industry

The FDA publishes guidances for the industry to provide recommendations to pharmaceutical manufacturers for the development and manufacture of drug substances and drug products (www.fda.gov/cder/guidance/index.htm). The International Conference on Harmonisation of Technical Requirements for registration of Pharmaceuticals for Human Use (ICH) is composed of the regulatory authorities of Europe, Japan, and the United States and experts from the pharmaceutical industry. The ICH is interested in the global development and availability of new medicines while maintaining safeguards on quality, safety and efficacy, and regulatory obligations to protect public health (www.ifpma.org/ich1.html).

Quality Standards

Public standards are necessary to assure that drug substances and drug products have consistent and reproducible quality. The *United States Pharmacopeia* National Formulary, USP-NF (www.usp.org), is legally recognized by the U.S. Food, Drug and Cosmetic Act and sets public standards for drug products and drug substances. The USP-NF contains monographs for drug substances and drug products that include standards for strength, quality, and purity. In addition, the USP-NF contains general chapters that describe specific procedures that support the monographs. The tests in the monographs may provide *acceptance criteria*, i.e., numerical limits, ranges, or other criteria for the test for the drug substance or drug product. An

TABLE 16.2   Current Good Manufacturing Practice for Finished Pharmaceuticals

Subpart A—General Provisions
  Scope, Definitions
Subpart B—Organization and Personnel
  Responsibilities of quality control unit, Personnel qualifications,
    Personnel responsibilities, Consultants
Subpart C—Buildings and Facilities
  Design and construction features, Lighting, Ventilation, air filtration, air heating and cooling,
    Plumbing, Sewage and refuse, Washing and toilet facilities, Sanitation, Maintenance
Subpart D—Equipment
  Equipment design, size, and location, Equipment construction, Equipment cleaning and
    maintenance, Automatic, mechanical, and electronic equipment, Filters
Subpart E—Control of Components and Drug Product Containers and Closures
  General requirements, Receipt and storage of untested components, drug product containers, and
    closures, Testing and approval or rejection of components, drug product, containers, and closures,
    Use of approved components, drug product containers, and closures, Retesting of approved
    components, drug product containers, and closures, Rejected components, drug product
    containers, and closures, Drug product containers and closures
Subpart F—Production and Process Controls
  Written procedures; deviations, Charge in of components, Calculation of yield, Equipment
    identification, Sampling and testing of in-process materials and drug products, Time limitations on
    production, Control of microbiological contamination, Reproccessing
Subpart G—Packaging and Labeling Controls
  Materials examination and usage criteria, Labeling issuance, Packaging and labeling operations,
    Tamper-resistant packaging requirements for over-the-counter human drug products, Drug product
    inspection, Expiration dating
Subpart H—Holding and Distribution
  Warehousing procedures, Distribution procedures
Subpart I—Laboratory Controls
  General requirements, Testing and release for distribution, Stability testing, Special testing
    requirements, Reserve samples, Laboratory animals, Penicillin contamination
Subpart J—Records and Reports
  General requirements, Equipment cleaning and use log, Component, drug product, container,
    closure, and labeling records, Master production and control records, Batch production and control
    records, Production record review, Laboratory records.
  Distribution, Complaint files
Subpart K—Returned and Salvaged Drug Products
  Returned drug products, Drug product salvaging

Source: U.S. Code of Federal Regulations (CFR), 21 CFR Part 211.

impurity is defined as any component of the drug substance that is not the entity defined as the drug substance. Drugs with a USP or NF designation that do not conform to the USP monograph may be considered adulterated. *Specifications* are the standards a drug product must meet to ensure conformance to predetermined criteria for consistent and reproducible quality and performance.

RISK MANAGEMENT

Regulatory and Scientific Considerations

The FDA develops rational, science-based regulatory requirements for drug substances and finished drug products. The FDA establishes quality standards and acceptance criteria for each component used in the manufacture of a drug product. Each component must meet an appropriate quality and performance objective.

Drug Manufacturing Requirements

Assurance of product quality is derived from careful attention to a number of factors, including selection of quality parts and materials, adequate product and process design, control of the process, and in-process and end-product testing. Because of the complexity of today's medical products, routine end-product testing alone often is not sufficient to assure product quality. The *Chemistry, Manufacturing Controls* (CMC) section of a Drug Application describes the composition, manufacture, and specifications of the drug substance and drug product (Table 16.3).

Process Validation

Process validation is the process for establishing documented evidence to provide a high degree of assurance that a specific process will consistently produce a product meeting its predetermined specifications and quality characteristics. Process validation is a key element in assuring that these quality assurance goals are met. Proof of validation is obtained through collection and evaluation of data, preferably beginning at the process development phase and continuing through the production phase.

The product's end use should be a determining factor in the development of product (and component) characteristics and specifications. All pertinent aspects

TABLE 16.3 Guideline for the Format and Content of the Chemistry, Manufacturing, and Controls Section of an Application

I. Drug Substance
   A. Description, including physical and chemical characteristics and stability
      1. Name(s)
      2. Structural formula
      3. Physical and chemical characteristics
      4. Elucidation of Structure
      5. Stability
   B. Manufacturer(s)
   C. Method(s) of manufacturer and packaging
      1. Process controls
      2. Container-closure system
   D. Specifications and analytical methods for the drug substance
   E. Solid-state drug substance forms and their relationship to bioavailability
II. Drug Product
   A. Components
   B. Composition
   C. Specifications and analytical methods for inactive components
   D. Manufacturer(s)
   E. Method(s) of manufacture and packaging
      1. Process controls
      2. Container closure system
III. Methods validation package
IV. Environmental assessment

Source: FDA Guidance (1999).

of the product that may affect safety and effectiveness should be considered. These aspects include performance, reliability, and stability. Acceptable ranges or limits should be established for each characteristic to set up allowable variations. *Specifications* are the quality standards (ie, tests, analytical procedures, and acceptance criteria) that confirm the quality of drug substances, drug products, intermediates, raw material reagents, components, in-process material, container closure systems, and other materials used in the production of the drug substance or drug product.

Through careful design and validation of both the process and process controls, a manufacturer can establish with a high degree of confidence that all manufactured units from successive lots will be acceptable. Successfully validating a process may reduce the dependence on intensive in-process and finished product testing. In most cases, end-product testing plays a major role in assuring that quality assurance goals are met; ie, validation and end-product testing are not mutually exclusive.

Drug Recalls and Withdrawals

The FDA coordinates drug recall information and prepares health hazard evaluations to determine the risk to public health by products being recalled. The FDA classifies recall actions in accordance to the level of risk. The FDA and the manufacturer develop recall strategies based on the potential health hazard and other factors, including distribution patterns and market availability. The FDA also determines the need for public warnings and assists the recalling firm with public notification. Table 16.4 lists some of the major reasons for drug recalls.

SCALE-UP AND POSTAPPROVAL CHANGES (SUPAC)

A *postapproval change* is any change in a drug product after it has been approved for marketing by the FDA. A change to a marketed drug product can be initiated for a number of reasons, including a revised market forecast, change in an active pharmaceutical ingredient source, change in excipients, optimization of the manufacturing process, and upgrade of the packaging system. A change within a given parameter can have varied effect on different types of products. For example, a change in the container closure/system of a solid oral dosage form may have little impact for an oral tablet dosage form unless the primary packaging component is critical to the shelf life of the finished product.

TABLE 16.4   *Major Reasons for Drug Recalls*

Failure or inability to validate drug analysis methods
Subpotency
Stability data failing to support expiration date
Failure or inability to validate manufacturing processes
Deviations from good manufacturing practices
Failure of drug to dissolve properly
Labeling mix-ups
Marketed without a new or generic approval
Lack of assurance of sterility
Cross-contamination with other products

If a pharmaceutical manufacturer makes any change in the drug formulation, scales up the formulation to a larger batch size, or changes the process, equipment, or manufacturing site, the manufacturer should consider whether any of these changes will affect the identity, strength, purity, quality, safety, and efficacy of the approved drug product. Moreover, any changes in the raw material (ie, active pharmaceutical ingredient), excipients (including a change in grade or supplier), or packaging (including container closure system) should also be shown not to affect the quality of the drug product. The manufacturer should assess the effect of the change on the identity, strength (eg, assay, content uniformity), quality (eg, physical, chemical, and biological properties), purity (eg, impurities and degradation products), or potency (eg, biological activity, bioavailability, bioequivalence) of a product as they may relate to the safety or effectiveness of the product.

The FDA has published several SUPAC guidances, including *Changes to an Approved NDA or ANDA* (www.fda.gov/cder/guidance/index.htm) for the pharmaceutical industry. These guidances address the following issues:

- Components and composition of the drug product
- Manufacturing site change
- Scale-up of drug product
- Manufacturing equipment
- Manufacturing process
- Packaging
- Active pharmaceutical ingredient

These documents describe (1) the level of change, (2) recommended chemistry, manufacturing and controls tests for each level of change, (3) *in-vitro* dissolution tests and/or bioequivalence tests for each level of change, and (4) documentation that should support the change. The level of change is classified as to the likelihood that a change in the drug product as listed above might affect the quality of the drug product. The levels of change as described by the FDA are listed in Table 16.5.

As noted in Table 16.5, a Level 1 change, which could be a small change in the excipient amount (eg, starch, lactose), would be unlikely to alter the quality or performance of the drug product, whereas a Level 3 change, which may be a qualitative or quantitative change in the excipients beyond an allowable range, particularly for drug products containing a narrow therapeutic window might require an *in-vivo* bioequivalence study to demonstrate that drug quality and performance were not altered by the change.

TABLE 16.5 FDA Definitions of Level of Changes That May Affect the Quality of an Approved Drug Product

CHANGE LEVEL	DEFINITION OF LEVEL
Level 1	Changes that are unlikely to have any detectable impact on the formulation quality and performance.
Level 2	Changes that could have a significant impact on formulation quality and performance.
Level 3	Changes that are likely to have a significant impact on formulation quality and performance.

Assessment of the Effects of the Change

Assessment of the effect of a change should include a determination that the drug substance intermediates, drug substance, in-process materials, and/or drug product affected by the change conform to the approved specifications. A *specification* is a quality standard (ie, tests, analytical procedures, and acceptance criteria) provided in an approved application to confirm the quality of drug substances, drug products, intermediates, raw materials, reagents, and other components, including container closure systems and their components and in-process materials. *Acceptance criteria* are numerical limits, ranges, or other criteria for the tests described. *Conformance* to a specification means that the material, when tested according to the analytical procedures listed in the specification, will meet the listed acceptance criteria. Additional testing may be needed to confirm that the material affected by manufacturing changes continues to meet its specification. The assessment may include, as appropriate, evaluation of any changes in the chemical, physical, microbiological, biological, bioavailability, and/or stability profiles. This additional assessment may involve testing of the postchange drug product itself or, if appropriate, the component directly affected by the change. The type of additional testing depends on the type of manufacturing change, the type of drug substance and/or drug product, and the effect of the change on the quality of the product. Examples of additional tests include:

- Evaluation of changes in the impurity or degradant profile
- Toxicology tests to qualify a new impurity or degradant or to qualify an impurity that is above a previously qualified level
- Evaluation of the hardness or friability of a tablet
- Assessment of the effect of a change on bioequivalence (may include multipoint and/or multimedia dissolution profiles and/or an *in-vivo* bioequivalence study)
- Evaluation of extractables from new packaging components or moisture permeability of a new container closure system

Equivalence

The manufacturer usually assesses the extent to which the manufacturing change has affected the identity, strength, quality, purity, or potency of the drug product by comparing test results from *pre-* and *postchange* material and then determining if the test results are equivalent. The drug product after any changes should be equivalent to the product made before the change. An exception to this general approach is that when bioequivalence should be redocumented for certain Abbreviated New Drug Application (ANDA) postapproval changes, the comparator should be the reference listed drug. Equivalence does not necessarily mean identical. Equivalence may also relate to maintenance of a quality characteristic (eg, stability) rather than a single performance of a test.

Critical Manufacturing Variables

Critical manufacturing variables (CMVs) include changes in the formulation, process, equipment, materials and methods for the drug product that can significantly affect *in-vitro* dissolution. If possible, the manufacturer should determine whether there is a relationship between CMV, *in-vitro* dissolution and *in-vivo* bioavailability. The goal is to develop product specifications that will assure bioequivalence of future batches prepared within limits of acceptable dissolution specifications. One approach to obtaining this relationship is to compare the bioavailability of test products with slowest and fastest dissolution characteristics to the bioavailability of the marketed drug product. Dissolution specifications for the drug product are then established so that future production batches do not fall outside the bioequivalence of the marketed drug product.

Adverse Effect

Sometimes manufacturing changes have an adverse effect on the identity, strength, quality, purity, or potency of the drug product. For example, a type of process change could cause a new degradant to be formed that requires qualification and/or quantification. The manufacturer must show that the new degradant will not affect the safety or efficacy of the product. Changes in the qualitative or quantitative formulation, including inactive ingredients, are considered major changes and are likely to have a significant impact on formulation quality and performance. However, the deletion or reduction of an ingredient intended to affect only the color of a product is considered to be a minor change that is unlikely to affect the safety of the drug product.

Bulk Actives Postapproval Changes (BACPACs)

Manufacturing changes of the *active pharmaceutical ingredient* (API)—also known as the drug substance or bulk active—may change its quality attributes. These quality attributes include chemical purity, solid-state properties, and residual solvents. Chemical purity is dependent on the synthetic pathway and purification process. Solid-state properties include particle size, polymorphism, hydrate/solvate, and solubility. Small amounts of residual solvents such as dichloromethane may remain in the API after extraction and/or purification. Changes in the solid-state properties of the API may affect the manufacture of the dosage form or product performance. For example, a change in particle size may affect API bulk density and tablet hardness, whereas different polymorphs may affect API solubility and stability. Changes in particle size and/or polymorph may affect the drug's bioavailability *in vivo*. Moreover, the excipient(s) and vehicle functionality and possible pharmacologic properties may affect product quality and performance.

 PRACTICAL FOCUS

Quantitative Change in Excipients

A manufacturer would like to increase the amount of starch by 2% (w/w) in an immediate-release drug product. Would you consider this change in an excipient to be a Level 1, 2, or 3 change?

The FDA has determined that small changes in certain excipients for immediate-release drug products may be considered Level 1 changes (see Table 16.5). Table 16.6 lists the changes in excipients, expressed as percentage (w/w) of the total formulation, less than or equal to the following percent ranges that are considered as Level 1 changes. According to this table, a 2% increase in starch would be considered a Level 1 change.

The total additive effect of all excipient changes should not be more than 5%. For example, a drug product containing the active ingredient lactose, mirocrystalline cellulose, and magnesium stearate, the lactose and microcrystalline cellulose should not vary by more than an absolute total of 5% (eg, lactose increases 2.5% and microcrystalline cellulose decreases by 2.5%) relative to the target dosage form weight if it is to stay within the Level 1 range.

It should be noted that a small change in the amount of excipients is less likely to affect the bioavailability of a highly soluble, highly permeable drug in an immediate-release drug product compared to a drug that has low soluble and low permeability.

Changes in Batch Size (Scale-up/Scale-down)

For commercial reasons, a manufacturer may increase the batch size of a drug product from 100,000 units to 5 million units. Even though similar equipment is used and the same Standard Operating Procedures (SOPs) are used, there may be problems in manufacturing a very large batch. This problem is similar to a chef's problem of cooking the main entrée for two persons versus cooking the same entrée for a banquet of 200 persons using the same recipe. The FDA has generally considered that a change in batch size greater than 10-fold is a Level 2 change and requires the manufacturer to notify the FDA and provide documentation for all testing before marketing this product.

TABLE 16.6 Level 1—Allowable Changes in Excipients

EXCIPIENT	PERCENT EXCIPIENT (W/W) OUT OF TOTAL TARGET DOSAGE FORM WEIGHT
Filler	±5
Disintegrant	
Starch	±3
Other	±1
Binder	±0.5
Lubricant	
Calcium stearate	±0.25
Magnesium stearate	±0.25
Other	±1
Glidant	
Talc	±1
Other	±0.1
Film coat	±1

These percentages are based on the assumption that the drug substance in the product is formulated to 100% of label/potency.

Source: FDA Guidance: Immediate release solid oral dosage forms: Scale-up and postapproval changes (1995).

TABLE 16.7   Quality Attributes and Criteria for Certain Approved Drug Substances and Drug Products

DRUG SUBSTANCES		DRUG PRODUCTS	
Attribute	**Criteria**	**Attribute**	**Criteria**
Chemical structure	Well characterized	Dosage form	Oral (immediate release), simple solutions, others
Synthetic process	Simple process		
Quality	No toxic impurities; adequate specifications	Manufacturing process	Easy to manufacture (TBD)
		Quality	Adequate specifications
Physical properties	Polymorphic forms, particle size are well controlled	Biopharmaceutic Classification Systems (BCS)	Highly permeable and highly soluble drugs
Stability	Stable drug substance	Stability	Stable drug product (TBD)
Manufacturing history	TBD		
Others	TBD	Manufacturing history	TBD
		Others	TBD

TBD, to be defined.

Adopted from Yuan-yuan Chui, CMC Initiative: Risk-based CMC reviews, *PhRMA-Dialog*, October 27, 2000 (http://www.fda.gov/cder/ondc/).

PRODUCT QUALITY PROBLEMS

The FDA and industry are working together to establish a set of quality attributes and acceptance criteria for certain approved drug substances and drug products that would indicate less manufacturing risk. Table 16.7 summarizes some of the quality attributes for these products. However, all approved drug products must be manufactured under current Good Manufacturing Practices.

Drug substances and drug products that have more quality risk are generally those products that are more complex to synthesize or manufacture (Fig. 16-2). For example, biotechnology-derived drugs (eg, proteins) made by fermentation may have more quality risk than chemically synthesized small molecules. Extended-release and delayed-release drug products may also present a greater quality risk

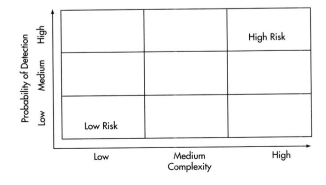

Figure 16-2 General principles to define low-risk drugs.
(*Source:* Adapted from Yuan-yuan Chui, Risk based CMC review, Advisory Committee for Pharmaceutical Sciences, FDA, October 21, 2002.)

than an immediate-release drug product. Drug products that have a very small ratio of active drug substance to excipients are more difficult to blend uniformly and thus may have a greater quality risk. Good Manufacturing Practices and control of the critical manufacturing operations help maintain the quality of the finished product. Complex operations can have consistent outcome quality as long as the manufacturer maintains control of the process and builds in quality during the manufacturing operations.

 PRACTICAL FOCUS

BSE in Gelatin

Gelatin may be produced from bones and hides obtained from cattle. In the early 1990s, the FDA became concerned about transmissible spongiform encephalopathies (TSEs) in animals and Creutzfeldt-Jakob disease in humans. In 1993, the FDA recommended against the use of materials from cattle that had resided in, or originated from, countries in which *bovine spongiform encephalopathy* (BSE, or "mad cow disease") had occurred. The FDA organized a Transmissible Spongiform Encephalopathies Advisory Committee to help assess the safety of imported and domestic gelatin and gelatin by-products in FDA-regulated products with regard to the risk posed by BSE. The FDA published a Guidance to industry concerning the sourcing and processing of gelatin used in pharmaceutical products to assure the safety of gelatin as it relates to the potential risk posed by BSE (www.fda.gov/opacom/morechoices/industry/guidance/gelguide.htm).

Gelatin Capsules Stability

Soft and hard gelatin capsules show a decrease in the dissolution rate over time in simulated gastric fluid (SGF) with and without pepsin or in simulated intestinal fluid (SIF) without pancreatin. This has been attributed to pellicle formation. When the dissolution of aged or slower-releasing capsules was carried out in the presence of an enzyme (pepsin in SGF or pancreatin in SIF), a significant increase in dissolution was observed. In this setting, multiple dissolution media may be necessary to assess product quality adequately.

Excipient Effects

Excipients can sometimes affect the rate and extent of drug absorption. In general, using excipients that are currently in FDA-approved immediate-release solid oral dosage forms will not affect the rate or extent of absorption of a highly soluble and highly permeable drug substance that is formulated in a rapidly dissolving immediate-release product.

When new excipients or atypically large amounts of commonly used excipients are included in an immediate solid dosage form, additional information documenting the absence of an impact on bioavailability of the drug may be requested by the FDA. Such information can be provided with a relative bioavailability study using a simple aqueous solution as the reference product. Large quantities of certain excipients, such as surfactants (eg, polysorbate 80) and sweeteners (eg, mannitol or sorbitol) may be problematic.

POSTMARKETING SURVEILLANCE

Pharmaceutical manufacturers are required to file periodic Post-Market Reports for an approved ANDA to the FDA through its *Postmarketing Surveillance Program.* The main component of the requirement is the reporting of adverse drug experiences. This is accomplished by reassessing drug risks based on data learned after the drug is marketed. In addition, labeling changes may occur after market approval. For example, a new adverse reaction discussed by postmarketing surveillance is required for both branded and generic drug products.

FREQUENTLY ASKED QUESTIONS

1. Three batches of ibuprofen tablets, 200 mg, are manufactured by the same manufacturer using the same equipment. Each batch meets the same specifications. Does meeting specifications mean that each batch of drug product contains the identical amount of ibuprofen?

2. What should a manufacturer of a modified-release tablet consider when making a qualitative or quantitative change in an excipient?

LEARNING QUESTIONS

1. For solid oral drug products, a change in the concentration of which the following excipients is more likely to influence the bioavailability of a drug? Why?

   Starch
   Magnesium stearate
   Microcrystalline cellulose
   Talc
   Lactose

2. How does the polymorphic form of the active drug substance influence the bioavailability of a drug? Can two different polymorphs of the same active drug substance have the same bioavailability?

REFERENCES

CMC Initiative: Risk-based CMC Reviews, PhRMA-Dialog, Oct 27, 2000 (www. fda.gov/cder/ondc/

FDA, CDER Report to the Nation: 2001 (www.fda.gov/cder/reports/rtn/2001/rtn2001-3.htm)

FDA Guidance for Industry: Changes to an Approved NDA or ANDA, FDA/CDER, November 1999 (www.fda.gov/cder/guidance/index.htm)

Risk-Based CMC Review; Advisory Committee for Pharmaceutical Sciences, FDA, Oct 21, 2002

17

MODIFIED-RELEASE DRUG PRODUCTS

Most conventional oral drug products, such as tablets and capsules, are formulated to release the active drug immediately after oral administration, to obtain rapid and complete systemic drug absorption. Such *immediate-release products* result in relatively rapid drug absorption and onset of accompanying pharmacodynamic effects. However, after absorption of the drug from the dosage form is complete, plasma drug concentrations decline according to the drug's pharmacokinetic profile. Eventually, plasma drug concentrations fall below the minimum effective plasma concentration (MEC), resulting in loss of therapeutic activity. Before this point is reached, another dose is usually given if a sustained therapeutic effect is desired. An alternative to administering another dose is to use a dosage form that will provide sustained drug release, and therefore maintain plasma drug concentrations, beyond what is typically seen using immediate-release dosage forms. In recent years, various modified-release drug products have been developed to control the release rate of the drug and/or the time for drug release.

The term *modified-release drug product* is used to describe products that alter the timing and/or the rate of release of the drug substance. A modified-release dosage form is defined "as one for which the drug-release characteristics of time course and/or location are chosen to accomplish therapeutic or convenience objectives not offered by conventional dosage forms such as solutions, ointments, or promptly dissolving dosage forms as presently recognized" (USP Subcommittee on Biopharmaceutics, 1988). Several types of modified-release drug products are recognized:

1. *Extended-release drug products.* A dosage form that allows at least a twofold reduction in dosage frequency as compared to that drug presented as an immediate-release (conventional) dosage form. Examples of extended-release dosage forms include controlled-release, sustained-release, and long-acting drug products.
2. *Delayed-release drug products.* A dosage form that releases a discrete portion or portions of drug at a time or at times other than promptly after administration, although one portion may be released promptly after administration. Enteric-coated dosage forms are the most common delayed-release products.

515

3. *Targeted-release drug products.* A dosage form that releases drug at or near the intended physiologic site of action. Targeted-release dosage forms may have either immediate- or extended-release characteristics.

The term *controlled-release drug product* was previously used to describe various types of oral extended-release-rate dosage forms, including sustained-release, sustained-action, prolonged-action, long-action, slow-release, and programmed drug delivery. Other terms, such as ER, SR, XL, XR, and CD, are also used to indicate an extended-release drug product. Many of these terms for modified-release drug products were introduced by drug companies to reflect either a special design for an extended-release drug product or for use as a marketing term.

Modified-release drug products are designed for different routes of administration based on the physicochemical, pharmacologic, and pharmacokinetic properties of the drug and on the properties of the materials used in the dosage form (Table 17.1). Several different terms are now defined to describe the available types of modified-release drug products based on the drug release characteristics of the products.

EXAMPLES OF MODIFIED-RELEASE ORAL DOSAGE FORMS

An enteric-coated tablet is an example of a delayed-release type of modified-release dosage form designed to release drug in the small intestine. For example, aspirin irritates the gastric mucosal cells of the stomach. An enteric coating on the aspirin tablet prevents the tablet from dissolving and releasing its contents at the low pH in the stomach. The coating and the tablet later dissolve and release the drug in the higher pH of the duodenum, where the drug is rapidly absorbed with less irritation to the mucosal cells. Mesalamine (5-aminosalicylic acid) tablets (Asacol, Proctor & Gamble) is a delayed-release tablet coated with an acrylic-based resin that delays the release of mesalamine until it reaches the terminal ileum and colon. Mesalamine tablets could also be considered a targeted-release dosage form.

Various other unofficial terms are used to describe modified-release drug products. A *repeat-action tablet* is a type of modified-release drug product that is designed to release one dose of drug initially, followed by a second dose of drug at a later time. A *prolonged-action drug product* is designed to release the drug slowly and to provide a continuous supply of drug over an extended period. The prolonged-action drug product prevents very rapid absorption of the drug, which could result in extremely high peak plasma drug concentration. Most prolonged-release products extend the duration of action but do not release drug at a constant rate. A *sustained-release drug product* can be designed to deliver an initial therapeutic dose of the drug (loading dose), followed by a slower and constant release of drug. The rate of release of the maintenance dose is designed so that the amount of drug loss from the body by elimination is constantly replaced. With the sustained-release product, a constant plasma drug concentration is maintained with minimal fluctuations. Figure 17-1 shows the dissolution rate of three sustained-release products without loading dose. The plasma concentrations resulting from the sustained-release products are shown in Figure 17-2.

A prolonged-action tablet is similar to a first-order-release product except that the peak is delayed differently. A prolonged-action tablet typically results in peak

TABLE 17.1 Modified Drug Delivery

ROUTE OF ADMINISTRATION	DRUG PRODUCT	EXAMPLES	COMMENTS
Oral drug products	Extended release	Diltiazem HCl extended release	Once-a-day dosing.
	Delayed release	Diclofenac sodium delayed-release	Enteric-coated tablet for drug delivery into small intestine.
		Mesalamine delayed-release	Coated for drug release in terminal ileum.
	Oral mucosal drug delivery	Oral transmucosal fentanyl citrate	Fentanyl citrate is in the form of a flavored sugar lozenge that dissolves slowly in the mouth.
Transdermal drug delivery systems	Transdermal therapeutic system (TTS)	Clonidine transdermal therapeutic system	Clonidine TTS is applied every 7 days to intact skin on the upper arm or chest.
	Iontophoretic drug delivery		Small electric current moves charged molecules across the skin.
Ophthalmic drug delivery	Insert	Controlled-release pilocarpine	Elliptically shaped insert designed for continuous release of pilocarpine following placement in the cul-de-sac of the eye.
Intravaginal drug delivery	Insert	Dinoprostone vaginal insert	Hydrogel pouch containing prostaglandin within a polyester retrieval system.
Parenteral drug delivery	Intramuscular drug products	Depot injections	Lyophylized microspheres containing leuprolide acetate for depot suspension.
		Water-immiscible injections (eg, oil)	Medroxyprogesterone acetate (Depo-Provera®)
	Subcutaneous drug products	Controlled-release insulin	Basulin is a controlled-release, recombinant human insulin delivered by nanoparticulate technology.
Targeted delivery systems	IV injection	Daunorubicin citrate liposome injection	Liposomal preparation to maximize the selectivity of daunorubicin for solid tumors *in situ*.
Implants	Brain tumor	Polifeprosan 20 with carmustine implant (Gliadel wafer)	Implant designed to deliver carmustine directly into the surgical cavity when a brain tumor is resected.

and trough drug levels in the body. The product releases drug without matching the rate of drug elimination, resulting in uneven plasma drug levels in the body.

The use of these various terms for extended-release drug products does not mean that the drug is released at a constant or zero-order drug release rate. Many of these drug products release the drug at a first-order rate. Some modified-release

Figure 17-1. Drug dissolution rates of three different extended-release products *in vitro*.

Figure 17-2. Simulated plasma–drug concentrations resulting from three different sustained-release products in Figure 17.1

drug products are formulated with materials that are more soluble at a specific pH, and the product may release the drug depending on the pH of a particular region of the gastrointestinal (GI) tract. Ideally, an extended-release drug product should release the drug at a constant rate, independent of both the pH and the ionic content within the entire segment of the gastrointestinal tract.

An extended-release dosage form with zero- or first-order drug absorption is compared to drug absorption from a conventional dosage form given in multiple doses in Figures 17-3 and 17-4, respectively. Drug absorption from conventional (immediate-release) dosage forms generally follows first-order drug absorption.

BIOPHARMACEUTIC FACTORS

The major objective of an extended-release drug product is to achieve a prolonged therapeutic effect while minimizing unwanted side effects due to fluctuating plasma drug levels. Ideally, the extended-release drug product should release the drug at

Figure 17-3. Plasma level of a drug from a conventional tablet containing 50 mg of drug given at 0, 4, and 8 hours (A) compared to a single 150-mg drug dose given in an extended-release dosage form (B). The drug absorption rate constant from each drug product is first order. The drug is 100% bioavailable and the elimination half-life is constant.

Figure 17-4. Bioavailability of a drug from an immediate-release tablet containing 50 mg of drug given at 0, 4, and 8 hours compared to a single 150-mg drug dose given in an extended-release dosage form. The drug absorption rate constant from the immediate-release drug product is first order, whereas the drug absorption rate constant from the extended-release drug product is zero order. The drug is 100% bioavailable and the elimination half-life is constant.

a constant, or zero-order, rate. After release from the drug product, the drug is rapidly absorbed, and the drug absorption rate should follow zero-order kinetics similar to an intravenous drug infusion. In all cases, the drug product is designed so that the rate of systemic drug absorption is limited by the rate of drug release via the drug delivery system. Unfortunately, most extended-release drug products that release a drug by zero-order kinetics *in vitro* do not demonstrate zero-order drug absorption when given *in vivo*. The lack of zero-order drug absorption from these extended-release drug products after oral administration may be due to a number of unpredictable events happening in the gastrointestinal tract during absorption.

Extended-release oral drug products remain in the GI tract longer than conventional, immediate-release drug products intended for rapid absorption. Thus, drug release from an extended-release drug product is more affected by the anatomy and physiology of the gastrointestinal tract and its contents compared to an immediate-release oral drug product. The physiologic characteristics of the GI tract, such as variations in pH, blood flow, GI motility, presence of food, enzymes, bacteria, etc, affects the position of the extended-release drug product within the GI tract and may affect the drug release rate from the product. In some cases, there may be a specific absorption site or location within the GI tract in which the extended-release drug product should release the drug.

Stomach

The stomach is a "mixing and secreting" organ, where food is mixed with digestive juices and emptied periodically into the small intestine. However, the movement of food or drug product in the stomach and small intestine is very different depending on the physiologic state. In the presence of food, the stomach is in the *digestive phase*; in the absence of food, the stomach is in the *interdigestive phase* (Chapter 13). During the digestive phase, the food particles or solids larger than 2 mm are retained in the stomach, whereas smaller particles are emptied through the pyloric sphincter at a first-order rate depending on the content and size of the meals. During the interdigestive phase, the stomach rests for a period of up to 30 to 40 minutes, coordinated with an equal resting period in the small intestine. Peristaltic contractions then occur, which ends with strong *housekeeper contractions* that move everything in the stomach through to the small intestine. Similarly, large particles in the small intestine are moved along only in the housekeeper contraction period.

A drug may remain for several hours in the stomach if it is administered during the digestive phase. Fatty material, nutrients, and osmolality may further extend the time the drug stays in the stomach. When the drug is administered during the interdigestive phase, the drug may be swept along rapidly into the small intestine. Dissolution of drugs in the stomach may also be affected by the presence or absence of food. When food is present, HCl is secreted and the pH is about 1–2. Although some food and nutrients can neutralize the acid and raise stomach pH, the fasting pH of the stomach is about 3–5. The release rates of some drugs are affected by food. For example, the extended-release drug product Theo-24 was shown to release drug at a higher rate in the presence of food (Chapter 13). Whether this more rapid drug release rate is related to a change in pH, the stomach-emptying rate, or a food–drug interaction is not known. A longer time of retention in the stomach may expose the drug to stronger agitation in the acid environment. The stomach has been described as having "jet mixing" action, which sends mixture at up to 50 mm Hg pressure toward the pyloric sphincter, causing it to open and periodically release chyme to the small intestine.

Small Intestine and Transit Time

The small intestine is about 10 to 14 feet in length. The duodenum is sterile, while the terminal part of the small intestine that connects the cecum contains some bacteria. The proximal part of the small intestine has a pH of about 6, because of neutralization of acid by bicarbonates secreted by the duodenal mucosa and the pancreas. The small intestine provides an enormous surface area for drug absorption because of the presence of microvilli. The small-intestine transit time of a solid preparation has been concluded to be about 3 hours or less in 95% of the population (Hofmann et al, 1983). Transit time for meals from mouth to cecum (beginning of large intestine) has been reviewed by Shareef et al, 2003. Various investigators have used the lactulose hydrogen test, which measures the appearance of hydrogen in a patient's breath, to estimate transit time. Lactulose is metabolized rapidly by bacteria in the large intestine, yielding hydrogen that is exhaled. Hydrogen is normally absent in a person's breath. These results and the use of gamma-scintigraphy studies confirm a relatively short GI transit time from mouth to cecum of 4 to 6 hours.

This transit time interval was concluded to be too short for extended-release dosage forms that last up to 12 hours, unless the drug is to be absorbed in the colon. The colon has little fluid and the abundance of bacteria may make drug absorption erratic and incomplete. The transit time for pellets has been studied in both disintegrating and nondisintegrating forms using both insoluble and soluble radiopaques. Most of the insoluble pellets were released from the capsule within 15 minutes. Scattering of pellets were seen in the stomach and along the entire length of the small intestine at 3 hours. At 12 hours most of the pellets were in the ascending colon, and at 24 hours the pellets were all in the descending colon, ready to enter the rectum. With the disintegrating pellets, there was more scattering of the pellets along the GI tract. The pellets also varied widely in their rate of disintegration *in vivo* (Galeone et al, 1981).

Large Intestine

The large intestine is about 4 to 5 feet long. It consists of the cecum, the ascending and descending colons, and eventually ends at the rectum. Little fluid is in the colon, and drug transit is slow. Not much is known about drug absorption in this area, although unabsorbed drug that reaches this region may be metabolized by bacteria. Incompletely absorbed antibiotics may affect the normal flora of the bacteria. The rectum has a pH of about 6.8–7.0 and contains more fluid compared to the colon. Drugs are absorbed rapidly when administered as rectal preparations. However, the transit rate through the rectum is affected by the rate of defecation. Presumably, drugs formulated for 24 hours' duration must remain in this region to be absorbed.

Several extended-release and delayed-release drug products, such as mesalamine delayed-release tablets (Asacol), are formulated to take advantage of the physiologic conditions of the GI tract (Shareef et al, 2003). Enteric-coated beads have been found to release drug over 8 hours when taken with food, because of the gradual emptying of the beads into the small intestine. Specially formulated "floating tablets" that remain in the top of the stomach have been used to extend the residence time of the product in the stomach. None of these methods, however, is consistent enough to perform reliably for potent medications. More experimental research is needed in this area.

DOSAGE FORM SELECTION

The properties of the drug and required dosage are important in formulating an extended-release product. For example, a drug with low aqueous solubility generally should not be formulated into a nondisintegrating tablet, because the risk of incomplete drug dissolution is high. Instead, a drug with low solubility at neutral pH should be formulated, so that most of the drug is released before it reaches the colon, since the lack of fluid in the colon may make complete dissolution difficult. Erosion tablets are more reliable for these drugs because the entire tablet eventually dissolves.

A drug that is highly water soluble in the acid pH in the stomach but very insoluble at intestinal pH may be very difficult to formulate into an extended-release product. Too much coating protection may result in low bioavailability, while too little protection may result in dose dumping in the stomach. A moderate extension of duration with enteric-coated beads may be possible. However, the risk of erratic performance is higher than with a conventional dosage form. The osmotic type of controlled system may be more suitable for this type of drug.

In addition, with most single-unit dosage forms, there is a risk of erratic performance due to variable stomach emptying and GI transit time. Selection of a pellet or bead dosage form may minimize the risk of erratic stomach emptying, because pellets are usually scattered soon after ingestion. Disintegrating tablets have the same advantages because they break up into small particles soon after ingestion.

ADVANTAGES AND DISADVANTAGES OF EXTENDED-RELEASE PRODUCTS

Extended-release drug products offer several important advantages over immediate-release dosage forms of the same drug. Extended release allows for sustained therapeutic blood levels of the drug; sustained blood levels provide for a prolonged and consistent clinical response in the patient. Moreover, if the drug input rate is constant, the blood levels should not fluctuate between a maximum and minimum, as in a multiple-dose regimen with an immediate-release drug product (Chapter 8). Highly fluctuating blood concentrations of drug may produce unwanted side effects in the patient if the drug level is too high, or may fail to exert the proper therapeutic effect if the drug level is too low. Another advantage of extended release is patient convenience, which leads to better patient compliance. For example, if the patient needs to take the medication only once daily, he or she will not have to remember to take additional doses at specified times during the day. Furthermore, because the dosage interval is longer, the patient's sleep may not be interrupted to take another drug dose. With the longer-available dose, the patient awakes without having subtherapeutic drug levels. The patient may also derive an economic benefit in using a extended-release drug product. A single dose of an extended-release product may cost less than an equivalent drug dose given several times a day in rapid-release tablets. For patients under nursing care, the cost of nursing time required to administer medication is decreased if only one drug dose is given to the patient each day.

For some drugs which have long elimination half-lives, such as chlorpheniramine, the inherent duration of pharmacologic activity is long. Moreover, minimal fluctuations in blood concentrations of these drugs are observed after multiple doses are administered. Therefore, there is no rationale for extended-release formulations of these drugs. However, such drug products are marketed with the justification that extended-release products minimize toxicity, decrease adverse reactions, and provide patients with more convenience and, thus, better compliance. In contrast, drugs with very short half-lives need to be given at frequent dosing intervals to maintain therapeutic efficacy. For drugs with very short elimination half-lives, an extended-release drug product maintains the efficacy over a longer duration.

There are also a number of disadvantages in using extended-release medication. If the patient suffers from an adverse drug reaction or accidentally becomes intoxicated, the removal of drug from the system is more difficult with an extended-release drug product. Orally administered extended-release drug products may yield erratic or variable drug absorption as a result of various drug interactions with the contents of the GI tract and changes in GI motility. The formulation of extended-release drug products may not be practical for drugs that are usually given in large doses (e.g., 500 mg) in conventional dosage forms. Because the extended-release drug product may contain two or more times the dose given at more frequent intervals, the size of the extended-release drug product may have to be quite large, too large for the patient to swallow easily.

The extended-release dosage form contains the equivalent of two or more drug doses given in a conventional dosage form. Therefore, failure of the extended-release dosage form may lead to dose dumping. *Dose dumping* can be defined either as the release of more than the usual fraction of drug or as the release of drug at a greater rate than the customary amount of drug per dosage interval, such that potentially adverse plasma levels may be reached (Dighe and Adams, 1988; Skelly and Barr, 1987). With delayed release or enteric drug products, two possible problems may occur if the enteric coating is poorly formulated. First, the enteric coating may become degraded in the stomach, allowing for early release of the drug, possibly causing irritation to the gastric mucosal lining. Second, the enteric coating may fail to dissolve at the proper site, and therefore the tablet may be lost prior to drug release, resulting in incomplete absorption.

In recent years, pharmaceutical manufacturers have made new extended-release drug products of branded drugs that are losing patent protection. Although these extended-release drug products may have some of the advantages stated above, the cost of the medication may be much higher than that of the generic drug in a conventional drug product given several times a day.

KINETICS OF EXTENDED-RELEASE DOSAGE FORMS

The amount of drug required in an extended-release dosage form to provide a sustained drug level in the body is determined by the pharmacokinetics of the drug, the desired therapeutic level of the drug, and the intended duration of action. In general, the total dose required (D_{tot}) is the sum of the maintenance dose (D_m) and the initial dose (D_I) released immediately to provide a therapeutic blood level.

$$D_{tot} = D_I + D_m \tag{17.1}$$

In practice, D_m (mg) is released over a period of time and is equal to the product of t_d (the duration of drug release) and the zero-order rate k_r^0 (mg/hr). Therefore, Equation 17.1 can be expressed as

$$D_{tot} = D_I + k_r^0 t_d \tag{17.2}$$

Ideally, the maintenance dose (D_m) is released after D_I has produced a blood level equal to the therapeutic drug level (C_p). However, due to the limits of formulations, D_m actually starts to release at $t = 0$. Therefore, D_I may be reduced from the calculated amount to avoid "topping." (Figure 17.8)

$$D_{tot} = D_I - k_r^0 t_p + k_r^0 t_d \tag{17.3}$$

Equation 17.3 describes the total dose of drug needed, with t_p representing the time needed to reach peak drug concentration after the initial dose.

For a drug that follows a one-compartment open model, the rate of elimination (R) needed to maintain the drug at a therapeutic level (C_p) is

$$R = kV_D C_p \tag{17.4}$$

where k_r^0 must be equal to R in order to provide a stable blood level of the drug. Equation 17.4 provides an estimation of the release rate (k_r^0) required in the formulation. Equation 17.4 may also be written as

$$R = C_p Cl_T \tag{17.5}$$

where Cl_T is the clearance of the drug. In designing an extended-release product, D_I would be the loading dose that would raise the drug concentration in the body to C_p, and the total dose needed to maintain therapeutic concentration in the body would be simply

$$D_{tot} = D_I + C_p Cl_T \tau \tag{17.6}$$

For many sustained-release drug products, there is no built-in loading dose (ie, $D_I = 0$). The dose needed to maintain a therapeutic concentration for τ hours is

$$D_0 = C_p \tau Cl_T \tag{17.7}$$

where τ is the dosing interval.

EXAMPLE

What dose is needed to maintain a therapeutic concentration of 10 μg/mL for 12 hours in a sustained-release product? (**a**) Assume that $t_{1/2}$ for the drug is 3.46 hours and V_D is 10 L. (**b**) Assume that $t_{1/2}$ of the drug is 1.73 hours and V_D is 5 L.

a. $k = \dfrac{0.693}{3.46} = 0.2/\text{hr}$

$Cl_T = kV_D = 0.2 \times 10 = 2 \text{ L/hr}$

From Equation 17.7,

$$D_0 = (10 \ \mu\text{g/mL})(1000 \ \text{mL/L})(12 \ \text{hr})(2 \ \text{L/hr}) = 240{,}000 \ \mu\text{g} \quad \text{or} \quad 240 \ \text{mg}$$

b. $k = \dfrac{0.693}{1.73} = 0.4 \text{ hr}$

$Cl_T = 0.4 \times 5 = 2 \text{ L/hr}$

From Equation 17.8,

$$D_0 = 10 \times 2 \times 1000 \times 12 = 240{,}000 \ \mu\text{g} \quad \text{or} \quad 240 \ \text{mg}$$

In this example, the amount of drug needed in a sustained-release product to maintain therapeutic drug concentration is dependent on both V_D and the elimination half-life. In part **b** of the example, although the elimination half-life is shorter, the volume of distribution is also smaller. If the volume of distribution is constant, then the amount of drug needed to maintain C_p is dependent simply on the elimination half-life.

Table 17.2 shows the influence of $t_{1/2}$ on the amount of drug needed for an extended-release drug product. Table 17.2 was constructed by assuming that the drug has a desired serum concentration of 5 μg/mL and an apparent volume of distribution of 20,000 mL. The release rate R decreases as the elimination half-life increases. Because elimination is slower for a drug with a long half-life, the input rate should be slower. The total amount of drug needed in the extended-release drug product is dependent on both the release rate R and the desired duration of activity for the drug. For a drug with an elimination half-life of 4 hours and a release rate of 17.3 mg/hr, the extended-release product must contain 207.6 mg to provide a duration of activity of 12 hours. The bulk weight of the extended-release product will be greater than this amount, due to the presence of excipients needed in the formulation. The values in Table 17.2 show that, in order to achieve a long duration of activity ($\geq$12 hours) for a drug with a very short half-life (1–2 hours), the extended-release drug product becomes quite large and impractical for most patients to swallow.

TABLE 17.2 Release Rates for Extended-Release Drug Products as a Function of Elimination Half-Life[a]

$t_{1/2}$ (hr)	k (hr^{-1})	R (mg/hr)	TOTAL (mg) TO ACHIEVE DURATION			
			6 hr	8 hr	12 hr	24 hr
1	0.693	69.3	415.8	554.4	831.6	1663
2	0.347	34.7	208.2	277.6	416.4	832.8
4	0.173	17.3	103.8	138.4	207.6	415.2
6	0.116	11.6	69.6	92.8	139.2	278.4
8	0.0866	8.66	52.0	69.3	103.9	207.8
10	0.0693	6.93	41.6	55.4	83.2	166.3
12	0.0577	5.77	34.6	46.2	69.2	138.5

[a] Assume $C_{desired}$ is 5 μg/mL and the V_D is 20,000 mL; $R = kV_DC_p$: no immediate-release dose.

PHARMACOKINETIC SIMULATION OF EXTENDED-RELEASE PRODUCTS

The plasma drug concentration profiles of many extended-release products fit an oral one-compartment model assuming first-order absorption and elimination. Compared to an immediate-release product, the extended-release product typically shows a smaller absorption rate constant, because of the slower absorption of the extended-release product. The time for peak concentration (t_{max}) is usually longer (Fig. 17-5), and the peak drug concentration (C_{max}) is reduced. If the drug is properly formulated, the area under the plasma drug concentration curve should be the same. Parameters such as C_{max}, t_{max}, and area under the curve (AUC) conveniently show how successfully the extended-release product performs *in vivo*. For example, a product with a t_{max} of 3 hours would not be very satisfactory if the product is intended to last 12 hours. Similarly, an excessively high C_{max} is a sign of dose

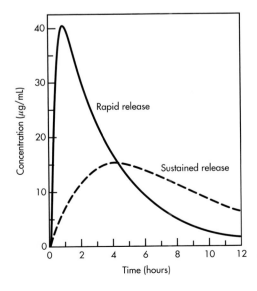

Figure 17-5. Plasma drug concentration of a sustained-release and a regular-release product. Note the difference of peak time and peak concentration of the two products.

dumping due to inadequate formulation. The pharmacokinetic analysis of single- and multiple-dose plasma data has been used by regulatory agencies to evaluate many sustained-release products. The analysis is practical because many products can be fitted to this model even though the drug is not released in a first-order manner. The limitation of this type of analysis is that the absorption rate constant may not relate to the rate of drug dissolution *in vivo*. If the drug strictly follows zero-order release and absorption, the model may not fit the data.

Various other models have been used to simulate plasma drug levels of extended-release products (Welling, 1983). The plasma drug levels from a zero-order, extended-release drug product may be simulated with Equation 17.8.

$$C_p = \frac{D_s}{V_D k} (1 - e^{-kt}) \tag{17.8}$$

where D_s = maintenance dose or rate of drug release (mg/min), C_p = plasma drug concentration, k = overall elimination constant, and V_D = volume of distribution. In the absence of a loading dose, the drug level in the body rises slowly to a plateau with minimum fluctuations (Fig. 17-6). This simulation assumes that (1) rapid drug release occurs without delay, (2) perfect zero-order release and absorption of the drug takes place, and (3) the drug is given exactly every 12 hours. In practice, the above assumptions are not precise, and fluctuations in drug level do occur.

When a sustained-release drug product with a loading dose (rapid release) and a zero-order maintenance dose is given, the resulting plasma drug concentrations are described by

$$C_p = \frac{D_i k_a}{V_D(k_a - k)} (e^{-kt} - e^{-k_a t}) + \frac{D_s}{V_D k} (1 - e^{-kt}) \tag{17.9}$$

where D_i = immediate-release (loading dose) dose and D_s = maintenance dose (zero-order). This expression is the sum of the oral absorption equation (first part) and the intravenous infusion equation (second part). An example of a zero-order release product with loading dose is shown in Figure 17-7. The contribution due to the loading and maintenance dose is shown by the dashed lines. The inclusion of a built-in loading dose in the extended-release product has only limited use.

With most extended-release products, the patient is given more than one dose, and there is no need for a built-in loading dose with subsequent doses. Putting a loading dose in the subsequent dosing would introduce more drug into the body than necessary, because of the "topping" effect (Fig. 17-8). In situations where a loading dose is necessary, the rapid-release product is used to titrate a loading dose that will bring the plasma drug level to therapeutic level.

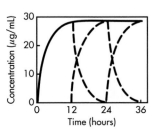

Figure 17-6. Simulated plasma drug level of a extended-release product administered every 12 hours. The plasma level shows a smooth rise to steady-state level with no fluctuations.

Figure 17-7. Simulated plasma drug level of a extended-release product with a fast-release component (A), and a maintenance component (B). The solid line represents total plasma drug level due to the two components.
(From Welling, 1983, with permission.)

A pharmacokinetic model that assumes first-order absorption of the loading and maintenance dose has also been proposed. This model predicts spiking peaks due to loading dose when the drug is administered continuously (Fig. 17-8) in multiple doses.

TYPES OF EXTENDED-RELEASE PRODUCTS

General approaches to manufacturing an extended-release drug product include the use of a matrix structure in which the drug is suspended or dissolved, the use of a rate-controlling membrane through which the drug diffuses, or a combination of both. Among the many types of commercial preparations available, none works by a single drug-release mechanism. Most extended-release products release drug by a combination of processes involving dissolution, permeation, and diffusion. The single most important factor is water permeation, without which none of the product release mechanisms would operate. Controlling the rate of water influx into the product generally dictates the rate at which the drug dissolves. Once the drug is dissolved, the rate of drug diffusion may be further controlled to a desirable rate. Table 17.3 shows some common extended-release product examples and the mechanisms for controlling drug release, and Table 17.4 lists the compositions for some drugs.

Drug Release from Matrix

A *matrix* is an inert solid vehicle in which a drug is uniformly suspended. A matrix may be formed by compressing or fusing the drug and the matrix material

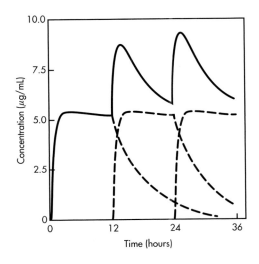

Figure 17-8. Simulated plasma level for a extended-release product given every 12 hours. The product has a built-in loading dose of 160 mg and a maintenance rate of 27.2 mg/hr. The plateau level was achieved rapidly after the first dose. Note the spiking peak following each dose due to the topping of the loading dose.
(From Welling, 1983, with permission.)

TABLE 17.3 *Examples of Oral Extended-Release Products*

TYPE	TRADE NAME	RATIONALE
Erosion tablet	Constant-T	Theophylline
	Tenuate Dospan	Diethylpropion HCl dispersed in hydrophilic matrix
	Tedral SA	Combination product with a slow-erosion component (theophylline, ephedrine HCl) and an initial-release component theophylline, ephedrine HCl, phenobarbital)
Waxy matrix tablet	Kaon *Cl*	Slow release of potassium chloride to reduce GI irritation
Coated pellets in capsule	Ornade spansule	Combination phenylpropanolamine HCl and chlorpheniramine with initial- and extended-release component
Pellets in tablet	Theo-Dur	Theophylline
Leaching	Ferro-Gradumet (Abbott)	Ferrous sulfate in a porous plastic matrix that is excreted in the stool; slow release of iron decreases GI irritation
	Desoxyn gradumet tablet (Abbott)	Methamphetamine methylacrylate methylmethacrylate copolymer, povidone, magnesium stearate; the plastic matrix is porous
Coated ion exchange	Tussionex	Cation ion-exchange resin complex of hydrocodone and phenyltoloxamine
Flotation–diffusion	Valrelease	Diazapam
Osmotic delivery	Acutrim	Phenylpropanolamine HCl (Oros delivery system)
	Procardia-XL	GITS—gastrointestinal therapeutic system with NaCl-driven (osmotic pressure) delivery system for nifedipine
Microencapsulation	Bayer timed-release	Aspirin
	Nitrospan	Microencapsulated nitroglycerin
	Micro-K Extencaps	Potassium chloride microencapsulated particles

together. Generally, the drug is present in a small percentage, so that the matrix protects the drug from rapid dissolution and the drug diffuses out slowly over time. Most matrix materials are water insoluble, although some matrix materials may swell slowly in water. Drug release using a matrix dosage form may be achieved using tablets or small beads, depending on the formulation composition and therapeutic objective. Figure 17-9 shows three common approaches by which matrix mechanisms are employed. In Figure 17-9A, the drug is coated with a soluble coating, so drug release relies solely on the regulation of drug release by the matrix material. If the matrix is porous, water penetration will be rapid and the drug will diffuse out rapidly. A less porous matrix may give a longer duration of release. Unfortunately, drug release from a simple matrix tablet is not zero order. The *Higuchi equation* describes the release rate of a matrix tablet:

$$Q = DS\left(\frac{P}{\lambda}\right)(A - 0.5SP)^{1/2}\sqrt{t} \tag{17.10}$$

TABLE 17.4 Composition and Examples of Some Modified-Release Products

K-Tab (Abbott)	750 mg or 10 mEq of potassium chloride in a film-coated matrix tablet. The matrix may be excreted intact, but the active ingredient is released slowly without upsetting the GI tract.
	Inert ingredients: Cellulosic polymers, castor oil, colloidal silicon dioxide, polyvinyl acetate, paraffin. The product is listed as a waxy/polymer matrix tablet for release over 8–10 hr.
Toprol-XL tablets (Astra)	Contains metoprolol succinate for sustained release in pellets, providing stable beta-blockade over 24 hr with one daily dose. Exercise tachycardia was less pronounced compared to immediate-release preparation. Each pellet separately releases the intended amount of medication.
	Inert ingredients: Paraffin, PEG, povidone, acetyltributyl citrate, starch, silicon dioxide, and magnesium stearate.
Quinglute Dura tablets (Berlex)	Contains 320 mg quinidine gluconate in a prolonged-action matrix tablet lasting 8–12 hr and provides PVC protection.
	Inert ingredients: Starch, confection's sugar, and magnesium stearate.
Brontil Slow-Release capsules (Carnrick)	Phendimetrazine tartrate 105 mg sustained pellet in capsule.
Slow Fe tablets (Ciba)	Slow-release iron preparation (OTC medication) with 160 mg ferrous sulfate for iron deficiency.
	Inert ingredients: HPMC, PEG shellac, and cetostearyl alcohol.
Tegretol-XR tablets (Ciba Geneva)	Carbamazepine extended-release tablet.
	Inert ingredients: Zein, cetostearyl alcohol, PEG, starch, talc, gum tragacanth, and mineral oil.
Sinemed CR tablets (Dupont pharma)	Contains a combination of carbidopa and levodopa for sustained release delivery. This is a special erosion polymeric tablet for Parkinson's disease treatment.
Pentasa capsules (Hoechst Marion/Roussel)	Contains mesalamine for ulcerative colitis in a sustained-release mesalamine coated with ethylcellulose. For local effect mostly, about 20% absorbed versus 80% otherwise.
Isoptin SR (Knoll)	Verapamil HCl sustained-release tablet.
	Inert ingredients: PEG, starch, PVP, alginate, talc, HPMC, methylcellulose, and microcrystalline cellulose.
Pancrease capsules (McNeil)	Enteric-coated microspheres of pancrelipase. Protects the amylase, lipase, and protease from the action of acid in the stomach.
	Inert ingredients: CAP, diethyl phthalate, sodium starch glycolate, starch, sugar, gelatin and talc.
Cotazym-S (Organon)	Enteric-coated microspheres of pancrelipase.
Eryc (erythromycin delayed-release capsules) (Warner-Chilcott)	Erythromycin enteric-coated tablet that protects the drug from instability and irritation.
Dilantin Kapseals (Parke-Davis)	Extended-release phenytoin capsule which contains beads of sodium phenytoin, gelatin, sodium lauryl sulfate, glyceryl monooleate, PEG 200, silicon dioxide, and talc.
Micro-K Extencaps (Robbins)	Ethylcellulose forms semipermeable film surrounding granules by microencapsulation for release over 8–10 hr without local irritation.
	Inert ingredients: Gelatin, and sodium lauryl sulfate.
Quinidex Extentabs (Robbins)	300 mg dose, 100 mg release immediately in the stomach and is absorbed in the small intestine. The rest is absorbed later over 10–12 hr in a slow-dissolving core as it moves down the GI tract.

(Continued)

TABLE 17.4   *Composition and Examples of Some Modified-Release Products (continued)*

Compazine Spansules (GSK)	Inert ingredients: White wax, carnauba wax, acacia, acetylated monoglyceride, guar gum, edible ink, calcium sulfate, corn derivative, and shellac. Initial dose of prochlorperazine release first, then release slowly over several hours.
Slo-bid Gyrocaps (Rhone-Poulenc Rorer)	Inert ingredients: Glycerylmonostearate, wax, gelatin, sodium lauryl sulfate. A controlled-release 12–24-hr theophylline product.
Theo-24 capsules (UCB Pharma)	A 24-hr sustained-release theophylline product. Inert ingredients: Ethylcellulose, edible ink, talc, starch, sucrose, gelatin, silicon dioxide, and dyes.
Sorbitrate SA (Zeneca)	The tablet contains isosorbide dinitrate 10 mg in the outer coat and 30 mg in the inner coat. Inert ingredients: Carbomer 934P, ethylcellulose, lactose magnesium stearate, and Yellow No. 10.

where Q = amount of drug release per cm^2 of surface at time t, S = solubility of drug in g/cm^3 in the dissolution medium, A = content of drug in insoluble matrix, P = porosity of matrix, D = diffusion coefficient of drug, and λ = tortuosity factor.

Figure 17-9B represents a matrix enclosed by an insoluble membrane, so the drug release rate is regulated by the permeability of the membrane as well as the matrix. Figure 17-9C represents a matrix tablet enclosed with a combined film. The film becomes porous after dissolution of the soluble part of the film. An example of this is the combined film formed by ethylcellulose and methylcellulose. Close to zero-order release has been obtained with this type of release mechanism.

Gum-Type Matrix Tablets

Some excipients have a remarkable ability to swell in the presence of water and form a substance with a gel-like consistency. When this happens, the gel provides a natural barrier to drug diffusion from the tablet. Because the gel-like material is quite viscous and may not disperse for hours, this provides a means for sustaining the drug for hours until all the drug has been completely dissolved and has diffused into the intestinal fluid. A common gelling material is gelatin. However, gelatin dissolves rapidly after the gel is formed. Drug excipients such as methylcellulose, gum tragacanth, Veegum, and alginic acid form a viscous mass and provide a useful matrix for controlling drug dissolution. Drug formulation with these excipients provides sustained drug release for hours. The drug diazepam, for example, has been formulated using methylcellulose to provide sustained release. In the case of

Figure 17-9.   *Examples of three different types of modified matrix-release mechanisms.*

sustained-release diazepam, claims were made that the hydrocolloid (gel) floated in the stomach to give sustained release. In other studies, however, materials of various densities were emptied from the stomach without any difference as to whether the drug product was floating on top or sitting at the bottom of the stomach.

The most important consideration in this type of formulation appears to be the gelling strength of the gum material and the concentration of gummy material. Modification of the release rates of the product may further be achieved with various amounts of talc or other lipophilic lubricant.

Polymeric Matrix Tablets

The use of polymeric material in prolonging the release rate of drug has received increased attention. The most important characteristic of this type of preparation is that the prolonged release may last for days or weeks rather than for a shorter duration (as with other techniques). The first example of an oral polymeric matrix tablet was Gradumet (Abbott Laboratories), which is marketed as an iron preparation. The plastic matrix provides a rigid geometric surface for drug diffusion, so that a relatively constant rate of drug release is obtained. In the case of the iron preparation, the matrix reduces the exposure of the irritating drug to the GI mucosal tissues. The matrix is usually expelled unchanged in the feces after all the drug has leached out.

Polymeric matrix tablets for oral use are generally quite safe. However, for certain patients with reduced GI motility caused by disease, polymeric matrix tablets should be avoided, because accumulation or obstruction of the GI tract by matrix tablets has been reported. As an oral sustained-release product, the matrix tablet has not been popular. In contrast, the use of the matrix tablet in implantation has been more popular.

The use of biodegradable polymeric material for extended release has been the focus of intensive research. One such example is the use of polylactic acid copolymer, which degrades to natural lactic acid and eliminates the problem of retrieval after implantation.

The number of polymers available for drug formulations is increasing and includes polyacrylate, methacrylate, polyester, ethylene–vinyl acetate copolymer (EVA), polyglycolide, polylactide, and silicone. Of these, the hydrophilic polymers, such as polylactic acid and polyglycolic acid, erode in water and release the drug gradually over time. A hydrophobic polymer such as EVA releases the drug over a longer duration time of weeks or months. The rate of release may be controlled by blending two polymers and increasing the proportion of the more hydrophilic polymer, thus increasing the rate of drug release. The addition of a low-molecular-weight polylactide to a polylactide polymer formulation increased the release rate of the drug and enabled the preparation of an extended-release system (Bodmeier et al, 1989). The type of plasticizer and the degree of cross-linking provide additional means for modifying the release rate of the drug. Many drugs are incorporated into the polymer as the polymer is formed chemically from its monomer. Light, heat, and other agents may affect the polymer chain length, degree of cross-linking, and other properties. This may provide a way to modify the release rate of the polymer matrices prepared. Drugs incorporated into polymers may have release rates that last over days, weeks, or even months. These vehicles have been often recommended for protein and peptide drug administration. For example, EVA is biocompatible and was shown to prolong insulin release in rats.

Hydrophobic polymers with water-labile linkages are prepared so that partial breakdown of the polymers allows for desired drug release without deforming the matrix during erosion. For oral drug delivery, the problem of incomplete drug release from the matrix is a major hurdle that must be overcome with the polymeric matrix dosage form. Another problem is that drug release rates may be affected by the amount of drug loaded. For implantation and other uses, the environment is more stable compared to oral routes, so a stable drug release from the polymer matrix may be attained for days or weeks.

Pellet-Type Sustained-Release Products

The pellet type of sustained-release drug product is also often referred to as a bead-type dosage form. In general, the beads are prepared by coating drug powder onto preformed cores called *nonpareil seeds*. The nonpareil seeds are made from slurry of starch, sucrose, and lactose. Preparation of the cores is tedious. The rough core granules are rounded for hours on a coating pan and then classified according to size. The drug-coated beads generally provide a rapid-release carrier for the drug depending on the coating solution used. Coatings may be aqueous or nonaqueous. Aqueous coatings are preferred. Nonaqueous coatings may leave residual solvents in the product, and removal of solvents during manufacture presents danger to workers and the environment. Cores are coated by either sprayed pan coating or by air-suspension coating. Once the drug beads are prepared, they may be further coated with a protective coating to allow a sustained or prolonged release of the drug.

The use of various amounts of coating solution can provide beads with various coating protection. A careful blending of beads may achieve any release profile desired. Alternatively, a blend of beads coated with materials of different solubility may also provide a means of controlling dissolution of the drug.

Some products take advantage of bead blending to provide two doses of drug in one formulation. For example, a blend of rapid-release beads with some pH-sensitive enteric-coated material may provide a second dose of drug release when the drug reaches the intestine.

The pellet dosage form can be prepared as a capsule or tablet. When pellets are prepared as tablets, the beads must be compressed lightly so that they do not break. Usually, a disintegrant is included in the tablet, causing the beads to be released rapidly after administration. Formulation of a drug into pellet form may reduce gastric irritation, because the drug is released slowly over a period of time, therefore avoiding high drug concentration in the stomach. Dextroamphetamine sulfate timed-release pellets (Dexedrine Spansule) is an early example of a beaded dosage form. Another older product is a pellet-type extended-release product of theophylline (Gyrocap). Table 17.5 shows the frequency of adverse reactions after theophylline is administered as solution versus pellets. If theophylline is administered as a solution, a high drug concentration may be reached in the body due to rapid drug absorption. Some side effects may be attributed to the high concentration of theophylline. Pellet dosage form allows drug to be absorbed gradually, therefore reducing the incidence of side effects by preventing a high C_{max}.

TABLE 17.5   Incidence of Adverse Effects of Sustained-Release Theophylline Pellet versus Theophylline Solution[a]

SIDE EFFECTS	VOLUNTEERS SHOWING SIDE EFFECTS	
	Using Solution	Using Sustained-Release Pellets
Nausea	10	0
Headache	4	0
Diarrhea	3	0
Gastritis	2	0
Vertigo	5	0
Nervousness	3	1

[a]After 5-day dosing at 600 mg theophylline/24 hr, adverse reaction points on fifth day: solution, 135; pellets, 18.

From Breimer and Dauhof (1980), with permission.

A second example involves the drug bitolterol mesylate (Tornalate). A study in dogs indicated that the incidence of tachycardia was reduced using an extended-release bead preparation, whereas the bronchodilation effect was not reduced. Administering the drug as extended-release pellets apparently reduced excessively high drug concentration in the body and avoided stimulated increase in heart rate. Studies also reported reduced gastrointestinal side effects of the drug potassium chloride in pellet or microparticulate form. Potassium chloride is irritating to the GI tract. Formulation in pellet form reduces the chance of exposing high concentrations of potassium chloride to the mucosal cells in the GI tract.

Many extended-release cold products also employ the bead concept. A major advantage of the pellet dosage form is that the pellets are less affected by the effect of stomach emptying. Because numerous pellets are within a capsule, some pellets will gradually reach the small intestine each time the stomach empties, whereas a single extended-release tablet may be delayed in the stomach for a long time as a result of erratic stomach emptying. Stomach emptying is particularly important in the formulation and *in-vivo* behavior of enteric-coated products. Enteric-coated tablets may be delayed for hours by the presence of food in the stomach, whereas enteric-coated pellets are relatively unaffected by the presence of food.

Prolonged-Action Tablets

An approach to prolong the action of a drug is to reduce the aqueous solubility of the drug, so that the drug dissolves slowly over a period of several hours. The solubility of a drug is dependent on the salt form used, and an examination of the solubility of the various salt forms of the drug should be the first step in drug development. In general, the base or acid form of the drug is usually much less soluble than the corresponding salt. For example, sodium phenobarbital is more water soluble than phenobarbital, the acid form of the drug. Diphenhydramine hydrochloride is more soluble than the base form, diphenhydramine.

In cases where it is inconvenient to prepare a less soluble form of the drug, the drug may be granulated with an excipient to slow dissolution of the drug. Often, fatty or waxy lipophilic materials are employed in formulations. Stearic acid, castor wax, high-molecular-weight polyethylene glycol (Carbowax), glyceryl monosterate, white wax, and spermaceti oil are useful ingredients in providing an oily barrier to slow water penetration and the dissolution of the tablet. Many of the lubricants used in tableting may also be used as lipophilic agents to slow dissolution. For example, magnesium stearate and hydrogenated vegetable oil (Sterotex) are actually used in high percentages to cause sustained drug release in a preparation. The major disadvantage of this type of preparation is the difficulty in maintaining a reproducible drug release from patient to patient, because oily materials may be subjected to digestion, temperature, and mechanical stress, which may affect the release rate of the drug.

Ion-Exchange Products

Ion-exchange preparations usually involve an insoluble resin capable of reacting with either an anionic or cationic drug. An anionic resin is negatively charged so that a positively charged cationic drug may react with the resin to form an insoluble nonabsorbable resin–drug complex. Upon exposure in the GI tract, cations in the gut, such as potassium and sodium, may displace the drug from the resin, releasing the drug, which is absorbed freely. The main disadvantage of ion-exchange preparations is that the amount of cation–anion in the GI tract is not easily controllable and varies among individuals, making it difficult to provide a consistent mechanism or rate of drug release. A further disadvantage is that resins may provide a potential means of interaction with nutrients and other drugs.

Ion exchange may be used in extended-release liquid preparations. An added advantage is that the technique provides some protection for very bitter or irritating drugs. Ion exchange has been combined with a coating to obtain a more effective sustained-release product. For example, the drug dextromethorphan (Tussionex) was formulated using the ion-exchange principle to mask the bitter taste and to prolong the duration of action of the drug. In the past, amphetamine was formulated with ion-exchange resins to provide prolonged release as an appetite suppressant in weight reduction.

A general mechanism for the formulation of cationic drugs is

$$H^+ + resin\text{–}SO_3^- drug^+ \rightleftharpoons resin\text{–}SO_3^- H^+ + drug^+$$

$$\text{Insoluble drug complex} \qquad\qquad \text{Soluble drug}$$

For anionic drugs, the corresponding mechanism is

$$Cl^- + resin\text{–}N^+(CH_3)_3 drug^- \rightleftharpoons resin\text{–}N^+(CH_3)_3 Cl^- + drug^-$$

$$\text{Insoluble drug complex} \qquad\qquad \text{Soluble drug}$$

The insoluble drug complex containing the resin and drug dissociates in the GI tract in the presence of the appropriate counter ions. The released drug dissolves in the fluids of the GI tract and is rapidly absorbed.

Core Tablets

A core tablet is a tablet within a tablet. The core is usually used for the slow-drug-release component, and the outside shell contains a rapid-release dose of drug. Formulation of a core tablet requires two granulations. The core granulation is usually compressed lightly to form a loose core and then transferred to a second die cavity, where a second granulation containing additional ingredients is compressed further to form the final tablet.

The core material may be surrounded by hydrophobic excipients so that the drug leaches out over a prolonged period of time. This type of preparation is sometimes called a *slow-erosion core tablet*, because the core generally contains either no disintegrant or insufficient disintegrant to fragment the tablet. The composition of the core may range from wax to gum or polymeric material. Numerous slow-erosion tablets have been patented and are sold commercially under various trade names.

The success of core tablets depends very much on the nature of the drug and the excipients used. As a general rule, this preparation is very much hardness dependent in its release rate. Critical control of hardness and processing variables are important in producing a tablet with a consistent release rate.

Core tablets are occasionally used to avoid incompatibility in preparations containing two physically incompatible ingredients. For example, buffered aspirin has been formulated into a core and shell to avoid a yellowing discoloration of the two ingredients upon aging.

Microencapsulation

Microencapsulation is a process of encapsulating microscopic drug particles with a special coating material, therefore making the drug particles more desirable in terms of physical and chemical characteristics. A common drug that has been encapsulated is aspirin. Aspirin has been microencapsulated with ethylcellulose, making the drug superior in its flow characteristics; when compressed into a tablet, the drug releases more gradually compared to a simple compressed tablet.

Many techniques are used in microencapsulating a drug. One process used in microencapsulating acetaminophen involves suspending the drug in an aqueous solution while stirring. The coating material, ethylcellulose, is dissolved in cyclohexane, and the two liquids are added together with stirring and heating. As the cyclohexane is evaporated by heat, the ethylcellulose coats the microparticles of the acetaminophen. The microencapsulated particles have a slower dissolution rate because the ethylcellulose is not water soluble and provides a barrier for diffusion of drug. The amount of coating material deposited on the acetaminophen determines the rate of drug dissolution. The coating also serves as a means of reducing the bitter taste of the drug. In practice, microencapsulation is not consistent enough to produce a reproducible batch of product, and it may be necessary to blend the microencapsulated material in order to obtain a desired release rate.

Osmotic Extended-Release Products

The osmotic pump represents a newer concept in extended-release preparations. Drug delivery is controlled by the use of an osmotically controlled device that promotes a constant amount of water into the system, either by dissolving and releasing a constant amount of drug per unit time or by the use of a "push–pull" system that pushes the drug out at a constant rate as water flows into an expandable osmotic compartment. Drug is released via a single laser-drilled hole in the tablet.

Figure 17-10. Cross-sectional diagram of simple osmotic delivery system (gastrointestinal therapeutic system).
(From Shaw and Chandrasekaran, 1978, with permission.)

One preparation consists of an outside layer of semipermeable membrane filled with a mixture of drug and osmotic agent (Fig. 17-10). When the device is placed in water, osmotic pressure generated by the osmotic agent within the core causes water to move into the device, which forces the dissolved drug to move out of the drug delivery orifice. The rate of drug delivery is relatively constant and unaffected by the pH of the environment. A similar osmotic product available for implantation is the osmotic *minipump.* Another osmotic oral drug product is the "push–pull" system called Gastrointestinal Therapeutic System (GITS), developed by Alza Corporation for nifedipine (Procardia XL) and other drugs. The system consists of a semipermeable membrane and a two-layer core of osmotic ingredient and active drug. As water enters the system, the osmotic pressure builds up from the inner layer, pushing the drug out through a laser-drilled orifice in the drug layer. An example of GITS uses acetazolamide for the treatment of ocular hypertension in glaucoma. The drug was delivered from the system at zero-order rate for 12 hours at 15 mg/hr, as shown in Figure 17-11.

The frequency of side effects experienced by patients using GITS was considerably less than that with conventional tablets (Fig. 17-12). When the therapeutic system was compared to the regular 250-mg tablet given twice daily, ocular pressure was effectively controlled by the osmotic system. The blood level of acetazolanine using GITS, however, was considerably below that from the tablet. In fact, the therapeutic index of the drug was measurably increased by using the therapeutic system. The use of extended-release drug products, which release drug consistently, may provide promise for administering many drugs that previously had frequent adverse side effects because of the drug's narrow therapeutic index. The osmotic

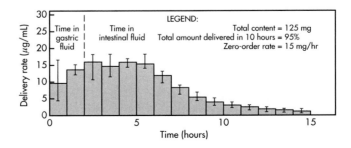

Figure 17-11. Pattern of delivery of acetazolamide from elementary osmotic pump therapeutic system delivering 70% of the total content (125 mg) at specified rate of 15 mg/hr in 6 hours and 80% in 8 hours.
(From Shaw and Chandrasekaran, 1978, with permission.)

Figure 17-12. Incidence of drowsiness and confusion on acetazolamide given in three regimens. More frequent incidence of side effects were seen with the tablet over the osmotic system.
(From Shaw and Chandrasekaran, 1978, with permission.)

drug delivery system has become a popular drug vehicle for many products that require extended period of drug delivery for 12 to 24 hours (Table 17.6).

A newer osmotic delivery system is the L-Oros Softcap (Alza), which claims to enhance bioavailability of poorly soluble drug by formulating the drug in a soft gelatin core and then providing extended drug delivery through an orifice drilled

TABLE 17.6 OROS Osmotic Therapeutic Systems[a]

TRADE NAME	MANUFACTURER	GENERIC NAME	DESCRIPTION
Acutrim	Ciba	Phenylpropanolamine	Once-daily, over-the-counter appetite suppressant
Covera-HS	Searle	Verapamil	Controlled-Onset Extended-Release (COER-24) system for hypertension and angina pectoris
DynaCirc CR	Sandoz Pharmaceuticals	Isradipine	Treatment of hypertension
Efidac 24	Ciba Self-Medication		Over-the-counter, 24-hour extended-release tablets providing relief of allergy and cold symptoms, containing either chlorpheniramine maleate, pseudoephedrine hydrochloride, or a combination of pseudoephedrine hydrochloride/ brompheniramine maleate
Glucotrol XL	Pfizer	Glipizide	Extended-release tablets indicated as an adjunct to diet for the control of hyperglycemia in patients with non-insulin-dependent diabetes
Minipress XL	Pfizer	Prazosin	Extended-release tablets for treatment of hypertension
Procardia XL	Pfizer	Nifedipine	Extended-release tablets for treatment of angina and hypertension
Adalat CR	Bayer AG	Nifedipine	An Alza-based OROS system of nifedipine introduced internationally
Volmax	Glaxo-Wellcome	Albuterol	Extended-release tablets for the relief of bronchospasm in patients with reversible obstructive airway disease

[a]Alza's OROS Osmotic Therapeutic Systems use osmosis to deliver drug continuosly at controlled rates for up to 24 hr.

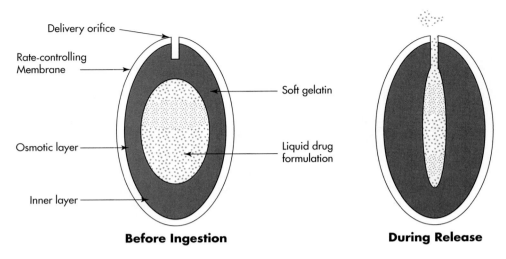

Figure 17-13. Configuration of L-OROS SOFTCAP.
(From Dong et al, 2002, with permission.)

into an osmotic driven shell (Fig 17.13). The soft gelatin capsule is surrounded by the barrier layer, the expanding osmotic layer, and the release-rate-controlling membrane. A delivery orifice is formed through the three outer layers but not through the gelatin shell. When the system is administered, water permeates through the rate-controlling membrane and activates the osmotic engine. As the engine expands, hydrostatic pressure inside the system builds up, thereby forcing the liquid formulation to break through the hydrated gelatin capsule shell at the delivery orifice and be pumped out of the system. At the end of the operation, liquid drug fill is squeezed out, and the gelatin capsule shell becomes flattened. The osmotic layer, located between the inner layer and the rate-controlling membrane, is the driving force for pumping the liquid formulation out of the system. This layer can gel when it hydrates. In addition, the high osmotic pressure can be sustained to achieve a constant release. This layer should comprise, therefore, of a high-molecular-weight hydrophilic polymer and an osmotic agent. It is a challenge to develop a coating solution for a high-molecular-weight hydrophilic polymer. A mixed solvent of water and ethanol was used for this coating composition.

Transdermal Drug Delivery Systems

A transdermal drug delivery system (or patch) is a drug-dosage form intended for delivering a dose of medication across the skin for systemic drug absorption. The transdermal delivery system is popular with patients because it delivers the drug dose through the skin in a controlled rate over an extended period of time. Transdermal products allow a unique route of administration for drugs (Chapter 14, Table 14.12). More examples are listed in Tables 17.7 and 17.8. Transdermal products vary in patch design, but many units consist of drugs impregnated on a reservoir layer supported by a backing. Drug diffusion is controlled by a semipermeable membrane next to the reservoir layer. In general, the patch (Fig. 17-14) contains several parts: (1) a backing or support layer, (2) a drug layer (reservoir

TABLE 17.7 Examples of Transdermal Delivery Systems

TYPE	TRADE NAME	RATIONALE
Membrane-controlled system	Transderm-Nitro (Novartis)	Drug in reservoir, drug release through a rate-controlling polymeric membrane
Adhesive diffusion-controlled system	Deponit system (PharmaSchwartz)	Drug dispersed in an adhesive polymer and in a reservoir
Matrix dispersion system	Nitro-Dur (Key)	Drug dispersed into a rate-controlling hydrophilic or hydrophobic matrix molded into a transdermal system
Microreservoir system	Nitro-Disc (Searle)	Combination reservoir and matrix-dispersion system

containing the dose), (3) a release-controlling layer (usually a semipermeable film), (4) a pressure-sensitive adhesive (PSA), and (5) a protective strip, which must be removed before application.

Nitroglycerin is commonly administered by transdermal delivery. Transdermal delivery systems of nitroglycerin may provide hours of protection against angina, whereas the duration of nitroglycerin given in a sublingual tablet may be only a few minutes. Several commercial transdermal preparations are available, including Nitro-Disc (Searle), Transderm-Nitro (Novartis), and Nitro-Dur (Key Pharmaceuticals). These preparations are placed over the chest area and provide up to 12 hours of angina protection. In a study comparing these three dosage forms in patients, no

TABLE 17.8 Transdermal Delivery Systems

TRADE NAME	MANUFACTURER	GENERIC NAME	DESCRIPTION
Catapres-TTS	Boehringer Ingelheim	Clonidine	Once-weekly product for the treatment of hypertension
Duragesic	Janssen Pharmaceutical	Fentanyl	Management of chronic pain in patients who require continuous opioid analgesia for pain that cannot be managed by lesser means
Estraderm	Ciba Geigy	Estradiol	Twice-weekly product for treating certain postmenopausal symptoms and preventing osteoporosis
Nicoderm CQ	Hoechst Marion	Nicotine	An aid to smoking cessation for the relief of nicotine-withdrawal symptoms
Testoderm	Alza	Testosterone	Replacement therapy in males for conditions associated with a deficiency or absence of endogenous testosterone
Transderm-Nitro	Novartis	Nitroglycerin	Once-daily product for the prevention of angina pectoris due to coronary artery disease; contains nitroglycerin in a proprietary, transdermal therapeutic system
Transderm Scop		Scopolamine	Prevention of nausea and vomiting associated with motion sickness

Figure 17-14.   *The four basic configurations for transdermal drug delivery systems.*

substantial difference was observed among the three preparations. In all cases, the skin was found to be the rate-limiting step in nitroglycerin absorption. There were fewer variations among products than of the same product among different patients.

The skin is a natural barrier to prevent the influx of foreign chemicals (including water) into the body and the loss of water from the body (Guy, 1996). To be a suitable candidate for transdermal drug delivery, the drug must possess the right combination of physicochemical and pharmacodynamic properties. The drug must be highly potent so that only a small systemic drug dose is needed and the size of the patch (dose is also related to surface area) need not be exceptionally large, not greater than 50 cm^2 (Guy, 1996). Physicochemical properties of the drug include a small molecular weight (<500 Da), and high lipid solubility. The elimination half-life should not be too short, to avoid having to apply the patch more frequently than once a day.

After the application of a transdermal patch, there is generally a lag time before the onset of the drug action, because of the drug's slow diffusion into the dermal layers of the skin. When the patch is removed, diffusion of the drug from the dermal layer to the systemic circulation may continue for some time until the drug is depleted from the site of application. The solubility of drug in the skin rather than the concentration of drug in the patch layer is the most important factor controlling the rate of drug absorption through the skin. Humidity, temperature, and other factors have been shown to affect the rate of drug absorption through the skin. With most drugs, transdermal delivery provides a more stable blood level of the drug than oral dosing. However, with nitroglycerin, the sustained blood level of the drug provided by transdermal delivery is not desirable, due to induced tolerance to the drug not seen with sublingual tablets.

Transdermal Therapeutic Systems (TTS, Alza) consist of a thin, flexible composite of membranes, resembling a small adhesive bandage, which is applied to the skin and delivers drug through intact skin into the bloodstream. Other examples of products delivered using this system are shown in Table 17.8. Transderm Nitro consists of several layers: (1) an aluminized plastic backing that protects nitroglycerin from loss through vaporization; (2) a drug reservoir containing nitroglycerin adsorbed onto lactose, colloidal silicon dioxide, and silicone medical fluid; (3) a diffusion-controlling membrane consisting of ethylene–vinyl acetate copolymer; (4) a layer of silicone adhesive; and (5) a protective strip.

Other transdermal delivery manufacturers have made transdermal systems in which the adhesive functions both as a pressure-sensitive adhesive and as a controlling matrix. Dermaflex (Elan) is a uniquely passive transdermal patch system that employs a hydrogel matrix into which the drug is incorporated. Dermaflex regulates both the availability and absorption of the drug in a manner that allows for controlled and efficient systemic delivery of many drugs.

An important limitation of transdermal preparation is the amount of drug that is needed in the transdermal patch to be absorbed systemically to provide the optimum therapeutic response. The amount of drug absorbed transdermally is related to the amount of drug in the patch, the size of the patch, and the method of manufacture. A dose–response relationship is obtained by applying a proportionally larger transdermal patch that differs only in surface area. For example, a 5-cm^2 transdermal patch will generally provide twice as much drug absorbed systemically as a 2.5-cm^2 transdermal patch.

In general, drugs given at a dose of over 100 mg would require too large a patch to be used practically. However, new advances in pharmaceutic solvents may provide a mechanism for an increased amount of drug to be absorbed transdermally. Azone, a *permeation enhancer*, is a solvent that increases the absorption of many drugs through the skin. This solvent is relatively nontoxic.

For ionic drugs, absorption may be enhanced transdermally by *iontophoresis*, a method in which an electric field is maintained across the epidermal layer with special miniature electrodes. Some drugs, such as lidocaine, verapamil, insulin, and peptides, have been absorbed through the skin by iontophoresis. A process in which transdermal drug delivery is aided by high-frequency sound is called *sonophoresis*. Sonophoresis has been used with hydrocortisone cream applied to the skin to enhance penetration for treating "tennis elbow" and other mild inflammatory muscular problems. Many such novel systems are being developed by drug delivery companies.

Panoderm XL patch technology (Elan) is a new system that delivers a drug through a concealed miniature probe which penetrates the stratum corneum. Panoderm XL is fully disposable and may be programmed to deliver drugs as a preset bolus, in continuous or pulsed regimen. The complexity of the device is hidden from the patient and is simple to use. Panoderm (Elan) is an electrotransdermal drug delivery system that overcomes the skin diffusion barriers through the use of low-level electric current to transport the drug through the skin. Several transdermal products, such as fentanyl, hydromorphone, calcitonin, and LHRH (luteinizing hormone–releasing hormone), are in clinical trials. More improvements in absorption enhancers and delivery systems will be available in the future for transdermal preparations.

Combination Products

Combination products consist of the drug in combination with a device and or biologic that is physically, chemically, or otherwise combined or mixed and produced as a single entity. Possible combinations include drug/device, biologic/device, drug/biologic, or drug/device/biologic. The device and/or biologic is intended for use with the approved drug and influences the route of administration and pharmacokinetics of the drug. For example, designs for metered-dose inhalers for inhalation therapy greatly influence the delivery of the drug into the lungs.

Implants and Inserts

Polymeric drug implants can deliver and sustain drug levels in the body for an extended period of time. Both biodegradable and nonbiodegradable polymers can be impregnated with drugs in a controlled drug delivery system. For example, levo-norgestrel implants (Norplant system, Wyeth-Ayerst) is a set of six flexible closed capsules made of silastic (dimethylsiloxane/methylvinylsiloxane copolymer), each containing 36 μg of the progestin levonorgestrel. The capsules are sealed with silastic adhesive and sterilized. The Norplant system is available in an insertion kit to facilitate subdermal insertion of all six capsules in the mid-portion of the upper arm. The dose of levonorgestrel is about 85 μg/day, followed by a decline to about 50 μg/day by 9 months and to about 35 μg/day by 18 months, declining further to about 30 μg/day (Facts and Comparisons, 1997). The levonorgestrel implants are effective for up to 5 years for contraception and then must be replaced. An intrauterine progesterone contraceptive system (Progestasert, Alza) is a T-shaped unit that contains a reservoir of 38 μg of progesterone. Contraceptive effectiveness for Progestasert is enhanced by continuous release of progesterone into the uterine cavity at an average rate of 65 μg/day for 1 year.

A dental insert available for the treatment of peridontitis is the doxycycline hyclate delivery system (Atrigel). This is a subgingival controlled-release product consisting of two syringe mixing systems that, when combined, form a bioabsorbable, flowable polymeric formulation. After administration under the gum, the liquid solidifies and then allows for controlled release of doxycycline for a period of 7 days.

CONSIDERATIONS IN THE EVALUATION OF MODIFIED-RELEASE PRODUCTS

The two important requirements for preparing extended-release products are (1) demonstration of safety and efficacy and (2) demonstration of controlled drug release.

For many drugs, data are available demonstrating the safety and efficacy for those drugs given in a conventional dosage form. Bioavailability data demonstrating comparable blood levels to an approved extended-release product are acceptable. The bioavailability data requirements are specified in the Code of Federal Regulations, 21 CFR 320.25(f). The important points are as follows.

1. The product should demonstrate sustained release, as claimed, without dose dumping (abrupt release of a large amount of the drug in an uncontrolled manner).
2. The drug should show steady-state levels comparable to those reached using a conventional dosage form given in multiple doses, and which was demonstrated to be effective.
3. The drug product should show consistent pharmacokinetic performance between individual dosage units.
4. The product should allow for the maximum amount of drug to be absorbed while maintaining minimum patient-to-patient variation.
5. The demonstration of steady-state drug levels after the recommended doses are given should be within the effective plasma drug levels for the drug.
6. An *in-vitro* method and data that demonstrate the reproducible extended-release nature of the product should be developed. The *in-vitro* method usually consists of a suitable dissolution procedure that provides a meaningful *in-vitro–in-vivo* correlation.

7. *In-vivo* pharmacokinetic data consist of single and multiple dosing comparing the extended-release product to a reference standard (usually an approved non-sustained-release or a solution product).

The pharmacokinetic data usually consist of plasma drug data and/or drug excreted into the urine. Pharmacokinetic analyses are performed to determine such parameters as $t_{1/2}$, V_D, t_{max}, AUC, and k.

Pharmacodynamic and Safety Considerations

Pharmacokinetic and safety issues must be considered in the development and evaluation of a modified-release dosage form. The most critical issue is to consider whether the modified-release dosage form truly offers an advantage over the same drug in an immediate-release (conventional) form. This advantage may be related to better efficacy, reduced toxicity, or better patient compliance. However, because the cost of manufacture of a modified-release dosage form is generally higher than the cost for a conventional dosage form, economy or cost savings for patients also may be an important consideration.

Ideally, the extended-release dosage form should provide a more prolonged pharmacodynamic effect compared to the same drug given in the immediate-release form. However, an extended-release dosage form of a drug may have a different pharmacodynamic activity profile compared to the same drug given in an acute, intermittent, rapid-release dosage form. For example, transdermal patches of nitroglycerin, which produce prolonged delivery of the drug, may produce functional tolerance to vasodilation that is not observed when nitroglycerin is given sublingually for acute angina attacks. Certain bactericidal antibiotics such as penicillin may be more effective when given in intermittent (pulsed) doses compared to continuous dosing. The continuous blood level of a hormone such as a corticosteroid might suppress adrenocorticotropic hormone (ACTH) release from the pituitary gland, resulting in atrophy of the adrenal gland. Furthermore, drugs that act indirectly or cause irreversible toxicity may be less efficacious when given in an extended-release rather than in conventional dosage form.

Because the modified-release dosage form may be in contact with the body for a prolonged period, the recurrence of sensitivity reactions or local tissue reactions due to the drug or constituents of the dosage form are possible. For oral modified-release dosage forms, prolonged residence time in the GI tract may lead to a variety of interactions with GI tract contents, and the efficiency of absorption may be compromised as the drug moves distally from the duodenum to the large intestine.

Moreover, dosage form failure due to either dose dumping or to the lack of drug release may have important clinical implications. Another possible unforeseen problem with modified-release dosage forms is an alteration in the metabolic fate of the drug, such as nonlinear biotransformation or site-specific disposition.

Design and selection of extended-release products are often aided by dissolution tests carried out at different pH units for various time periods to simulate the condition of the GI tract. Topographical plots of the dissolution data may be used to graph the percent of drug dissolved versus two variables (time, pH) that may affect dissolution simultaneously. For example, Skelly and Barr (1987) have shown that extended-release preparations of theophylline, such as Theo-24, have a more rapid dissolution rate at a higher pH of 8.4 (Fig. 17-15), whereas Theo-Dur is less

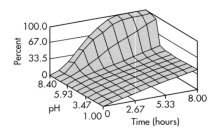

Figure 17-15. Topographical dissolution characterization of theophylline controlled release. Topographical dissolution characterization (as a function of time and pH) of Theo-24, a theophylline controlled-release preparation, which has been shown to have a greater rate and extent of bioavailability when dosed after a high-fat meal than when dosed under fasted conditions.

(From Skelly and Barr, 1987, with permission.)

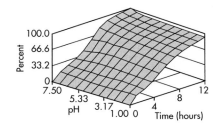

Figure 17-16. Topographical dissolution characterization of theophylline extended release. Topographical dissolution characterization (as a function of time and pH) of Theo-Dur, a theophylline controlled-release preparation, the bioavailability of which was essentially the same whether administered with food or under fasted conditions. *(From Skelly and Barr, 1987, with permission.)*

affected by pH (Fig. 17-16). These dissolution tests *in vitro* may help to predict the *in-vivo* bioavailability performance of the dosage form.

EVALUATION OF MODIFIED-RELEASE PRODUCTS

Dissolution Studies

Dissolution requirements for each of the three types of modified-release dosage form are published in the USP-NF. Some of the key elements for the *in-vitro* dissolution/drug release studies are listed in Table 17.9. Dissolution studies may be used together with bioavailability studies to predict *in-vitro–in-vivo* correlation of the drug release rate of the dosage forms.

In-Vitro–In-Vivo Correlations

A general discussion of correlating dissolution data to blood-level data for immediate-release oral drug products is presented in Chapter 14. Ideally, the *in-vitro* drug release of the extended-release product should relate to the bioavailability of the drug *in vivo*, so that changes in drug dissolution rates will be correlated directly to changes in drug bioavailability. Methods for establishing *in-vitro–in-vivo correlation* are discussed by Skelly et al (1990) and in the USP-NF. The following is a brief summary of the various categories of dissolution showing different degrees of correlation to *in-vivo* data.

Correlation Level A

Level A is the highest level of correlation, in which a 1:1 relationship between *in-vitro* dissolution and *in-vivo* bioavailability is demonstrated. Included in Level A are extended-release dosage forms that demonstrate an *in-vitro* drug release essentially independent of the dissolution medium. In this case, the *in-vitro*

TABLE 17.9 Suggested Dissolution/Drug Release Studies for Modified-Release Dosage Forms

Dissolution studies
1. Reproducibility of the method.
2. Proper choice of medium.
3. Maintenance of sink conditions.
4. Control of solution hydrodynamics.
5. Dissolution rate as a function of pH, ranging from pH 1 to pH 8 and including several intermediate values.
6. Selection of the most discriminating variables (medium, pH, rotation speed, etc) as the basis for the dissolution test and specification.

Dissolution procedures
1. Lack of dose dumping, as indicated by a narrow limit on the 1-hr dissolution specification.
2. Controlled-release characteristics obtained by employing additional sampling windows over time. Narrow limits with an appropriate Q value system will control the degree of first-order release.
3. Complete drug release of the drug from the dosage form. A minimum of 75–80% of the drug should be released from the dosage form at the last sampling interval.
4. The pH dependence/independence of the dosage form as indicated by percent dissolution in water, appropriate buffer, simulated gastric juice, or simulated intestinal fluid.

Adapted from Skelly and Barr (1987), with permission.

dissolution curve is compared directly to the percentage of drug absorbed calculated from the plasma drug concentration–time curve using a pharmacokinetic model or a model-independent method.

Generally, the percentage of drug absorbed may be calculated by the Wagner–Nelson or Loo–Riegelman procedures or by direct mathematical deconvolution, a process of mathematical resolution of blood level into an input (absorption) and an output (disposition) component (Chapter 7). The main advantage of a Level A correlation is that the quality control procedure of the *in-vitro* dissolution/drug release test is predictive of drug product performance *in vivo*.

Correlation Level B
Correlation Level B is based on the principle of statistical moment analysis (see Chapter 22). The mean residence time of the drug in the body and mean dissolution time *in vitro* are determined and correlated. This level of correlation is less than a Level A 1:1 correlation because the complete *in-vivo* plasma drug concentration–time curve is not fully described by the mean residence time.

Correlation Level C
Correlation Level C uses a single point in the dissolution curve to correlate to plasma drug concentration–time data. For example, a single dissolution time at $t_{50\%}$, $t_{90\%}$, and so forth, may be selected and correlated to pharmacokinetic parameters, such as AUC, t_{max}, or C_{max}. This is the weakest level of correlation because only partial relationship between absorption and dissolution is evident. Some examples of this correlation are given in Chapter 14.

Pharmacokinetic Studies

Various types of pharmacokinetic studies may be required by the Food and Drug Administration (FDA) for marketing approval of the modified-release drug product, depending on knowledge of the drug, its clinical pharmacokinetics, and its biopharmaceutics (Skelly et al, 1990). Furthermore, the extended-release dosage form should be available in several dosage strengths to allow flexibility for the clinician to adjust the dose for the individual patient.

Both single- and multiple-dose steady-state crossover studies using the highest strength of the dosage form may be performed. The reference dosage form may be a solution of the drug or the full NDA-approved conventional, immediate-release dosage form given in an equal daily dose as the extended-release dosage form. If the dosage strengths differ from each other only in the amount of the drug–excipient blend, but the concentration of the drug–excipient blend is the same in each dosage form, then the FDA may approve the NDA or ANDA on the basis of single- and multiple-dose studies of the highest dosage strength, whereas the other lower-strength dosage forms may be approved on the basis of comparative *in-vitro* dissolution studies (Chapter 14). The latest FDA Guidance for Industry should be consulted for regulatory requirements (www.fda.gov/cder/guidance/index.htm). Skelly et al, 1990b have described several types of such pharmacokinetic studies.

Case One

The first case involves the extended-release oral dosage form of a modified immediate-release drug for which extensive pharmacodynamic or pharmacokinetic data exist. Both single- and multiple-dose steady-state crossover studies are required. In the case of the single-dose study, a well-controlled pharmacokinetic study must also be performed to define the effects of a concurrent high-fat meal on the extended-release dosage form. This food study, comparing fasting versus fed subjects, is to determine (1) whether there is any need for labeling specifications of special conditions for administration of the dosage form with respect to meals, and (2) whether the absorption pattern of the extended-release dosage compares to that for the immediate-release (conventional) form of the same drug.

Case Two

The second case concerns nonoral extended-release dosage forms. Pharmacokinetic studies for the evaluation of extended-release dosage forms designed for an alternate route of administration would require studies similar to case 1, but would not need a food-effect study. However, when the route of administration is changed from the oral route, other factors may require consideration. An alternative route of administration may alter the biotransformation pattern of active or inactive metabolites. For example, isoproterenol given orally forms a sulfate conjugation as a result of metabolism within the cells of the small intestine, whereas after IV administration, isoproterenol forms a 3-O-methylated metabolite via catechol O-methyltransferase (COMT). Clinical efficacy may be altered by an alternative route of administration when a drug is switched from the oral to the parenteral or transdermal route. In this case, possible risk factors, such as irritation or sensitivity at the site of application, must also be studied.

Case Three

In case 3, studies involve the generic equivalent of an NDA-approved, extended-release product. The same bioequivalence studies are required to establish the equivalence of the formulation used in efficacy studies if the formula is different from the one intended for marketing and generic approval. The establishment of bioequivalence is based on both pharmacokinetic and statistical analyses.

Case Four

Finally, case 4 addresses an extended-release dosage form as an NDA. For an NDA, the studies required for new extended-release dosage forms are clinical and pharmacokinetic studies including dose linearity, bioavailability, food effects, fluctuation of the plasma drug concentrations, and characterizations of the plasma drug concentration–time profile.

The FDA's Center for Drug Evaluation and Research (CDER) maintains a website (www.fda.gov/cder) that lists regulatory guidances to provide the public with the FDA's latest submission requirements for NDAs and ANDAs.

EVALUATION OF *IN-VIVO* BIOAVAILABILITY DATA

A properly designed *in-vivo* bioavailability study is performed. The data are then evaluated using both pharmacokinetic and statistical analysis methods. The evaluation may include a pharmacokinetic profile, steady-state plasma drug concentrations, rate of drug absorption, occupancy time, and statistical evaluation of the computed pharmacokinetic parameters.

Pharmacokinetic Profile

The plasma drug concentration–time curve should adequately define the bioavailability of the drug from the dosage form. The bioavailability data should include a profile of the fraction of drug absorbed (Wagner–Nelson) and should rule out dose dumping or lack of a significant food effect. The bioavailability data should also demonstrate the extended-release characteristics of the dosage form compared to the reference or immediate-release drug product.

Steady-State Plasma Drug Concentration

The fluctuation between the C_{max}^{∞} (peak) and C_{min}^{∞} (trough) concentrations should be calculated:

$$\text{Fluctuation} = \frac{C_{max}^{\infty} - C_{min}^{\infty}}{C_{av}^{\infty}} \qquad (17.11)$$

where C_{av}^{∞} is equal to $[\text{AUC}]/\tau$

An ideal extended-release dosage form should have minimum fluctuation between C_{max} and C_{min}. A true zero-order release will have no fluctuation. In practice, the fluctuation in plasma drug levels after the extended-release dosage form should be less than the fluctuation after the same drug given in an immediate-release dosage form.

Rate of Drug Absorption

For the extended-release drug product to claim zero-order absorption, an appropriately calculated input function such as used in the Wagner–Nelson approach should substantiate this claim. The difference between first-order and zero-order

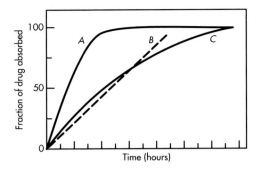

Figure 17-17. The fraction of drug absorbed using the Wagner–Nelson method may be used to distinguish between the first-order drug absorption rate of a conventional (immediate-release) dosage form (A) and *an* extended-release dosage form (C). Curve B represents *an* extended-release dosage form with zero-order absorption rate.

absorption of a drug is shown in Figure 17-17. The rate of drug absorption from the conventional or immediate-release dosage form is generally first order, as shown by Fig. 17-17A. Drug absorption after an extended-release dosage form may be zero order (Fig. 17-17B), first order (Fig. 17-17A), or an indeterminate order (Fig. 17-17C). For many extended-release dosage forms, the rate of drug absorption is first order, with an absorption rate constant k_a smaller than the elimination rate constant k. The pharmacokinetic model when $k_a > k$ is termed *flip-flop pharmacokinetics* and is discussed in Chapter 7.

Occupancy Time

For drugs for which the therapeutic window is known, the plasma drug concentrations should be maintained above the minimum effective drug concentration (MEC) and below the minimum toxic drug concentration (MTC). The time required to obtain plasma drug levels within the therapeutic window is known as *occupancy time* (Fig. 17-18).

Bioequivalence Studies

Bioequivalence studies for extended-release drug products are discussed in detail in Chapter 15. Bioequivalence studies may include (1) a fasting study, (2) a

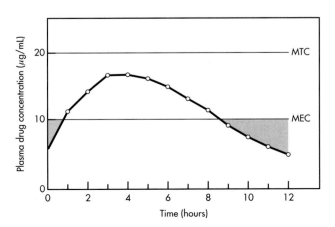

Figure 17-18. Occupancy time.

food-intervention study, and (3) a multiple dose study. The FDA's Center for Drug Evaluation and Research (CDER) maintains a website (www.fda.gov/cder) that lists regulatory guidances to provide the public with the FDA's latest submission requirements for NDAs and ANDAs.

Statistical Evaluation

Variables subject to statistical analysis generally include plasma drug concentrations at each collection time, AUC (from zero to last sampling time), AUC (from zero to time infinity), C_{max}, t_{max}, and elimination half-life $t_{1/2}$. Statistical testing may include an analysis of variance (ANOVA), computation of 90% and 95% confidence intervals on the difference in formulation means, and the power of ANOVA to detect a 20% difference from the reference mean.

FREQUENTLY ASKED QUESTIONS

1. Are extended-release drug products always more efficacious than immediate-release drug products containing the same drug?

2. What are the advantages and disadvantages of a zero-order rate for drug absorption?

LEARNING QUESTIONS

1. The design for most extended-release or sustained-release oral drug products allows for the slow release of the drug from the dosage form and subsequent slow absorption of the drug from the gastrointestinal tract.

   a. Why does the slow release of a drug from an extended-release drug product produce a longer-acting pharmacodynamic response compared to the same drug prepared in a conventional, oral, immediate-release drug product?

   b. Why do manufacturers of sustained-release drug products attempt to design this dosage form to have a zero-order rate of systemic drug absorption?

2. The dissolution profiles of three drug products are illustrated in Figure 17-19.

   a. Which of the drug products in Figure 17-19 release drug at a zero-order rate of about 8.3% every hour?

   b. Which of the drug products does not release drug at a zero-order rate?

   c. Which of the drug products has an almost zero-rate of drug release during certain hours of the dissolution process?

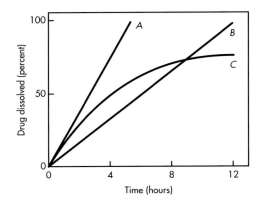

Figure 17-19. Dissolution profile of three different drug products. Drug dissolved (percent).

    d. Suggest a common cause of slowing drug dissolution rate of many rapid-release drug products toward the end of dissolution.

    e. Suggest a common cause of slowing drug dissolution of a sustained-release product toward the end of a dissolution test.

3. A drug is normally given at 10 mg four times a day. Suggest an approach for designing a 12-hour zero-order release product.

    a. Calculate the desired zero-order release rate.

    b. Calculate the concentration of the drug in an osmotic pump type of oral dosage form that delivers 0.5 mL/hr of fluid.

4. An industrial pharmacist would like to design a sustained-release drug product to be given every 12 hours. The active drug ingredient has an apparent volume of distribution of 10 L, an elimination half-life of 3.5 hours, and a desired therapeutic plasma drug concentration of 20 μg/mL. Calculate the zero-order release rate of the sustained-release drug product and the total amount of drug needed, assuming no loading dose is required.

REFERENCES

Bodmeier R, Oh KH, Chen H: The effect of the addition of low molecular weight poly(DL-lactide) on drug release from biodegradable poly(DL-lactide) drug delivery systems. *Int J Pharm* **51**:1–8, 1989

Breimer DD, Dauhof M: *Towards Better Safety of Drugs and Pharmaceutical Products.* Amsterdam, Elsevier/North-Holland, 1980, pp 117–142

Dighe SV, Adams WP: Bioavailability and bioequivalence of oral extended-release products: A regulatory perspective. In Welling PG, Tse FLS (eds), *Pharmacokinetics: Regulatory, Industrial, Academic Perspectives.* New York, Marcel Dekker, 1988

Dong L, Shafi K, Wong P, Wan J: L-OROS® SOFTCAP™ for controlled release of non-aqueous liquid formulation. *Drug Delivery Technol* **2**(1), 2002

Galeone M, Nizzola L, Cacioli D, Moise G: *In vivo* demonstration of delivery mechanisms sustained-release pellets. *Curr Ther Res* **29**:217–234, 1981

Guy RH: Current status and future prospects of transdermal drug delivery. *Pharm Res* **13**:1765–1769, 1996

Hofmann FF, Pressman JH, Code CF, Witztum KF: Controlled entry of orally administered drugs: Physiological considerations. *Drug Dev Ind Pharm* **9:**1077, 1983

Shareef MA, Ahuja A, Ahmad FJ, Raghava S: Colonic drug delivery: An updated review, *AAPS PharmSci* **5:**161–186, 2003

Shaw JE, Chandrasekaran SK: Controlled topical delivery systems for systemic action. *Drug Metab Rev* **8:**223–233, 1978

Skelly JP, Amidon GL, Barr WH, et al: *In vitro* and *in vivo* testing and correlation for oral controlled/modified-release dosage forms. Workshop report. *Pharm Res* **7:**975–982, 1990. Also published in *J Pharm Sci* **79:**849–854, 1990; *J Control Release* **14:**95, 1990.

Skelly JP, Barr WH: Regulatory assessment. In Robinson JR, Lee VHL (eds), *Controlled Drug Delivery: Fundamentals and Applications*, 2nd ed. New York, Marcel Dekker, 1987

Skelly JP, Van Buskirk GA, Arbit HM, et al: Workshop report; Scaleup of oral extended-release dosage forms. *Pharm Res* **10**, 1800 (1993)

Welling PG: Pharmacokinetic considerations of controlled release drug products. *Drug Dev Ind Pharm* **9:**1185–1225, 1983

BIBLIOGRAPHY

Akala EO, Collett JH: Influence of drug loading and gel structure on in-vitro release kinetics from photopolymerized gels. *Ind Pharm* **13:**1779–1798, 1987

Arnon R: In Gregoriadis G, Senior J, Trouet A (eds), *Targeting of Drugs*. New York, Plenum, 1982, pp 31–54

Arnon R, Hurwitz E: In Goldberg EP (ed), *Targeted Drugs*. New York, Wiley, 1983, pp 23–55

Bayley H, Gasparro F, Edelson R: Photoactive drugs. *TIPS* **8:**138–144, 1987

Boxenbaum HG: Physiological and pharmacokinetic factors affecting performance of sustained release dosage forms. *Drug Dev Ind Pharm* **8:**1–25, 1982

Brodsky FM: Monoclonal antibodies as magic bullets. *Pharm Res* **5:**1–9, 1988

Bruck S (ed): *CRC Controlled Drug Delivery*. Boca Raton, FL, CRC Press, 1983

Cabana BE: Bioavailability regulations and biopharmaceutic standard for controlled release drug delivery. *Proceedings of 1982 Research and Scientific Development Conference*. Washington, DC, The Proprietary Association, 1983, pp 56–69

Chien YW: *Novel Drug Delivery Systems*. New York, Marcel Dekker, 1982

Chien YW: Oral controlled drug administration. *Drug Dev Ind Pharm* **9**, 1983

Chien YW, Siddiqui O, Shi WM, et al: Direct current iontophoretic transdermal delivery of peptide and protein drugs. *J Pharm Sci* **78:**376–383, 1989

Chu BCF, Whiteley JM: High molecular weight derivatives of methotrexate as chemotherapeutic agents. *Mol Pharmacol* **13:**80, 1980

Fiume L, Busi C, Mattioli A: Targeting of antiviral drugs by coupling with protein carriers. *FEBS Lett* **153:**6, 1983

Fiume L, Busi C, Mattioli A, et al: In Gregoriadis G, Senior J, Trouet A (eds), *Targeting of Drugs*. New York, Plenum, 1982

Friend DR, Pangburn S: Site-specific drug delivery. *Medicinal Res Rev* **7:**53–106, 1987

Gros L, Ringsdorf H, Schupp H: *Angew Chem Int Ed Engl* **20:**312, 1981

Heller J: Controlled drug release from monolithic bioerodible polymer devices. *Pharm Int* **7:**316–318, 1986

Hunter E, Fell JT, Sharma H: The gastric emptying of pellets contained in hard gelatin capsules. *Drug Dev Ind Pharm* **8:**151–157, 1982

Joshi HN: Recent advances in drug delivery systems: Polymeric prodrugs. *Pharm Technol* **12:**118–125, 1988

Langer R: New methods of drug delivery. *Science* **249:**1527–1533, 1990

Levy G: Targeted drug delivery: Some pharmacokinetic considerations. *Pharm Res* **4:**3–4, 1987

Malinowski HJ: Biopharmaceutic aspects of the regulatory review of oral controlled release drug products. *Drug Dev Ind Pharm* **9:**1255–1279, 1983

Miyazaki S, Ishii K, Nadai T: Controlled release of prednisolone from ethylene-vinyl acetate copolymer matrix. *Chem Pharm Bull* **29:**2714–2717, 1981

Mueller-Lissner SA, Blum AL: The effect of specific gravity and eating on gastric emptying of slow-release capsules. *N Engl J Med* **304:**1365–1366, 1981

Okabe K, Yamoguchi H, Kawai Y: New ionotophoretic transdermal administration of the beta-blocker metoprolol. *J Control Release* **4:**79–85, 1987

Park H, Robinson JR: Mechanisms of mucoadhesion of poly(acrylic acid) hydrogels. *Pharm Res* **4:**457–464, 1987

Pozansky MJ, Juliano RL: Biological approaches to the controlled delivery of drugs: A critical review. *Pharmacol Rev* **36:**277–336, 1984

Robinson JR: *Sustained and Controlled Release Drug Delivery Systems.* New York, Marcel Dekker, 1978

Robinson JR: Oral drug delivery systems. *Proceedings of 1982 Research and Scientific Development Conference.* Washington, DC, The Proprietary Association, 1983, pp 54–69

Robinson JR, Eriksen SP: Theoretical formulation of sustained release dosage forms. *J Pharm Sci* **53:**1254–1263, 1966

Robinson JR, Lee VHL (eds): *Controlled Drug Delivery: Fundamentals and Applications,* 2nd ed. New York, Marcel Dekker, 1987

Rosement TJ, Mansdorf SZ: *Controlled Release Delivery Systems.* New York, Marcel Dekker, 1983

Schechter B, Wilchek M, Arnon R: Increased therapeutic efficacy of cis-platinum complexes of poly L-glutamic acid against a murine carcinoma. *Int J Cancer* **39:**409–413, 1987

Urquhart J: *Controlled-Release Pharmaceuticals.* Washington, DC, American Pharmaceutical Association, 1981

USP Subcommittee on Biopharmaceutics: *In-vitro/in-vivo* correlation for extended-release oral dosage forms. *Pharm Forum* 4160–4161, 1988

18

TARGETED DRUG DELIVERY SYSTEMS AND BIOTECHNOLOGICAL PRODUCTS

Many diseases occur as a result of defects or errors in the genes involved in producing essential enzymes or proteins in the body. The genes are coded in *deoxyribonucleic acid* (DNA), helical double-stranded molecules folded into chromosomes in the nucleus of cells. The Human Genome Project was created several years ago to sequence the human genome. This national effort is now yielding information on the role of genetics in congenital defects, cancer, disorders involving the immune system, and other diseases that have a genetic link.

The emerging genetic basis of disease will provide novel opportunities for the development of new drugs to treat these disorders, particularly in the field of biotechnology. The discovery of recombinant DNA (rDNA) technology and its application to new drug development has revolutionized the biopharmaceutical industry. Previously, the pharmaceutical industry relied on the use of relatively simple small drug molecules to treat disease. Modern molecular techniques have changed the face of new drug development to include larger, more sophisticated and complex drug molecules. These large biopharmaceuticals have enormous potential to treat disease in novel ways previously unavailable to small drug molecules. As a result, *biotechnology,* or the use of biological materials to create a specific drug product, has become an important sector of the pharmaceutical industry and accounts for the fastest-growing class of new drugs in the market. Nucleic acid, protein and peptide drugs, and diagnostics are the main drug products emerging from the biopharmaceutical industry.

BIOTECHNOLOGY

Protein Drugs

The human genome produces thousands of gene products that prevent disease and maintain health. Many may have therapeutic applications if supplemented to normal or supraphysiologic levels in the body. Most of the biologic molecules listed in Table 18.1 are normally present in the body in small concentrations but are used for certain therapeutic indications. For example, some diseases such as insulin-dependent diabetes result from insufficient production of a natural product, in this case insulin. For these patients, the treatment is to supplement the patient's own insulin production with recombinant human insulin (eg, Humulin). Similarly, human recombinant growth hormone (Protropin, Nutropin) and glucocerebrocidase (Ceredase, Cerezyme) are used to treat growth hormone deficiency and Gaucher's disease, respectively.

In contrast, *interferons* are proteins produced by the immune system in response to viral infection and other biologic inducers. When infection or cancer surpasses the capacity of the body's immune system, recombinant interferons (Roferon-A, Intron A, Alferon N, Actimmune, Infergen, Rebif) or other immune-enhancing molecules can be used to boost immunity. Recombinant interferons and interleukins (Proleukin, Neumega) are therefore used to strengthen the immune system during infection, immunosuppression, cancer, and multiple sclerosis. Erythropoetin and derivatives (Epogen, Procrit, Aronesp) and growth factors (Prokine, Leukine, Neupogen, Becaplermin) are also used to stimulate red and white cell production for anemia or immune suppression following chemotherapy. These molecules were originally available only by purification from human or animal sources. Biotechnology, bioengineering, and the use of cell banks have enabled the large-scale and reproducible production of these naturally occurring biologically derived drugs (Table 18.1).

The size and complexity of protein and nucleic acid drugs require extensive design and engineering of the manufacturing and control processes to produce the drug in large quantities with consistent quality. The size of a protein or peptide drug can range from a few hundred to several hundred thousand daltons. The three-dimensional structure of a protein or peptide drug is important for its pharmacodynamic activity, so the corresponding specific primary amino acid, secondary (alpha or beta helix), tertiary (special relationship of secondary structures), or even quaternary orientation of subunits must be considered. A biotechnology-derived drug (also referred to as a *biologic drug* or *biopharmaceutical*) must be designed such that the structure is stable, reproducible, and accurate during manufacture, storage, and administration. The manufacturing process and product are intricately linked. Small changes in the manufacturing process may affect the sequence of the resulting protein, but are more likely will affect the structure, yield, or activity of the protein. Therefore, pharmaceutical controls and testing must be carefully designed, controlled, and monitored, and must also be able to distinguish minor chemical or structural changes that could affect the safety or efficacy in the product during each of these stages.

Drug delivery of biologics can be a problem for therapeutic use because the protein drug must reach the site of action physically and structurally intact. Biologic drugs are notoriously unstable in plasma and the gastrointestinal tract,

TABLE 18.1   A Sample of Approved Recombinant Drugs

DRUG	INDICATION	PHARMACOKINETICS	YEAR INTRODUCED, COMPANY (TRADE NAME)
Aldesleukin; interleukin-2	Renal cell carcinoma	Half-life = 85 min; Cl = 268 mL/min	1992 Chiron (Proleukin)
Alteplase	Acute myocardial infarction Acute pulmonary embolism	Half-life < 5 min; Cl = 380–570 mL/min; $V_d \approx$ plasma volume	1987 Genentech (Activase) 1990 Genentech (Activase)
Antihemophilic factor	Hemophilia B		1992 Armour (Mononine)
Antihemophilic factor	Hemophilia A	Half-life = 13 hr	1992 Genetics Institute, Baxter Healthcare, Bayer (ReFacto, Recombinate, Kogenate, Helixate FS)
Agalsidase-beta; α-galactosidase A	Fabry's disease	Half-life = 45–102 min; nonlinear kinetics	2003 Genzyme (Fabrazyme)
Anakinara; IL-1 receptor antagonist	Rheumatoid arthritis	Half-life = 4–6 hr	2001 Amgen (Kineret)
β-Glucocerebrosidase;	Type I Gaucher's disease		1991 Genzyme (Ceredase)
Glucocerebrocidase	Type I Gaucher's disease		1994 Genzyme (Cerezyme)
CMV immune globulin	CMV prevention in kidney transplant		1990 Medimmune (CytoGam)
DNase	Cystic fibrosis		1993 Genentech (Pulmozyme)
Drotrecogin-α; activated protein C	Severe sepsis	Cl = 40 L/hr	2001 Lilly (Xigris)
Erythropoietin	Anemia associated with chronic renal failure Anemia associated with AIDS/AZT Anemia associated with cancer and chemotherapy	Half-life = 4–13 hr	1989 Amgen; Johnson & Johnson; Kirin (Epogen); 1990 Ortho Biotech (Procrit) 1990 Amgen; Ortho Biotech (Procrit) 1993 Amgen; Ortho Biotech (Procrit)
Factor VIII	Hemophilia A		1993 Genentech; Miles (Kogenate)
Filgrastim; G-CSF	Chemotherapy-induced neutropenia Bone marrow transplant	Half-life = 3.5 hr; V_d = 150 mL/kg; Cl = 0.5–0.7 mL/kg/min	1991 Amgen (Neupogen) 1994 Amgen (Neupogen)
Human insulin	Diabetes		1982 Eli Lilly, Genentech (Humulin)
Interferon-α-2a	Hairy cell leukemia; AIDS-related Kaposi's sarcoma	Half-life = 5.1 hr; V_d = 0.4 L/kg; Cl = 2.9 mL/min/kg	1986 Hoffmann-La Roche (Roferon-A) 1988 Hoffmann-La Roche (Roferon-A)
Interferon-α-2b	Hairy cell leukemia; AIDS-related Kaposi's sarcoma	Half-life = 2–3 hr	1986 Schering-Plough; Biogen (Intron A) 1991 Schering-Plough; Biogen (Intron A)
Interferon-α-n3	Genital warts		1989 Interferon Sciences (Alferon N injection)

(Continued)

TABLE 18.1 A Sample of Approved Recombinant Drugs (continued)

DRUG	INDICATION	PHARMACOKINETICS	YEAR INTRODUCED, COMPANY (TRADE NAME)
Interferon-β 1b	Relapsing/remitting multiple sclerosis	Half-life = 8 min–4.3 hr; Cl = 9.4–28.9 mL/kg/min; V_d = 0.25–2.9 L/kg	1993 Chiron; Berlex (Betaseron)
Interferon-β1a	Multiple sclerosis	Half-life = 8.6–10 hr	1996 Biogen (Avonex); 2002 Serano (Rebif)
Interferon-γ-1b	Management of chronic granulomatous disease		1990 Genentech (Actimmune)
Human growth hormone	Short stature caused by human growth hormone deficiency		1994 Genentech (Nutropin)
Hepatitis B vaccine, MSD	Hepatitis B prevention		1986 Merck; Chiron (Recombivax HB) Smith Kline 1989 Beecham; Biogen (Engerix-B)
Laronidase; α-L-iduronidase	Mucopolysaccharidosis I	Half-life = 1.5–3.6 hr; Cl = 1.7–2.7 mL/min/kg; V_d = 0.24–0.6 L/kg	2003 Biomarin (Aldurazyme)
Pegadamase (PEG-adenosin)	ADA-deficient SCID		1990 Enzon; Eastman Kodak (Adagen)
PEG-L-asparaginase	Refractory childhood acute lymphoblastic leukemia		1994 Enzon (Oncaspar)
Reteplase; plasminogen activator	Acute myocardial infarction	Half-life = 0.2–0.3 hr; Cl = 7.5–9.7 mL/min/kg	1996 Boehringer Mannheim (Retavase)
Sargramostim (GM-CSF)	Autologous bone marrow transplantation Neutrophil recovery following bone marrow transplantation		1991 Hoechst-Roussel; Immunex (Prokine) 1991 Immunex; Hoechst-Roussel (Leukine)
Somatropin Somatrem	hGH deficiency in children		1987 Eli Lilly (Humatrope) 1985 Genentech (Protropin)
Tenecteplase	Acute myocardial infarction	Half-life = 90–130 min; Cl = 99–119 mL/min; $V_d \approx$ plasma vol.	2002 Genentech (TNKase)

From Yu and Fong (1997), with permission, and www.fda.gov/cber/appr2003.

so modifications to improve drug delivery or stability are often required. Currently, most biologic drugs are generally too unstable for oral delivery and must usually be administered by parenteral routes. However, other, nonparenteral routes of administration, such as intranasal and inhalation, are being investigated for biologic drug delivery. Fortunately, because many of these recombinant protein drugs are designed to act extracellularly, transmembrane delivery may not be required once the drug reaches the plasma.

Monoclonal Antibodies

Another new class of protein drugs is *monoclonal antibodies* (mAbs). Antibodies are produced by the body's immune system for specific recognition and removal of

TABLE 18.2   Applications of Monoclonal Antibodies

Cancer treatment

mAbs against leukemia and lymphomas have been used in treatment with variable results. Regression of tumor is produced in about 25%, although mostly transient.

Imaging diagnosis

mAbs may be used together with radioactive markers to locate and visualize the location and extent of the tumors.

Target-specific delivery

mAbs may be conjugated to drugs or other delivery systems such as liposomes to allow specific delivery to target sites. For example, urokinase was conjugated to an antifibrin mAb to dissolve fibrin clots. The carrier system would seek fibrin sites and activate the conversion of plasmogen to plasmin to cause fibrin to degrade.

Transplant rejection suppression

In kidney transplants, a mAb against CD3, a membrane protein of cytotoxic T cells that causes a rejection reaction, was very useful in suppressing rejection and allowing the transplant to function. The drug was called OKT3. mAbs are also used for kidney and bone marrow transplants.

foreign bodies. The power of mAbs lies in their highly specific binding of only one antigenic determinant. As a result, mAb drugs, targeting agents, and diagnostics are creating new ways to treat and diagnose previously untreatable diseases and to detect extraordinarily low concentrations of protein or other molecules (Table 18.2).

Theoretically, an almost infinite amount and number of antibodies can be produced by the body to respond immunologically to foreign substances containing antigenic sites. These antigenic sites are usually on protein molecules, but nonprotein material or *haptens* may be conjugated to a protein to form an antigen. Periodic injections of an antigen into an animal result in production of antibodies that bind a site or sites on that antigen. The serum of the animal will also contain antibodies to antigens to which the animal has been previously exposed. Though these mixtures of antibodies in the serum (*polyclonal antibodies*) are too impure for therapeutic use, they can be used for diagnostic immunoassays.

In contrast to polyclonal antibodies, mAbs are preparations that contain many copies of a single antibody that will therefore bind to and only detect one antigenic site. The purity of these preparations make them very useful as both diagnostics and as new therapeutic agents. However, the techniques for the preparation of mAbs are quite complicated. In mAb production, normal antibody-producing cells, such as a mouse spleen cell, are fused with a myeloma cell and allow the hybrid cells (*hybridoma*) to grow in a test tube. The nonfused cells will die, the myeloma cells will be selectively destroyed with an antitumor drug such as aminopterin (Fig. 18-1), whereas the hybridoma cells will continue to grow. Each hybridoma cell is then separated into a separate growth chamber or well in which they are allowed to multiply. Each cell and its clones in the respective growth chamber will make antibodies to only one antigen (mAb). The cells producing the desired antibody are selected by testing each well for mAb binding to the desired antigen. The desired cells (clones) are then expanded for mAb production. Since the resulting mAb is of murine origin, often genetic engineering is used to "humanize" the mAb, thus minimizing an immune response to the therapeutic mAb.

Monoclonal antibodies may be used therapeutically to neutralize unwanted cells or molecules. Several mAbs with proven indications are listed in Tables 18.1, 18.2, and 18.3. Monoclonal antibodies are used as antivenoms (CroFab), for overdose of digoxin (DigiFab), or to neutralize endotoxin (Nebacumab, investigative) or viral

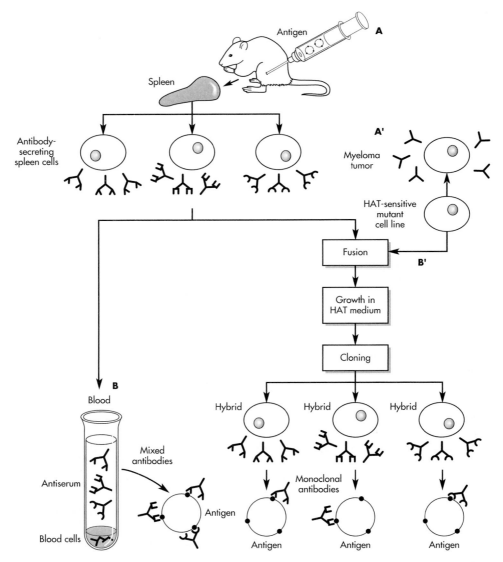

Figure 18-1. Monoclonal antibody production. **A.** A mouse is immunized with an antigen bearing three antigenic determinants (distinct sites that can be recognized by an antibody). Antibodies to each determinant are produced in the spleen. One spleen cell produces a single type of antibody. A spleen cell has a finite lifetime and cannot be cultured indefinitely *in vitro.* **B.** In the mouse, the antibody-producing cells from the spleen secrete into the blood. The liquid portion of the blood (serum) therefore contains a mixture of antibodies reacting with all three sites on the antigen (antiserum). **A'.** A mutant cell derived from a mouse myeloma tumor of an antibody-producing cell that has stopped secreting antibody and is selected for sensitivty to the drug aminopterin (present in HAT medium). This mutant tumor cell can grow indefinitely *in vitro* but is killed by HAT medium. **B'.** The mutant myeloma cell is fused by chemical means with spleen cells from an immunized mouse. The resulting hybrid cells can grow indefinitely *in vitro* due to properties of the myeloma cell parent and can grow in HAT medium because of an enzyme provided by the spleen cell parent. The unfused myeloma cells die because of their sensitivity to HAT, and unfused spleen cells cannot grow indefinitely *in vitro.* The hybrid cells are cloned so that individual cultures are grown from a single hybrid cell. These individual cells produce a single type of antibody because they derive from a single spleen cell. The monoclonal antibody isolated from these cultures is specific for only one antigenic determinant on the original antigen. (From Milstein, 1980, and Brodsky, 1988, with permission.)

TABLE 18.3   Approved Monoclonal Antibody Drugs and In-Vivo Diagnostics

mAb PRODUCT (TRADE NAME)	TARGET		INDICATION
Abciximab (ReoPro)	Platelet surface glycoprotein	Half-life < 10 min	Unstable angina Coronary angioplasty or atherectomy (PCTA) Antiplatelet prevention of blood clots
Adalimumab (Humira)	Tumor necrosis factor	V_d = 4–6 L; Cl = 12 mL/hr; half-life = 2 wk	Rheumatoid arthritis
Alefacept (Amevive)	CD2 (LFA) on lymphocytes	Half-life = 270 hr; Cl = 0.25 mL/kg/hr; V_d = 94 mL/kg	Psoriasis
Alemtuzumab (Campath)	CD52 on blood cells	Half-life = 12 d	B-cell chronic lymphocytic leukemia
Antithymocyte globulin (rabbit) thymoglobulin	T-lymphocyte antigens	Half-life = 2–3 d	Acute rejection in renal transplant patients
Basiliximab (Simulect)	Interleukin-2	Half-life = 7.2 d; V_d = 8.6 L; Cl = 41 mL/hr	Renal transplantation immunosuppression
Capromab pendetide (ProstaScint)	Prostate glycoprotein	Half-life = 67 hr; Cl = 42 mL/hr; V_d = 4 L	Diagnosing imaging agent in prostate cancer
Daclizumab (Zenapax)	Interleukin-2 receptor	Half-life = 20 d; Cl = 15 mL/hr; V_d = 6 L	Renal transplants immunosuppression
Denileukin diftitox (Ontak)	Interleukin-2 mAb conjugate to diptheria toxin	Half-life = 70–80 min; Cl = 1.5–2 mL/min/kg; V_d = 0.06–0.08 L/kg	Cutaneous T-cell lymphoma
Digoxin Immune Fab—Ovine (DigiFab)	Digoxin	Half-life = 15–20 hr; V_d = 0.3–0.4 L/kg	Digoxin toxicity or overdose
Etanercept (Enbrel)	Tumor necrosis factor receptor	Half-life = 115 hr; Cl = 89 mL/hr	Rheumatoid arthritis
Hepatitis B immune globulin—human (Nabi-HB)	Hepatitis B	Half-life = 25 d; Cl = 0.4 L/d; V_d = 15 L	Acute exposure to hepatitis B
Ibritumomab tiuxetan (Zevalin)	CD28 on B cells	Half-life = 30 hr	Follicular or transformed B-cell non-Hodgkin's lymphoma
Imciromab pentetate (Myoscint)	Myosin	Half-life = 20 hr	Imaging agent for detecting myocardial injury
Infliximab (Remicade)	Tumor necrosis factor	Half-life = 9.5 d; V_d = 3 L	Crohn's disease Rheumatoid arthritis
Nofetumomab (Verluma)	Carcinoma-associated antigen, Tc^{99m} labeled	Half-life = 10.5 hr	Detection of small cell lung cancer
Muromonab-CD3 (Orthoclone OKT3)	CD3 on T cells		Reversal of acute kidney transplant rejection
Palivizumab (Synagis)	RSV antigens	Half-life = 197 hr; Cl = 0.33 mL/hr/kg; V_d = 90 mL/kg	RSV disease
Rituximab (Rituxan)	CD20 on B cells	Half-life = 60 hr	Follicular, B-cell non-Hodgkin's lymphoma
Trastuzumab (Herceptin)	Human epidermal growth factor receptor	Half-life = 1.7–12 d; V_d = 44 mL/kg	Metastatic breast cancer whose tumors overexpress the HER2 protein

antigen (Nabi-HB). Nebacumab is a human IgM mAb (HA-1A) with specificity for the lipid designed for septic shock treatment. Monoclonal antibodies (mAb) are named by a source identifier preceding "-mab," e.g., -**u**mab (human), -**o**mab (mouse), -**zu**mab (humanized), and -**xi**mab (cl.meric). Other common indications for mAb drugs include imaging (ProstaScint, Myocint, Verluma), cancer (Campath, Ontak, Zevalin, Rituxan, Herceptin), rheumatoid arthritis (Humira, Remicade), and transplant immunosuppression (Simulect, Thymoglobulin). Monoclonal antibodies are also used for more novel indications. For example, Abciximab (c7E3 Fab, ReoPro) is a chimeric mAb Fab (humanized) fragment specific for platelet glycoprotein IIb-IIIa receptors. This drug is extremely effective in reducing fatalities (0.50%) in subjects with unstable angina after angioplasty treatment.

Monoclonal antibodies can also target and deliver toxins specifically to cancer cells and destroy them while sparing normal cells (see below), and they are important detectors used in laboratory diagnostics.

Gene Therapy

Gene therapy refers to a pharmaceutical product that delivers a recombinant gene to somatic cells *in vivo* (Ledley, 1996). In turn, the gene within the patients' cell produces a protein that has therapeutic benefit to the patient. The therapeutic approach in gene therapy is often the restoration of defective biologic function within cells, as is frequently seen in inherited disorders and cancer.

Gene therapy has been applied to the inherited disorder cystic fibrosis, in which patients have a defective chloride ion channel gene, resulting in chloride ion channel abnormalities. Although improved therapy has transformed cystic fibrosis from a disease characterized by death in early childhood to a chronic illness, there still is no cure for the disease and most patients eventually succumb to infections of the airways and lung failure. The aim of gene therapy for these patients is to deliver a "normal" chloride ion channel gene to the cells of cystic fibrosis patients and restore chloride transport in cells. More information on gene therapy of cystic fibrosis has been published by the National Institutes of Health (www.niddk.nih.gov/health/endo/pubs/cystic/cystic.htm).

Gene therapy faces several challenges despite over a decade of research and development. These challenges include gene delivery, sufficient extent and duration of stable gene expression, and safety. Because the gene coding the therapeutic protein (*transgene*) must also contain gene control regions such as the promoter, the actual rDNA (*recombinant DNA*) to be delivered to target cells' nucleus can easily be 10–20 kilobases (kb) in size.

Two main approaches have been used for *in-vivo* delivery of rDNA. The first is a virus-based approach that involves replacing viral replicative genes with the transgene, then packaging the rDNA into the viral particle. The recombinant virus can then infect target cells, and the transgene is expressed, though the virus is not capable of replicating. Both retroviruses, RNA viruses that have the ability to permanently insert their genes into the chromosomes of the host cells, and DNA viruses (which remain outside host chromosomes) have been used successfully in viral gene delivery. Most of the gene therapy trials worldwide involve the use of such viral delivery systems.

In addition to viral delivery systems (*vectors*), nonviral approaches have been used with some success for *in-vivo* gene delivery. The transgene is engineered into a plasmid vector, which contains gene-expression control regions. These naked DNA molecules may enter cells and express product in some cell types, such as muscle cells. This naked DNA delivery technique is being tested as possible DNA vaccines, in which the muscle cells produce small amounts of antigen that stimulate immunity to the antigen. However, usually either cationic or a fusogenic liposome delivery systems (see below) is required in most other cell types to produce measurable levels of transgene expression. Both types of lipid vesicles or particles result in intracellular delivery of DNA to cells.

An alternative to direct *in-vivo* delivery is a cell-based approach that involves the administration of transgenes to cells that have been removed from a patient. For example, cells (usually bone marrow cells) are removed from the patient; genes encoding a therapeutic product are then introduced into these cells *ex vivo* using a viral or nonviral delivery system, and then the cells are returned into the patient. The advantage of *ex-vivo* approaches is that systemic toxicity of viral or nonviral delivery systems is avoided.

Effective gene therapy depends on several conditions. The vector must be able to enter the target cells efficiently and deliver the corrective gene without damaging the target cell. The corrective gene should be stably expressed in the cells, to allow continuous production of the functional protein. Neither the vector nor the functional protein produced from it should cause an immune reaction in the patient. It is also difficult to control the amount of functional protein produced after gene therapy, and excess production of the protein could cause side effects, although insufficient production is more typically observed. Additional problems in gene therapy include the physical and chemical properties of DNA and RNA molecules, such as size, shape, charge, surface characteristics, and the chemical stability of these molecules and delivery systems. *In-vivo* problems may include bioavailability, distribution, and uptake of these macromolecules into cells. Moreover, naked DNA molecules are rapidly degraded in the body (Ledley, 1996).

Antisense Drugs

Antisense drugs are drugs that seek to block DNA transcription or RNA translation in order to moderate many disease processes. Antisense drugs consist of nucleotides linked together in short DNA or RNA sequences known as *oligonucleotides*. Oligonucleotides are designed knowing the target DNA/RNA to bind to specific DNA or RNA sequences or regions (eg, messenger RNA) to block transcription or translation of that targeted protein. An oligonucleotide that binds complementary ("sense") mRNA sequences and blocks translation is referred to as *antisense*. To further stabilize the drug, many chemical modifications have been made to the oligonucleotide structure. The most common modification used involves substitution of a nonbridging oxygen in the phosphate backbone with sulfur, resulting in a phosphorothioate-derived antisense oligonucleotide. Some of these drugs have been designed to target viral disease and cancer cells in the body. Vitravene (ISIS Pharmaceuticals), an oligonucleotide targeted to cytomegalovirus, was the first antisense oligonucleotide drug approved by the U.S. Food and Drug Administration (FDA).

For this approach to be useful, the etiology and genetics of the disease must be known. For example, in the case of viral infection, known sequences belonging to vital genes can be targeted and inhibited by antisense drugs. Many antisense sequences are usually tested to find the best candidate, since intra- and intermolecular interactions can affect oligonucleotide activity and delivery. Though oligonucleotides are relatively well internalized compared to rDNA molecules, cellular uptake is often low enough to require delivery systems, such as liposomes. Antisense and gene therapy approaches have also been combined using viral vectors to deliver an antisense sequence. In this case, the transgene is transcribed into an mRNA molecule that is antisense and therefore binds to the target mRNA. The resulting RNA:RNA interaction is high affinity and results in inhibition of translation of that mRNA molecule.

DRUG CARRIERS AND TARGETING

Formulation and Delivery of Protein Drugs

Advances in biotechnology have resulted in the commercial production of naturally produced active drug substances for drug therapy (Table 18.1). These substances hold great potential for more specific drug action with fewer side effects. However, many naturally produced substances are complex molecules, such as large-molecular-weight proteins and peptides. Conventional delivery of protein and peptide drugs is generally limited to injectables and implantable dosage forms. Insulin pumps for implantation have been developed for diabetes, for precise control of sugar levels.

Formulating protein drugs for systemic use by oral, or even any extravascular, route of administration is extremely difficult due to drug degradation and absorption from the site of administration. There are several requirements for effective oral drug delivery of protein and peptide drugs: (1) protection of the drug from degradation while in the harsh environment of the digestive tract, (2) consistent absorption of the drug in a manner that meets bioavailability requirements, (3) consistent release of the drug so that it enters the bloodstream in a reproducible manner, (4) nontoxicity, and (5) delivery of the drug through the GI tract and maintenance of pharmacologic effect similar to IV injection.

Designing, evaluating, and improving protein and peptide drug stability is considerably more complex than for small conventional drug molecules. A change in quaternary structure, such as aggregation or deaggregation of the protein, may result in loss of activity. Changes in primary structure of proteins frequently occur and include deamidation of the amino acid chains, oxidation of chains with sulfhydryl groups, and cleavage by proteolytic enzymes present throughout the body and that may be present due to incomplete purification. Because of protein drugs' complex structures, impurities are much harder to detect and quantify. In addition, proteins may be recognized as foreign substances in the body and become actively phagocytized by the reticuloendothelial system (RES), resulting in the inability of these proteins to reach the intended target. Proteins may also have a high allergenic or immunogenic potential, particularly when nonhuman genes or production cells are used.

Because of the many stability and delivery problems associated with protein and nucleic acid drugs, new delivery systems are being tested to improve their *in-vivo* properties. Carriers can be used to protect the drug from degradation, improve transport or delivery to cells, decrease clearance, or a combination of the above. In this chapter, carriers used for both small traditional drug and biopharmaceutical drug delivery are reviewed. Carriers may be covalently bound to the drug, where drug release is usually required for pharmacologic activity. Noncovalent drug carriers such as liposomes typically require uncoating of the drug for biologic activity to occur.

Polymeric Carriers and Conjugates

Polymers can be designed to include a wide range of physical and chemical properties and are popularly used in drug formulations because of their versatility. Polymers initially were used to prolong drug release in controlled-release dosage forms. The development of site-specific polymer or macromolecular carrier systems is a more recent extension of earlier research. The basic components of site-specific polymer carriers are (1) the polymeric backbone (Fig. 18-2), (2) a site-specific component (homing device) for recognizing the target, (3) the drug covalently attached to the polymer chain, and (4) functional chains to enhance the physical characteristics of the carrier system. Improved physical characteristics may include improved aqueous solubility. In the case of polymeric prodrugs, a spacer group may be present, bridging the drug and the carrier. The spacer chain may influence the rate at which the drug will hydrolyze from the prodrug system. At present, most site-specific polymeric drug carriers are limited to parenteral administration and primarily utilize soluble polymers.

Positively charged polymers such as polyethylenediamine (PEI), polylysine, and chitosan (Fig. 18-3) are used in noncovalent complexes for macromolecular drugs, such as gene or oligonucleotide therapy. For example, polymer:DNA complexes improve DNA delivery to cells in part by providing some protection from nuclease degradation *in vivo*. An added advantage of complexed cationic polymers is that targeting agents such as receptor ligands can be covalently attached to the polymer rather than the drug to provide cell-specific targeting. Cationic polymer use is limited because of toxicity of the polymer and dissociation of the complex *in vivo*.

Polymers may also be covalently conjugated to drugs to improve their solubility or pharmacokinetic properties. Polymers with molecular weights greater than 30–50 kDa bypass glomerular filtration, thereby extending the duration of drug circulation in the body. Polyethylene glycol (PEG) is used to improve the clearance of some drugs, such as adenosine deaminase (PEG-ADA), filgrastim (Neulasta), interferon (PEG-Intron and PEGASYS), and asparaginase (Oncospar). Daunomycin has been linked to dextran, resulting in improved drug activity in

Figure 18-2. Site-specific polymeric carrier.

Figure 18-3. A = solubilizer, IG = immunoglobulin; polyglutamic acid [PGA]; B = Pharmacon, *p*-phenylenediamine [PDM]; C = homing device. (Adapted from Gros et al, 1981.)

animal studies (Levi-Shaffer, 1982). Dextrans are large polysaccharide molecules (MW 2000 to 1 million Da) with good water solubility, stability, and low toxicity. Drugs with a free amino or hydroxyl group may be linked chemically to hydroxyl groups in dextrans by activation of the dextran with periodate, azide, or other agents.

The molecular weight of the polymer carrier is an important consideration in designing these dosage forms. Generally, large-molecular-weight polymers have longer residence time and diffuse more slowly. However, large polymers are also more prone to capture by the reticuloendothelial system. To gain specificity, a monoclonal antibody, a recognized sugar moiety, or a small cell-specific ligand may be incorporated as a targeting agent into the delivery system. For example, exposed galactose residues are recognized by hepatocytes; whereas mannose or L-fructose is recognized by surface receptors in macrophages. HMPA [N-(2-hydroxypropyl)methacrylamide] is commonly used in drug conjugates because the polymer can be modified with monosaccharides that act as targeting agents for cells expressing the appropriate receptor (Joshi, 1988, Seymour, 1994). Similarly, a three-way conjugate consisting of mitomycin C, a monoclonal antibody (A7), and dextran (MW 70,000 Da) as the intermediate carrier resulted in a 10-fold increased activity against colon cancer cells due to improved target specificity (Joshi, 1988).

In addition to use as regular carriers, polymers may also be formulated into *microparticles* and *nanoparticles*. In such delivery systems, the therapeutic agent is encapsulated within a biodegradable polymeric colloidal particle that is in the micrometer or nanometer size range, respectively. Micro- and nanosphere formulations are useful for solubilizing poorly soluble drugs, improving oral bioavailability, protecting against degradation, or providing sustained drug delivery. The small size of nanospheres generally allows good tissue penetration while providing protection or sustained release.

The size of the microsphere and nanosphere has a profound impact on an encapsulated drugs' *in-vivo* properties and disposition. At over 12 μm, particles are lodged in the capillary bed at the site of the injection. From 2 to 12 μm, particles are retained at the lung, spleen, or liver. Particles less than 0.5 μm (500 nm) deposit into the spleen and bone marrow. In gene therapy, particles smaller than 100 nm demonstrate higher gene expression *in vitro* compared to larger particles (Panyam and Labhasetwar, 2003). Though some peptides and nucleic acids have been successfully formulated into nanospheres, protein denaturation and degradation can be significant during encapsulation.

Cyclodextrins (CDs) are also used to improve stability, delivery, and water solubility of drugs. The lipophilic cavity of CDs typically contains the therapeutic agent, while the exterior of the CD molecule is hydrophilic and allows solubilization of the complex. Many folded proteins and nucleic acids are too large to be completely included into the CD cavity and can result in protein denaturation. However, CDs have been used to solubilize and stabilize several proteins and peptides (Irie and Uekama, 1999).

Albumin

Albumin is a large protein (MW 69,000 Da) that is distributed in the plasma and extracellular water. Albumin has been experimentally conjugated with many drugs to improve site-specific drug delivery. Methotrexate, cytosine arabinoside, and 6-fluorodeoxyuridine have each been conjugated with albumin. Methotrexate albumin conjugates may increase the duration of drug action after conjugation (Chu and Whiteley, 1980). In general, the distribution of albumin is not site specific. Because albumin will concentrate in the liver, 5-fluorodeoxyuridine (Amanitin) albumin complex has been used experimentally to deliver drug to the Kupffer cells in the liver for treatment of ectromelia virus (Fiume et al, 1983).

Lipoproteins

Lipoproteins are lipid protein complexes in the blood involved in the circulation and distribution of lipids in the body. The lipid components are polar phospholipids and cholesterol. Because of their various sizes, lipoproteins have been classified according to molecular weight based on centrifugation: (1) high-density lipoprotein (HDL, MW 300,000–600,000 Da), (2) low-density lipoprotein (LDL, MW 2.3×10^6 Da), (3) very-low-density lipoprotein (VLDL, MW 10×10^6 Da), and (4) chylomicrons (MW 10^9 Da). Low-density lipoproteins enter the cell by a receptor-mediated pathway through the process of endocytosis. Endocytosis is a potential means of transporting drugs into the cell in which the lipoprotein–drug complex is hydrolyzed by intracellular lysosomal enzymes, releasing the active drug within the vesicle.

More research is needed on the use of lipoproteins for drug targeting. For example, lipophilic drugs may be dissolved within the core of the lipoprotein. After oral administration, fatty substances incorporated into the chylomicron formed in the gastrointestinal tract may be absorbed into the lymphatic system.

Liposomes

Liposomes have an aqueous, drug-containing interior surrounded by an exterior lipid bilayer, and typically range in size from 0.5 to 100 μm. Liposomes have been used successfully to reduce side effects of antitumor drugs and antibiotics. For example, doxorubicin liposomes have reduced cardiotoxicity and emetic side effects. Amphotericin B may have reduced nephrotoxicity side effects when formulated with liposomes. An innovative liposome-related product (Abelcet) consists of amphotericin B complexed with two phospholipids, L-a-dimyristoyl-phosphatidylcholine and L-a-dimyristoylphosphatidylglycerol (Liposome Company, www.lipo.com). The lipid drug complex releases the drug at the site of infection and reduces renal toxicity of amphotericin B without altering its antifungal activity. A more representative liposome product is AmBisome (NeXstar), which consists of very fine liposomes of amphotericin B. The product significantly reduces the side effects of amphotericin B. Other investigative liposomal products include TLC-C-53 (liposomal prostaglandin E1) for the treatment of acute respiratory distress syndrome (ARDS). Daunorubicin citrate liposomal (DaunoXome, NeXstar) is an aqueous solution of the citrate salt of the antineoplastic daunorubicin encapsulated within lipid vesicles. The distearoylphosphotidylcholine and cholesterol (2:1 molar ratio) liposome formulation in DaunoXome attempts to maximize the selectivity of daunorubicin into solid brain tumors. Once in the tumor, daunorubicin is released and exerts its antineoplastic activity. Liposome formulations have also been prepared with gentamicin, cisplatin, and other drugs.

There are three general ways of preparing conventional liposomes: (1) phase separation, (2) spray or shear method through orifice, and (3) coacervation. The choice of method depends on the drug, the yield requirements, and the nature of the lipids. Formation of the liposome bilayer depends on the hydrophobic and hydrophilic orientation of the lipids (Fig. 18-4).

Liposomes have different electrical surface charges depending on the type of material used. Common anionic lipid materials are phosphatidyl choline and cholesterol. The phosphatidyl group is amphiphilic, with the choline being the polar group. This structure allows each molecule to attach to others through hydrophobic and hydrophilic interactions. Thermodynamically, liposomes are in equilibrium between different membrane conformations or structures (lipid polymorphism). Thus, some seemingly stable liposome systems exhibit leakage and generally do not have long shelf lives.

Liposomes can be engineered to be site specific. Generally, site specificity is conferred by the type of lipid or by inclusion of a targeting agent, such as a monoclonal antibody, into the liposome bilayer (see Targeted Drug Delivery, below). Liposomes may be used to improve intracellular delivery, in which case the liposome must also be designed to fuse with the plasma or endosome membrane. Lipids or fusogenic peptides that facilitate membrane fusion, such as phosphatidyl ethanolamine or GALA and KALA peptides, respectively, have been used to improve liposome intracellular delivery. Cationic lipids, such as N-[1-(2, 3 dioleyloxy)propyl]-N,N, N-trimethylammonium chloride (DOTMA) or oleoyl-phoshphatidylethanolamine (DOPE), are also commonly used for *in-vitro* delivery of DNA. When cationic lipids are mixed with DNA, a particle forms from DNA:lipid charge interactions. The

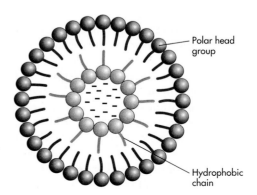

Polar head group

Hydrophobic chain

Figure 8-4. Diagrammatic representation of a liposome showing polar head group and hydrophobic chain.

cationic lipid is believed to destabilize biological membranes resulting in improved intracellular DNA delivery. The *in-vivo* use of cationic lipids is limited by systemic toxicity due to the positive charge of the lipid.

TARGETED DRUG DELIVERY

Most conventional dosage forms deliver drug into the body that eventually reaches the site of action by distribution and passive diffusion. In addition, the drug also distributes to nontarget site tissues. Because of nonselective distribution, a much larger dose is given to the patient to achieve therapeutic concentrations in the desired tissue. However, drug action at nontarget sites may result in toxicity or other adverse reactions. Delivery systems that target the drug only to the desired site of drug action allow for more selective therapeutic activity. For biopharmaceuticals, selective and targeted drug therapy could result in a significant reduction in dose and cost.

Targeted drug delivery or *site-specific drug delivery* refers to drug carrier systems that place the drug at or near the receptor site. Friend and Pangburn (1987) have classified site-specific drug delivery into three broad categories or drug targeting: (1) first-order targeting, which refers to drug delivery systems that deliver the drug to the capillary bed of the active site; (2) second-order targeting, which refers to the specific delivery of drug to a special cell type such as the tumor cells and not to the normal cells; and (3) third-order targeting, which refers to drug delivery specifically to the internal (intracellular) site of cells. An example of third-order drug targeting is the receptor-mediated entry of a drug complex into the cell by endocytosis followed by lysosomal release of the lysosomally active drug. Numerous techniques have been developed for site-specific delivery. Ideally, site-specific carriers guide the drug to the intended target site (tissues or organ) in which the receptor is located without exposing the drug to other tissues, thereby avoiding adverse toxicity. Much of the research in targeted drug delivery has been in cancer chemotherapy.

Site-specific drug delivery has also been characterized as passive or active targeting (Takakura and Hashida, 1996). *Passive targeting* refers to the exploitation of the natural (passive) disposition profiles of a drug carrier, which are passively determined by its physicochemical properties relative to the anatomic and physiologic characteristics of the body. *Active targeting* refers to alterations of the natural disposition of a drug carrier, directing it to specific cells, tissues, or organs. One approach to active targeting is the use of ligands or monoclonal antibodies which can target specific cells. Monoclonal antibodies were discussed more fully earlier in this chapter. Active targeting employing receptor-mediated endocytosis is a saturable, nonlinear process that depends on the drug–carrier concentration, whereas passive targeting is most often a linear process over a large range of doses.

General Considerations in Targeted Drug Delivery

Considerations in the development of site-specific or targeted drug delivery systems include: (1) the anatomic and physiologic characteristics of the target site, including capillary permeability to macromolecules and cellular uptake of the drug (Molema et al, 1997); (2) the physicochemical characteristics of the therapeutically active drug; (3) the physical and chemical characteristics of the carrier; (4) the selectivity of the drug–carrier complex; (5) any impurities introduced during the conjugation reaction linking the drug and the carrier that may be immunogenic, toxic, or produce other adverse reactions.

Target Site

The accessibility of the drug–carrier complex to the target site may present bioavailability and pharmacokinetic problems, which also include anatomic and/or physiologic considerations. For example, targeting a drug into a brain tumor requires a different route of drug administration (intrathecal injection) than targeting a drug into the liver or spleen. Moreover, the permeability of the blood vessels or biologic membranes to macromolecules or drug carrier complex may be a barrier preventing delivery and intracellular uptake of these drugs (Molema et al, 1997).

Site-Specific Carrier

To target a drug to an active site, one must consider whether there is a unique property of the active site that makes the target site differ from other organs or tissue systems in the body. The next consideration is to take advantage of this unique difference so that the drug goes specifically to the site of action and not to other tissues in which adverse toxicity may occur. In many cases the drug is complexed with a carrier that targets the drug to the site of action. The successful application of these delivery systems requires the drug–carrier complex to have both affinity for the target site and favorable pharmacokinetics for delivery to the organ, cells, and subcellular target sites. An additional problem, particularly in the use of protein carriers, is the occurrence of adverse immunological reactions—an occurrence that is partially overcome by designing less immunoreactive proteins (Takakura and Hashida, 1996).

Drugs

Most of the drugs used for targeted drug delivery are highly reactive drugs that have potent pharmacodynamic activities with a narrow therapeutic range. These drugs are often used in cancer chemotherapy. Many of these drugs may be derived from biologic sources, made by a semisynthetic process using a biologic source as a precursor, or produced by recombinant DNA techniques. The drugs may be large macromolecules, such as proteins, and are prone to instability and inactivation problems during processing, chemical manipulation, and storage.

Targeting Agents

Properly applied, drug targeting can improve the therapeutic index of many toxic drugs. However, monoclonal antibodies (see discussion above) are not the "magic bullet" for drug targeting that many people had hoped. One difficulty encountered is that the large molecule reduces the total amount of active drug that can be easily dosed (ie, the ratio of drug to carrier). In contrast, conventional carriers that are not specific are often many orders of magnitude smaller in size, and a larger effective drug dose may be given more efficiently.

In addition to employing monoclonal antibodies in liposomes and other delivery systems as described above, mAbs may be conjugated directly to drugs. The resulting conjugate can theoretically deliver the drug directly to a cell that expresses a unique surface marker. For example, a tumor cell may overexpress the interleukin-2 receptor. In this case, a cytotoxic molecule such as recombinant diptheria toxin is coupled to a mAb specific for the interleukin-2 receptor (Ontak). The conjugate delivers the toxin preferentially to these tumor cells. An overall tumor response rate for Ontak is 38%, with side effects including acute hypersensitivity reaction (69%) and vascular leak syndrome (27%). Zolimomab aritox (Orthozyme-CD5, Xoma/Ortho Biotech) is an investigational immunoconjugate of monoclonal anti-CD5 murine IgG and the ricin A-chain toxin. This conjugate is used in the treatment of steroid-resistant graft-versus-host disease after allogeneic bone marrow transplants for hematopoietic neoplasms, such as acute myelogenous leukemia. Myoscint is an ^{111}In-labeled mAb targeted to myosin that is used to image myocardial injury in patients with suspected myocardial infarction. An immune response to mAb drugs may develop, since mAbs are produced in mouse cells. Recent efforts to engineer or "humanize" mAbs have produced a new generation of molecules that are less immunogenic.

Oral Immunization

Antigens or fragmented antigenic protein may be delivered orally and stimulate gut-associated lymphoid tissue (GALT) in the gastrointestinal tract. This represents a promising approach for protecting many secretory surfaces against a variety of infectious pathogens. Immunization against salmonella and *Escherichia coli* in chickens was investigated for agricultural purpose. Particulate antigen delivery systems, including several types of microspheres, have been shown to be effective orally inducing various types of immune response. Encapsulation of antigens with mucosal adjuvants can protect both the antigen and the adjuvant against gastric degradation and increase the likelihood that they will reach the site of absorption.

PHARMACOKINETICS OF BIOPHARMACEUTICALS

The unusual nature of biopharmaceuticals compared to traditional drugs presents new development challenges for scientists in the biotechnology industry. Because of the size and complexity of biopharmaceuticals, stability and delivery are major developmental issues with these new drugs. The prerequisite of the maintenance of higher-order structure adds a new dimension to formulation, drug delivery, and stability testing of biologic drugs. Pharmacokinetic studies are often complicated by bioanalytic challenges, since preservation of primary structure or an isotope label alone does not necessarily coincide with biologic activity.

Once in the body, protein and nucleic acid drugs are subject to rapid degradation by endogenous proteases and nucleases that are present in the serum, tissues, and cells. Unmodified phosphodiester DNA and RNA are extremely labile in the body, with half-lives of the order of a few minutes. Houk et al (2001) report that naked DNA clearance in rats is rapid and depends on the conformation of the plasmid: supercoiled, open circular, versus linear. Many of the early recombinant protein drugs also have half-lives of the order of a few minutes, such as Alteplase (Activase) and interleukin-2 (Proleukin) (Table 18.1). However, if immediate stability or immunigenicity concerns can be remedied by chemical modification or bioengineering, the biopharmaceutical may be large enough to escape glomerular filtration and enjoy a prolonged circulation in the body (Table 18.1).

The size and generally hydrophilic nature of the nucleic acid and protein molecules also often precludes the use of diffusional and paracellular transport pathways available to small drug molecules. The capillary wall in most organs and tissues limits passage of macromolecules such as albumin. A typical vector is 20–150 nm, and monoclonal antibodies are composed of four polypeptide chains (over 1200 amino acids total). Such compounds would be expected to have limited diffusional access to most tissues, except the liver, spleen, bone marrow, and tumor tissues, which have higher vascular permeability. As a result, the volume of drug distribution is often smaller for the larger protein and nucleic acid drugs because of vascular confinement or binding to specific tissues. Indeed, the volume of distribution for some of these drugs approximates plasma volume: the apparent volume of distribution at steady state of the mAb Nebacumab is 0.11 ± 0.03 L/kg (Romano et al, 1993), and of Simulect is approximately 7.5 L.

Because of the stability and distribution limitations of large biologic drugs, delivery systems such as conjugates, nanoparticles, liposomes, and viral vectors as described above have been used to improve activity and delivery. The pharmacokinetics of recombinant viral gene delivery systems have been difficult to measure because of the relatively low doses given and often inefficient transgene expression. As a result, gene expression and transgene persistence in tissues are used to determine pharmacokinetic profiles (NIH Report, 2002). Nonviral and naked DNA delivery systems are relatively well characterized in comparison to viral delivery systems. Hengge et al (2001), using polymerase chain reaction (PCR), demonstrate that intramuscular or cutaneous injection of a DNA vaccine resulted in gene expression primarily in surrounding tissues unless extremely high doses were administered. Nomura et al (1998) similarly showed that intratumoral injection of plasmid complexed with cationic lipid resulted in primarily local expression.

Liposome delivery systems are fairly well characterized in terms of their pharmacokinetic properties. Liposome encapsulation may reduce the V_D (Minchin et al, 2001), and may (Houk et al, 2001) or may not (Minchin et al, 2001) improve upon DNA half-life by several hours. However, lipid delivery systems are also rapidly cleared by the mononuclear phagocyte system (spleen and liver) unless injected intratumorally (Nomura et al, 1997). In addition, liposomes may enhance an immune response to the drug and complement activation, also resulting in rapid clearance.

Alternatively, liposomes can be designed to evade phagocyte detection and improve circulation time by coating with polyethylene glycol (PEG), which minimizes opsonin-dependent clearance. *In vivo,* the PEG provides a "bulky" headgroup that serves as a barrier to prevent interaction with the plasma opsonins. The hydrated groups sterically inhibit hydrophobic and electrostatic interaction of a variety of blood components at the liposome surface, thereby evading recognition by the reticuloendothelial system. An example of this concept is the Stealth liposome, which led to the marketing of the PEG-ylated liposomal doxorubicin, Doxil in the United States. Liposomal PEG-ylation can reduce the volume of distribution and extend the half-life of a drug such as doxorubicin (Gabizon et al, 2003). Optimal formulation of a PEG-ylated liposome can improve liposome stability from 1% to 31% of dose remaining in the body at 24 hours postinjection (Allen et al, 2002).

The pharmacokinetics of a liposomal formulation can be different from those of a nonliposomal product given by the same route of administration. For new liposome products, the FDA (draft document, see www.fda.gov/cder/guidance/2191dft.pdf) recommends a comparative mass balance study be performed to assess the differences in systemic exposure and pharmacokinetics between liposome and nonliposome drug products when (1) the two products have the same active moiety, (2) the two products are given by the same route of administration, and (3) one of the products is already approved for marketing. If satisfactory mass balance information is already available for the approved drug product, a limited mass balance study can be undertaken for the new drug product. Comparison of the absorption, distribution, metabolism, and excretion (ADME) of the liposome and nonliposome drug product forms should be made, using a crossover or a parallel noncrossover study design that employs an appropriate number of subjects.

BIOEQUIVALENCE OF BIOTECHNOLOGY-DERIVED DRUG PRODUCTS

The dosage form or formulation of a drug product may change during the course of drug development. The initial drug formulation used in early clinical studies (eg, Phase I/II) may not be the same formulation as the drug formulation used in later clinical trials (Phase III) or the marketed formulation. The demonstration of the bioequivalence of biotechnology products may be difficult (Mordenti et al, 1996). After patent expiration, pharmaceutical manufacturers may develop a generic equivalent. Currently, there is no general scientific agreement as to how to demonstrate bioequivalence of biotechnology-derived drug products (generic biologics). See Chapter 15 for a more detailed on bioequivalence.

 # FREQUENTLY ASKED QUESTIONS

1. What is the most frequent route of administration of biologic compounds?
2. What is the effect of glycosylation on the activity of a biologic compound? Give an example.
3. What are the major differences in drug distribution and elimination between conventional molecules and biotechnological compounds?
4. What is meant by targeted drug delivery? How does gene therapy differ from targeted drug delivery?

5. Why are macromolecular carrier systems used for targeted drug delivery?

6. What are monoclonal antibodies? What advantages do monoclonal antibodies have as carriers for site-specific drug delivery?

 # LEARNING QUESTIONS

1. Explain why most drugs produced by biotechnology cannot be given orally. What routes of drug administration would you recommend for these drugs? Why?

2. What is meant by site-specific drug delivery? Describe several approaches that have been used to target a drug to a specific organ.

3. Doxorubicin (Adriamycin) is available as a conventional solution and as a liposomal preparation. What effect would the liposomal preparation have on the distribution of doxorubicin compared to an injection of the conventional doxorubicin injection?

REFERENCES

Allen C, Dos Santos N, Gallagher R: Controlling the physical behavior and biological performance of liposome formulations through use of surface grafted poly(ethylene glycol). *Biosci Rep* **22**:225–250, 2002

Chu BCF, Whiteley JM: High molecular weight derivatives of methotrexate as chemotherapeutic agents. *Mol Pharm* **13**:80, 1980

Fiume L, Busi C, Mattioli A, et al: In Gregoriadis G, Senior J, Trouet A (eds), *Targeting of Drugs.* New York, Plenum, 1982

Foss FM, Bacha P, Osann KE, Demicre MF, Bell T, Kuzel T: Biological correlates of acute hypersensitivity events with DAB(389) IL-2(deni leukin diftitox, ONJAK) in cutaneous T-cell lymphoma: decreased frequency & severity with steroid premedication. *Clin Lymphoma* March 1:298–302, 2001

Friend DR, Pangburn S: Site-specific drug delivery. *Med Res Rev* **7**:53–106, 1987

Gabizon A, Shmeeda H, Barenholz Y, et al: Pharmacokinetics of pegylated liposomal doxorubicin—Review of animal and human studies. *Clin Pharmacokinet* **42**(45):419–436, 2003

Gros L, Ringsdorf H, Schupp H: Polymeric Antitumor Agents on a Molecular & Cellular Level *Angew Chem Int Ed Engl* **20**:312, 1981

Hengge UR, Dexling B, Mirmohammadsadegh A: Safety and pharmacokinetics of naked plasmid DNA in the skin: Studies on dissemination and ectopic expression. *J Invest Dermatol* **116**:979, 2001

Houk BE, Martin R, Hochhaus G, Hughes JA: Pharmacokinetics of plasmid DNA in the rat. *Pharm Res* **18**:67–74, 2001

Irie T, Uekama K: Cyclodextrins in peptide and protein delivery. *Adv Drug Delivery Rev* **36**:101–123, 1999

Joshi HN: Recent advances in drug delivery systems: Polymeric prodrugs. *Pharm Technol* **12**:118–125, 1988

Ledley, FD: Pharmaceutical approaches to somatic cell therapy. *Pharm Res* **13**:1595–1614, 1996

Levi-Shaffer F, Bernstein A, Meshorer A, Arnon R: Reduced toxicity of daunomycin by confusurtion to dextran Cancer Treat Ref 1982 Jan. **66**:107–14

Minchin RF, Carpenter D, Orr RJ: Polyinosinic acid and polycationic liposomes attenuate the hepatic clearance of circulating plasmid DNA. *J Pharmacol Exp Ther* **296**:1006–1012, 2001

Molema G, de Leij LFMH, Meijer DKE: Tumor vascular endothelium: Barrier or target in tumor directed drug delivery and immunotherapy. *Pharm Res* **14**:2–10, 1997

Mordenti J, Cavagnaro JA, Green JD: Design of biological equivalence programs for therapeutic biotechnology products in clinical development: A perspective. *Pharm Res* **13**:1427–1437, 1996

NIH Report: Assessment of adenoviral vector safety and toxicity: Report of the National Institutes of Health Recombinant DNA Advisory Committee. *Hum Gene Ther* **13**:3–13, 2002

Nomura T, Nakajima S, Kawabata K, et al: Intratumoral pharmacokinetics and *in vivo* gene expression of naked plasmid DNA and its cationic liposome complexes after direct gene transfer. *Cancer Res* **57**:2681–2686, 1997

Panyam J, Labhasetwar V: Biodegradable nanoparticles for drug and gene delivery to cells and tissue. *Adv Drug Del Rev* **55**:329–347, 2003

Romano MJ, Kearns GL, Kaplan SL, et al: Single-dose pharmacokinetics and safety of HA-1A, a human IgM anti-lipid-A monoclonal antibody, in pediatric patients with sepsis syndrome. *J Pediatr* **122**(6):974–984, 1993

Seymour LW: Soluble polymers for lectin-mediated drug targeting. *Adv Drug Delivery Rev* **14**:89–111, 1994

Takakura Y, Hashida M: Macromolecular carrier systems for targeted drug delivery: Pharmacokinetic considerations on biodistribution. *Pharm Res* **13**:820–831, 1996

Yu ABC, Fong GW: Biotechnologic products. In Shargel L, Mutnick AH, Souney PF and Swanson LN (eds) *Comprehensive Pharmacy Review*, 3rd ed. Baltimore, Williams & Wilkins, 1997, chap 10

BIBLIOGRAPHY

Akala EO, Collett JH: Influence of drug loading and gel structure on in-vitro release kinetics from photopolymerized gels. *Ind Pharm* **13**:1779–1798, 1987

Bayley H, Gasparro F, Edelson R: Photoactive drugs. *TIPS* **8**:138–144, 1987

Body A, Aarons L: Pharmacokinetic and pharmacodynamic aspects of site specific drug delivery. *Adv Drug Delivery Rev* **3**:155–163, 1989

Borchardt RT, Repta AJ, Stella VJ (eds): *Directed Drug Delivery*. Clifton, NJ, Humana, 1985

Boxenbaum HG: Physiological and pharmacokinetic factors affecting performance of sustained release dosage forms. *Drug Dev Ind Pharm* **8**:1–25, 1982

Breimer DD, Dauhof M: *Towards Better Safety of Drugs and Pharmaceutical Products.* Amsterdam, Elsevier/North-Holland, 1980, pp 117–142

Brester ME, Hora MS, Simpkins JW, Bodor N: Use of 2-hydroxypropyl-b-cyclodextrin as a solubilizing and stabilizing excipient for protein drugs. *Pharm Res* **8**:792–795, 1991

Brodsky FM: Monoclonal antibodies as magic bullets. *Pharm Res* **5**:1–9, 1988

Bruck S (ed): *CRC Controlled Drug Delivery.* Boca Raton, FL, CRC Press, 1983

Chien YW: *Novel Drug Delivery Systems.* New York, Marcel Dekker, 1982

Dighe SV, Adams WP: Bioavailability and bioequivalence of oral controlled-release products: A regulatory perspective. In Welling PG, Tse FLS (eds), *Pharmacokinetics: Regulatory, Industrial, Academic Perspectives.* New York, Marcel Dekker, 1988

Eckhardt BM, Oeswein JQ, Bewley TA: Effect of freezing on aggregation of human growth hormone. *Pharm Res* **8**:1360–1364, 1991

Emisphere literature: Mucosal immunization with derivatized μ- and non-μ-amino acid delivery agents. Presented at the American Association of Pharmaceutical Scientists (AAPS) Annual Meeting, Seattle, WA, October 1996

Emisphere literature: Oral delivery of interferon in rats and primates. Presented at the American Association of Pharmaceutical Scientists (AAPS) Annual Meeting, San Diego, CA, 1994. *Pharm Res* **11**(10):S-298, 1994

Galeone M, Nizzola L, Cacioli D, Moise G: *In vivo* demonstration of delivery mechanisms from sustained-release pellets. *Curr Ther Res* **29**:217–234, 1981

Heller J: Controlled drug release from monolithic bioerodible polymer devices. *Pharm Int* **7**:316–318, 1986

Jensen JD, Jensen LW, Madsen JK, Poulsen L: The metabolism of erythropoietin in liver cirrhosis patients compared with healthy volunteers. *Eur J Haematol* **54**(2):111–116, 1995

Langer R: New methods of drug delivery. *Science* **249**:1527–1533, 1990

Le-Cotonnec JY, Porchet HC, Betrami V, et al: Comprehensive pharmacokinetics of urinary human follicle stimulating hormone in healthy female volunteers. *Pharm Res* **12**(6):844–850, 1995

Lee VH, Hashida M, Mizushima Y: *Trends and Future Perspectives in Peptide and Protein Drug Development.* Langhorne, PA, Harwood Academic, 1995

Levy G: Targeted drug delivery: Some pharmacokinetic considerations. *Pharm Res* **4:**3–4, 1987

Oeswein JA: Formulation considerations in polypeptide delivery. Presented at Biotech 87. Pinner, UK, Online Publications, 1987

Ostro MJ: *Liposome: From Biophysics to Therapeutics.* New York, Marcel Dekker, 1987

Park H, Robinson JR: Mechanisms of mucoadhesion of poly(acrylic acid) hydrogels. *Pharm Res* **4:**457–464, 1987

Pozansky MJ, Juliano RL: Biological approaches to the controlled delivery of drugs: A critical review. *Pharmacol Rev* **36:**277–336, 1984

Robinson JR: Oral drug delivery systems. *Proceedings of 1982 Research and Scientific Development Conference.* Washington, DC, The Proprietary Association, 1983, pp 54–69

Rodwell JD (ed): *Antibody Mediated Delivery Systems.* New York, Marcel Dekker, 1988

Salmonson T, Danielson BG, Wikstrom B: The pharmacokinetics of recombinant erythropoietin after intravenous and subcutaneous administration to healthy subjects. *Br J Clin Pharm* **29:**709, 1990

Silverman HS, Becker LC, Siddoway LA, et al: Pharmacokinetics of human recombinant superoxide dismutase. *J Am Coll Cardiol* **11:**164A, 1988

Sobel BE, Fields LE, Robinson AK, et al: Coronary thrombolysis with facilitated absorption of intramuscular injected tissue-type plasminogen activator. *Proc Natl Acad Sci USA* **82:**4258, 1985

Spenlehauer G, Vert M, Benoit JP, et al: Biodegradable cisplatin microspheres prepared by the solvent evaporation method: Morphology and release characteristics. *J Control Release* **7:**217–229, 1988

19

RELATIONSHIP BETWEEN PHARMACOKINETICS AND PHARMACODYNAMICS

PHARMACODYNAMICS AND PHARMACOKINETICS

Previous chapters in this book have discussed the importance of using pharmacokinetics to develop dosing regimens that will result in plasma concentrations in the therapeutic window and yield the desired therapeutic or pharmacologic response. The interaction of a drug molecule with a receptor causes the initiation of a sequence of molecular events resulting in a pharmacodynamic or pharmacologic response. The term *pharmacodynamics* refers to the relationship between drug concentrations at the site of action (receptor) and pharmacologic response, including the biochemical and physiologic effects that influence the interaction of drug with the receptor. Early pharmacologic research demonstrated that the pharmacodynamic response produced by the drug depends on the chemical structure of the drug molecule. Drug receptors interact only with drugs of specific chemical structure, and the receptors were classified according to the type of pharmacodynamic response induced.

Since most pharmacologic responses are due to noncovalent interaction between the drug and the receptor, the nature of the interaction is generally assumed to be reversible and conforms to the *Law of Mass Action*. One or several drug molecules may interact simultaneously with the receptor to produce a pharmacologic response. Typically, a single drug molecule interacts with a receptor with a single binding site to produce a pharmacologic response, as illustrated below.

$$[\text{Drug}] + [\text{receptor}] \Leftrightarrow [\text{drug–receptor complex}] \rightarrow \text{response}$$

where the brackets [ ] denote molar concentrations. This scheme illustrates the *occupation theory* and the interaction of a drug molecule with a receptor molecule. The following assumptions are made in this model.

1. The drug molecule combines with the receptor molecule as a bimolecular association, and the resulting drug–receptor complex disassociates as a unimolecular entity.
2. The binding of drug with the receptor is fully reversible.
3. The basic model assumes a single type of receptor binding site, with one binding site per receptor molecule. It is also assumed that a receptor with multiple sites may be modeled after this (Taylor and Insel, 1990).

It is assumed that the occupancy of the drug molecule at one receptor site does not change the affinity of more drug molecules to complex at additional receptor sites. However, the model is not suitable for drugs with *allosteric* binding to receptors, in which the binding of one drug molecule to the receptor affects the binding of subsequent drug molecules, as in the case of oxygen molecules binding to iron in hemoglobin. As more receptors are occupied by drug molecules, a greater pharmacodynamic response is obtained until a maximum response is reached.

The receptor occupancy concept was extended to show how drugs elicit a pharmacologic response as an *agonist,* or produce an opposing pharmacologic response as an *antagonist* through drug–receptor interactions. Basically, three types of related responses may occur at the receptor: (1) a drug molecule that interacts with the receptor and elicits a maximal pharmacologic response is referred to as an *agonist;* (2) a drug that elicits a partial (below maximal) response is termed a *partial agonist;* and (3) an agent that elicits no response from the receptor, but inhibits the receptor interaction of a second agent, is termed an *antagonist.* An antagonist may prevent the action of an agonist by competitive (reversible) or noncompetitive (irreversible) inhibition.

Spare, unoccupied receptors are assumed to be present at the site of action, because a maximal pharmacologic response may be obtained when only a small fraction of the receptors are occupied by drug molecules. Equimolar concentrations of different drug molecules that normally bind to the same receptor may give different degrees of pharmacologic response. The term *intrinsic activity* is used to distinguish the relative extent of pharmacologic response between different drug molecules that bind to the same receptor. The *potency* of a drug is the concentration of drug needed to obtain a specific pharmacologic effect, such as the EC_{50} (see $E_{\max}$ model, below).

The receptor occupation theory, however, was not consistent with all kinetic observations. An alternative theory, known as the *rate theory,* essentially states that the pharmacologic response is not dependent on drug–receptor complex concentration but rather depends on the rate of association of the drug and the receptor. Each time a drug molecule "hits" a receptor, a response is produced, similar to a ball bouncing back and forth from the receptor site. The rate theory predicts that an agonist will associate rapidly to form a receptor complex, which dissociates rapidly to produce a response. An antagonist associates rapidly to form a receptor–drug complex and dissociates slowly to maintain the antagonist response.

Both theories are consistent with the observed saturation (*sigmoidal*) drug–dose response relationships, but neither theory is sufficiently advanced to give a detailed description of the "lock-and-key" or the more recent "induced-fit" type of drug interactions with enzymatic receptors. Newer theories of drug action are based on *in-vitro* studies on isolated tissue receptors and on observation of the conformational and binding changes with different drug substrates. These *in-vitro* studies show that other types of interactions between the drug molecule and the receptor are possible. However, the results from the *in-vitro* studies are difficult to extrapolate to *in-vivo* conditions. The pharmacologic response in drug therapy is often a product of physiologic adaptation to a drug response. Many drugs trigger the pharmacologic response through a cascade of enzymatic events highly regulated by the body.

Unlike pharmacokinetic modeling, pharmacodynamic modeling can be more complex because the clinical measure (change in blood pressure or clotting time) is often a surrogate for the drug's actual pharmacologic action. For example, after the drug is systemically absorbed, it is then transported to site of action where the pharmacologic receptor resides. Drug–receptor binding may then cause a secondary response, such as signal transduction, which then produces the desired effect. Clinical measurement of drug response may only occur after many such biologic events, such as transport or signal transduction (an *indirect effect*), so pharmacodynamic modeling must account for biologic processes involved in eliciting drug-induced responses.

The complexity of the molecular events triggering a pharmacologic response is less difficult to describe using a pharmacokinetic approach. Pharmacokinetic models allow very complex processes to be simplified. The process of pharmacokinetic modeling continues until a model is found that describes the real process quantitatively. The understanding of drug response is greatly enhanced when pharmacokinetic modeling techniques are combined with clinical pharmacology, resulting in the development of *pharmacokinetic–pharmacodynamic models*. Pharmacokinetic–pharmacodynamic models use data derived from the plasma drug concentration-versus-time profile and from the time course of the pharmacologic effect to predict the pharmacodynamics of the drug. Pharmacokinetic–pharmacodynamic models have been reported for antipsychotic medications, anticoagulants, neuromuscular blockers, antihypertensives, anesthetics, and many antiarrhythmic drugs (the pharmacologic responses of these drugs are well studied because of easy monitoring).

RELATION OF DOSE TO PHARMACOLOGIC EFFECT

The onset, intensity, and duration of the pharmacologic effect depend on the dose and the pharmacokinetics of the drug. As the dose increases, the drug concentration at the receptor site increases, and the pharmacologic response (effect) increases up to a maximum effect. A plot of the pharmacologic effect to dose on a linear scale generally results in a hyperbolic curve with maximum effect at the plateau (Fig. 19-1). The same data may be compressed and plotted on a log–linear scale and results in a sigmoid curve (Fig. 19-2).

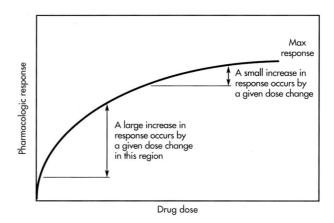

Figure 19-1. Plot of pharmacologic response versus dose on a linear scale.

For many drugs, the graph of log dose–response curve shows a linear relationship at a dose range between 20% and 80% of the maximum response, which typically includes the therapeutic dose range for many drugs. For a drug that follows one-compartment pharmacokinetics, the volume of distribution is constant; therefore, the pharmacologic response is also proportional to the log plasma drug concentration within a therapeutic range, as shown in Figure 19-3.

Mathematically, the relationship in Figure 19-3 may be expressed by the following equation, where m is the slope, e is an extrapolated intercept, and E is the drug effect at drug concentration C:

$$E = m \log C + e \tag{19.1}$$

Solving for $\log C$ yields

$$\log C = \frac{E - e}{m} \tag{19.2}$$

Figure 19-2. Typical log dose versus pharmacologic response curve.

Figure 19-3. Graph of log drug concentration versus pharmacologic effect. Only the linear portion of the curve is shown.

However, after an intravenous dose, the concentration of a drug in the body in a one-compartment open model is described as follows:

$$\log C = \log C_0 - \frac{kt}{2.3} \tag{19.3}$$

By substituting Equation 19.2 into Equation 19.3, we get Equation 19.4, where E_0 = effect at concentration C_0:

$$\frac{E - e}{m} = \frac{E_0 - e}{m} - \frac{kt}{2.3}$$

$$E = E_0 - \frac{kmt}{2.3} \tag{19.4}$$

The theoretical pharmacologic response at any time after an intravenous dose of a drug may be calculated using Equation 19.4. Equation 19.4 predicts that the pharmacologic effect will decline linearly with time for a drug that follows a one-compartment model, with a linear log dose–pharmacologic response. From this equation, the pharmacologic effect declines with a slope of $km/2.3$. The decrease in pharmacologic effect is affected by both the elimination constant k and the slope m. For a drug with a large m, the pharmacologic response declines rapidly and multiple doses must be given at short intervals to maintain the pharmacologic effect.

The relationship between pharmacokinetics and pharmacologic response can be demonstrated by observing the percent depression of muscular activity after an IV dose of (+)-tubocurarine. The decline of pharmacologic effect is linear as a function of time (Fig. 19-4). For each dose and resulting pharmacologic response, the slope of each curve is the same. Because the values for each slope, which include km (Eq. 19.4), are the same, the sensitivity of the receptors for (+)-tubocurarine is assumed to be the same at each site of action. Note that a plot of the log concentration of drug versus time yields a straight line.

A second example of the pharmacologic effect declining linearly with time was observed with lysergic acid diethylamide, or LSD (Fig. 19-5). After an IV dose of the drug, log concentrations of drug decreased linearly with time except for a brief distribution period. Furthermore, the pharmacologic effect, as measured by the performance score of each subject, also declined linearly with time. Because the

Figure 19-4. Depression of normal muscle activity as a function of time after IV administration of 0.1–0.2 mg (+)-tubocurarine per kilogram to unanesthetized volunteers, presenting mean values of 6 experiments on 5 subjects. Circles represent head lift; squares, hand grip; and triangles, inspiratory flow. (Adapted from Johansen et al, 1964, with permission.)

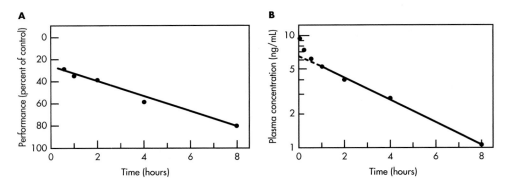

Figure 19-5. Mean plasma concentrations of LSD and performance test scores as a function of time after IV administration of 2 μg LSD per kilogram to 5 normal human subjects. (Adapted from Aghajanian and Bing, 1964, with permission.)

slope is governed in part by the elimination rate constant, the pharmacologic effect declines much more rapidly when the elimination rate constant is increased as a result of increased metabolism or renal excretion. Conversely, a longer pharmacologic response is experienced in patients when the drug has a longer half-life.

RELATIONSHIP BETWEEN DOSE AND DURATION OF ACTIVITY (t_{eff}), SINGLE IV BOLUS INJECTION

The relationship between the duration of the pharmacologic effect and the dose can be inferred from Equation 19.3. After an intravenous dose, assuming a one-compartment model, the time needed for any drug to decline to a concentration C is given by the following equation, assuming the drug takes effect immediately:

$$t = \frac{2.3\,(\log C_0 - \log C)}{k} \tag{19.5}$$

Using C_{eff} to represent the minimum effective drug concentration, the duration of drug action can be obtained as follows:

$$t_{eff} = \frac{2.3[\log(D_0/V_D) - \log C_{eff}]}{k} \tag{19.6}$$

Some practical applications are suggested by this equation. For example, a doubling of the dose will not result in a doubling of the effective duration of pharmacologic action. On the other hand, a doubling of $t_{1/2}$ or a corresponding decrease in k will result in a proportional increase in duration of action. A clinical situation is often encountered in the treatment of infections in which C_{eff} is the bacteriocidal concentration of the drug, and, in order to double the duration of the antibiotic, a considerably greater increase than simply doubling the dose is necessary.

PRACTICE PROBLEM

The minimum effective concentration (MEC) in plasma for a certain antibiotic is 0.1 $\mu g/mL$. The drug follows a one-compartment open model and has an apparent volume of distribution, V_D, of 10 L and a first-order elimination rate constant of 1.0 hr^{-1}.

a. What is the t_{eff} for a single 100-mg IV dose of this antibiotic?

b. What is the new t_{eff} or t'_{eff} for this drug if the dose were increased 10-fold, to 1000 mg?

Solution

a. The t_{eff} for a 100-mg dose is calculated as follows. Because $V_D = 10,000$ mL,

$$C_0 = \frac{100 \text{ mg}}{10,000 \text{ mL}} = 10 \ \mu g/mL$$

For a one-compartment-model IV dose, $C = C_0 e^{-kt}$. Then

$$0.1 = 10e^{-(1.0)t_{eff}}$$

$$t_{eff} = 4.61 \text{ hr}$$

b. The t'_{eff} for a 1000-mg dose is calculated as follows (prime refers to a new dose). Because $V_D = 10,000$ mL,

$$C'_0 = \frac{1000 \text{ mg}}{10,000 \text{ mL}} = 100 \ \mu g/mL$$

and

$$C'_{eff} = C'_0 e^{-kt'_{eff}}$$

$$0.1 = 100e^{-(1.0)t'_{eff}}$$

$$t'_{eff} = 6.91 \text{ hr}$$

The percent increase in t_{eff} is therefore found as

$$\text{Percent increase in } t_{eff} = \frac{t'_{eff} - t_{eff}}{t_{eff}} \times 100$$

$$\text{Precent increase in } t_{eff} = \frac{6.91 - 4.61}{4.61} \times 100$$

$$\text{Percent increase in } t_{eff} = 50\%$$

This example shows that a 10-fold increase in the dose increases the duration of action of a drug (t_{eff}) by only 50%.

EFFECT OF BOTH DOSE AND ELIMINATION HALF-LIFE ON THE DURATION OF ACTIVITY

A single equation can be derived to describe the relationship of dose (D_0) and the elimination half-life ($t_{1/2}$) on the effective time for therapeutic activity (t_{eff}). This expression is derived below.

$$\ln C_{eff} - \ln C_0 - k t_{eff}$$

Because $C_0 = D_0/V_D$,

$$\ln C_{eff} = \ln\left(\frac{D_0}{V_D}\right) - k t_{eff}$$

$$k t_{eff} = \ln\left(\frac{D_0}{V_D}\right) - \ln C_{eff} \tag{19.7}$$

$$t_{eff} = \frac{1}{k}\ln\left(\frac{D_0/V_D}{C_{eff}}\right)$$

Substituting $0.693/t_{1/2}$ for k,

$$t_{eff} = 1.44 t_{1/2} \ln\left(\frac{D_0}{V_D C_{eff}}\right) \tag{19.8}$$

From Equation 19.8, an increase in $t_{1/2}$ will increase the t_{eff} in direct proportion. However, an increase in the dose, D_0, does not increase the t_{eff} in direct proportion. The effect of an increase in V_D or C_{eff} can be seen by using generated data. Only the positive solutions for Equation 19.8 are valid, although mathematically a negative t_{eff} can be obtained by increasing C_{eff} or V_D. The effect of changing dose on t_{eff} is shown in Figure 19-6 using data generated with Equation 19.8. A nonlinear increase in t_{eff} is observed as dose increases.

EFFECT OF ELIMINATION HALF-LIFE ON DURATION OF ACTIVITY

Because elimination of drugs is due to the processes of excretion and metabolism, an alteration of any of these elimination processes will effect the $t_{1/2}$ of the drug. In certain disease states, pathophysiologic changes in hepatic or renal function will

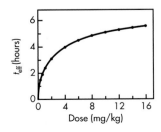

Figure 19-6. Plot of t_{eff} versus dose.

decrease the elimination of a drug, as observed by a prolonged $t_{1/2}$. This prolonged $t_{1/2}$ will lead to retention of the drug in the body, thereby increasing the duration of activity of the drug (t_{eff}) as well as increasing the possibility of drug toxicity.

To improve antibiotic therapy with the penicillin and cephalosporin antibiotics, clinicians have intentionally prolonged the elimination of these drugs by giving a second drug, probenecid, which competitively inhibits renal excretion of the antibiotic. This approach to prolonging the duration of activity of antibiotics that are rapidly excreted through the kidney has been used successfully for a number of years. Similarly, Augmentin is a combination of amoxicillin and clavulanic acid; the latter is an inhibitor of β-lactamase. This β-lactamase is a bacterial enzyme that degrades penicillin-like drugs. The data in Table 19.1 illustrate how a change in the elimination $t_{1/2}$ will affect the t_{eff} for a drug. For all doses, a 100% increase in the $t_{1/2}$ will result in a 100% increase in the t_{eff}. For example, for a drug whose $t_{1/2}$ is 0.75 hour and that is given at a dose of 2 mg/kg, the t_{eff} is 3.24 hours. If the $t_{1/2}$ is increased to 1.5 hours, the t_{eff} is increased to 6.48 hours, an increase of 100%. However, the effect of doubling the dose from 2 to 4 mg/kg (no change in elimination processes) will only increase the t_{eff} to 3.98 hours, an increase of 22.8%. The effect of prolonging the elimination half-life has an extremely important effect on the treatment of infections, particularly in patients with high metabolism, or clearance, of the antibiotic. Therefore, antibiotics must be dosed with full consideration of the effect of alteration of the $t_{1/2}$ on the t_{eff}. Consequently, a simple proportional increase in dose will leave the patient's blood concentration below the effective antibiotic level most of the time during drug therapy. The effect of a prolonged t_{eff} is shown in lines *a* and *c* in Figure 19-7, and the disproportionate increase in t_{eff} as the dose is increased 10-fold is shown in lines *a* and *b*.

TABLE 19.1   Relationship between Elimination Half-Life and Duration of Activity

DOSE (mg/kg)	$t_{1/2} = 0.75$ hr t_{eff} (hr)	$t_{1/2} = 1.5$ hr t_{eff} (hr)
2.0	3.24	6.48
3.0	3.67	7.35
4.0	3.98	7.97
5.0	4.22	8.45
6.0	4.42	8.84
7.0	4.59	9.18
8.0	4.73	9.47
9.0	4.86	9.72
10	4.97	9.95
11	5.08	10.2
12	5.17	10.3
13	5.26	10.5
14	5.34	10.7
15	5.41	10.8
16	5.48	11.0
17	5.55	11.1
18	5.61	11.2
19	5.67	11.3
20	5.72	11.4

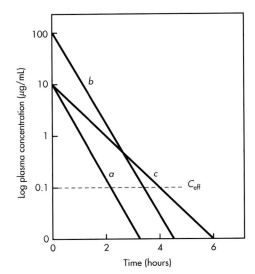

Figure 19-7. Plasma level–time curves describing the relationship of both dose and elimination half-life on duration of drug action. C_{eff} = effective concentration. Curve a = single 100-mg IV injection of drug; k = 1.0 hr^{-1}. Curve b = single 1000-mg IV injection; k = 1.0 hr^{-1}. Curve c = single 100-mg IV injection; k = 0.5 hr^{-1}. V_D is 10 L.

CLINICAL EXAMPLES

Pharmacokinetic/Pharmacodynamic Relationships and Efficacy of Antibiotics

In the previous section, the time above the effective concentration, t_{eff}, was shown to be important in optimizing the therapeutic response of many drugs. This concept has been applied to antibiotic drugs (Drusano, 1988; Craig, 1995; Craig and Andes, 1996; Scaglione, 1997). For example, Craig and Andes (1996) discussed the antibacterial treatment of otitis media. Using the minimum inhibitory antibiotic concentration (MIC) for the microorganism in serum, the percent time for the antibiotic drug concentration to be above the MIC was calculated for several antibacterial classes, including cephalosporins, macrolides, and trimethoprim-sulfamethoxazole (TMP/SMX) combination (Table 19.2). Although the drug concentration in the

TABLE 19.2 Middle Ear Fluid-to-Serum Ratios for Common Antibiotics

ANTIBIOTIC	MIDDLE EAR FLUID (MEF)/SERUM RATIO
Cephalosporins	
Cefaclor	0.18–0.28
Cefuroxime	0.22
Macrolide antibiotic	
Erythromycin	0.49
Sulfa drug	
Sulfisoxazole	0.20

From Craig and Andes (1996).

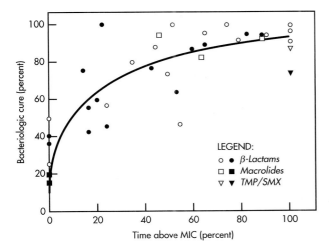

Figure 19-8. Relationship between the percent time above MIC$_{90}$ of the dosing interval during therapy and percent of bacteriologic cure in otitis media caused by *S. pneumoniae* (open symbols) and β-lactamase-positive and -negative *H. influenzae* (closed symbols). (Circles, closed and open = β-lactams; squares, closed and open = macrolides; triangles, closed and open = TMP/SMX.) (From Craig and Andres, 1996, with permission.)

middle ear fluid (MEF) is important, once the ratio (MEF/serum) is known, the serum drug level may be used to project MEF drug levels. The percent time above MIC of the dosing interval during therapy correlated well to the percent of bacteriologic cure (Figure 19-8). An almost 100% cure was attained by maintaining the drug concentration above the MIC for 60–70% of the dosing interval; an 80–85% cure was achieved with 40–50% of the dosing interval above MIC. When the percent of time above MIC falls below a critical value, bacteria will regrow, thereby prolonging the time for eradication of the infection. The pharmacokinetic model was further supported by experiments from a mouse infection model in which an infection in the thigh due to *Pseudomonas aeruginosa* was treated with ticarcillin and tobramycin.

In another study, Craig (1995) compared the AUC/MIC, the time above MIC, and drug peak concentration over MIC and found that the best fit was obtained when colony-forming units (CFUs) were plotted versus time above MIC for cefotaxime in a mouse infection model (Fig. 19-9).

Both Drusano (1988) and Craig (1995) reviewed the relationship of pharmacokinetics and pharmacodynamics in the therapeutic efficacy of antibiotics. For some antibiotics, such as the aminoglycosides and fluoroquinolones, both the drug concentration and the dosing interval have an influence on the antibacterial effect. For some antibiotics, such as the β-lactams, vancomycin, and the macrolides, the duration of exposure (time-dependent killing) or the time the drug levels are maintained above the MIC (t_{eff}) is most important for efficacy. For many antibiotics (eg, fluoroquinolones), there is a defined period of bacterial growth suppression after short exposures to the antibiotic. This phenomenon is known as the *postantibiotic effect* (PAE). Other influences on antibiotic activity include the presence of active metabolite(s), plasma drug protein binding, and the penetration of the antibiotic into the tissues. In addition, the MIC for the antibiotic depends on the infectious microorganism and the resistance of the microorganism to the antibiotic. In the case of ciprofloxacin, a quinolone, the percent of cure of infection at various doses was better related to AUIC, which is the product of area under the curve and the

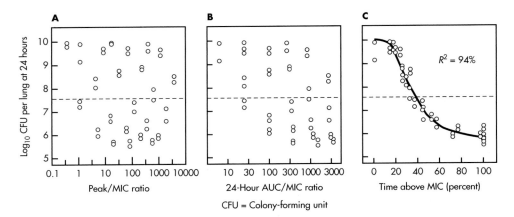

Figure 19-9. Relationship among three pharmacodynamic parameters and the number of *Klebsiella pneumoniae* in the lungs of neurotroponic mice after 24-hour therapy with cefotaxime. Each point represents one mouse.
(From Craig WA, 1995, with permission.)

reciprocal of minimum inhibition concentration, MIC (Forrest et al, 1993). Interestingly, quinolones inhibit bacterial DNA gyrase, quite different from the β-lactam antibiotics, which involve damage to bacterial cell walls.

Relationship between Systemic Exposure and Response—Anticancer Drugs

Plasma drug concentrations for drugs that have highly variable drug clearance in patients fluctuate widely even after intravenous infusion (Rodman and Evans, 1991). For highly variable drugs, there is no apparent relationship between the therapeutic response and the drug dose. For example, the anticancer drug teniposide at three different doses give highly variable steady-state drug concentrations and therapeutic response (Fig. 19-10). In some patients, single-point drug concentrations were variable and even higher with lower doses. Careful pharmacokinetic–pharmacodynamic analysis showed that a graded response curve may be obtained when responses are plotted versus systemic exposure as

Figure 19-10. Steady-state concentration and response after three levels of teniposide administered by intravenous infusion.
(From Rodman and Evans, 1991, with permission.)

Figure 19-11. Relationship between systemic exposure for teniposide and toxicity and efficacy, shown as proportions of patients. (From Rodman and Evans, 1991, with permission.)

measured by "concentration × time" (Fig. 19-11). This is one example showing that anticancer response may be better correlated to total area under the drug concentration curve (AUC), even when no apparent dose–response relationship is observed. Undoubtedly, the cytotoxic effect of the drug involves killing cancer cells with multiple-resistance thresholds that require different time exposures to the drug. The objective of applying pharmacokinetic–pharmacodynamic principles is to achieve therapeutic efficacy without triggering drug toxicity. This relationship is illustrated by the sigmoid curves for response and toxicity (Fig. 19-11), both of which lie close to each other and intensify as concentration increases.

RATE OF DRUG ABSORPTION AND PHARMACODYNAMIC RESPONSE

The rate of drug absorption influences the rate in which the drug gets to the receptor and the subsequent pharmacologic effect. For drugs that exert an acute pharmacologic effect, usually a direct-acting drug agonist, extremely rapid drug absorption may have an intense and possibly detrimental effect. For example, niacin (nicotinic acid) is a vitamin given in large doses to decrease elevated plasma cholesterol and triglycerides. Rapid systemic absorption of niacin when given in an immediate-release tablet will cause vasodilation, leading to flushing and postural hypertension. Extended-release niacin products are preferred because the more slowly absorbed niacin allows the baroreceptors to adjust to the vasodilation and hypotensive effects of the drug. Phenylpropanolamine was commonly used as a nasal decongestant in cough and cold products or as an anorectant in weight-loss products. Phenylpropanolamine acts as a pressor, increasing the blood pressure much more intensely when given as an immediate-release product compared to an extended-release product.

Equilibration Pharmacodynamic Half-Life

For some drugs, the half-time for drug equilibration has been estimated by observing the onset of response. A list of drug half-times reported by Lalonde (1992) is shown in Table 19.3. The factors that affect this parameter include perfusion of

TABLE 19.3   Equilibration Half-Times Determined Using the Effect Compartment Method

DRUG	EQUILIBRATION $t_{1/2}$ (min)	PHARMACOLOGIC RESPONSE
d-Tubocurarine	4	Muscle paralysis
Disopyramide	2	QT prolongation
Quinidine	8	QT prolongation
Digoxin	214	LVET shortening
Terbutaline	7.5	FEV_1
Terbutaline	11.5	Hypokalemia
Theophylline	11	FEV_1
Verapamil	2	PR prolongation
Nizatidine	83	Gastric pH
Thiopental	1.2	Spectral edge
Fentanyl	6.4	Spectral edge
Alfentanil	1.1	Spectral edge
Ergotamine	595	Vasoconstriction
Vercuronium	4	Muscle paralysis
N-Acetylprocainamide	6.4	QT prolongation

From Lalonde (1992), with permission.

the effect compartment, blood–tissue partitioning, drug diffusion from capillaries to the effect compartment, protein binding, and elimination of the drug from the effect compartment.

Substance Abuse Potential

The rate of drug absorption has been associated with the potential for substance abuse. Drugs taken by the oral route have the lowest abuse potential. For example, cocoa leaves containing cocaine alkaloid have been chewed by South American Indians for centuries (Johanson and Fischman, 1989). Cocaine abuse has become a problem as a result of the availability of cocaine alkaloid ("crack" cocaine) and because of the use of other routes of drug administration (intravenous, intranasal, or smoking) that allow a very rapid rate of drug absorption and onset of action (Cone, 1995). Studies on diazepam (deWit et al, 1993) and nicotine (Henningfield and Keenan, 1993) have shown that the rate of drug delivery correlates with the abuse liability of such drugs. Thus, the rate of drug absorption influences the abuse potential of these drugs, and the route of drug administration that provides faster absorption and more rapid onset leads to greater abuse.

DRUG TOLERANCE AND PHYSICAL DEPENDENCY

The study of drug tolerance and physical dependency is of particular interest in understanding the actions of abused drug substances, such as opiates and cocaine. Drug *tolerance* is a quantitative change in the sensitivity of the drug and is demonstrated by a decrease in pharmacodynamic effect after repeated exposure to the same drug. The degree of tolerance may vary greatly (Cox, 1990). Drug tolerance has been well described for organic nitrates, opioids, and other drugs. For example, the nitrates relax vascular smooth muscle and have been used for both acute angina (eg, nitroglycerin sublingual spray or transmucosal tablet) or angina prophylaxis (eg, nitroglycerin transdermal, oral controlled-release isosorbide dinitrate). Well-controlled clinical studies have shown that tolerance to the vascular and antianginal effects of nitrates may develop. For nitrate therapy, the use of a low nitrate or nitrate-free periods has been advocated as part of the therapeutic approach. The magnitude of drug tolerance is a function of both the dosage and the frequency of drug administration. *Cross tolerance* can occur for similar drugs that act on the same receptors. Tolerance does not develop uniformly to all the pharmacologic or toxic actions of the drug. For example, patients who show tolerance to the depressant activity of high doses of opiates will still exhibit "pinpoint" pupils and constipation.

The mechanism of drug tolerance may be due to (1) disposition or pharmacokinetic tolerance or (2) pharmacodynamic tolerance. *Pharmacokinetic tolerance* is often due to enzyme induction (discussed in earlier chapters), in which the hepatic drug clearance increases with repeated drug exposure. *Pharmacodynamic tolerance* is due to a cellular or receptor alteration in which the drug response is less than what is predicted in the patient given subsequent drug doses. Measurement of serum drug concentrations may differentiate between pharmacokinetic tolerance and pharmacodynamic tolerance. Acute tolerance, or *tachyphylaxis*, which is the rapid development of tolerance, may occur due to a change in the sensitivity of the receptor or depletion of a cofactor after only a single or a few doses of the drug. Drugs that work indirectly by releasing norepinephrine may show tachyphylaxis. Drug tolerance should be differentiated from genetic factors which account for normal variability in the drug response.

Physical dependency is demonstrated by the appearance of withdrawal symptoms after cessation of the drug. Workers exposed to volatile organic nitrates in the workplace may initially develop headaches and dizziness followed by tolerance with continuous exposure. However, after leaving the workplace for a few days, the workers may demonstrate nitrate withdrawal symptoms. Factors that may affect drug dependency may include the dose or amount of drug used (intensity of drug effect), the duration of drug use (months, years, and peak use) and the total dose (amount of drug × duration). The appearance of withdrawal symptoms may be abruptly precipitated in opiate-dependent subjects by the administration of naloxone (Narcan), an opioid antagonist that has no agonist properties.

HYPERSENSITIVITY AND ADVERSE RESPONSE

Many drug responses, such as hypersensitivity and allergic responses, are not fully explained by pharmacodynamics and pharmacokinetics. Allergic responses generally are not dose related, although some penicillin-sensitive patients may respond to threshold skin concentrations, but, otherwise, no dose–response relationship has been established. Skin eruption is a common symptom of drug allergy. Allergic reactions can occur at extremely low drug concentrations. Some urticaria episodes in patients have been traced to penicillin contamination in food or to penicillin contamination during dispensing or manufacturing of other drugs. Allergic reactions are important data that must be recorded in the patient's profile along with other adverse reactions. Penicillin allergic reaction in the population is often detected by skin test with benzylpenicilloyl polylysine (PPL). The incidence of penicillin allergic reaction occurs in about 1–10% of patients. The majority of these reactions are minor cutaneous reactions such as urticaria, angioedema, and pruritus. Serious allergic reactions, such as anaphylaxis, are rare, with an incidence of 0.021–0.106% for penicillins (Lin, 1992). For cephalosporins, the incidence of anaphylactic reaction is less than 0.02%. Anaphylactic reaction for cefaclor was reported to be 0.001% in a postmarketing survey. There are emerging trends showing that there may be a difference between the original and the new generations of cephalosporins (Reisman and Reisman, 1995). Cross sensitivity to similar chemical classes of drugs can occur.

Allergic reactions may be immediate or delayed and have been related to IgE mechanisms. In β-lactam (penicillin) drug allergy, immediate reactions occur in about 30 to 60 minutes, but delayed reaction, or accelerated reaction, may occur from 1 to 72 hours after administration. Anaphylactic reaction may occur in both groups. Although some early evidence of cross hypersensitivity between penicillin and cephalosporin was observed, the incidence in patients sensitive to penicillin show only a twofold increase in sensitivity to cephalosporin compared with that of the general population. The report rationalized that it is safe to administer cephalosporin to penicillin-sensitive patients and that the penicillin skin test is not useful in identifying patients who are allergic to cephalosporin, because of the low incidence of cross reactivity (Reisman and Reisman, 1995). In practice, the clinician should evaluate the risk of drug allergy against the choice of alternative medication. Some earlier reports showed that cross sensitivity between penicillin and cephalosporin was due to the presence of trace penicillin present in cephalosporin products.

DRUG DISTRIBUTION AND PHARMACOLOGIC RESPONSE

After systemic absorption, the drug is carried throughout the body by the general circulation. Most of the drug dose will reach unintended target tissues, in which the drug may be passively stored, produce an adverse effect, or be eliminated. A fraction of the dose will reach the target site and establish an equilibrium. The receptor site is unknown most of the time, but, kinetically, it is known as the *effect compartment*. The time course of drug delivery to the effect compartment will determine whether the onset of pharmacologic response is immediate or delayed. The delivery of drug to the effect compartment is affected by the rate of blood flow, diffusion, and partition properties of the drug and the receptor molecules.

At the receptor site, the onset, duration, and intensity of the pharmacologic response are controlled by receptor concentration and the concentration of the drug and/or its active metabolites. The ultimate pharmacologic response (*effect*) may depend largely on the stereospecific nature of the interaction of the drug with the receptor and the rates of association and dissociation of the drug–receptor complex. Depending on their location and topography, not all receptor molecules are occupied by drug molecules when a maximum pharmacologic response is produced. Other variables, such as age, sex, genetics, nutrition, and tolerance, may also modify the pharmacologic response, making it difficult to relate the pharmacologic response to plasma drug concentration. To control data fluctuation and simplify pharmacodynamic fitting, the pharmacologic response is often expressed as a percent of response above a baseline or percent of maximum response. By combining pharmacokinetics and pharmacodynamics, some drugs with relatively complex pharmacologic responses have been described by pharmacodynamic models that account for their onset, intensity, and duration of action.

After the pharmacodynamics of a drug are characterized, the time course of pharmacologic response may be predicted after drug administration. Also, from these data, it is possible to determine from the pharmacokinetic parameters whether an observed change in pharmacologic response is due to pharmacodynamic factors, such as tachyphylaxis or tolerance, or to pharmacokinetic factors, such as a change in drug absorption, elimination, or distribution.

Drug–Receptor Theory Relating Pharmacologic Effect and Dose

The relationship between pharmacologic effect and dose was advanced by Wagner (1968), who derived a kinetic expression that relates drug concentration to pharmacologic effect. This theoretical development transformed the semiempirical dose–effect relationship (the hyperbolic or log sigmoid profile) into a theoretical equation that relates pharmacologic effect to pharmacokinetics (ie, a pharmacokinetics/pharmacodynamic, PK/PD model). Because the equation was developed for a drug receptor with either single or multiple drug binding, many drugs with a sigmoid concentration effect profile may be described by this model. The slope of the profile also provides some insight into the drug–receptor interaction.

The basic equation mimics somewhat the kinetic equation for protein drug binding (Chapter 10). One or more drug molecules may interact with a receptor to form a complex that in turn elicits a pharmacodynamic response, as illustrated in Figure 19-12. The rate of change in the number of drug–receptor complexes is expressed as db/dt. From Figure 19-12, a differential equation is obtained as shown:

$$\frac{db}{dt} = k_1 c^s (a - b) - bk_2 \tag{19.9}$$

where $k_1 c^s (a - b)$ = rate of receptor complex formation and bk_2 = rate of dissociation of the receptor complex.

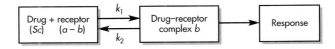

Figure 19-12. Model of the drug–receptor theory: a = total number of drug receptors, c = concentration of drug, S = number of moles of drug that combine with one receptor (constant for each drug), and b = number of drug–receptor complexes.

At steady state, $db/dt = 0$ and Equation 19.9 reduces to

$$k_1 c^s a - k_1 c^s b - bk_2 = 0$$

$$\frac{b}{a} = \frac{k_1 c^s}{k_1 c^s + k_2} = \frac{1}{1 + (k_2/k_1 c^s)} \tag{19.10}$$

For many drugs, the pharmacologic response (R) is proportional to the number of receptors occupied:

$$R \propto \frac{b}{a} \tag{19.11}$$

The pharmacologic response (R) is related to the maximum pharmacologic response (R_{max}), concentration of drug, and rate of change in the number of drug receptor complexes occupied:

$$R = \frac{R_{max}}{1 + (k_2/k_1 c^s)} \tag{19.12}$$

A graph of Equation 19.12 constructed from the percent pharmacologic response, $(R/R_{max}) \times 100$, versus the concentration of drug gives the response–concentration curve (Fig. 19-13). This type of theoretical development explains that the pharmacologic response–dose curve is not completely linear over the entire dosage range, as is frequently observed.

The total pharmacologic response elicited by a drug is difficult to quantitate in terms of the intensity and the duration of the drug response. The *integrated pharmacologic response* is a measure of the total pharmacologic response and is expressed mathematically as the product of these two factors (ie, duration and intensity of drug action) summed up over a period of time. Using Equation 19.12, an integrated pharmacologic response is generated if the drug plasma concentration–time curve can be adequately described by a pharmacokinetic model.

Table 19.4 is based on a hypothetical drug that follows a one-compartment open model. The drug is given intravenously in divided doses. With this drug, the total integrated response increases considerably when the total dose is given in a greater number of divided doses. By giving the drug in a single dose, two doses, four doses, and eight doses, an integrated response was obtained that ranged from 100% to 138.9%, using the single-dose response as a 100% reference. It should be noted that when the bolus dose is broken into a smaller number of doses, the largest percent increase in the integrated response occurs when the bolus dose is divided into two doses. Further division will cause less of an increase, proportionally. The

Figure 19-13. Graph of drug concentration versus pharmacologic response.

TABLE 19.4   Hypothetical Drug Given Intravenously in Single and Divided Doses[a]

DOSE NUMBER	SINGLE DOSE	DOSE GIVEN INITIALLY AND AT 12th hr	DOSE GIVEN AT 0, 6, 12, 18 hr	DOSE GIVEN AT 0, 3, 6, 9, 12, 15, 18, 21 hr
1	422	272	139.4	62.53
2		276	148.2	71.46
3			148.5	74.41
4			149.0	75.61
5				76.27
6				76.44
7				76.71
8				76.81
Total response	422	548	585.1	590.2
Percent response	100	130	138.7	138.9

[a]The drug follows a one-compartment open model. Each value represents a unit of integrated pharmacologic response.

Adapted with permission from Wagner (1968).

actual percent increase in integrated response depends on the $t_{1/2}$ of the drug as well as the dosing interval.

The values in Table 19.4 were generated from theory. However, these data illustrate that the pharmacologic response depends on the dosing schedule. A large total dose given in divided doses may produce a pharmacologic response quite different from that obtained by administering the drug in a single dose.

Correlation of pharmacologic response to pharmacokinetics is not always possible with all drugs. Sometimes intermediate steps are involved in the mechanism of drug action that are more complex than is assumed in the model. For example, warfarin (an anticoagulant) produces a delayed response, and there is no direct correlation of the anticoagulant activity to the plasma drug concentration. The plasma warfarin level is correlated with the inhibition of the prothrombin complex production rate. However, many correlations between pharmacologic effect and plasma drug concentration are performed by proposing models that may be discarded after more data are collected. The process of pharmacokinetic modeling can greatly enhance our understanding of the way drugs act in a quantitative manner.

PHARMACODYNAMIC MODELS

No unified general pharmacodynamic model based on detailed drug–receptor theory that relates pharmacologic response to pharmacokinetics is available. Most of the drug–receptor-based models are descriptive and lack quantitative details. Successful modeling of pharmacologic response has been achieved with semiempirically based assumptions and usually with some oversimplification of the real process. Many of the classic pharmacodynamic models were developed without detailed knowledge of the drug–receptor interaction. The successful modeling of the degree of muscle paralysis of *d*-tubocurarine to plasma concentrations is an

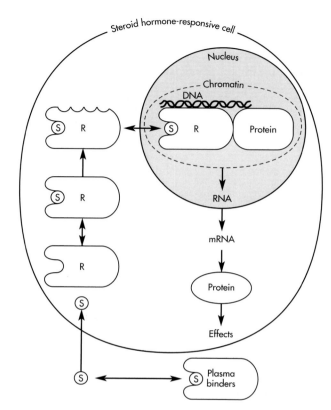

Figure 19-14. Receptor-mediated (R) mechanism of action of corticosteroid (S) hormones.
(From Baxter and Funder, 1979, with permission. Cited by Boudinot et al, 1986.)

interesting example in which the exact mechanism of the drug–receptor interaction was not considered. One of the few pharmacodynamic models that takes into account the interaction between the receptor and the drug molecule leading to a pharmacologic effect was described by Boudinot et al (1986) using the drug prednisolone as an example. Prednisolone is a corticosteroid that binds to cytosolic receptors within the cell (Fig. 19-14). The bound steroid receptor complex is activated and translocated into the nucleus of the cell. Within the cell, the drug–receptor complex associates with specific DNA sequences and modulates the transcription of RNA, which ultimately initiates protein synthesis (Boudinot et al, 1986). Tyrosine aminotransferase (TAT) is an enzyme protein that is increased (induced) by the action of prednisolone. In the liver cell, the prednisolone concentration, drug–receptor concentration, and TAT enzyme were measured with respect to time.

The pharmacodynamic model accounted for the delayed response of prednisolone, a characteristic of corticosteroid response. In this model, prednisolone is first bound to plasma protein, and free drug must leave the plasma compartment and enter the cell to form a drug–receptor complex; creation of this complex then triggers the pharmacologic events leading to an increase in intracellular TAT concentration. A decrease in free receptor or an increase in bound receptor complexes after drug administration was observed. Plasma prednisolone concentrations were

Figure 19-15.   A. Prednisolone levels in plasma (□) and liver (△) fall exponentially after 50 mg/kg of drug IV during the first 10 hours, as described by a pharmacokinetic model. **B.** Free cytosolic glucocorticoid receptor (CGR) concentration fell from control level (●) after 5- (○) and 50-mg/kg (□) IV doses of prednisolone. Free CGR fell as prednisolone interacted with receptor to form receptor complex. The free CGR returned to baseline level after about 10 hours.
(From Boudinot et al, 1986, with permission.)

described by a triexponential equation, and a time lag was built into the model to account for the delay between TAT increase and the drug–receptor–DNA complex formation (Figs. 19-15 and 19-16). A review on PK/PD modelling has been published by Meibohm and Derendorf, 1997.

Maximum Effect (E_{max}) Model

The *maximum effect model* (E_{max}) is an empirical model that relates pharmacologic response to drug concentrations. This model incorporates the observation known as the *law of diminishing return,* which shows that an increase in drug concentration near the maximum pharmacologic response produces a disproportionately smaller increase in the pharmacologic ressponse (Fig. 19-17). The E_{max} model describes drug action in terms of maximum effect (E_{max}) and EC$_{50}$, the drug concentration that produces 50% maximum pharmacologic effect.

$$E = \frac{E_{max}C}{EC_{50} + C}$$

$$(19.13)$$

where C is the plasma drug concentration and E is the pharmacologic effect.

Equation 19.13 is a saturable process resembling Michaelis–Menton enzyme kinetics. As the plasma drug concentration C increases, the pharmacologic effect

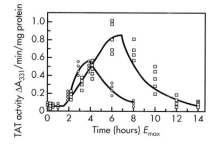

Figure 19-16.   Tyrosine aminotransferase (TAT) activity in liver was described by a pharmacodynamic model (solid line) after 5 (○) and 50 mg/kg (□) IV prednisolone. The pharmacodynamic model accounts for the delay of TAT activity.
(From Boudinot et al, 1986, with permission.)

Figure 19-17.   Plot of pharmacologic response versus plasma drug concentration in a hyperbolic model.

E approaches E_{max} asymptotically. A double-reciprocal plot of Equation 19.13 may be used to linearize the relationship, similar to a Lineweaver–Burke equation.

E_{max} is the maximum pharmacologic effect that may be obtained by the drug. EC_{50} is the drug concentration that produces one-half (50%) of the maximum pharmacologic response. In this model, both E_{max} and EC_{50} can be measured. For example, the bronchodilator activity of theophylline may be monitored by measuring FEV_1 (forced expiratory volume) at various plasma drug concentrations (Fig. 19-18). For theophylline, a small gradual increase in FEV_1 is obtained as the plasma drug concentrations are increased higher than 10 mg/L. Only a 17% increase in FEV_1 is observed when the plasma theophylline concentration is doubled from 10 to 20 mg/L. The EC_{50} for theophylline is 10 mg/L. The E_{max} is equivalent to 63% of normal FEV_1. A further increase in the plasma theophylline concentration will not yield an improvement in the FEV_1 beyond E_{max}. Either drug saturation of the receptors or other limiting factors prevent further improvement in the pharmacologic response.

The E_{max} model describes two key features of the pharmacologic response: (1) the model mimics the hyperbolic shape of the pharmacologic response–drug concentration curve, and (2) a maximum pharmacologic response (E_{max}) may be induced by a certain drug concentration, beyond which no further increase

Figure 19-18.   Use of E_{max} model to describe the effects of theophylline on change in normalized forced expiratory volume (FEV_1); E_{max} = 63%, EC_{50} = 10 mg/L.
(From Mitenko and Ogilvie, 1973, and Holford and Sheiner, 1981, with permission.)

in pharmacologic response is obtained (Fig. 19-17). The drug concentration that produces a 50% maximum pharmacologic response (EC_{50}) is useful as a guide for achieving drug concentration that lies within the therapeutic range.

In many cases, the measured pharmacologic effect has some value when drug is absent (eg, blood pressure, heart rate, respiration rate). E_0 is the measured pharmacologic effect (baseline activity) at zero drug concentration in the body. The measurement for E_0 may be variable due to intra- and intersubject differences. Using E_0 as a baseline constant-effect term, Equation 19.13 may be modified as follows:

$$E = E_0 + \frac{E_{max}C}{EC_{50} + C} \tag{19.14}$$

Sigmoid E_{max} Model

The *sigmoid E_{max} model* describes the pharmacologic response–drug concentration curve for many drugs that appear to be S-shaped (ie, sigmoidal) rather than hyperbolic as described by the simpler E_{max} model. The model was first used by Hill (1910) to describe the association of oxygen with hemoglobin, in which the association with one oxygen molecule influences the association of the hemoglobin with the next oxygen molecule. The equation for the sigmoid E_{max} model is an extension of the E_{max} model:

$$E = \frac{E_{max}C^n}{EC_{50} + C^n} \tag{19.15}$$

where n is an exponent describing the number of drug molecules that combine with each receptor molecule. When n is equal to unity ($n = 1$), the sigmoidal E_{max} model reduces to the E_{max} model. A value of $n > 1$ influences the slope of the curve and the model fit.

The sigmoidal E_{max} model has been used to describe the effect of tocainamide on the suppression of ventricular extrasystoles (Winkle et al, 1976). As shown in Figure 19-19, the very steep slope of the tocainamide concentration–response curve

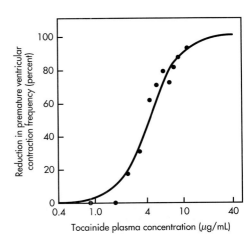

Figure 19-19. Steep concentration response curve for tocainide requiring use of the sigmoid E_{max} model. (From Winkle et al, 1976, with permission.)

required that $n = 20$ in order to fit the model. Although this model was developed empirically, the mathematical equation describing the model is similar to the one elaborated by Wagner (1968) and discussed earlier in this chapter.

In the sigmoid E_{max} model, the slope is influenced by the number of drug molecules bound to the receptor. Moreover, a very large n value may indicate *allosteric* or *cooperative effects* in the interaction of the drug molecules with the receptor.

Pharmacokinetic Pharmacodynamic Models with an Effect Compartment

Many pharmacokinetic models describe the time course for drug and metabolite concentrations in the body. Using either the sigmoid E_{max} or one of the other pharmacodynamic models described earlier, the pharmacologic response may be obtained at various time periods. This simple approach has worked for some neuromuscular blockers and anesthetic agents, whose activities are related to plasma drug concentrations.

For some drugs, the time course for the pharmacologic response may not directly parallel the time course of the plasma drug concentration. The maximum pharmacologic response produced by the drug may be observed before or after the plasma drug concentration has peaked. Moreover, other drugs may produce a delayed pharmacologic response unrelated to the plasma drug concentration.

A pharmacokinetic/pharmacodynamic model with an effect compartment is used to describe the pharmacokinetics of the drug in the plasma and the time course of a pharmacologic effect of a drug in the site of action. To account for the pharmacodynamics of an indirect or delayed drug response, a hypothetical *effect compartment* has been postulated (Fig. 19-20). This effect compartment is not part of the pharmacokinetic model but is a hypothetical pharmacodynamic compartment that links to the plasma compartment containing drug. Drug transfers from the plasma compartment to the effect compartment, but no significant amount of drug moves from the effect compartment to the plasma compartment. Only free drug will diffuse into the effect compartment, and the transfer rate constants are usually first order. The pharmacologic response is determined from the rate constant, k_{e0}, and the drug concentration in the effect compartment (Fig. 19-20).

The amount of drug in the hypothetical effect compartment after a bolus IV dose may be obtained by writing a differential describing the rate of change in drug amounts in each compartment:

$$\frac{dD_e}{dt} = k_{1e}D_1 - k_{e0}D_e \qquad \qquad (19.16)$$

Figure 19-20. Pharmacokinetic–pharmacodynamic model with an effect compartment.

where D_e is the amount of drug in the effect compartment, D_1 is the amount of drug in the central compartment, k_{1e} is the transfer rate constant for drug movement from the central compartment into the effect compartment, and k_{e0} is the transfer rate constant out of the effect compartment.

Integrating Equation 19.16 yields the amount of drug in the effect compartment D_e:

$$D_e = \frac{D_0 k_{1e}}{(k_{e0} - k)}(e^{-kt} - e^{-k_{e0}t}) \tag{19.17}$$

Dividing Equation 19.17 by V_e, the volume of the effect compartment, yields the concentration C_e of the effect compartment:

$$C_e = \frac{D_0 k_{1e}}{V_e(k_{e0} - k)}(e^{-kt} - e^{-k_{e0}t}) \tag{19.18}$$

where D_0 is the dose, V_e is the volume of the effect compartment, and k is the elimination rate constant from the central compartment. Equation 19.18 is not very useful because the parameters V_e and k_{1e} are both unknown and cannot be obtained from plasma drug concentration data. Several assumptions were made to simplify this equation.

The pharmacodynamic model assumes that even though an effect compartment is present in addition to the plasma compartment, this hypothetical effect compartment takes up only a negligible amount of the drug dose, so that plasma drug level still follows a one-compartment equation. After an IV bolus dose, the rate of drug entering and leaving the effect compartment is controlled by the incoming rate constant k_{1e} and the elimination rate constant k_{e0}. (There is no diffusion of drug from the effect compartment into the plasma compartment.) At steady state, both the input and output rates from the effect compartment are equal,

$$k_{1e}D_1 = D_e k_{e0} \tag{19.19}$$

Rearranging,

$$D_1 = \frac{k_{e0}D_e}{k_{1e}} \tag{19.20}$$

Dividing by V_D yields the steady-state plasma drug concentration C_1:

$$C_1 = \frac{k_{e0}D_e}{k_{1e}V_D} \tag{19.21}$$

$$D_e = \frac{D_0 k_{1e}}{(k_{e0} - k)}(e^{-kt} - e^{-k_{e0}t}) \tag{19.22}$$

Substituting for D_e into Equation 19.21 yields

$$C_1 = \frac{k_{e0}D_0 k_{1e}}{k_{1e}V_D(k_{e0} - k)}(e^{-kt} - e^{-k_{e0}t}) \tag{19.23}$$

Cancelling the common term k_{1e},

$$C_1 = \frac{k_{e0}D_0}{V_D(k_{e0} - k)}(e^{-kt} - e^{-k_{e0}t}) \qquad (19.24)$$

At steady state, C_1 is unaffected by k_{1e} and is controlled only by the elimination constant k and k_{e0}. C_1 is called C_{pss}, or steady-state drug concentration, and has been used successfully to relate the pharmacodynamics of many drugs, including some with delayed equilibration between the plasma and the effect compartment. Thus, k and k_{e0} jointly determine the pharmacodynamic profile of a drug. In fitting the pharmacokinetic–pharmacodynamic model, the IV bolus equation is fitted to the plasma drug concentration–time data to obtain k and V_D, while C_{pss}, or C_1 from Equation 19.24, is used to substitute into the concentration in Equation 19.15 to fit the pharmacologic response.

Many drug examples have been described by this type of pharmacokinetic–pharmacodynamic model. The key feature of this model is its dynamic flexibility and adaptability to pharmacokinetic models that account for drug distribution and pharmacologic response. The aggregate effects of drug elimination, binding, partitioning, and distribution in the body are accommodated by the model. The basic assumptions are practical and pragmatic, although some critics of the model (Colburn, 1987) believe the hypothetical effect compartment may oversimplify more complex drug–receptor events. On the positive side, the model represents elegantly an *in-vivo* pharmacologic event relating to the plasma drug concentrations that a clinician can monitor and adjust.

Until more information is known about the effect compartment, a pharmacokinetic–pharmacodynamic model is proposed to describe these kinetic processes combining some of the variables. A good fit of the data to the model is useful but does not necessarily describe the actual pharmacodynamic process. The process of model development evolves until a better model replaces an inadequate one. Several examples of drugs incorporating the effect compartment concept cited in the next section support the versatility of this model. The model accommodates some difficult drug response–concentration profiles, such as the puzzling hysteresis profile of some drug responses (eg, responses to cocaine and ajmaline).

Pharmacodynamic Models Using an Effect Compartment

The antiarrhythmic drug ajmaline slows the heart rate by delaying the depolarization of the heart muscle in the atrium and the ventricle. The pharmacologic effect of the drug is observed in the ECG by measuring the prolongation of the PQ and QRS interval after an IV infusion of ajmaline. A two-compartment model with binding described the pharmacokinetics of the drug and a pharmacodynamic model with an effect compartment was linked to the central compartment in which free drug may diffuse into the effect compartment. The effect compartment was necessary because the plasma ajmaline concentration did not correlate well with changes in recorded ECG events. When the effect-compartment drug concentration was used instead, drug activity was well described by the model (Figs. 19-21 and 19-22).

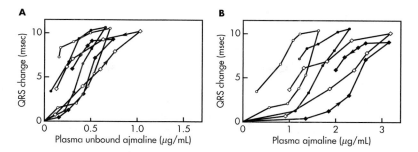

Figure 19-21.   Plot of ajmaline concentration versus change in QRS interval for four dogs: (◆) 1, (◇) 2, (●) 3, (O) 4. **A.** Unbound plasma ajmaline versus response. **B.** Plasma ajmaline versus response. (From Yasuhara et al, 1987, with permission.)

Hysteresis of Pharmacologic Response

Many pharmacologic responses are complex and do not show a direct relationship between pharmacologic effect and plasma drug concentration. Some drugs have a plasma drug concentration–pharmacologic response that resembles a *hysteresis loop* (Fig. 19-23). For these drugs, an identical plasma concentration can result in significantly different pharmacologic responses, depending on whether the plasma drug concentration is on the ascending or descending phase of the loop. The time-dependent nature of a pharmacologic response may be due to tolerance, induced metabolite deactivation, reduced response, or translocation of receptors at the site of action. This type of time-dependent pharmacologic response is characterized by a clockwise profile when pharmacologic response is plotted versus plasma drug concentrations over time (Fig. 19-23).

For example, fentanyl (a lipid-soluble, opioid anesthetic) and alfentanil (a closely related drug) display *clockwise* hysteresis, apparently due to rapid lipid partition. β-Adrenoreceptors, such as isoproterenol, apparently have no direct relationship between response and plasma drug concentration and show hysteresis features. The diminished pharmacologic response was speculated to be a result of cellular response and physiologic adaptation to intense stimulation of the drug. A decrease in the number of receptors as well as translocation of receptors was proposed as the explanation for the observation. The euphoria produced by cocaine also displayed a clockwise profile when responses were plotted versus plasma cocaine concentration (Fig. 19-24).

Figure 19-22.   Plot of change in QRS interval versus ajmaline concentration in the effect compartment in dog 2. The lines were generated based on the effect compartment model. (From Yasuhara et al, 1987, with permission.)

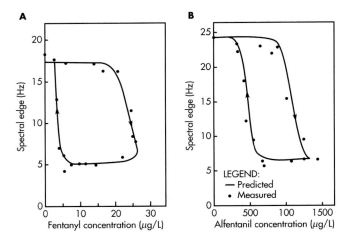

Figure 19-23.   Response of the EEG spectral edge to changing fentanyl **(A)** and alfentanil **(B)** serum concentrations. Plots are data from single patients after rapid drug infusion. Time is indicated by arrows. The clockwise hysteresis indicates a significant time lag between blood and effect site. (From Scott and Stanski, 1985, with permission.)

A second type of pharmacologic response shows a *counterclockwise* hysteresis profile (Fig. 19-25). The pharmacologic response increases with time as the pharmacologic response is plotted versus plasma drug concentrations. An example of a counterclockwise hysteresis loop is the antiarrhythmic drug ajmaline. When the QRS interval changes in dogs were plotted versus plasma ajmaline concentration in each dog, an interesting counterclockwise hysteresis loop was seen (Fig. 19-21). Yasuhara and co-workers (1987) developed a pharmacodynamic model to analyze the molecular events between drug concentration and change in ECG parameters such as QRS. A relationship was established between pharmacologic response and drug concentration in the effect-compartment drug level (Fig. 19-22). The hysteresis profile (Fig. 19-21) is the result of the drug being highly bound to the plasma protein (α_1-acid glycoprotein), and of a slow initial diffusion of drug into the effect compartment.

Counterclockwise hysteresis curves may also result when the measured pharmacodynamic response is not the primary effect of the drug, ie, there is an *indirect*

Figure 19-24.   Clockwise hysteresis loop typical of tolerance is seen after intranasal administration of cocaine when related to degree of euphoria experienced in volunteers. (From van Dyke et al, 1978.)

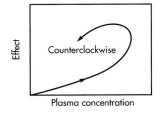

Figure 19-25.   Counterclockwise hysteresis loop indicating equilibration delay between plasma concentration and the effect site producing the effect. (From Holford and Sheiner, 1981.)

effect. For example, warfarin inhibits hepatic synthesis of clotting factors II, VII, IX, and X, but prothrombin time is measured as a surrogate for warfarin activity and clotting factor concentration.

To predict the time course of drug response using a pharmacodynamic model, a mathematical expression is developed to describe the drug concentration–time profile of the drug at the receptor site. This equation is then used to relate drug concentrations to the time course and intensity of the pharmacologic response. Most pharmacodynamic models assume that pharmacologic action is due to a drug–receptor interaction, and the magnitude of the response is related quantitatively to the drug concentration in the receptor compartment. In the simplest case, the drug receptor lies in the plasma compartment and pharmacologic response is established through a one-compartment model with drug response proportional to log drug concentration (Eq. 19.1). A more complicated model involving a receptor compartment that lies outside the central compartment was proposed by Sheiner and associates (1979). This model locates the receptor in an effect compartment in which a drug equilibrates from the central compartment by a first-order rate constant k_{1e}. There is no back diffusion of drug away from the effect compartment, thereby simplifying the complexity of the equations. This model was applied successfully to monitor the pharmacologic effects of the drug trimazosin (Meredith et al, 1983).

The pharmacokinetics of trimazosin are described as a two-compartment open model with conversion to a metabolite by a first-order rate constant k_{1m}. The pharmacokinetics of the metabolite are described by a one compartment model with a first-order elimination constant k_{m0}. The drug effect may be described by two pharmacodynamic models, either model A or B. Model A assumes that the drug effect in the effect compartment is produced by the drug only. Model B assumes that both the drug and a metabolite produce drug effect (Fig. 19-26).

The following equation describes the pharmacokinetics and pharmacodynamics of the drug:

$$C_p = Ae^{-at} - Be^{-bt} \tag{19.25}$$

where C_p is the concentration of the drug in the central compartment.

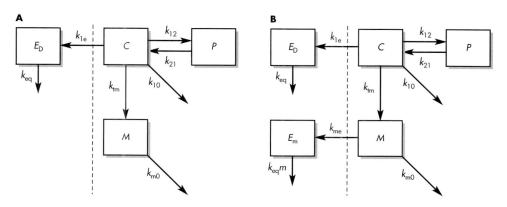

Figure 19-26. Two proposed pharmacodynamic models for describing the hypotensive effect of trimazosin. **A** assumes an effect compartment (left of dashed line) for the drug. **B** assumes an effect compartment for the drug as well as the metabolite.
(From Meredith et al, 1983, with permission.)

$$C_m = \frac{V_1 k_{1m}}{V_m} \left[\frac{A}{(k_{m0} - a)} (e^{-at} - e^{-k_{m0}t}) + \frac{B}{(k_{m0} - b)} (e^{-bt} - e^{-k_{m0}t}) \right] \tag{19.26}$$

where C_m is the concentration of the metabolite in the body, V_m is the volume of distribution of the metabolite, V_1 is the volume of the central compartment of the body, k_{1m} is the first-order constant for converting drug to metabolite, k_{m0} is the elimination rate constant of the metabolite, A and B are two-compartment model coefficients for the drug (see Chapter 4), and k_{10} is the elimination rate constant of the drug.

The drug concentration in the effect compartment is calculated by assuming that at equilibrium the concentration of the drug in the effect compartment and the central compartment are equal,

$$k_{1e} V_1 = k_{eq} V_e \tag{19.27}$$

where V_e is volume of the effect compartment and k_{eq} is the elimination rate constant of the drug from the effect compartment. Therefore, the drug concentration in the effect compartment $C(e, d)$ is calculated as

$$C(e, d) = \frac{A K_{eq}}{(k_{eq} - a)} (e^{-at} - e^{-k_{eq}t}) + \frac{B k_{eq}}{(k_{eq} - b)} (e^{-bt} - e^{-k_{eq}t}) \tag{19.28}$$

The effect due to drug is assumed to be linear,

$$E = M_d C(e, d) + i \tag{19.29}$$

where M_d is the *sensitivity slope* to the drug (ie, the effect per unit of drug concentration in the effect compartment). The parameters M_d, i, and k_{eq} are determined by least-squares fitting of the data. For the metabolite, the concentration of metabolite in the effect compartment is $C(e, m)$.

$$C(e, m) = \frac{A V_1 k_{1m} k_{eq} m}{V_m} \tag{19.30}$$

$$\times \left[\frac{e^{-at}}{(a - k_{m0})(a - k_{eq}m)} + \frac{e^{-k_{m0}t}}{(a - k_{m0})(k_{eq}m - k_{m0})} \right.$$

$$- \frac{e^{-k_{eq}mt}}{(a - k_{eq}m)(k_{eq}m - k_{m0})}$$

$$+ \frac{B V_1 k_{1m} k_{eq} m}{V_m} \frac{e^{-bt}}{(b - k_{m0})(b - k_{eq}m)}$$

$$+ \left. \frac{e^{-k_{m0}t}}{(b - k_{m0})(k_{eq}m - k_{m0})} - \frac{e^{-k_{eq}mt}}{(b - k_{eq}m)(k_{eq}m - k_{m0})} \right]$$

Figure 19-27.   Diagram showing the agreement between recorded hypotensive effect (solid line) and hypotensive effect as projected by model B (broken line). (From Meredith et al, 1983, with permission.)

The concentration of the metabolite in the effect compartment is in turn related to drug effect as for the parent drug. The total effect produced is

$$E = M_d C(e, d) + M_m C(e, m) + i \tag{19.31}$$

The five parameters M_d, M_m, i, k_{eq}, k_{eqm} may be estimated from Equation 19.31 by fitting the data to an appropriate model. Figure 19-27 shows the observed decline in systolic blood pressure compared with the theoretical decline in blood pressure predicted by the model. An excellent fit of the data was obtained by assuming that both drug and metabolite are active. This example illustrates that, for a dose of a drug, the drug concentration in the effect compartment and others may be described by a mathematical model. These equations were further developed to describe the time course of a pharmacologic event. In this case, Meredith and associates (1983) demonstrated that both the drug and the metabolite formed in the body may affect the time course of the pharmacologic action of the drug in the body.

Simulation of *In-Vitro* Pharmacodynamic Effect Involving Hysteresis

An *in-vitro* model simulation of the sum of pharmacologic effect contributed by a drug and its active metabolite may explain the observation of the hysteresis response curve *in vivo*. Gupta et al (1993) discussed the factors that affect the shape of the response curve. In the simplest case, pharmacokinetic equations are developed to calculate C_p, the drug concentration, and C_m, the metabolite concentration. To estimate the pharmacologic effect due to both the drug and active metabolite, the potency of the drug is defined as P, the potency of the metabolite is P_m, and

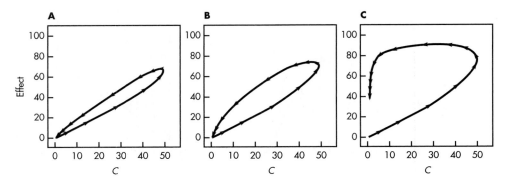

Figure 19-28.   Simulated *in-vitro* pharmacodynamic response versus concentration (*C*) contributed by a drug and a metabolite. Potency of parent drug and metabolite are equal, but **(A)** k_{m0} = large, **(B)** k_{m0} = medium, and **(C)** k_{m0} = small.
(From Gupta et al, 1993, with permission.)

the sum of the pharmacologic effect is as shown below. (In their first simulation, Gupta et al assumed that the effect is linearly related to drug and metabolite concentrations.)

$$E = PC_p + P_m C_m \tag{19.32}$$

The shape of hysteresis simulated is very dependent on P_m and k_{m0}, the rate constant of metabolite elimination. If k_{m0} is given a high, medium, or low value, the effect on the shape of the hysteresis loop is changed dramatically, as shown in Figure 19-28. A temporal effect causes a counterclockwise loop. In the case of a metabolite that acts as an antagonist, the hysteresis loop is clockwise. The more elaborate features of an E_{max} model were simulated by Gupta et al (1993) in their paper.

CLINICAL EXAMPLE

Lorazepam Pharmacodynamics—Example of an In-Vivo Hysteresis Loop

Many drugs that act on the central nervous systems (CNS) have a lag time before the tissues and the plasma are equilibrated with drug. The pharmacokinetics of lorazepam after oral absorption were fitted to a two-compartment model with lag time. Lorazepam was studied because the drug accounts for all the activity, such that the counterclockwise response profile may be attributed to equilibration rather than to metabolism (Gupta et al, 1990).

The description of the plasma drug concentrations, C_p, is obtained by conventional pharmacokinetic equations, whereas the pharmacodynamic effect, E, is

Figure 19-29. Plot of responses of lorazepam versus plasma drug concentration showing counterclockwise hysteresis.
(From Gupta et al, 1990, with permission.)

described by a sigmoid E_{max} model similar to Equation 19.15, except that the baseline effect is also included. Gupta et al (1990) monitored three pharmacodynamic effects due to lorazepam. The monitored pharmacodynamic effects were mental impairment processes evaluated by the cognitive and psychomotor performance of the subjects, including (A) subcritical tracking, (B) sway open (a measurement of gross body movements), and (C) digital symbol substitution. When the time course of each effect was plotted versus plasma drug concentration, a counterclockwise loop was observed (Fig. 19-29). When the same pharmacodynamic responses were plotted versus lorazepam concentration in the effect compartment accounting for the equilibration lag, a classical sigmoid relation was observed (Fig. 19-30). The observations showed that the temporal response of many drugs may be the result of pharmacodynamic and distributional factors interacting with each other. Thus, a model with an effect compartment can more fully help to understand the time course of the drug response.

Figure 19-30. Plot of responses to lorazepam versus effect compartment concentration showing sigmoid relationship between effect and concentration without hysteresis.
(From Gupta et al, 1990, with permission.)

FREQUENTLY ASKED QUESTIONS

1. Explain why doubling the dose of a drug does not double the pharmacodynamic effect of the drug.

2. What is meant by a hysteresis loop? Why do some drugs follow a clockwise hysteresis loop and other drugs follow a counterclockwise hysteresis loop?

3. What is meant by an effect compartment? How does the effect compartment differ from pharmacokinetic compartments, such as the central compartment and the tissue compartment?

LEARNING QUESTIONS

1. On the basis of the graph in Figure 19-31, answer "true" or "false" to statements (a)–(e) and state the reason for each answer.

   a. The plasma drug concentration is more related to the pharmacodynamic effect of the drug compared to the dose of the drug.

   b. The pharmacologic response is directly proportional to the log plasma drug concentration.

   c. The volume of distribution is not changed by uremia.

   d. The drug is exclusively eliminated by hepatic biotransformation.

   e. The receptor sensitivity is unchanged in the uremic patient.

2. What do clavulanate, sulbactam, and tazobactam have in common? Why are they used together with antibiotics?

3. Explain why subsequent equal doses of a drug do not produce the same pharmacodynamic effect as the first dose of a drug.

   a. Provide an explanation based on pharmacokinetic considerations.

   b. Provide an explanation based on pharmacodynamic considerations.

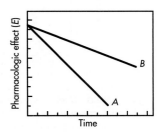

Figure 19-31. Graph of pharmacologic response *E* as a function of time for the same drug in patients with normal **(A)** and uremic **(B)** kidney function, respectively.

4. How are the parameters AUC and t_{eff} used in pharmacodynamic models?

5. What class of drug tends to have a lag time between the plasma and the effect compartment?

6. Name an example of a pharmacodynamic response that does not follow a drug dose–response profile?

7. When an antibiotic concentration falls below the MIC, there is a short time period in which bacteria fail to regrow because of postantibiotic effect (PAE). This time period is referred to as PAT. What is PAT?

8. What is AUIC with regard to an antibiotic?

REFERENCES

Aghajanian OK, Bing OHL: Persistence of lysergic acid diethylamide in the plasma of human subjects. *Clin Pharmacol Ther* **5**:611–614, 1964

Baxter JD, Funder JW: Hormone receptors. *N Engl J Med* **301**:1149–1161, 1979

Boudinot FD, D'Ambrosio R, Jusko WJ: Receptor-mediated pharmacodynamics of prednisolone in the rat. *J Pharmacokinet Biopharm* **14**:469–493, 1986

Colburn WA: Perspectives in pharmacokinetics: Pharmacokinetic/pharmacodynamic modeling: What is it? *J Pharmacokinet Biopharm* **15**:545–553, 1987

Cone EJ: Pharmacokinetics and pharmacodynamics of cocaine. *J Anal Toxicol* **19**:459–478, 1995

Cox, BM: Drug tolerance and physical dependence. In WB Pratt, P Taylor (eds): *Principles of Drug Action. The Basis of Pharmacology.* New York, Churchill Livingstone, 1990, chap 10

Craig, WA: Interrelationship between pharmacokinetics and pharmacodynamics in determining dosage regimens for broad-spectrum cephalosporins. *Diag Microbiol Infect Dis* **22**:89–96, 1995

Craig WA, Andes D: Pharmacokinetics and pharmacodynamics of antibiotics in otitis media. *J Pediatr Infect Dis* **15**:255–259, 1996

deWit H, Dudish S, Ambre J: Subjective behavioral effects of diazepam depend upon its rate of onset. *Psychopharmacology* **112**:324–330, 1993

Drusano GL: Minireview: Role of pharmacokinetics in the outcome of infections. *Antimicrob Agents Chemother* **32**(3):289–297, 1988

Forrest A, Nix DE, Ballow CH, Goss TF, Birmingham MC, Schentag JJ: Pharmacodynamics of intravenous ciprofloxacin in seriously ill patients. *Antimicrob Agents Chemother* **37**(5):1073–1081, 1993

Gupta SK, Ellinwood EH, Nikaido AM, Heatherly DG: Simultaneous modeling of the pharmacokinetic and pharmacodynamic properties of benzodiazepines I: Lorazepam. *J Pharmacokinet Biopharm* **18**:89–102, 1990

Gupta SK, Hwang SS, Benet LZ, Gumbleton M: Interpretation and utilization of effect and concentration data collected in an *in vivo* pharmacokinetic and in vitro pharmacodynamic study. *Pharm Res* **10**:889–894, 1993

Henningfield JE, Keenan RM: Nicotine delivery kinetics and abuse liability. *J Consult Clin Pharmacol* **61**:743–750, 1993

Hill AV: The possible effects of the aggregation of the molecules of haemoglobin on its dissociation curves. *J Physiol* **40**:4–7, 1910

Holford NHG, Sheiner LB: Understanding the dose–effect relationship. Clinical application of pharmacokinetic–pharmacodynamic models. *Clin Pharmacokinet* **6**:429–453, 1981

Holford NHG, Sheiner LB: Kinetics of pharmacologic response. *Pharm Ther* **16**:143–166, 1982

Johanson C-E, Fischman MW: The pharmacology of cocaine related to its abuse. *Pharmacol Rev* **41**:3–52, 1989

Johansen SH, Jorgensen M, Molbech S: Effect of tubocurarine on respiratory and nonrespiratory muscle power in man. *J Appl Physiol* **19**:990–991, 1964

Lalonde RL: Pharmacodynamics. In Evans WE et al. (eds): *Applied Pharmacokinetics,* 3rd ed. Vancouver, WA, Applied Therapeutics, 1992, chap 4

Lin RY: A perspective on penicillin allergy. *Arch Intern Med* **152**:930–937, 1992

Meredith PA, Kelman AW, Eliott HL, Reid JL: Pharmacokinetic and pharmacodynamic modeling of trimazosin and its major metabolite. *J Pharmacokinet Biopharm* **11**:323–334, 1983

Meibohm B, Derendorf H: Basic concepts of pharmacokinetic/pharmacodynamic (PK/PD) modelling. *Int J Clin Pharmacol* **35**(10):401–413, 1997

Mitenko PA, Ogilvie RI: Rational intravenous doses of theophylline. *N Engl J Med* **289**:600–603, 1973

Reisman AS, Reisman RE: Risk of administering cephalosporin antibiotics to patients with histories of penicillin allergy. *Ann Aller Asthma Immunol* **74**:167–170, 1995

Rodman JH, Evans WE: Targeted systemic exposure for pediatric cancer therapy. In D'Argenio (ed): *Advanced Methods of Pharmacokinetic and Pharmacodynamic Systems Analysis.* New York, Plenum Press, 1991, pp 177–183

Scaglione F: Predicting the clinical efficacy of antibiotics: Toward definitive criteria. *Pediatr Infect Dis J* **3**:S56–S59, 1997

Scott JC, Stanski DR: Decreased fentanyl/alfentanil dose requirement with increasing age: A pharmacodynamic basis. *Anesthesiology* **63**:A374, 1985

Sheiner LB, Stanski DR, Vozeh S, et al: Simultaneous modeling of pharmacokinetics and pharmacodynamics: Application to d-tubocurarine. *Clin Pharmacol Ther* **25**:358–370, 1979

Taylor P, Insel PA: Molecular basis of pharmacologic selectivity. In Pratt WB, Taylor P (eds): *Principles of Drug Action. The Basis of Pharmacology,* 3rd ed. New York, Churchill Livingstone, 1990

van Dyke C, Jatlow P, Ungerer J, et al: Oral cocaine: Plasma concentration and central effects. *Science* **200**:211–213, 1978

Wagner JG: Kinetics of pharmacologic response: 1. Proposed relationship between response and drug concentration in the intact animal and man. *J Theor Biol* **20**:173–201, 1968

Winkle RA, Meffin PJ, Fitzgerald JW, Harrison DC: Clinical efficacy and pharmacokinetics of a new orally effective antiarrhythmic tocainide. *Circulation* **54**:884–889, 1976

Yasuhara M, Hashimoto Y, Okumura K, et al: Kinetics of ajmaline disposition and pharmacologic response in beagle dogs. *J Pharmacokinet Biopharm* **15**:39–56, 1987

BIBLIOGRAPHY

Derendorf H, Meibohm B: Modeling of pharmacokinetic/pharmacodynamic (PK/PD) relationships: Concepts and perspectives. *Pharm Res* **6**:176–185, 1999

Drusano GL: Human pharmacodynamics of beta-lactams, aminoglycosides and their combination. *Scand J Infect Dis* **74**(suppl):235–248, 1991

Drusano GL, Craig WA: Relevance of pharmacokinetics and pharmacodynamics in the selection of antibiotics for respiratory tract infections. *J Chemother* **9**(suppl 3):38–44, 1997

Galeazzi RL, Benet LZ, Sheiner LB: Relationship between the pharmacokinetics and pharmacodynamics of procainamide. *Clin Pharmacol Ther* **20**:278–289, 1976

Gibaldi M, Levy G, Weintraub H: Drug distribution and pharmacologic effects. *Clin Pharmacol Ther* **12**:734, 1971

Gunderson BW, Ross GH, Ibrahim KH, Rotschafer JC: What do we really know about antibiotic pharmacodynamics? *Pharmacotherapy* **21**(11s):302s–318s, 2001

Harron DWG: Digoxin pharmacokinetic modeling—10 years later. *Int J Pharm* **53**:181–188, 1989

Hochhaus G, Barrett JS, Derendorf H: Evolution of pharmacokinetics and pharmacokinetic/dynamic correlations during the 20th century. *J Clin Pharmacol* **40**(9):908–917, 2000

Holford NHG: Clinical pharmacokinetics and pharmacodynamics of warfarin. Understanding the dose–effect relationship. *Clin Pharmacokinet* **11**:583–604, 1986

Jusko WJ: Pharmacodynamics of chemotherapeutic effects: Dose–time–response relationship for phase-nonspecific agents. *J Pharm Sci* **60**:892, 1971

Levy G: Kinetics of pharmacologic effects. *Clin Pharmacol Ther* **1**:362, 1966

Meffin PJ, Winkle RA, Blaschke RF, et al: Response optimization of drug dosage: Antiarrhythmic studies with tocainide. *Clin Pharmacol Ther* **22**:42–57, 1977

Meibohm B, Derendorf H: Pharmacokinetic/pharmacodynamic studies in drug product development. *J Pharm Sci* **91**:18–31, 2002

Mueller M, de la Pena A, Derendorf H: Issues in pharmacokinetics and pharmacodynamics of anti-infective agents: Kill curves versus MIC. *Antimicrob Agents Chemother* **48**(2):369–377, 2004

Packer M, Carver JR, Rodeheffer RJ, et al: Effect of oral milrinone on mortality in severe chronic heart failure. *N Engl J Med* **21**:1468, 1991

Schwinghammer TL, Kroboth PD: Basic concepts in pharmacodynamic modeling. *J Clin Pharmacol* **28**:388–394, 1988

Seeman P, Lee T, Chau-Wong M, Wong K: Antipsychotic drug doses and neuroleptic/dopamine receptors. *Nature* **261**:717–719, 1976

Sheiner LB: Commentary to pharmacokinetic/pharmacodynamic modeling: What it is! *J Pharmacokinet Biopharm* **15**:553–555, 1987

Suresh A, Reisman RE: Risk of administering cephalosporin antibiotics to patients with histories of penicillin allergy. *Ann Allergy Asthma Immunol* **74**:167–170, 1995

Swerdlow BN, Holley FO: Intravenous anaesthetic agents. Pharmacokinetic/pharmacodynamic relationships. *Clin Pharmacokinet* **12**:79–110, 1987

Verrijk R, Vleeming W, Hans H, et al: Plasma elimination of milrinone in rats in relation to its hemodynamic effects. *J Pharm Sci* **79**:236–239, 1990

Whiting B, Holford NHG, Sheiner LB: Quantitative analysis of the disopyramide concentration–effect relationship. *Br J Clin Pharmacol* **9**:67–75, 1980

20

APPLICATION OF PHARMACOKINETICS TO CLINICAL SITUATIONS

The success of drug therapy is highly dependent on the choice of the drug and drug product and on the design of the dosage regimen. The choice of the drug and drug product, eg, immediate release versus modified release, is based on the patient's characteristics and the known pharmacokinetics of the drug as discussed in earlier chapters. A properly designed dosage regimen tries to achieve a specified concentration of the drug at a receptor site to produce an optimal therapeutic response with minimum adverse effects. Individual variation in pharmacokinetics and pharmacodynamics makes the design of dosage regimens difficult. Therefore, the application of pharmacokinetics to dosage regimen design must be coordinated with proper clinical evaluation of the patient and monitoring.

INDIVIDUALIZATION OF DRUG DOSAGE REGIMENS

Not all drugs require rigid individualization of the dosage regimen. Many drugs have a large margin of safety (ie, exhibit a wide therapeutic window), and strict individualization of the dose is unnecessary. The U.S. Food and Drug Administration (FDA) has approved an *over-the-counter* (OTC) classification for drugs that the public may buy without prescription. In the past few years, many prescription drugs, such as ibuprofen, loratidine, omeprazole, naproxen, nicotine patches, and others, have been approved by the FDA for OTC status. These OTC drugs and certain prescription drugs, when taken as directed, are generally safe and effective for the labeled indications without medical supervision. For drugs that are relatively safe and have a broad safety-dose range, such as the penicillins, cephalosporins, and tetracyclines, the antibiotic dosage is not dose titrated precisely but is based rather on the clinical judgment of the physician to maintain an effective plasma antibiotic concentration above a minimum inhibitory concentration.

For drugs with a narrow therapeutic window, such as digoxin, aminoglycosides, antiarrhythmics, anticonvulsants, and some antiasthmatics, such as theophylline, individualization of the dosage regimen is very important. The objective of the dosage regimen design for these drugs is to produce a safe plasma drug concentration that does not exceed the minimum toxic concentration or fall below a critical minimum drug concentration below which the drug is not effective. For this reason, the dose of these drugs is carefully individualized to avoid plasma drug concentration fluctuations due to intersubject variation in drug absorption, distribution, or elimination processes. For drugs such as phenytoin that follow nonlinear pharmacokinetics at therapeutic plasma drug concentrations, a small change in the dose may cause a huge increase in the therapeutic response, leading to possible adverse effects.

The monitoring of plasma drug concentrations is valuable only if a relationship exists between the plasma drug concentration and the desired clinical effect or between the plasma drug concentration and an adverse effect. For those drugs in which plasma drug concentration and clinical effect are not related, other pharmacodynamic parameters may be monitored. For example, clotting time may be measured directly in patients on warfarin anticoagulant therapy. For asthmatic patients, the bronchodilator, albuterol, is given by inhalation via a metered-dose inhaler and the patient's FEV_1 (forced expiratory volume) may be used as a measure of drug efficacy. In cancer chemotherapy, dose adjustment for individual patients may depend on the severity of side effects and the patient's ability to tolerate the drug. For some drugs that have large inter- and intrasubject variability, clinical judgment and experience with the drug is needed to dose the patient properly.

THERAPEUTIC DRUG MONITORING

The therapeutic range for a drug is an approximation of the average plasma drug concentrations that are safe and efficacious in most patients. When using published therapeutic drug concentration ranges, such as those in Table 20.1, the clinician

TABLE 20.1   Therapeutic Range for Commonly Monitored Drugs

Amikacin	20–30 μg/mL
Carbamazepine	4–12 μg/mL
Digoxin	1–2 ng/mL
Gentamicin	5–10 μg/mL
Lidocaine	1–5 μg/mL
Lithium	0.6–1.2 mEq/L
Phenytoin	10–20 μg/mL
Procainamide	4–10 μg/mL
Quinidine	1–4 μg/mL
Theophylline	10–20 μg/mL
Tobramycin	5–10 μg/mL
Valproic acid	50–100 μg/mL
Vancomycin	20–40 μg/mL

From Schumacher (1995), with permission.

Figure 20-1. Correlation between the frequency and severity of adverse effects and plasma concentration of theophylline (mean ± SD) in 50 adult patients. Mild symptoms of toxicity included nausea, vomiting, headache, and insomnia: a potentially serious effect was sinus tachycardia, and severe toxicity was defined as the occurrence of life-threatening cardiac arrhythmias and seizures. (Adapted from Hendeles and Weinberger, 1980, with permission.)

must realize that the therapeutic range is essentially a probability concept and should never be considered as absolute values (Evans et al, 1992; Schumacher, 1995). For example, the accepted therapeutic range for theophylline is 10–20 μg/mL. Some patients may exhibit signs of theophylline intoxication such as central nervous system excitation and insomnia at serum drug concentrations below 20 μg/mL (see Fig. 20.1, below) whereas other patients may show drug efficacy at serum drug concentrations below 10 μg/mL.

In administering potent drugs to patients, the physician must maintain the plasma drug level within a narrow range of therapeutic concentrations (Table 20.1). Various pharmacokinetic methods may be used to calculate the initial dose or dosage regimen. Usually, the initial dosage regimen is calculated based on body weight or body surface after a careful consideration of the known pharmacokinetics of the drug, the pathophysiologic condition of the patient, and the patient's drug history.

Because of interpatient variability in drug absorption, distribution, and elimination as well as changing pathophysiologic conditions in the patient, *therapeutic drug monitoring* (TDM) or clinical pharmacokinetic (laboratory) services (CPKS) have been established in many hospitals to evaluate the response of the patient to the recommended dosage regimen. The improvement in the clinical effectiveness of the drug by therapeutic drug monitoring may decrease the cost of medical care by preventing untoward adverse drug effects. The functions of a TDM service are listed below.

- Select drug.
- Design dosage regimen.
- Evaluate patient response.
- Determine need for measuring serum drug concentrations.
- Assay for drug concentration in biological fluids.
- Perform pharmacokinetic evaluation of drug concentrations.

- Readjust dosage regimen, if necessary.
- Monitor serum drug concentrations.
- Recommend special requirements.

Drug Selection

The choice of drug and drug therapy is usually made by the physician. However, many practitioners consult with the clinical pharmacist in drug product selection and dosage regimen design. Increasingly, clinical pharmacists in hospitals and nursing care facilities are closely involved in prescribing, monitoring, and substitution of medications. The choice of drug and the drug product is made not only on the basis of therapeutic consideration, but also based on cost and therapeutic equivalency. Pharmacokinetics and pharmacodynamics are part of the overall considerations in the selection of a drug for inclusion into the drug formulary (DF). New pharmacokinetic and pharmacodynamic data are periodically reviewed and updated by Institutional Pharmacy and Therapeutic Committees (IPTCs).

Drugs with similar therapeutic indications may differ in dose and pharmacokinetics. The pharmacist may choose one drug over another based on cost, therapeutic, and pharmacokinetic considerations. Other factors include patient-specific information such as medical history, pathophysiologic states, concurrent drug therapy, known allergies, drug sensitivities, and drug interactions; all are important considerations in drug selection (Table 20.2).

Dosage Regimen Design

The overall objective of dosage regimen design is to achieve a *target* drug concentration at the receptor site. Once the proper drug is selected for the patient, a number of factors must be considered when designing a therapeutic dosage regimen. First, the usual pharmacokinetics of the drug—including its absorption, distribution, and elimination profile—are considered in the patient. Some patients have unusual first-pass metabolism and bioavailability may be reduced. Second, the physiology of the patient, age, weight, gender, and nutritional status will affect the disposition of the drug and should be considered. Third, any pathophysiologic conditions, such as renal dysfunction, hepatic disease, or congestive heart failure, may change the normal pharmacokinetic profile of the drug, and the dose must be carefully adjusted. For some patients, the hidden effect of exposure to long-term medication or drug abuse are important. Personal lifestyle factors, such as cigarette smoking, alcohol abuse, and obesity are known to alter the pharmacokinetics of drugs.

TABLE 20.2   *Factors Producing Variability in Drug Response*

PATENT FACTORS	DRUG FACTORS
Age	Bioavailability and biopharmaceutics
Weight	Pharmacokinetics (including absorption, distribution, and elimination)
Pathophysiology	Drug interactions
Nutritional status	Receptor sensitivity
Genetic variability	Rapid or slow metabolism
Gender	

Optimal dosing design can greatly improve the safety and efficacy of the drug, including reduced side effects and a decrease in frequency of therapeutic drug monitoring and its associated costs. For some drugs, TDM will be necessary because of the unpredictable nature of their pharmacodynamics and pharmacokinetics. Changes in drug or drug dose may be required after careful assessment by the pharmacist of the patient, including changes in the drug's pharmacokinetics, drug tolerance, cross sensitivity, or history of unusual reactions to related drugs. The pharmacist must develop competency and experience in clinical pharmacology and therapeutics in addition to the necessary pharmacokinetic skills. Several mathematical approaches to dosage regimen design are given in later sections of this chapter and in Chapter 21.

Pharmacokinetics of the Drug

Various popular drug references list pharmacokinetic parameters such as clearance, bioavailability, and elimination half-life. The values for these pharmacokinetic parameters are often obtained from small clinical studies. Therefore, it is difficult to determine whether these reported pharmacokinetic parameters are reflected in the general population or in specific patient groups. Differences in study design, patient population, and data analysis may lead to conflicting values for the same pharmacokinetic parameters. For example, values for the apparent volume of distribution and clearance can be estimated by different methods, as discussed in previous chapters.

Ideally, the target drug concentration and the therapeutic window for the drug should be obtained, if available. In using the target drug concentration in the development of a dosage regimen, the clinical pharmacist should know whether the reported target (effective) drug concentration represents an average steady-state drug concentration, a peak drug concentration, or a trough concentration.

Drug Dosage Form (Drug Product)

The dosage form of the drug will affect drug bioavailability and the rate of absorption and thus the subsequent pharmacodynamics of the drug in the patient. The route of drug administration and the desired onset and duration of the clinical response will affect the choice of drug dosage form. In addition, the selection of an extended-release drug product instead of an immediate-release drug product may affect both the cost of the drug and patient compliance. These biopharmaceutic factors have been discussed in Chapter 14.

Patient Compliance

Factors that may affect patient compliance include the cost of the medication, complicated instructions, multiple daily doses, difficulty in swallowing, adverse drug reactions, and ambulatory versus institutionalized status. Institutionalized patients may have very little choice as to the prescribed drug and drug dosage form. Moreover, patient compliance in institutions is dictated by the fact that medication is provided by the medical personnel. Ambulatory patients must remember to take the medication as prescribed to obtain the optimum clinical effect of the drug. Therefore, it is very important that the clinician or clinical pharmacist consider the patient's lifestyle and needs when developing a drug dosage regimen.

Evaluation of Patient's Response

After the drug and drug product are chosen and the patient receives the initial dosage regimen, the practitioner should evaluate the patient's response clinically. If the patient is not responding to drug therapy as expected, then the drug and dosage regimen should be reviewed. The dosage regimen should be reviewed for adequacy, accuracy, and patient compliance to the drug therapy. In many situations, sound clinical judgment may preclude the need for measuring serum drug concentrations.

Measurement of Serum Drug Concentrations

Before blood samples are taken from the patient, the practitioner needs to determine whether serum drug concentrations in the patient need to be measured. In some cases, the patient's response may not be related to the serum drug concentration. For example, allergy or mild nausea may not be dose related. In other cases, the response of a drug may be related to its chronopharmacology (see examples in Chapter 9).

A major assumption made by the practitioner is that serum drug concentrations relate to the therapeutic and/or toxic effects of the drug. For many drugs, clinical studies have demonstrated a therapeutically effective range of serum concentrations. Knowledge of the serum drug concentration may clarify why a patient is not responding to the drug therapy or why the drug is having an adverse effect. In addition, the practitioner may want to verify the accuracy of the dosage regimen.

When ordering serum drug concentrations to be measured, a single serum drug concentration may not yield useful information unless other factors are considered. For example, the dosage regimen of the drug should be known, including the size of the dose and the dosage interval, the route of drug administration, the time of sampling (peak, trough, or steady state), and the type of drug product (eg, immediate release or extended release).

In many cases, a single blood sample gives insufficient information. Several blood samples are often needed to clarify the adequacy of the dosage regimen. In practice, trough serum concentrations are easier to obtain than peak or C_{av}^{∞} samples under a multiple-dose regimen. In addition, limitations in terms of the number of blood samples that may be taken, total volume of blood needed for the assay, and time to perform the drug analysis may exist. Schumacher (1985b) has suggested that blood sampling times for therapeutic drug monitoring should be taken during the postdistributive phase for loading and maintenance doses, but at steady state for maintenance doses. After distribution equilibrium has been achieved, the plasma drug concentration during the postdistributive phase is better correlated with the tissue concentration and, presumably, the drug concentration at the site of action. In some cases, the clinical pharmacist may want an early-time sample that approximates the peak drug level, whereas a blood sample taken at three or four elimination half-lives will approximate the steady-state drug concentration. The practitioner who orders the measurement of serum concentrations should also consider the cost of the assays, the risks and discomfort for the patient, and the utility of the information gained.

Assay for Drug

Drug analyses are usually performed by either a clinical chemistry laboratory or a clinical pharmacokinetics laboratory. A variety of analytic techniques are available for drug measurement, including high-pressure liquid chromatography, gas chromatography, spectrophotometry, fluorometry, immunoassay, and radioisotopic methods. The methods used by the analytic laboratory may depend on such factors as the physicochemical characteristics of the drug, target concentration for measurement, amount and nature of the biologic specimen (serum, urine), available instrumentation, cost for each assay, and analytical skills of the laboratory personnel. The laboratory should have a standard operating procedure (SOP) for each drug analysis technique and follow good laboratory practices. Moreover, analytic methods used for the assay of drugs in serum should be validated with respect to specificity, linearity, sensitivity, precision, accuracy, stability, and ruggedness.

Because of cost and equipment constraints, most clinical pharmacokinetic services routinely analyze drugs by immunoassay. Various immunoassay methods are currently available that may differ in assay specificity for the drug, the cost of analyses, and the time to perform the assay and obtain the results. The Abbott TDx system is a fluorescence polarization immunoassay (FPI), which measures most of the antiarrhythmics and aminoglycosides and other drugs of abuse (Table 20.3). TDxFLx is a newer system that allows flexible handling of samples. Other dedicated systems routinely used in hospitals include the Autocarousel (Syva Corp., which markets many EMIT test kits for many drugs). Other makers of instruments or kits for drug testing include Syntex, Eastman Kodak, Hoffman-LaRoche, and Miles Laboratories.

Specificity

Chromatographic evidence should be used to demonstrate that the analytic method is specific for detection of the drug. The method should demonstrate that there is

TABLE 20.3   Common Drugs Monitored in Hospitals

ANTIARRHYTHMICS	ANTIBIOTICS	ANTICONVULSANTS
Disopyramide	Amikacin	Carbamazepine, free carbamazepine
Flecainide	Gentamicin	Valproic acid, free valproic acid
Lidocaine	Netilmicin	Ethosuximide
N-acetylprocainamide	Tobramycin	Phenobarbital
Procainamide	Vancomycin	Phenytoin, free phenytoin
Quinidine		Primidone

OTHERS	TOXICOLOGY ASSAYS	DRUG SCREENING ASSAYS
Digoxin	Acetaminophen	Amphetamine
Digitoxin	Ethanol	Barbiturates
Methotrexate	Salicylate	Salicylate
Benzodiazepines	Tricyclic antidepressants	Cannabinoids
Theophylline		Cocaine
		Methadone
		Opiates
		Phencyclidine
		Propoxyphene

no interference between the drug and its metabolites and endogenous or exogenous substances. In addition, the internal standard should be resolved completely and also demonstrate no interference with other compounds. Immunoassays depend on an antibody and antigen (usually the drug to be measured) reaction. The antibody may not be specific for the drug analyte, but may also cross-react with drugs that have similar structures, including related compounds (endogenous or exogenous chemicals) and metabolites of the drug. Colorimetric and spectrophotometric assays are usually less specific. Interference from other materials may inflate the results.

Sensitivity

Sensitivity is the minimum detectable level or concentration of drug in serum that may be approximated as that lowest drug concentration that is two to three times the background noise. A *minimum quantifiable level* (MQL) is a statistical method for the determination of the precision of the lower level.

Linearity and Dynamic Range

Dynamic range refers to the relationship between the drug concentration and the instrument response (or signal) used to measure the drug. Many assays show a linear drug concentration-versus-instrument response relationship. Immunoassays generally have a nonlinear dynamic range. High serum drug concentrations, above the dynamic range of the instrument response, must be diluted before assay. The dynamic range is determined by using serum samples that have known (standard) drug concentrations (including a blank serum sample or zero drug concentration). Extrapolation of the assay results above or below the measured standard drug concentrations may be inaccurate if the relationship between instrument response and extrapolated drug concentration is unknown.

Precision

Precision is a measurement of the variability or reproducibility of the data. Precision measurements are obtained by replication of various drug concentrations and by replication of standard concentration curves prepared separately on different days. A suitable statistical measurement of the dispersion of the data, such as standard deviation or coefficient of variation, is then performed.

Accuracy

Accuracy refers to the difference between the average assay values and the true or known drug concentrations. Control (known) drug serum concentrations should be prepared by an independent technician using such techniques to minimize any error in their preparation. These samples, including a "zero" drug concentration, are assayed by the technician assigned to the study along with a suitable standard drug concentration curve.

Stability

Standard drug concentrations should be maintained under the same storage conditions as the unknown serum samples and assayed periodically. The stability study should continue for at least the same length of time as the patient samples are to be stored. Freeze–thaw stability studies are performed to determine the effect of thawing and refreezing on the stability of the drug in the sample. On occasion, a previously frozen biologic sample must be thawed and reassayed if the first assay result is uncertain.

Serum samples obtained from subjects on a drug study are usually assayed along with a minimum of three standard processed serum samples containing known standard drug concentrations and a minimum of three control serum samples whose concentrations are unknown to the analyst. These control serum samples are randomly distributed in each day's run. Control samples are replicated in duplicate to evaluate both within-day and between-day precision. The concentration of drug in each serum sample is based on each day's processed standard curve.

Ruggedness

Ruggedness is the degree of reproducibility of the test results obtained by the analysis of the same samples by different analytical laboratories. The determination of ruggedness measures the reproducibility of the results under normal operational conditions from laboratory to laboratory and from analyst to analyst.

Because each method for drug assay may have differences in sensitivity, precision, and specificity, the pharmacokineticist should be aware of which drug assay method the laboratory used.

Pharmacokinetic Evaluation

After the serum or plasma drug concentrations are measured, the pharmacokineticist must evaluate the data. Most laboratories report total drug (free plus bound drug) concentrations in the serum. The pharmacokineticist should be aware of the usual therapeutic range of serum concentrations from the literature. However, the literature may not indicate whether the reported values were trough or peak serum levels. Moreover, the assay used in reporting the methodology may be different in terms of specificity and precision.

The assay results from the laboratory may show that the patient's serum drug levels are higher, lower, or similar to the expected serum levels. The pharmacokineticist should evaluate these results while considering the patient and the patient's pathophysiologic condition. Table 20.4 lists a number of factors the pharmacokineticist should consider when intepreting drug serum concentration. Often, other data, such as a high serum creatinine and high blood urea nitrogen (BUN), may help verify that an observed high serum drug concentration in a patient is due to lower renal drug clearance because of compromised kidney function. In another case, a complaint by the patient of overstimulation and insomnia might collaborate the laboratory's finding of higher-than-anticipated serum concentrations of theophylline. Therefore, the clinician or pharmacokineticist should evaluate the data using sound medical judgment and observation. The therapeutic decision should not be based solely on serum drug concentrations.

Dosage Adjustment

From the serum drug concentration data and patient observations, the clinician or pharmacokineticist may recommend an adjustment in the dosage regimen. Ideally, the new dosage regimen should be calculated using the pharmacokinetic parameters derived from the *patient's* serum drug concentrations. Although there may not be enough data for a complete pharmacokinetic profile, the pharmacokineticist

TABLE 20.4   *Pharmacokinetic Evaluation of Serum Drug Concentrations*

Serum Concentrations Lower than Anticipated
   Patient compliance
   Error in dosage regimen
   Wrong drug product (controlled-release instead of immediate-release)
   Poor bioavailability
   Rapid elimination (efficient metabolizer)
   Reduced plasma protein binding
   Enlarged apparent volume of distribution
   Steady state not reached
   Timing of blood sample
   Improving renal/hepatic function
   Drug interaction due to stimulation of elimination enzyme autoinduction
   Changing hepatic blood flow
Serum Concentrations Higher than Anticipated
   Patient compliance
   Error in dosage regimen
   Wrong drug product (immediate release instead of controlled release)
   Rapid bioavailability
   Smaller than anticipated apparent volume of distribution
   Slow elimination (poor metabolizer)
   Increased plasma protein binding
   Deteriorating renal/hepatic function
   Drug interaction due to inhibition of elimination
Serum Concentration Correct but Patient Does Not Respond to Therapy
   Altered receptor sensitivity (eg, tolerance)
   Drug interaction at receptor site
   Changing hepatic blood flow

should still be able to derive a new dosage regimen based on the available data and the pharmacokinetic parameters in the literature that are based on average population data.

Monitoring Serum Drug Concentrations

In many cases, the patient's pathophysiology may be unstable, either improving or deteriorating further. For example, proper therapy for congestive heart failure will improve cardiac output and renal perfusion, thereby increasing renal drug clearance. Therefore, continuous monitoring of serum drug concentrations is necessary to ensure proper drug therapy for the patient. For some drugs, an acute pharmacologic response can be monitored in lieu of actual serum drug concentration. For example, prothrombin clotting time might be useful for monitoring anticoagulant therapy and blood pressure monitoring for hypotensive agents.

Special Recommendations

At times, the patient may not be responding to drug therapy because of other factors. For example, the patient may not be following instructions for taking the medication (patient noncompliance). The patient may be taking the drug after a meal instead of before, or may not be adhering to a special diet (eg, low salt). Therefore, the patient may need special instructions that are simple and easy to follow.

DESIGN OF DOSAGE REGIMENS

Several methods may be used to design a dosage regimen. Generally, the initial dosage of the drug is estimated using average population pharmacokinetic parameters obtained from the literature. The patient is then monitored for the therapeutic response by physical examination and, if necessary, by measurement of serum drug levels. After evaluation of the patient, adjustment of the dosage regimen using the patient's individual pharmacokinetic parameters may be indicated, with further therapeutic drug monitoring.

Many versions of clinical pharmacokinetic software are available for dose calculations of drugs with narrow therapeutic index (eg, DataKinetics [ASHSP], and the Abbottbase pharmacokinetic system). The dosing strategies are based generally on basic pharmacokinetic principles that have been estimated manually. Computer automation and pharmacokinetic software packages improve the accuracy of the calculation, make the calculations "easier," and have an added advantage of maintaining proper documentation (see Appendix B).

Individualized Dosage Regimens

The most accurate approach to dosage regimen design is to calculate the dose based on the pharmacokinetics of the drug in the individual patient. This approach is not feasible for calculation of the initial dose. However, once the patient has been medicated, the readjustment of the dose may be calculated using pharmacokinetic parameters derived from measurement of the serum drug levels from the patient after the initial dose. Most dosing programs record the patient's age and weight and calculate the individual dose based on creatinine clearance and lean body weight.

Dosage Regimens Based on Population Averages

The method most often used to calculate a dosage regimen is based on average pharmacokinetic parameters obtained from clinical studies published in the drug literature. This method may be based on a fixed or an adaptive model (Greenblatt, 1979; Mawer, 1976).

The *fixed model* assumes that population average pharmacokinetic parameters may be used directly to calculate a dosage regimen for the patient, without any alteration. Usually, pharmacokinetic parameters such as absorption rate constant k_a, bioavailability factor F, apparent volume of distribution V_D, and elimination rate constant k, are assumed to remain constant. Most often the drug is assumed to follow the pharmacokinetics of a one-compartment model. When a multiple-dose regimen is designed, multiple-dosage equations based on the principle of superposition (Chapter 8) are used to evaluate the dose. The practitioner may use the usual dosage suggested by the literature and then make a small adjustment of the dosage based on the patient's weight and/or age.

The *adaptive model* for dosage regimen calculation uses patient variables such as weight, age, sex, body surface area, and known patient pathophysiology, such as renal disease, as well as the known population average pharmacokinetic parameters of the drug. In this case, calculation of the dosage regimen takes into consideration any changing pathophysiology of the patient and attempts to adapt or modify the dosage regimen according to the needs of the patient. The adaptive model generally assumes that pharmacokinetic parameters such as drug clearance do not change from one dose to the next. However, some adaptive models allow for continuously adaptive change with time in order to simulate more closely the changing process of drug disposition in the patient, especially during a disease state (Whiting et al, 1991).

Dosage Regimens Based on Partial Pharmacokinetic Parameters

For many drugs, the entire pharmacokinetic profile for the drug is unknown or unavailable. Therefore, the pharmacokineticist needs to make some assumptions in order to calculate the dosage regimen. For example, a common assumption is to let the bioavailability factor F equal 1 or 100%. Thus, if the drug is less than fully absorbed systemically, the patient will be undermedicated rather than overmedicated. Some of these assumptions will depend on the safety, efficacy, and therapeutic range of the drug. The use of population pharmacokinetics (discussed later in this chapter) uses average patient population characteristics and only a few serum drug concentrations from the patient. Population pharmacokinetic approaches to therapeutic drug monitoring have increased with the increased availability of computerized databases and the development of statistical tools for the analysis of observational data (Schumacher, 1985b).

Empirical Dosage Regimens

In many cases, the physician selects a dosage regimen for the patient without using any pharmacokinetic variables. In such a situation, the physician makes the decision based on empirical clinical data, personal experience, and clinical observations. The physician characterizes the patient as representative of a similar well-studied clinical population that has used the drug successfully.

CONVERSION FROM INTRAVENOUS INFUSION TO ORAL DOSING

After the patient's dosing is controlled by intravenous infusion, it is often desirable to continue to medicate the patient with the same drug using the oral route of administration. When intravenous infusion is stopped, the serum drug concentration decreases according to first-order elimination kinetics (Chapter 5). For most oral drug products, the time to reach steady state depends on the first-order elimination rate constant for the drug. Therefore, if the patient starts the dosage regimen with the oral drug product at the same time as the intravenous infusion is stopped, then the exponential decline of serum levels from the intravenous infusion should be matched by the exponential increase in serum drug levels from the oral drug product.

The conversion from intravenous infusion to a controlled-release oral medication given once or twice daily has become more common with the availability of more controlled-release drug products, such as theophylline (Stein et al, 1982) and quinidine. Computer simulation for the conversion of intravenous theophylline (aminophylline) therapy to oral controlled-release theophylline demonstrated that oral therapy should be started at the same time as intravenous infusion is stopped (Iafrate et al, 1982). With this method, minimal fluctuations are observed between the peak and trough serum theophylline levels. Moreover, giving the first oral dose when IV infusion is stopped may make it easier for the nursing staff or patient to comply with the dosage regimen.

Either of these methods may be used to calculate an appropriate oral dosage regimen for a patient whose condition has been stabilized by an intravenous drug infusion. Both methods assume that the patient's plasma drug concentration is at steady state.

Method 1

Method 1 assumes that the steady-state plasma drug concentration, C_{SS}, after IV infusion is identical to the desired C_{av}^{∞} after multiple oral doses of the drug. Therefore, the following equation may be used:

$$C_{av}^{\infty} = \frac{SFD_0}{kV_D\tau} \tag{20.1}$$

$$\frac{D_0}{\tau} = \frac{C_{av}^{\infty}kV_D}{SF} \tag{20.2}$$

where S is the salt form of the drug and D_0/τ is the dosing rate.

 # EXAMPLE

An adult male asthmatic patient (age 55, 78 kg) has been maintained on an intravenous infusion of aminophylline at a rate of 34 mg/hr. The steady-state theophylline drug concentration was 12 μg/mL and total body clearance was calculated as 3.0 L/hr. Calculate an appropriate oral dosage regimen of theophylline for this patient.

Solution

Aminophylline is a soluble salt of theophylline and contains 85% theophylline ($S = 0.85$). Theophylline is 100% bioavailable ($F = 1$) after an oral dose. Because total body clearance, $Cl_T = kV_D$, Equation 20.2 may be expressed as

$$\frac{D_0}{\tau} = \frac{C_{av}^{\infty}Cl_T}{SF} \tag{20.3}$$

The dose rate, D_0/τ (34 mg/hr), was calculated on the basis of aminophylline. The patient, however, will be given theophylline orally. To convert to oral theophylline, S and F should be considered.

$$\text{Theophylline dose rate} = \frac{SFD_0}{\tau} = \frac{(0.85)(1)(34)}{1} = 28.9 \text{ mg/hr}$$

The theophylline dose rate of 28.9 mg/hr must be converted to a reasonable schedule for the patient with a consideration of the various commercially available theophylline drug products. Therefore, the total daily dose is 28.9 mg/hr × 24 hr or 693.6 mg/day. Possible theophylline dosage schedules might be 700 mg/day, 350 mg every 12 hours, or 175 mg every 6 hours. Each of these dosage regimens would achieve the same C_{av}^{∞} but different C_{max}^{∞} and C_{min}^{∞}, which should be calculated. The dose of 350 mg every 12 hours could be given in sustained-release form to avoid any excessive high drug concentration in the body.

Method 2

Method 2 assumes that the rate of intravenous infusion (mg/hr) is the same desired rate of oral dosage.

 # EXAMPLE

Using the example in method 1, the following calculations may be used.

Solution

The aminophylline is given by IV infusion at a rate of 34 mg/hr. The total daily dose of aminophylline is 34 mg/hr × 24 hr = 816 mg. The equivalent daily dose in terms of theophylline is 816 × 0.85 = 693.6 mg. Thus, the patient should receive approximately 700 mg of theophylline per day or 350 mg controlled-release theophylline every 12 hours.

DETERMINATION OF DOSE

The drug dose is estimated to deliver a desirable (target) therapeutic level of the drug to the body. The dose of a drug is estimated with the objective of delivering a desirable therapeutic level of the drug in the body. For many drugs, the desirable therapeutic drug levels and pharmacokinetic parameters are available in the clinical literature. However, the literature in some cases may not yield complete drug information, or the information available may be partly equivocal. Therefore, the pharmacokineticist must make certain necessary assumptions in accordance with the best pharmacokinetic information available.

For a drug that is given in multiple doses for an extended period of time, the dosage regimen is usually calculated so that the average steady-state blood level is within the therapeutic range. The dose can be calculated with Equation 20.4, which expresses the C_{av}^{∞} in terms of dose (D_0), dosing interval (τ), volume of distribution

(V_D), and the elimination half-life of the drug. F is the fraction of drug absorbed and is equal to 1 for drugs administered intravenously.

$$C_{av}^\infty = \frac{1.44 D_0 t_{1/2} F}{V_D \tau}$$

(20.4)

PRACTICE PROBLEMS

1. Pharmacokinetic data for clindamycin were reported by DeHaan et al (1972) as follows:

$$k = 0.247 \ \text{hr}^{-1}$$
$$t_{1/2} = 2.81 \ \text{hr}$$
$$V_D = 43.9 \ \text{L}/1.73 \ \text{m}^2$$

What is the steady-state concentration of the drug after 150 mg of the drug is given orally every 6 hours for a week? (Assume the drug is 100% absorbed.)

Solution

$$C_{av}^\infty = \frac{1.44 \ D_0 t_{1/2} F}{V_D \tau}$$

$$= \frac{1.44 \times 150,000 \times 2.81 \times 1}{43,900 \times 6} \ \mu g/mL$$

$$= 2.3 \ \mu g/mL$$

2. According to Regamey et al (1973), the elimination half-life of tobramycin was reported to be 2.15 hours and the volume of distribution was reported to be 33.5% of body weight.
   a. What is the dose for an 80-kg individual if a steady-state level of 2.5 $\mu g/mL$ is desired?

Assume that the drug is given by intravenous bolus injection every 8 hours.

Solution

Assuming the drug is 100% bioavailable as a result of IV injection,

$$C_{av}^\infty = \frac{1.44 D_0 t_{1/2} F}{V_D \tau}$$

$$2.5 = \frac{1.44 \times 2.15 \times 1 \times D_0}{80 \times 0.335 \times 1000 \times 8}$$

$$D_0 = \frac{2.5 \times 80 \times 0.335 \times 1000 \times 8}{1.44 \times 2.15} \ \mu g$$

$$D_0 = 173 \ \text{mg}$$

The dose should be 173 mg every 8 hours.

b. The manufacturer has suggested that in normal cases, tobramycin should be given at a rate of 1 mg/kg every 8 hours. With this dosage regimen, what would be the average steady-state level?

Solution

$$C_{av}^\infty = \frac{1.44 \times 1 \times 1000 \times 2.15}{0.335 \times 1000 \times 8}$$

$$C_{av}^\infty = 1.16 \ \mu g/mL$$

Because the bacteriocidal concentration of an antibiotic varies with the organism involved in the infection, the dose prescribed may change. The average plasma drug concentration is used to indicate whether optimum drug levels have been reached. With certain antibiotics, the steady-state peak and trough levels are sometimes used as therapeutic indicators. (See Chapter 19 for discussion of time above minimum effective concentration (MIC). For example, the effective concentration of tobramycin was reported to be around 4–5 $\mu g/mL$ for peak level and around 2 $\mu g/mL$ for trough level when given intramuscularly every 12 hours (Table 20.1). Although peak and trough levels are frequently reported in clinical journals, these drug levels are only transitory in the body. Peak and trough drug levels are less useful pharmacokinetically, because peak and trough levels fluctuate more and are usually reported less accurately than average plasma drug concentrations. When the average plasma drug concentration is used as a therapeutic indicator, an optimum dosing interval must be chosen. The dosing interval is usually set at approximately one to two elimination half-lives of the drug, unless the drug has a very narrow therapeutic index. In this case the drug must be given in small doses more frequently or by IV infusion.

EFFECT OF CHANGING DOSE AND DOSING INTERVAL ON C_{max}^∞, C_{min}^∞, AND C_{av}^∞

During intravenous infusion, C_{SS} may be used to monitor the steady-state serum concentrations. In contrast, when considering therapeutic drug monitoring of serum concentrations after the initiation of a multiple-dosage regimen, the trough serum drug concentrations or C_{min}^∞ may be used to validate the dosage regimen. The blood sample withdrawn just prior to the administration of the next dose represents C_{min}^∞. To obtain C_{max}^∞, the blood sample must be withdrawn exactly at the time for peak absorption, or closely spaced blood samples must be taken and the plasma drug concentrations graphed. In practice, an approximate time for maximum drug absorption is estimated and a blood sample is withdrawn. Because of differences in rates of drug absorption, C_{max}^∞ measured in this manner is only an approximation of the true C_{max}^∞.

The C_{av}^{∞} is used most often in dosage calculation. The advantage of using C_{av}^{∞} as an indicator for deciding therapeutic blood level is that C_{av}^{∞} is determined on a set of points and generally fluctuates less than either C_{max}^{∞} or C_{min}^{∞}. Moreover, when the dosing interval is changed, the dose may be increased proportionally, to keep C_{av}^{∞} constant. This approach works well for some drugs. For example, if the drug diazepam is given either 10 mg TID (three times a day) or 15 mg BID (twice daily), the same C_{av}^{∞} is obtained, as shown by Equation 20.1. In fact, if the daily dose is the same, the C_{av}^{∞} should be the same. However, when monitoring serum drug concentrations, C_{av}^{∞} cannot be measured directly but may be obtained from AUC/τ during multiple-dosage regimens. As discussed in Chapter 8, the C_{av}^{∞} is not the arithmetic average of C_{min}^{∞} and C_{min}^{∞} because serum concentrations decline exponentially.

The dosing interval must be selected while considering the elimination half-life of the drug; otherwise, the patient may suffer the toxic effect of a high C_{max}^{∞} or subtherapeutic effects of a low C_{min}^{∞} even if the C_{av}^{∞} is kept constant. For example, using the same example of diazepam, the same C_{av}^{∞} is achieved at 10 mg TID or 60 mg every other day. Obviously, the C_{max}^{∞} of the latter dose regimen would produce a C_{max}^{∞} several times larger than that achieved with 10-mg-TID dose regimen. In general, if a drug has a relatively wide therapeutic index and a relatively long elimination half-life, then flexibility exists in changing the dose or dosing interval, τ, using C_{av}^{∞} as an indicator. When the drug has a narrow therapeutic index, C_{max}^{∞} and C_{min}^{∞} must be monitored to ensure safety and efficacy.

As the size of the dose or dosage intervals change proportionately, the C_{av}^{∞} may be the same but the steady-state peak, C_{max}^{∞}, and trough, C_{min}^{∞}, drug levels will change. C_{max}^{∞} is influenced by the size of the dose and the dosage interval. An increase in the size of the dose given at a longer dosage interval will cause an increase in C_{max}^{∞} and a decrease in C_{min}^{∞}. In this case C_{max}^{∞} may be very close or above the minimum toxic drug concentration (MTC). However, the C_{min}^{∞} may be lower than the minimum effective drug concentration (MEC). In this latter case the low C_{min}^{∞} may be subtherapeutic and dangerous for the patient, depending on the nature of the drug.

DETERMINATION OF FREQUENCY OF DRUG ADMINISTRATION

The size of a drug dose is often related to the frequency of drug administration. The more frequently a drug is administered, the smaller the dose must be to obtain the same C_{av}^{∞}. Thus, a dose of 250 mg every 3 hours could be changed to 500 mg every 6 hours without affecting the average steady-state plasma concentration of the drug. However, as the dosing intervals get longer, the size of the dose required to maintain the average plasma drug concentration gets correspondingly larger. When an excessively long dosing interval is chosen, the large dose may result in peak plasma levels that are above toxic drug concentration, even though C_{av}^{∞} will remain the same (see Chapter 8).

In general, the dosing interval for most drugs is determined by the elimination half-life. Drugs such as the penicillins, which have relatively low toxicity, may be given at intervals much longer than their elimination half-lives without any toxicity problems. Drugs having a narrow therapeutic range, such as digoxin and phenytoin, must be given relatively frequently to minimize excessive "peak-and-trough" fluctuations in blood levels. For example, the common maintenance schedule for digoxin is 0.25 mg/day and the elimination half-life of digoxin is 1.7 days. In contrast, penicillin G is given at 250 mg every 6 hours, while the elimination half-life of penicillin G is 0.75 hour. Penicillin is given at a dosage interval equal to 8 times its elimination half-life, whereas digoxin is given at a dosing interval only 0.59 times its elimination half-life. The toxic plasma concentration of penicillin G is over 100 times greater than its effective concentration, whereas digoxin has an effective concentration of 1–2 ng/mL and a toxicity level of 3 ng/mL. The toxic concentration of digoxin is only 1.5 times effective concentration. Therefore, a drug with a large therapeutic index (ie, a large margin of safety) can be given in large doses and at relatively long dosing intervals.

DETERMINATION OF BOTH DOSE AND DOSAGE INTERVAL

Both the dose and the dosage interval should be considered in the dosage regimen calculations. Ideally, the calculated dosage regimen should maintain the serum drug concentrations between C_{max}^{∞} and C_{min}^{∞}. For intravenous multiple-dosage regimens the ratio of $C_{max}^{\infty}/C_{min}^{\infty}$ may be expressed by

$$\frac{C_{max}^{\infty}}{C_{min}^{\infty}} = \frac{C_p^0/(1 - e^{-k\tau})}{C_p^0 e^{-k\tau}/(1 - e^{-k\tau})} \tag{20.5}$$

which can be simplified to

$$\frac{C_{max}^{\infty}}{C_{min}^{\infty}} = \frac{1}{e^{-k\tau}} \tag{20.6}$$

From Equation 20.6, a maximum dosage interval, τ, may be calculated that will maintain the serum concentration between C_{min}^{∞} and C_{max}^{∞}. After the dosage interval is calculated, then a dose may be calculated.

 # PRACTICE PROBLEM

The elimination half-life of an antibiotic is 3 hours with an apparent volume of distribution equivalent to 20% of body weight. The usual therapeutic range for this antibiotic is between 5 and 15 μg/mL. Adverse toxicity for this drug is often observed at serum concentrations greater than 20 μg/mL. Calculate a dosage regimen (multiple IV doses) that will just maintain the serum drug concentration between 5 and 15 μg/mL.

Solution

From Equation 20.6, determine the maximum possible dosage interval τ.

$$\frac{15}{5} = \frac{1}{e^{-(0.693/3)\tau}}$$

$$e^{-0.231\tau} = 0.333$$

Take the natural logarithm (ln) on both sides of the equation.

$$-0.231\tau = -1.10$$

$$\tau = 4.76 \text{ hr}$$

Then determine the dose required to produce C_{max}^{∞} from Equation 20.7 after substitution of $C_p^0 = D_0/V_D$:

$$C_{max}^{\infty} = \frac{D_0/V_D}{1 - e^{-k\tau}} \tag{20.7}$$

Solve for dose D_0, letting $V_D = 200$ mL/kg (20% body weight).

$$15 = \frac{D_0/200}{1 - e^{-(0.231)(4.76)}}$$

$$D_0 = 2 \text{ mg/kg}$$

To check this dose for therapeutic effectiveness, calculate C_{min}^{∞} and C_{av}^{∞}.

$$C_{min}^{\infty} = \frac{(D_0/V_D)e^{-k\tau}}{1 - e^{-k\tau}} = \frac{(2000/200)e^{-(0.231)(4.76)}}{1 - e^{-(0.231)(4.76)}}$$

$$C_{min}^{\infty} = 4.99 \ \mu g/mL$$

As a further check on the dosage regimen, calculate C_{av}^{∞}.

$$C_{av}^{\infty} = \frac{D_0}{V_D k\tau} = \frac{2000}{(200)(0.231)(4.76)}$$

$$C_{av}^{\infty} = 9.09 \ \mu g/mL$$

By calculation, the dose of this antibiotic should be 2 mg/kg every 4.76 hours to maintain the serum drug concentration between 5 and 15 μg/mL.

In practice, rather than a dosage interval of 4.76 hours, the dosage regimen and the dosage interval should be made as convenient as possible for the patient, and the size of the dose should take into account the commercially available drug formulation. Therefore, the dosage regimen should be recalculated to have a convenient value (below the maximum possible dosage interval) and the size of the dose adjusted accordingly.

NOMOGRAMS AND TABULATIONS IN DESIGNING DOSAGE REGIMENS

For ease of calculation of dosage regimens, many clinicians rely on nomograms to calculate the proper dosage regimen for their patients. The use of a nomogram

TABLE 20.5   Maintenance Dose of Theophylline When the Serum Concentration Is Not Measured[a]

AGE	DOSE	DOSE PER 12 HOURS
6–9 yrs	24 mg/kg/day	12.0 mg/kg
9–12 yrs	20 mg/kg/day	10.0 mg/kg
12–16 yrs	18 mg/kg/day	9.0 mg/kg
Over 16 yrs	13 mg/kg/day or 900 mg, *whichever is less*	6.5 mg/kg

[a]*Warning: Do not attempt to maintain a dose that is not tolerated.*

Adapted from product information for Theo-Dur Sprinkle (Theophylline Anhydrous Sustained Action Capsules, 1993) and *Facts and Comparisons* (1991).

may give a quick dosage regimen adjustment for patients with characteristics requiring adjustments, such as age, body weight, and physiologic state. In general, the nomogram of a drug is based on population pharmacokinetic data collected and analyzed using a specific pharmacokinetic model. In order to keep the dosage regimen calculation simple, complicated equations are often solved and the results displayed diagrammatically on special scaled axes to produce a simple dose recommendation based on patient information. Some nomograms make use of certain physiologic parameters, such as serum creatinine concentration, to help modify the dosage regimen according to renal function (Chapter 21).

For many marketed drugs, the manufacturer provides tabulated general guidelines for use in establishing a dosage regimen for patients, including loading and maintenance doses. For example, the initial doses and subsequent serum monitoring of theophylline anhydrous sustained-action capsules (Theo-Dur Sprinkle) and theophylline extended-release tablets (Theo-Dur tablets) are shown in Tables 20.5 and 20.6, respectively.

For drugs with a narrow therapeutic range, such as theophylline, a guide for monitoring serum drug concentrations is given. Another example is the aminoglycoside antibiotic, tobramycin sulfate USP (Nebcin, Eli Lilly), which is eliminated primarily by renal clearance. Thus, the dosage of tobramycin sulfate should be reduced in direct proportion to a reduction in creatinine clearance (see Chapter 21). The manufacturer provides a nomogram for estimating the percent of the normal dose of tobramycin sulfate assuming the serum creatinine level (mg/100 mL) has been obtained.

TABLE 20.6   Dosage Guidelines for Rapid Theophyllinization[a]

PATIENT GROUP	MAINTENANCE DOSE
Children 1–9 yrs	4 mg/kg every 6 hr
Children 9–16 and young adult smokers	3 mg/kg every 6 hr
Otherwise healthy nonsmoking adults	3 mg/kg every 8 hr
Older patients and patients with cor pulmonale	2 mg/kg every 8 hr
Patients with congestive heart failure	1–2 mg/kg every 8 hr

[a]In patients not receiving theophylline. The recommended loading dose for each patient group is 5 mg/kg.

Adapted from *Facts and Comparisons* (1991), with permission.

DETERMINATION OF ROUTE OF ADMINISTRATION

Selection of the proper route of administration is an important consideration in drug therapy. The rate of drug absorption and the duration of action are influenced by the route of drug administration. Moreover, the use of certain routes of administration is precluded by physiologic and safety considerations. For example, intra-arterial and intrathecal drug injections are less safe than other routes of drug administration and are used only when absolutely uecessary. Drugs that are unstable in the gastrointestinal tract or drugs that undergo extensive first-pass effect are not suitable for oral administration. For example, insulin is a protein that is degraded in the gastrointestinal tract by proteolytic enzymes. Drugs such as xylocaine and nitroglycerin are not suitable for oral administration because of first-pass effect. These drugs, therefore, must be given by an alternative route of administration.

Intravenous administration is the fastest and most reliable way of delivering a drug into the circulatory system. Drugs administered intravenously are removed more rapidly because the entire dose is subject to elimination immediately. Consequently, more frequent drug administration is required. Drugs administered extravascularly must be absorbed into the bloodstream, and the total absorbed dose is eliminated more slowly. The frequency of administration can be lessened by using routes of administration that give a sustained rate of drug absorption. Intramuscular injection generally provides more rapid systemic absorption than oral administration of drugs that are not very soluble.

Certain drugs are not suitable for administration intramuscularly because of erratic drug release, pain, or local irritation. Even though the drug is injected into the muscle mass, the drug must reach the circulatory system or other body fluid to become bioavailable. The anatomic site of drug deposition following intramuscular injection will affect the rate of drug absorption. A drug injected into the deltoid muscle is more rapidly absorbed than a drug injected similarly into the gluteus maximus, because there is better blood flow in the former. In general, the method of drug administration that provides the most consistent and greatest bioavailability should be used to ensure maximum therapeutic effect. The various routes of drug administration can be classified as either *extravascular* or *intravascular* and are listed in Table 20.7 (see also Chapter 13).

Precipitation of an insoluble drug at the injection site may result in slower absorption and a delayed response. For example, a dose of 50 mg of chlordiazepoxide

TABLE 20.7   Common Routes of Drug Administration

PARENTERAL	EXTRAVASCULAR
Intravascular	Enteral
Intravenous injection (IV bolus)	Buccal
Intravenous infusion (IV drip)	Sublingual
Intra-arterial injection	Oral
Intramuscular injection	Rectal
Intradermal injection	Inhalation
Subcutaneous injection	Transdermal
Intradermal injection	
Intrathecal injection	

(Librium) is more quickly absorbed after oral administration than after intramuscular injection. Some drugs, such as haloperidol decanoate, are very oil-soluble products that release very slowly after intramuscular injection (Chapter 14).

DOSING OF DRUGS IN INFANTS AND CHILDREN

Infants and children have different dosing requirements than adults. Dosing of drugs in this population requires a thorough consideration of the differences in the pharmacokinetics and pharmacology of a specific drug in the preterm newborn infant, newborn infant (birth to 28 days), infant (28 days to 23 months), young child (2 to 5 years), older child (6 to 11 years), adolescent (12 to 18 years), and the adult (*FDA Guidance for Industry,* 2000). Unfortunately, the pharmacokinetics and pharmacodynamics of most drugs are not well known in children under 12 years of age. The variation in body composition and the maturity of liver and kidney function are potential sources of differences in pharmacokinetics with respect to age. For convenience, "infants" are here arbitrarily defined as children 0 to 2 years of age. However, within this group, special consideration is necessary for infants less than 4 weeks (1 month) old, because their ability to handle drugs often differs from that of more mature infants.

In addition to different dosing requirements for the pediatric population, there is a need to consider the use of pediatric dosage forms that permit more accurate dosing and patient compliance. For example, liquid pediatric drug products may come with a calibrated dropper or a premeasured teaspoon (5 mL) for accurate dosing and have a cherry flavor for pediatric patient compliance. Pediatric drug formulations may also contain different drug concentrations compared to the adult drug formulation. Furthermore, alternative drug delivery such as an intramuscular antibiotic drug injection into the gluteus medius may be considered for a pediatric patient, as opposed to the deltoid muscle for an adult patient.

In general, complete hepatic function is not attained until the third week of life. Oxidative processes are fairly well developed in infants, but there is a deficiency of conjugative enzymes. In addition, many drugs exhibit reduced binding to plasma albumin in infants.

Newborns show only 30–50% of the renal activity of adults on the basis of activity per unit of body weight (Table 20.8). Drugs that are heavily dependent on renal excretion will have a sharply decreased elimination half-life. For example, the penicillins are excreted for the most part through the kidney. The elimination half-lives of such drugs are much reduced in infants, as shown in Table 20.9.

 PRACTICE PROBLEM

The elimination half-life of penicillin G is 0.5 hour in adults and 3.2 hours in neonates (0 to 7 days old). Assuming that the normal adult dose of penicillin G is 4 mg/kg every 4 hours, calculate the dose of penicillin G for an 11-pound infant.

TABLE 20.8   Comparison of Newborn and Adult Renal Clearances[a]

	AVERAGE INFANT	**AVERAGE ADULT**
Body weight (kg)	3.5	70
Body water		
(%)	77	58
(L)	2.7	41
Inulin clearance		
(mL/min)	Approx 3	130
k (min^{-1})	3/2700 = 0.0011	130/41,000 = 0.0032
$t_{1/2}$ (min)	630	220
PAH clearance		
(mL/min)	Approx 12	650
k (min^{-1})	12/2800 = 0.0043	650/41,000 = 0.016
$t_{1/2}$ (min)	160	43

[a]Computations are for a drug distributed in the whole body water, but any other V_D would give the same relative values.

Data for average infant from West et al (1948), with permission from Charles C Thomas and Cambridge University Press.

Solution

$$\frac{\tau_1}{\tau_2} = \frac{(t_{1/2})_1}{(t_{1/2})_2}$$

$$t_{1/2} = 0.5 \text{ hr}$$

$$\tau_2 = \frac{4 \times 3.2}{0.5} = 25.6 \text{ hr}$$

Therefore, this infant may be given the following dose:

$$\text{Dose} = 4 \text{ mg/kg} = \frac{11 \text{ lb}}{2.2 \text{ lb/kg}} = 20 \text{ mg every 24 hr}$$

Alternatively, 10 mg every 12 hours would achieve the same C_{av}^{∞}.

TABLE 20.9   Elimination Half-Lives of Drugs in Infants and Adults

DRUG	HALF-LIFE IN NEONATES[a] (hr)	HALF-LIFE IN ADULTS (hr)
Penicillin G	3.2	0.5
Ampicillin	4	1–1.5
Methicillin	3.3/1.3	0.5
Carbenicillin	5–6	1–1.5
Kanamycin	5–5.7	3–5
Gentamicin	5	2–3

[a]0–7 days old.

Various methods have been used in the past to estimate doses for a child. Methods such as Young's rule or Clark's rule for dose adjustment are at best crude approximations in that they take into account only body age and size change attributable to growth and do not consider the rate of drug elimination. Another dose adjustment method is based on body surface area. This approach has the advantage of avoiding bias due to obesity or unusual body weight, because the height and weight of the patient are both considered. The body surface area method gives only a rough estimation of the proper dose, because the pharmacokinetic differences of specific drugs are not considered.

DOSING OF DRUGS IN THE ELDERLY

Defining "elderly" is difficult. The geriatric population is often arbitrarily defined as patients who are older than 65 years, and many of these people live active and healthy lives. In addition, there is an increasing number of people who are living more than 85 years, who are often considered as the "older elderly" population. The aging process is more often associated with physiologic changes during aging rather than purely chronological age. Chronologically, the elderly have been classified as the *young old* (ages 65–75 years), the *old* (ages 75–85 years), and the *old old* (age > 85 years) (Abernethy, 2001).

Performance capacity and the loss of homeostatic reserve decreases with advanced age but occurs to a different degree in each organ and in each patient. Physiologic and cognitive functions tend to change with the aging process and can affect compliance and the therapeutic safety and efficacy of a prescribed drug. The elderly also tend to be on multiple drug therapy due to concomitant illness. Decreased cognitive function in some geriatric patients, complicated drug dosage schedules, and/or the high cost of drug therapy may result in poor drug compliance, resulting in lack of drug efficacy, possible drug interactions, and/or drug intoxication.

Several vital physiologic functions related to age as measured by markers show that renal plasma flow, glomerular filtration, cardiac output, and breathing capacity can drop from 10% to 30% in elderly subjects compared to those at age 30. The physiologic changes due to aging may necessitate special considerations in administering drugs in the elderly. For some drugs, an age-dependent increase in adverse drug reactions or toxicity may be observed. This apparent increased drug sensitivity in the elderly may be due to pharmacodynamic and/or pharmacokinetic changes (Mayersohn, 1994; Schmuker, 1985a).

The pharmacodynamic hypothesis assumes that age causes alterations in the quantity and quality of target drug receptors, leading to enhanced drug response. Quantitatively, the number of drug receptors may decline with age, whereas qualitatively, a change in the affinity for the drug may occur. Alternatively, the pharmacokinetic hypothesis assumes that age-dependent increases in adverse drug reactions are due to physiologic changes in drug absorption, distribution, and elimination, including renal excretion and hepatic clearance.

In the elderly, age-dependent alterations in drug absorption may include a decline in the splanchnic blood flow, altered gastrointestinal motility, increase in gastric pH, and alteration in the gastrointestinal absorptive surface. The incidence of achlorhydria in the elderly may have an effect on the dissolution of certain drugs such as weak bases and certain dosage forms that require an acid environment for disintegration and release (Mayersohn, 1994). From a distribution consideration, drug protein binding in the plasma may decrease as a result of decrease in the albumin concentration, and the apparent volume of distribution may change due to a decrease in muscle mass and an increase in body fat. Renal drug excretion generally declines with age as a result of decrease in the glomerular filtration rate and/or active tubular secretion. Moreover, the activity of the enzymes responsible for drug biotransformation may decrease with age, leading to a decline in hepatic drug clearance.

Elderly patients may have several different pathophysiologic conditions that require multiple drug therapy that increases the likelihood for a drug interaction. Moreover, increased adverse drug reactions and toxicity may result from poor patient compliance. Both penicillin and kanamycin show prolonged $t_{1/2}$ in the aged patient, as a consequence of an age-related gradual reduction in the kidney size and function. The Gault–Cockroft rule for calculating creatinine clearance clearly quantitates a reduction in clearance with increased age (Chapter 21). Age-related changes in plasma albumin and α_1-acid glycoprotein may also be a factor in the binding of drugs in the body.

PRACTICE PROBLEMS

1. An aminoglycoside has a normal elimination half-life of 107 minutes in young adults. In patients 70 to 90 years old, the elimination half-life of the aminoglycoside is 282 minutes. The normal dose of the aminoglycoside is 15 mg/kg per day divided into two doses. What is the dose for a 75-year-old patient, assuming that the volume of distribution per body weight is not changed by the patient's age?

Solution

The longer elimination half-life of the aminoglycoside in elderly patients is due to a decrease in renal function. A good inverse correlation has been obtained of elimination half-life to the aminoglycoside and creatinine clearance. To maintain the same average concentration of the aminoglycoside in the elderly as in young adults, the dose may be reduced.

$$C_{av}^{\infty} = \frac{1.44 D_N (t_{1/2})_N}{\tau_N V_N} = \frac{1.44 D_0 (t_{1/2})_0}{\tau_0 V_0}$$

$$\frac{D_N (t_{1/2})_N}{\tau_N} = \frac{D_0 (t_{1/2})_0}{\tau_0}$$

Keeping the dose constant,

$$D_N = D_0$$

where D_N is the new dose and D_0 is the old dose.

$$\frac{\tau_0}{\tau_N} = \frac{(t_{1/2})_0}{(t_{1/2})_N}$$

$$\tau_0 = 12 \times \frac{282}{107} = 31.6 \text{ hr}$$

Therefore, the same dose of the aminoglycoside may be administered every 32 hours without affecting the average steady-state level of the aminoglycoside.

2. The clearance of lithium was determined to be 41.5 mL/min in a group of patients with an average age of 25 years. In a group of elderly patients with an average age of 63 years, the clearance of lithium was 7.7 mL/min. What percentage of the normal dose of lithium should be given to a 65-year-old patient?

Solution

The dose should be proportional to clearance; therefore,

$$\text{Dose reductions }(\%) = \frac{7.7 \times 100}{41.5} = 18.5\%$$

The dose of lithium may be reduced to about 20% of the regular dose in the 65-year-old patient without affecting the steady-state blood level.

CLINICAL EXAMPLE

Hypertension is common in elderly patients. The pharmacokinetics of felodipine (Plendil), a calcium channel antagonist for hypertension, was studied in young and elderly subjects. After a dose of 5 mg oral felodipine, the AUC and C_{max} in the elderly patients (67–79 years of age, mean weight 71 kg) were three times that of the young subjects (20–34 years of age, mean weight 75 kg), as shown in Figure 20-2. Side effects of felodipine in the elderly patients, such as flushing, were reported in 9 of 11 subjects, and palpitation was reported in 3 of 11 subjects, whereas, only 1 of 12 of the young subjects reported side effects. Systemic clearance in the elderly was 248 ± 108 L/hr compared to 619 ± 214 L/hr in the young subjects. The bioavailability of felodipine was reported to be about 15.5% in the elderly and 15.3% in the young subjects. (Concomitant medications included a diuretic and a β-blocker.)

    a. What is the main cause for the difference in the observed AUC between the elderly and young subjects?

    b. What would be the steady-state level of felodipine in the elderly if dose and dosing interval are unchanged?

    c. Can felodipine be given safely to elderly patients?

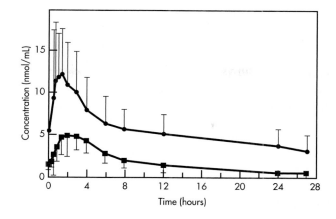

Figure 20-2. Plasma concentrations (mean ± SD) of felodipine after an oral dose during steady-state treatment with 5 mg twice daily in healthy subjects ($n = 12$) [■] and elderly hypertensive patients ($n = 1$) [●].
(From Landahl et al, 1988, with permission.)

Solution

a. The higher AUC in the elderly compared to young adults is due to the decreased drug clearance in the older subjects.

b. The elderly have more side effects with felodipine compared to young adults. Factors that may have increased side effects in the elderly could be (1) reduced hepatic blood flow, (2) potassium depletion in the body, (3) increased bioavailability, or (4) reduced clearance.

c.

$$C_{av}^{\infty} = \frac{FD_0}{Cl_\tau} \tag{20.8}$$

If D_0, F, and τ are the same, the steady-state drug concentration C_{av}^{∞} will be inversely proportional to clearance:

$$\frac{C_{av\ elderly}^{\infty}}{C_{av\ young}^{\infty}} = \frac{Cl_{young}}{Cl_{elderly}}$$

$$\frac{C_{av\ elderly}^{\infty}}{C_{av\ young}^{\infty}} = \frac{619}{248} = 2.5$$

(*Note:* Cl is in the denominator in Equation 20.8 and is inversely related to concentration.) The steady concentration of felodipine will be 250% or 2.5 times that in the young subjects.

Changes in Renal Function with Age

Many studies have shown a general decline in glomerular filtration rate (GFR) with age. Lindeman (1992) reported that the GFR as measured by creatinine clearance (see Chapter 21) decreases at a mean rate of 1% per year after 40 years of age. However, there is considerable variation in this rate of decline in normal healthy aging adults. In a previous study by Lindeman et al (1985), approximately two-thirds of the subjects (162 of 254) had declining creatinine clearances, whereas about one-third of the subjects (92 of 254) had no decrease in creatinine clearance. Since muscle mass and urinary creatinine excretion decrease at nearly the same rate in the elderly, mean serum concentrations may stay relatively constant. Creatinine clearance measured by serum creatinine concentrations only (see Chapter 21) may yield inaccurate GFR function if urinary creatinine excretion is not measured.

EXAMPLES

1. An elderly 85-year-old adult patient with congestive heart failure has a serum creatinine of 1.0 mg/dL. The 24-hour urinary creatinine excretion was 0.7 g. Based on the serum creatinine only, this patient has normal renal function, whereas based on both serum creatinine concentration and total 24-hour urinary creatinine excretion, the patient has a GFR of less than 50 mL/min. In practice, serum creatinine clearance is often estimated from serum creatinine concentration alone for dose adjustment. In elderly subjects, the clinician should carefully assess the patient, since substantial deviation from the true clearance may occur in some elderly subjects.

2. Diflunisal pharmacokinetics were studied in healthy young and old subjects. After a single dose of diflunisal, the terminal plasma half-life, mean residence time, and apparent volume of distribution were higher in elderly subjects than in young adults (Erikson et al, 1989). This study shows that renal function in elderly subjects is generally reduced somewhat compared to younger patients because of a diminished rate of glomerular filtration.

DOSING OF DRUGS IN THE OBESE PATIENT

Obesity is a major problem in the United States and is also becoming a problem in other countries. Obesity has been associated with increased mortality resulting from increases in the incidence of hypertension, atherosclerosis, coronary artery disease, diabetes, and other conditions compared to nonobese patients (Blouin and Warren, 1999; National Institutes of Health, 2003). A patient is considered obese if actual body weight exceeds ideal or desirable body weight by 20%, according to Metropolitan Life Insurance Company data (latest published tables). Ideal or desirable body weights are based on average body weights and heights for males and for females considering age. Athletes who have a greater body weight due to greater muscle mass are not considered obese. Obesity often is defined by *body mass index* (BMI), a value that normalizes body weight based on height. BMI is expressed as body weight (kg) divided by the square of the person's height (meters) or kg/m². BMI is calculated according to the following two equations:

$$BMI = \left[\frac{weight\ (lb)}{height\ (in)^2} \right] \times 703$$

$$BMI = \left[\frac{weight\ (kg)}{height\ (cm)^2} \right] \times 10,000$$

An extensive study on obesity has been published by the National Institutes of Health, National Heart, Lung and Blood Institute (2003), giving five weight classifications based on BMI:

	BMI
Underweight:	<18.5
Normal body weight:	18.5–24.9
Overweight:	25–29.9
Obese:	30–39.9
Extreme obesity	>40

The obese patient (BMI > 30) has a greater accumulation of fat tissue than is necessary for normal body functions. Adipose (fat) tissue has a smaller proportion of water compared to muscle tissue. Thus, the obese patient has a smaller proportion of total body water to total body weight compared to the patient of ideal body weight, which could affect the apparent volume of distribution of the drug. For example, Abernethy and Greenblatt (1982) showed a significant difference in the apparent volume of distribution of antipyrine in obese patients (0.46 L/kg) compared to ideal-body-weight patients (0.62 L/kg) based on actual total body weight. *Ideal body weight* (IBW) refers to the appropriate or normal weight for a male or female based on age, height, weight, and frame size; ideal body weights are generally obtained from the latest table of desirable weights for men and women compiled by the Metropolitan Life Insurance Company.

In addition to differences in total body water per kilogram body weight in the obese patient, the greatest proportion of body fat in these patients could lead to distributional changes in the drug's pharmacokinetics due to partitioning of the drug between lipid and aqueous environments (Blouin and Warren, 1999). Drugs such as digoxin and gentamicin are very polar and tend to distribute into water rather than into fat tissue. Although lipophilic drugs are associated with larger volumes of distribution in obese patients compared to hydrophilic drugs, there are exceptions and the effect of obesity on specific drugs must be considered for accurate dosing strategy.

Other pharmacokinetic parameters may be altered in the obese patient as a result of physiologic alterations, such as fatty infiltration of the liver affecting biotransformation and cardiovascular changes that may affect renal blood flow and renal excretion (Abernethy and Greenblatt, 1982).

Dosing by actual body weight may result in overdosing of drugs such as aminoglycosides (eg, gentamicin), which are very polar and are distributed in extracellular fluids. Dosing of these drugs is based on ideal body weight. *Lean body weight* has been estimated by several empirical equations based on the patient's height and actual (total) body weight. The following equations have been used for estimating lean body weight, particularly for adjustment of dosage in renally impaired patients:

$$\text{LBW (males)} = 50 \text{ kg} + 2.3 \text{ kg for each inch over 5 ft} \qquad \textbf{(20.9)}$$

$$\text{LBW (females)} = 45.5 \text{ kg} + 2.3 \text{ kg for each inch over 5 ft} \qquad \textbf{(20.10)}$$

where LBW is lean body weight.

EXAMPLE

Calculate the lean body weight for an adult male patient who is 5 ft 9 in (175.3 cm) tall and weighs 264 lb (120 kg).

Solution

Using Equation 20.9,

$$\text{LBW} = 50 + (2.3 \times 9) = 70.7 \text{ kg}$$

PHARMACOKINETICS OF DRUG INTERACTIONS

Drug interaction generally refers to a modification of the expected drug response in the patient as a result of exposure of the patient to another drug or substance. Some unintentional drug interactions produce adverse reactions in the patient, whereas some drug interactions may be intentional, to provide an improved therapeutic response or to decrease adverse drug effects. Drug interactions may include drug–drug interactions, food–drug interactions, or chemical–drug interactions, such as the interaction of a drug with alcohol or tobacco. A listing of food interactions is given in Chapter 13. A drug–laboratory test interaction pertains to an alteration in a diagnostic laboratory test result because of the drug.

The risk of a drug interaction increases with multiple drug therapy, multiple prescribers, poor patient compliance, and patient risk factors, such as predisposing illness (diabetes, hypertension, etc) or advancing age. Multiple drug therapy has become routine in most acute and chronic care settings. Elderly patients and patients with various predisposing illnesses tend to be a population using multiple drug therapy. A recent student survey found an average of 8 to 12 drugs per patient used in a group of hospital patients.

Screening for drug interactions should be performed whenever multiple drug uses are involved. Many computer programs will "flag" a potential drug interaction. However, the pharmacist needs to determine the clinical significance of the interaction. The determination of the clinical significance of a potential drug interaction should be documented in the literature. The likelihood of a drug interaction may be classified as an established drug interaction, probable drug interaction, possible drug interaction, or unlikely drug interaction. The size of the dose and the duration of therapy, the onset (rapid, delayed), the severity (major, minor) of the potential interaction, and extrapolation to related drugs should also be considered.

Preferably, drugs that interact should be avoided or given sufficiently far apart so that the interaction is minimized. In situations involving two drugs of choice that may interact, dose adjustment based on pharmacokinetic and therapeutic considerations of one or both of the drugs may be necessary. Dose adjustment may be based on clearance or elimination half-life of the drug. Assessment of the patient's renal function, such as serum creatinine concentration, and liver function indicators, such as alkaline phosphatase, alanine aminotransferase (ALT), aspartate aminotransferase (AST), or other markers of hepatic metabolism (Chapter 21), should be undertaken. In general, if the therapeutic response is predictable from serum drug concentration, dosing at regular intervals may be based on a steady-state concentration equation such as Equation 20.1. When the elimination half-life is changed by drug interaction, the dosing interval may be extended or the dose reduced according to Equation 20.4. Some examples of pharmacokinetic drug interactions are listed in Table 20.10. A more complete discussion of pharmacologic and therapeutic drug interactions of drugs is available in standard textbooks on clinical pharmacology.

TABLE 20.10 Pharmacokinetic Drug Interactions

DRUG INTERACTION	EXAMPLES (PRECIPITANT DRUGS)	EFFECT (OBJECT DRUGS)
Bioavailability		
Complexation/chelation	Calcium, magnesium, or aluminum and iron salts	Tetracycline complexes with divalent cations, causing a decreased bioavailability
Adsorption binding/ionic interaction	Cholestyramine resin (anion-exchange resin binding)	Decreased bioavailability of thyroxine, and digoxin; binds anionic drugs and reduces absorption
Adsorption	Antacids (adsorption) Charcoal, antidiarrheals	Decreased bioavailability of antibiotics Decreased bioavailability of many drugs
Increased GI motility	Laxatives, cathartics	Increases GI motility, decreases bioavailability for drugs which are absorbed slowly; may also affect the bioavailability of drugs from controlled-release products
Decreased GI motility	Anticholinergic agents	Propantheline decreases the gastric emptying of acetaminophen (APAP), delaying APAP absorption from the small intestine
Alteration of gastric pH	H-2 blockers, antacids	Both H-2 blockers and antacids increase gastric pH; the dissolution of ketoconazole is reduced, causing decreased drug absorption
Alteration of intestinal flora	Antibiotics (eg, tetracyclines, penicillin)	Digoxin has better bioavailability after erythromycin; erythromycin administration reduces bacterial inactivation of digoxin
Inhibition of drug metabolism in intestinal cells	Monoamine oxidase inhibitors (MAO-I) (eg, tranylcypromine, phenelzine)	Hypertensive crisis may occur in patients treated with MAO-I and foods containing tyramine

(Continued)

TABLE 20.10 Pharmacokinetic Drug Interactions (continued)

DRUG INTERACTION	EXAMPLES (PRECIPITANT DRUGS)	EFFECT (OBJECT DRUGS)
Distribution		
Protein binding	Warfarin–phenylbutazone	Displacement of warfarin from binding
	Phenytoin–valproic acid	Displacement of phenytoin from binding
Hepatic elimination		
Enzyme induction	Smoking (polycyclic aromatic hydrocarbons)	Smoking increases theophylline clearance
	Barbiturates	Phenobarbital increases the metabolism of warfarin
Enzyme inhibition Mixed-function oxidase	Cimetidine	Decreased theophylline, diazepam metabolism
	Fluvoxamine	Diazepam $t_{1/2}$ longer
	Quinidine	Decreased nifedipine metabolism
	Fluconazole	Increased levels of phenytoin, warfarin
Other enzymes	Monoamine oxidase inhibitors, MAO-I (eg, pargyline, tranylcypromine)	Serious hypertensive crisis may occur following ingestion of foods with a high content of tyramine or other pressor substances (eg, cheddar cheese, red wines)
Inhibition of biliary secretion	Verapamil	Decreased biliary secretion of digoxin causing increased digoxin levels
Renal clearance		
Glomerular filtration rate (GFR) and renal blood flow	Methylxanthines (eg, caffeine, theobromine)	Increased renal blood flow and GFR will decrease time for reabsorption of various drugs, leading to more rapid urinary drug excretion
Active tubular secretion	Probenecid	Probenecid blocks the active tubular secretion of penicillin and some cephalosporin antibiotics
Tubular reabsorption and urine pH	Antacids, sodium bicarbonate	Alkalinization of the urine increases the reabsorption of amphetamine and decreases its clearance
		Alkalinization of urine pH increases the ionization of salicylates, decreases reabsorption and increases its clearance
Diet		
Charcoal hamburgers	Theophylline	Elimination half-life of theophylline decreases due to increased metabolism
Grapefruit	Terfenadine, cyclosporin	Blood levels of terfenadine and cyclosporine increase due to decreased metabolism
Virus drug interactions		
Reye's syndrome	Aspirin	Aspirin in children exposed to certain viral infections such as influenza B virus leads to Reye's syndrome

Many drugs affect the cytochrome P-450 (CYP) family of hemoprotein enzymes that catalyze drug biotransformation (see also Chapters 11 and 12). Dr. David A. Flockhart, Indiana University School of Medicine, has compiled an excellent website that lists various drugs that may be substrates or inhibitors of cytochrome P-450 isozymes (http://medicine.iupui.edu/flockhart). Some examples of substrates of CYPs are

CYP1A2	Amitriptyline, fluvoxamine
CYP2B6	Cyclophosphamide
CYP2C9	Ibuprofen, fluoxetine, tolbutamide, amitriptyline
CYP2C19	Omeprazole, S-methenytoin, amitriptyline
CYP2D6	Propanolol, amitriptyline, fluoxetine, paroxetine
CYP2E1	Halothane
CYP3A4	Erythromycin, clarithromycin, midazolam, diazapam
CYP3A5	Clarithromycin, simvastatin, indinavir
CYP3A6	Erythromycin, clarithromycin, diltiazem

Many calcium channel blockers, macrolides, and protease inhibitors are substrates of CYP3A4, CYP3A5, or CYP3A6. An enzyme substrate may competitively interfere with other substrates metabolism if co-administered. Drug inducers of CYPs may also result in drug interactions by accelerating the rate of drug metabolism. When an unusually high plasma level is observed as a result of co-administration of a second drug, pharmacists should check whether the two drugs share a common CYP substrate. New substrates are still being discovered. For example, many proton inhibitors share the common CYP2C19 substrate, and many calcium channel blockers are CYP3A4 substrates. It is important to assess the clinical significance with the clinician before alarming the patient. It is also important to suggest an alternative drug therapy to the clinician if a clinically significant drug interaction is likely to be occurring.

Some examples of pharmacokinetic drug interactions are discussed in more detail below and in Chapter 12. Many side effects occur as a result of impaired or induced (stimulated) drug metabolism. Changes in pharmacokinetics due to impaired drug metabolism should be evaluated quantitatively. For example, acetaminophen is an OTC drug that has been used safely for decades, but incidences of severe hepatic toxicity leading to coma have occurred in some subjects with impaired liver function because of chronic alcohol use. Drugs that have reactive intermediates, active metabolites, and or metabolites with a longer half-life than the parent drug need to be considered carefully if there is a potential for a drug interaction. A polar metabolite may also distribute to a smaller fluid volume, leading to high concentration in some tissues. Drug interactions involving metabolism may be temporal, observed as a delayed effect. Temporal drug interactions are more difficult to detect in a clinical situation.

INHIBITION OF DRUG METABOLISM

Numerous clinical instances of severe adverse reactions as a result of drug interaction involving a change in the rate of drug metabolism have been reported. Knowledge of pharmacokinetics allows the clinical pharmacist to evaluate the clinical significance of the drug interaction. Pharmacokinetic models help to determine the need for dose reduction or discontinuing a drug. In assessing the situation, the pathophysiology of the patient and the effect of chronic therapy on drug disposition in the patient must be considered. A severe drug reaction in a patient with liver impairment has resulted in near-fatal reaction in subjects taking otherwise safe doses of acetaminophen. In some patients with injury or severe cardiovascular disease, blood flow may be impaired, resulting in delayed drug absorption and distribution. Many incidents of serious toxicity or accidents are caused by premature administration of a "booster dose" when the expected response is not immediately observed. Potent drugs such as morphine, midazolam, lidocaine, pentothal, and fentenyl can result in serious adverse reactions if the kinetics of multiple dosing are not carefully assessed.

 # EXAMPLES

1. *Fluvoxamine doubles the half-life of diazepam.* The effect of fluvoxamine on the pharmacokinetics of diazepam was investigated in healthy volunteers (Perucca et al, 1994). Concurrent fluvoxamine intake increased mean peak plasma diazepam concentrations from 108 to 143 ng/mL, and oral diazepam clearance was reduced from 0.40 to 0.14 mL/min/kg. The half-life of diazepam increased from 51 to 118 hours. The area under the plasma concentration–time curve for the diazepam metabolite N-desmethyldiazepam was also significantly increased during fluvoxamine treatment. These data suggest that fluvoxamine inhibits the biotransformation of diazepam and its active N-demethylated metabolite.

    In this example, the dosing interval, τ, may be increased twofold to account for the doubling of elimination half-life to keep average steady-state concentration unchanged based on Equation 20.4. The rationale for this recommendation may be demonstrated by sketching a diagram showing how the steady-state plasma drug level of diazepam differs after taking 10 mg orally twice a day with or without taking fluvoxamine for a week.

$$C_{av}^{\infty} = \frac{1.44 D_0 t_{1/2} F}{V_D \tau}$$

2. *Quinidine inhibits the metabolism of nifedipine and other calcium channel-blocking agents.* Quinidine co-administration significantly inhibited the aromatization of nifedipine to its major first-pass pyridine metabolite and prolonged the elimination half-life by about 40% (Schellens et al, 1991). The interaction between quinidine and nifedipine supports the involvement of a common cytochrome P-450 (P450 3A4) in the metabolism of the two drugs. Other calcium channel antagonists may also be affected by a similar interaction. What could be a potential problem if two drugs metabolized by the same isozyme are co-administered?

3. *Theophylline clearance is decreased by cimetidine.* Controlled studies have shown that cimetidine can decrease theophylline plasma clearance by 20–40% (apparently by inhibiting demethylation) (Loi et al., 1997). Prolongation of half-life by as much as 70% was found in some patients. Elevated theophylline plasma concentrations with toxicity may lead to nausea, vomiting, cardiovascular instability, and even seizure. What could happen to an asthmatic patient whose meals are

high in protein and low in carbohydrate, and who takes Tagamet 400 mg BID? (*Hint:* Check the effect of food on theophylline, below.)

4. *Interferon-β reduces metabolism of theophylline.* Theophylline pharmacokinetics were also examined before and after interferon treatment (Okuno et al, 1993). Interferon-β treatment reduced the activities of both O-dealkylases by 47%. The total body clearance of theophylline was also decreased (from 0.76 to 0.56 mL/kg/min) and its elimination half-life was increased (from 8.4 to 11.7 hr; $P < 0.05$). This study provided the first direct evidence that interferon-β can depress the activity of drug-metabolizing enzymes in the human liver. What percent of steady-state theophylline plasma concentration would be changed by the interaction? (Use Equation 20.8.)

5. *Torsades de pointes interaction.* A life-threatening ventricular arrhythmia associated with prolongation of the QT interval, known as torsades de pointes, caused the removal of the antihistamine terfenadine (Seldane) from the market because of drug interactions with cisapride, astemizole, and ketoconazole. Clinical symptoms of torsades de pointes include dizziness, syncope, irregular heartbeat, and sudden death. The active metabolite of terfenadine is not cardiac toxic and is now marked as fexofenadine (Allegra), a nonsedative antihistamine.

6. *Cimetidine and diazepam interaction.* The administration of 800 mg of cimetidine daily for 1 week increased the steady-state plasma diazepam and nordiazepam concentrations due to a cimetidine-induced impairment in microsomal oxidation of diazepam and nordiazepam. The concurrent administration of cimetidine caused a decrease in total metabolic clearance of diazepam and its metabolite, nordiazepam (Lima et al, 1991). How would the following pharmacokinetic parameters of diazepam be affected by the co-administration of cimetidine?

a. Area under the curve in the dose interval ($AUC_{0-24\ hr}$)

b. Maximum plasma concentration (C_{max})

c. Time to peak concentration (t_p)

d. Elimination rate constant (k)

e. Total body clearance (Cl_T)

INHIBITION OF BILIARY EXCRETION

The interaction between digoxin and verapamil (Hedman et al, 1991) was studied in six patients (mean age 61 ± 5 years) with chronic atrial fibrillation. The effects of adding verapamil (240 mg/day) on steady-state plasma concentrations of digoxin were studied. Verapamil induced a 44% increase in steady-state plasma concentrations of digoxin. The biliary clearance of digoxin was determined by a duodenal perfusion technique. The biliary clearance of digoxin decreased by 43%, from 187 ± 89 to 101 ± 55 mL/min, whereas the renal clearance was not significantly different (153 ± 31 versus 173 ± 51 mL/min).

INDUCTION OF DRUG METABOLISM

Cytochrome P-450 isozymes are often involved in the metabolic oxidation of many drugs (Chapter 11). Many drugs can stimulate the production of hepatic enzymes. Therapeutic doses of phenobarbital and other barbiturates accelerate the metabolism of coumarin anticoagulants such as warfarin and substantially reduce the hypoprothrombinemic effect. Fatal hemorrhagic episodes can result when phenobarbital is withdrawn and warfarin dosage maintained at its previous level. Other drugs known to stimulate drug metabolism include carbamazepine, rifampin, valproic acid, and phenytoin. Enzymatic stimulation can shorten the elimination half-life of the affected drug. For example, phenobarbital can result in lower levels of dexamethasone in asthmatic patients taking both drugs.

ALTERED RENAL REABSORPTION
DUE TO CHANGING URINARY PH

The normal adult urinary pH ranges from 4.8 to 7.5 but can increase due to chronic antacid use. This change in urinary pH affects the ionization and reabsorption of weak electrolyte drugs (Chapter 6). An increased ionization of salicylate due to an increase in urine pH reduces salicylate reabsorption in the renal tubule, resulting in increased renal excretion. Magnesium aluminum hydroxide gel (Maalox), 120 mL/day for 6 days, decreased serum salicylate levels from 19.8 to 15.8 mg/dL in six subjects who had achieved a control serum salicylate level of 0.10 mg/dL with the equivalent of 3.76 g/day aspirin (Hansten et al, 1980). Single doses of magnesium aluminum hydroxide gel did not alter urine pH significantly. Five milliliters of Titralac (calcium carbonate with glycine) 4 times a day or magnesium hydroxide for 7 days also increased urinary pH. In general, drugs with pK_a values within the urinary pH range are affected the most. Basic drugs tend to have longer half-lives when urinary pH is increased, especially near its pK_a.

 PRACTICAL FOCUS

Which of the following treatments would be most likely to decrease the $t_{1/2}$ of aspirin?

1. Calcium carbonate PO
2. Sodium carbonate PO
3. IV sodium bicarbonate

(*Hint:* Which drug can be absorbed and change urinary pH and the reabsorption of aspirin?)

INHIBITION OF DRUG ABSORPTION

Various drugs and dietary supplements can decrease the absorption of drugs from the gastrointestinal tract. Antacids containing magnesium and aluminum hydroxide often interfere with absorption of many drugs. Co-administration of magnesium and aluminum hydroxide caused a decrease of plasma levels of perfloxacin. The drug interaction is caused by the formation of chelate complexes and is possibly also due to adsorption of the quinolone to aluminum hydroxide gel. Perfloxacin should be given at least 2 hours before the antacid to ensure sufficient therapeutic efficacy of the quinolone.

Sucralfate is an aluminum glycopyranoside complex that is not absorbed but retards the oral absorption of ciprofloxacin. Sucralfate is used in the local treatment of ulcers. Cholestyramine is an anion-exchange resin that binds bile acid and many drugs in the gastrointestinal tract. Cholestyramine can bind digitoxin in the GI tract and shorten the elimination half-life of digitoxin by approximately 30–40%. Absorption of thyroxine may be reduced by 50% when it is administered closely with cholestyramine.

EFFECT OF FOOD ON DRUG DISPOSITION

Diet–Theophylline Interaction

Theophylline disposition is influenced by diet. A protein-rich diet will increase theophylline clearance. Average theophylline half-lives in subjects on a low-carbohydrate, high-protein diet increased from 5.2 to 7.6 hours when subjects were changed to a high-carbohydrate, low-protein diet. A diet of charcoal-broiled beef, which contains polycyclic aromatic hydrocarbons from the charcoal, resulted in a decrease in theophylline half-life of up to 42% when compared to a control non-charcoal-broiled-beef diet. Irregular intake of vitamin K may modify the anticoagulant effect of warfarin. Many foods, especially green, leafy vegetables such as broccoli and spinach, contain high concentrations of vitamin K. In one study, warfarin therapy was interfered with in patients receiving vitamin K, broccoli, or spinach daily for 1 week (Pedersen et al, 1991).

Grapefruit–Drug Interactions

Recent investigations have shown that the ingredients in a common food product, grapefruit juice, taken in usual dietary quantities, can significantly inhibit the metabolism by gut-wall cytochrome P-450 3A4 (CYP3A4) (Spence, 1997). For example, grapefruit juice increases average felodipine levels about threefold, increases cyclosporine levels, and increases the levels of terfenadine, a common antihistamine. In the case of terfenadine, Spence (1997) reported the death of a 29-year-old male who had been taking terfenadine and drinking grapefruit juice 2 to 3 times per week. Death was attributed to terfenadine toxicity. Grapefruit juice can also affect P-gp mediated efflux of some drugs.

ADVERSE VIRAL DRUG INTERACTIONS

Recent findings have suggested that some interactions of viruses and drugs may predispose individuals to specific disease outcomes (Haverkos et al, 1991). For example,

Reye's syndrome has been observed in children who had been taking aspirin and were concurrently exposed to certain viruses, including influenza B virus and varicella zoster virus. The mechanism by which salicylates and certain viruses interact is not clear. However, the publication of this interaction has led to the prevention of morbidity and mortality due to this complex interaction (Haverkos et al, 1991).

POPULATION PHARMACOKINETICS

Introduction to Bayesian Theory

Bayesian theory was originally developed to improve forecast accuracy by combining subjective prediction with improvement from newly collected data. In the diagnosis of disease, the physician may make a preliminary diagnosis based on symptoms and physical examination. Later, the results of laboratory tests are received. The clinician then makes a new diagnostic forecast based on both sets of information. Bayesian theory provides a method to weigh the prior information (eg, physical diagnosis) and new information (eg, results from laboratory tests) to estimate a new probability for predicting the disease.

In developing a drug dosage regimen, we assess the patient's medical history and then use average or population pharmacokinetic parameters appropriate for the patient's condition to calculate the initial dose. After the initial dose, plasma or serum drug concentrations are obtained from the patient that provide new information to assess the adequacy of the dosage. The dosing approach of combining old information with new involves a "feedback" process and is, to some degree, inherent in many dosing methods involving some parameter readjustment when new serum drug concentrations become known. The advantage of the Bayesian approach is the improvement in estimating the patient's pharmacokinetic parameters based on Bayesian probability versus an ordinary least-squares-based program. An example comparing the Bayesian method with an alternative method for parameter estimation from some simulated theophylline data will be shown in the next section. The method is particularly useful when only a few blood samples are available.

Because of inter- and intrasubject variability, the pharmacokinetic parameters of an individual patient must be estimated from limited data in the presence of unknown random error (assays, etc), known covariates and variables such as clearance, weight, and disease factor, etc, and possible structural (kinetic model) error. From knowledge of mean population pharmacokinetic parameters and their variability, Bayesian methods often employ a special *weighted least-squares* (WLS) approach and allow improved estimation of patient pharmacokinetic parameters when there is a lot of variation in data. The methodology is discussed in more detail under the Bayes estimator in the next section and also under pharmacokinetic analysis.

 # EXAMPLE

After diagnosing a patient, the physician gave the patient a probability of 0.4 of having a disease. The physician then ordered a clinical laboratory test. A positive laboratory test value had a probability of 0.8 of positively identifying the disease in patients with the disease (true positive) and a probability of 0.1 of positive identification of the disease in subjects without the disease (false positive). From the prior information (physician's diagnosis) and current patient-specific data (laboratory test), what is the posterior probability of the patient having the disease using the Bayesian method?

Solution

> Prior probability of having the disease (positive) = 0.4
> Prior probability of not having the disease (negative) = 1 − 0.4 = 0.6
> Ratio of disease positive/disease negative = 0.4/0.6 = 2/3, or, the physician's evaluation shows a 2/3 chance for the presence of the disease

The probability of the patient actually having the disease can be better evaluated by including the laboratory findings. For this same patient, the probability of a positive laboratory test of 0.8 for the detection of disease in positive patients (with disease) and the probability of 0.1 in negative patients (without disease) are equal to a ratio of 0.8/0.1 or 8/1. This ratio is known as the *likelihood ratio*. Combining with the prior probability of 2/3, the posterior probability ratio is

> Posterior probability ratio = (2/3)(8/1) = 16/3
>
> Posterior probability = 16/(16 + 3) = 84.2%

Thus, the laboratory test that estimates the likelihood ratio and the preliminary diagnostic evaluation are both used in determining the posterior probability. The results of this calculation show that with a positive diagnosis by the physician and a positive value for the laboratory test, the probability that the patient actually has the disease is 84.2%.

Bayesian probability theory when applied to dosing of a drug involves a given pharmacokinetic parameter (P) and plasma or serum drug concentration (C), as shown in Equation 20–11. The probability of a patient with a given pharmacokinetic parameter P, taking into account the measured concentration, is $\text{Prob}(P/C)$:

$$\text{Prob}(P/C) = \frac{\text{Prob}(P) \cdot \text{Prob}(C/P)}{\text{Prob}(C)} \qquad (20.11)$$

where $\text{Prob}(P)$ = the probability of the patient's parameter within the assumed population distribution, $\text{Prob}(C/P)$ = the probability of measured concentration within the population, and $\text{Prob}(C)$ = the unconditional probability of the observed concentration.

 EXAMPLE

Theophylline has a therapeutic window of 10–20 μg/mL. Serum theophylline concentrations above 20 μg/mL produce mild side effects, such as nausea and insomnia;

more serious side effects, such as sinus tachycardia, may occur at drug concentrations above 40 μg/mL; at serum concentrations above 45 μg/mL, cardiac arrhythmia and seizure may occur (Figure 20-1). However, the probability of some side effect occurring is by no means certain. Side effects are not determined solely by plasma concentration, as other known or unknown variables (called covariates) may affect the side-effect outcome. Some patients have initial side effects of nausea and restlessness (even at very low drug concentrations) that later disappear when therapy is continued. The clinician should therefore assess the probability of side effects in the patient, order a blood sample for serum theophylline determination, and then estimate a combined (or posterior) probability for side effects in the patient.

The decision process is illustrated graphically in Figure 20-3. The probability of initial (prior) estimation of side effects is plotted on the x axis, and the final (posterior) probability of side effects is plotted on the y axis for various serum theophylline concentrations. For example, a patient was placed on theophylline and the physician estimated the chance of side effects to be 40%, but therapeutic drug monitoring showed a theophylline level of 27 μg/mL. A vertical line of prior probability at 0.4 intersects curve a at about 0.78 or 78%. Hence, the Bayesian probability of having side effects is 78% taking both the laboratory and physician assessments into consideration. The curves (a–e in Fig. 20-3) for various theophylline concentrations are called *conditional probability curves*. Bayesian theory does not replace clinical judgment, but it provides a quantitative tool for incorporating subjective judgment (human) with objective (laboratory assay) in making risk decisions. When complex decisions involving several variables are involved, this objective tool can be very useful.

Bayesian probability is used to improve forecasting in medicine. One example is its use in the diagnosis of healed myocardial infarction (HMI) from a 12-lead electrocardiogram (ECG) by artificial neural networks using the Bayesian concept. Bayesian results were comparable to those of an experienced electrocardiographer (Heden et al, 1996). In pharmacokinetics, Bayesian theory is applied to "feed-forward neural networks" for gentamicin concentration predictions (Smith and Brier, 1996). A brief literature search of Bayesian applications revealed over 400

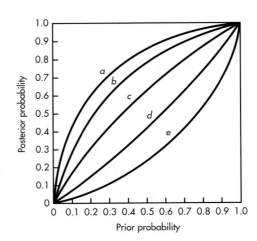

Figure 20-3. Conditional probability curves relating prior probability of toxicity to posterior probability of toxicity of STC, theophylline serum concentrations: (*a*) 27–28.9; (*b*) 23–24.9; (*c*) 19–20.9; (*d*) 15–16.9; and (*e*) 11–12.9 (all STC in μg/mL).
(From Schumacher, 1995, with permission.)

therapeutic applications between 1992 to 1996. Bayesian parameter estimations were most frequently used for drugs with narrow therapeutic ranges, such as the aminoglycosides, cyclosporin, digoxin, anticonvulsants (especially phenytoin), lithium, and theophylline. The technique has now been extended to cytotoxic drugs, factor VIII, and warfarin. Bayesian methods have also been used to limit the number of samples required in more conventional pharmacokinetic studies with new drugs (Thomson and Whiting, 1992). The main disadvantage of Bayesian methods is the subjective selection of prior probability. Therefore, it is not considered to be unbiased by many statisticians for drug approval purposes.

Adaptive Method or Dosing with Feedback

In dosing drugs with narrow therapeutic ratios, an initial dose is calculated based on mean population pharmacokinetic parameters. After dosing, plasma drug concentrations are obtained from the patient. As more blood samples are drawn from the patient, the calculated individualized patient pharmacokinetic parameters become increasingly more reliable. This type of approach has been referred to as *adaptive*, or *Bayesian adaptive method with feedback* when a spacial extended least-squares algorithm is used. Many ordinary least-squares computer software packages are available to clinical practice for parameter and dosage calculation (Appendix B). Some software packages record medical history and provide adjustments for weight, age, and in some cases, disease factors. A common approach is to estimate the clearance and volume of distribution from intermittent infusion (see Chapter 5). Abbottbase Pharmacokinetic Systems (1986 and 1992) is an example of patient-oriented software that records patient information and dosing history based on 24-hour clock time. An adaptive-type algorithm is used to estimate pharmacokinetic parameters. The average population clearance and volume of distribution of drugs are used for initial estimates and the program computes patient-specific Cl and V_D as serum drug concentrations are entered. The program accounts for renal dysfunction based on creatinine clearance, which is estimated from serum creatinine concentration using the Cockroft–Gault equation (see Chapter 21). The software package allows specific parameter estimation for digoxin, theophylline, and aminoglycosides, although other drugs can also be analyzed manually.

Many *least-squares* (LS) and *weighted-least-squares* (WLS) algorithms are available for estimating patient pharmacokinetic parameters. Their common objective involves estimating the parameters with minimum bias and good prediction, often as evaluated by mean predictive error. The advantage of the Bayesian method is the ability to input known information into the program, so that the search for the real pharmacokinetic parameter is more efficient and, perhaps, more precise. For example, a drug is administered by intravenous infusion at a rate, R, to a patient. The drug is infused over t hours (t may be 0.5 to 2 hours for a typical infusion). The patient's clearance, Cl_T, may be estimated from plasma drug concentration taken at a known time according to a one-compartment-model equation. Sheiner and Beal (1982) simulated a set of theophylline data and estimated parameters from the data using one- and two-serum concentrations, assuming different variabilities.

These investigators tested the method with a Bayesian approach and with an *ordinary least-squares method*, OBJ$_{OLS}$.

$$C_i = f(P, t_i) + \varepsilon_i \tag{20.12}$$

$$\text{OBJ}_{OLS} = \sum_{i=1}^{n} \frac{(C_i - \hat{C}_i)^2}{\sigma_i^2} \tag{20.13}$$

The Bayes Estimator

When the pharmacokinetic parameter, P, is estimated from a set of plasma drug concentration data (C_i) having several potential sources of error with different variance, the ordinary least-squares (OLS) method for parameter estimation is no longer adequate (it yields trivial estimates). The intersubject variation, intrasubject variance, and random error must be minimized properly to allow efficient parameter estimation. The weighted least-squares function in Equation 20.14 was suggested by Sheiner and Beal (1982). The equation represents the least-squares estimation of the concentration by minimizing deviation squares (first summation term of Eq. 20.14), and deviation of population parameter squares (second summation term). Equation 20.14 is called the *Bayes estimator*. This approach is frequently referred to as *extended least-squares* (ELS).

Intrasubject $C_i = f(P, X_i) + \varepsilon_i$

Intersubject $P_k = \hat{P}_k + \eta_k$ (20.14)

$$\text{OBJ}_{BAYES} = \sum_{i=1}^{n} \frac{(C_i - \hat{C}_i)^2}{\sigma_i^2} + \sum_{k=1}^{s} \frac{(P_k - \hat{P}_k)^2}{\omega_k^2}$$

For n number of drug plasma concentration data, i is an index to refer to each data item, C_i is the ith concentration, $\hat{c}_i$ is the ith model-estimated concentration, and σ^2 is the variance of random error, ε_i (assay errors, random intrasubject variation, etc). There is a series of population parameters in the model for the kth population parameter, P_k. $\hat{P}_k$ is the estimated population parameter and ηk is the kth parameter random error with variance of ω_k^2.

To compare the performance of the Bayesian method to other methods in drug dosing, Sheiner and Beal (1982) generated some theophylline plasma drug concentrations based on known clearance. They added various error levels to the data and divided the patients into groups with one and two plasma drug samples. The two pharmacokinetic parameters used were based on population pharmacokinetics for theophylline derived from the literature: (1) for P_1, a V_D of 0.5 L/kg and coefficient of variation of 32%; and (2) for P_2, clearance of 0.052 L/kg/hr and coefficient of variation of 44%.

The data were then analyzed using the Bayesian method and a second (alternative) approach in determining the pharmacokinetic parameter (Cl_T). In the presence of various levels of error, the Bayesian approach was robust and resulted in better estimation of clearance in both the one- and two-sample groups (Fig. 20-4 and Table 20.11). The success of the Bayesian approach is due to the ability of the

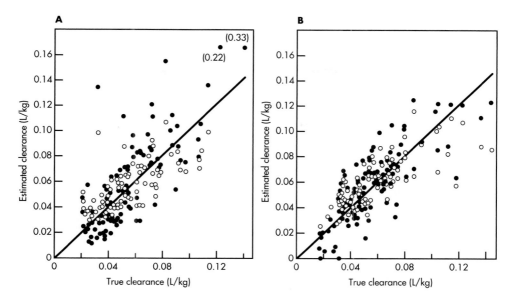

Figure 20-4. *Plots of predicted clearance versus true (simulated) clearance for predictions by the Bayesian (o) and alternative (●) methods. The diagonal line on each graph is the line of identity.* **A** *shows results for one-sample group;* **B** *shows results for two-sample group.* (From Sheiner and Beal, 1982, with permission.)

algorithm to minimize the total mean square terms of errors. A more precise clearance estimation will lead to more accurate dose estimation in the patient.

The implementation of the Bayesian (ELS) approach uses the NONMEM computer software, facilitated by response criteria defined through a first-order (FO) Taylor series expansion. Among other computer software packages available, the NPME2 (USC*PACK) is a nonparametric maximum expectation maximization

TABLE 20.11   Performance of Clearance Estimation Methods

METHOD	$\frac{\omega_{Cl}{}^a}{\sigma}$	$\frac{\omega_{V_D}{}^a}{\sigma}$	ERROR Example 1	ERROR Example 2	ABSOLUTE ERROR Example 1	ABSOLUTE ERROR Example 2
Alternative	—	—	−5.77(5.8)	−2.82(3.3)	37.1(4.5)	26.4(2.1)
Bayesian	1	1	−1.02(3.0)	−1.08(3.1)	22.2(2.0)[b]	21.7(2.2)[b]
	3/2	1	−4.94(3.4)	−3.77(3.0)	25.6(2.3)[b]	23.1(2.1)[b]
	2/3	1	5.02(3.2)	2.52(3.4)	23.7(2.2)[b]	23.5(2.4)
	1	3/2	0.44(3.0)	−0.26(3.1)	22.5(2.1)[b]	21.4(2.2)[b]
	1	2/3	−0.76(3.0)	−1.56(3.1)	22.5(1.9)[b]	21.7(2.2)

The header spanning ERROR/ABSOLUTE ERROR reads: **MEAN CLEARANCE ERROR (±SEM) AS PERCENT OF MEAN CLEARANCE**

[a]Ratio of standard deviation of clearance (or V_D) to σ used in the Bayesian method. All ratios are divided by the correct ratio so that a value of unity signifies that the correct ratio itself was used.
[b]Mean absolute error of Bayesian method less than that of alternative $(P < 0.05)$.

From Sheiner and Beal (1982), with permission.

method that makes no parametric assumptions about the mean and standard deviation of the distribution. The program can also discover unrecognized subpopulations. NONMEM also features FOEM, a first-order expectation maximization method. Generally, finding a set of best parameter estimates to describe the data involves minimizing the error terms; alternatively, another paradigm that maximizes the probability of the parameter estimates in the distribution serves the same purpose equally well or better. Thus, the first-order expectation maximization (FOEM) paradigm is also available in NONMEM and in other programs, such as P-PHARM (Mentre and Gomeni, 1995).

Comparison of Bayes, Least-Squares, Steady-State, and Chiou Methods

For theophylline dosing, the Bayes method and others, including the conventional steady-state method, were compared by Hurley and McNeil (1988). The Bayes method compared favorably with other methods (Tables 20.12 and 20.13). The steady-state method was also useful, but none of the methods was sufficiently accurate, probably due to other variables, such as saturation kinetics or use of an inappropriate compartment model.

Model fitting in pharmacokinetics often involves the search for a set of parameters that fits the data, a situation analogous to finding a point within a large geometric space. The ordinary least-squares (OLS) approach of iteratively minimizing the error terms may not be adequate when data are sparse, but are fine when sufficient data and good initial estimates are available. The Bayesian approach uses prior information, and, in essence, guides the search pointer to a proximity in the

TABLE 20.12 Pharmacokinetic Parameter Estimates (Mean ± SD)

METHOD	Cl^a (L/h/kg IBW)	k^b (hr^{-1})	V_D (L/kg IBW)
Least-squares			
Day 1	0.0383 ± 0.0129	0.105 ± 0.014	0.519 ± 0.291
Final	0.0391 ± 0.0117	0.095 ± 0.064	0.511 ± 0.239
Chiou			
1	0.0399 ± 0.0306		
2	0.0437 ± 0.0193		
3	0.0438 ± 0.0212		
Steady-state clearance			
	0.0408 ± 0.0174		
Bayesian			
1	0.0421 ± 0.0143	0.081 ± 0.030	0.534 ± 0.0745
2	0.0424 ± 0.0158	0.082 ± 0.035	0.532 ± 0.0802
3	0.0408 ± 0.0182	0.078 ± 0.037	0.531 ± 0.0820
4	0.0403 ± 0.0147	0.077 ± 0.027	0.530 ± 0.0787
Final	0.0372 ± 0.0113	0.070 ± 0.026	0.536 ± 0.0741

Cl = total body clearance, k = elimination rate constant, V_D = volume of distribution, IBW = ideal body weight.
[a]Calculated from least-squares estimates.
[b]Calculated by Bayesian estimates.

From Hurley and McNeil (1988), with permission.

TABLE 20.13   Predictive Accuracy at the End of Infusion 1[a]

METHOD	MEAN PREDICTION ERROR (mg/L)	MEAN PERCENT ABSOLUTE PREDICTION ERROR (%)
Least-squares		
Day 1	−0.06 (−1.1, 0.95)	17.6 (13.4, 21.7)
Chiou		
1	0.96 (−1.7, 3.60)	36.8 (27.3, 46.3)
2	−1.7 (−3.3, -0.08)	20.8 (14.1, 27.5)
3	−1.5 (−3.7, 0.80)	27.7 (17.8, 37.5)
Bayesian		
1	−0.61 (−1.7, 0.50)	18.8 (14.1, 23.6)
2	−0.65 (−2.0, 0.69)	22.7 (16.3, 29.2)
3	0.16 (−1.1, 1.40)	21.7 (16.1, 27.2)
4	−0.15 (−1.2, 0.96)	19.8 (15.6, 24.1)

[a]Figures in parentheses are 95% confidence intervals.

From Hurley and McNeil (1988), with permission.

geometric space where the estimates are more likely to be found (reducing variability but increasing subjectivity). Many algorithms use some form of gradient- or derivative-based method; other algorithms use a variable sequential simplex method. A discussion of the pharmacokinetic estimation methods was given by D'Argenio and Schumitzky (1979). Some common pharmacokinetic algorithms for parameter estimation are: (1) Newton–Raphson with first and second derivative, (2) Gauss–Newton method, (3) Levenberg–Marquardt method, and (4) Nelder–Mead simplex method. The Gauss–Newton method was used in the early versions of NONLIN. As discussed in relation to the mixed-effect models in later sections, assuming a relationship such as Cl_R proportional to Cl_{cr} (technically called linearization) reduces the minimum number of data necessary for parameter estimation.

Analysis of Population Pharmacokinetic Data

Traditional pharmacokinetic studies involve taking multiple blood samples periodically over time in a few individual patients, and characterizing basic pharmacokinetic parameters such as k, V_D, and Cl; because the studies are generally well designed, there are fewer parameters than data points (ie, that provide sufficient degree of freedom to reflect lack of fit of the model), and the parameters are efficiently estimated from the model with most least-squares programs. Traditional pharmacokinetic parameter estimation is very accurate, provided that enough samples can be taken for the individual patient. The disadvantage is that only a few relatively homogeneous healthy subjects are included in pharmacokinetic studies, from which dosing in different patients must be projected.

In the clinical setting, patients are usually not very homogeneous; patients vary in sex, age, body weight; they may have concomitant disease and may be receiving multiple drug treatments. Even the diet, lifestyle, ethnicity, and geographic location can differ from a selected group of "normal" subjects. Further, it is often not possible to take multiple samples from the same subject, and, therefore, no data are available to reflect intrasubject difference, so that iterative procedures for finding the maximum likelihood estimate can be complex and unpredictable due to incomplete or missing data. However, the vital information needed about the pharmacokinetics of drugs in patients at different stages of their disease with various therapies can only be obtained from the same population, or from a collection of pooled blood samples. The advantages of population pharmacokinetic analysis using pooled data were reviewed by Sheiner and Ludden (1992) and included a summary of population pharmacokinetics for dozens of drugs. Pharmacokinetic analysis of pooled data of plasma drug concentration from a large group of subjects may reveal much information about the disposition of a drug in a population. Unlike data from an individual subject collected over time, inter- and intrasubject variations must be considered. Both pharmacokinetic and nonpharmacokinetic factors, such as age, weight, sex, and creatinine concentration, should be examined in the model to determine the relevance to the estimation of pharmacokinetic parameters.

The *nonlinear mixed effect model* (or NONMEM) is so called because the model uses both fixed and random factors to describe data. Fixed factors such as patient weight, age, gender, and creatinine concentration are assumed to have no error, whereas random factors include inter- and intraindividual differences. NONMEM is a statistical program written in Fortran (see Appendix B) that allows Bayesian pharmacokinetic parameters to be estimated using an efficient algorithm called the *first-order* (FO) method. The parameters may now be estimated also with a *first-order conditional estimate* (FOCE) algorithm. In addition, to pharmacokinetic parameters, many examples of population plasma data have been analyzed to determine population factors. Multiplicative coefficients or parameters for patient factors may also be estimated.

NONMEM fits plasma drug concentration data for all subjects in the groups simultaneously and estimates the population parameter and its variance. The parameter may be clearance and/or V_D. The model may also test for other fixed effects on the drug due to factors such as age, weight, and creatinine concentration.

The model describes the observed plasma drug concentration (C_i) in terms of a model with:

1. P_k = fixed effect parameters, which include pharmacokinetic parameters or patient factor parameters. For example, P_1 is Cl, P_2 is the multiplicative coefficient including creatinine factor, and P_3 is the multiplicative coefficient for weight.
2. Random effect parameters, including (a) the variance of the structural (kinetic) parameter P_k or intersubject variability within the population ω_k^2; and (b) the residual intrasubject variance or variance due to measurement errors, fluctuations in individual parameter values, and all other errors not accounted for by the other parameters.

There are generally two reliable and practical approaches to population pharmacokinetic data analysis. One approach is the *standard two-stage* (STS) *method*, which estimates parameters from the plasma drug concentration data for an individual subject during the first stage. The estimates from all subjects are then combined to obtain an estimate of the parameters for the population. The method is useful because unknown factors that affect the response in one patient will not carry over and bias parameter estimates of the others. The method works well when sufficient drug concentration–time data are available.

A second approach, the *first-order* (FO) *method,* is also used but is perhaps less well understood. The estimation procedure is based on minimization of an extended least-squares criterion, which was defined through a first-order Taylor series expansion of the response vector about the fixed effects and which utilized a Newton–Raphson-like algorithm (Beal and Sheiner, 1980). This method attempts to fit the data and partition the unpredictable differences between theoretical and observed values into random error terms. When this model includes concomitant effects, it is called a *mixed-effect statistical model* (Beal and Sheiner, 1985).

The advantage of the first-order model is that it is applicable even when the amount of time–concentration data obtained from each individual is small, provided that the total number of individuals is sufficiently large. For example, in the example cited by Beal and Sheiner (1985), 116 plasma concentrations were collected from 39 patients with various weight, age, gender, serum creatinine, and congestive heart failure conditions. The two-stage method was not suitable, but the FO method was useful for analyzing this set of data. With a large number of factors and only limited data, and with hidden factors possibly affecting the pharmacokinetics of the drug, the analysis may sometimes be misleading. Beal and Sheiner (1985) suggested that the main concomitant factor should be measured whenever possible. Several examples of population pharmacokinetic data analysis using clinical data are listed below. Typically, a computer method is used in the data analysis based on a statistical model using either the weighted least-squares (WLS) or the extended least-squares (ELS) method in estimating the parameters. In the last few years, NONMEM has been regularly updated and improved. Many drugs have been analyzed with population pharmacokinetics to yield information not obtainable using the traditional two-stage method (Sheiner and Ludden, 1992). An added feature is the development of a population model involving both pharmacokinetics and pharmacodynamics, the so-called population PK/PD models.

One example involving analysis of population plasma concentration data involved the drug procainamide. The drug clearance of an individual in a group may be assumed to be affected by several factors (Whiting et al, 1986). These factors include body weight, creatinine clearance, and a clearance factor P_1 described in the following equation:

$$Cl_{\text{drug } j} = P_1 + P_2 \, (C_{\text{creatinine } j}) + P_3 \, (\text{weight}_j) + \eta_{Clj} \qquad \textbf{(20.15)}$$

where η_{Clj} is the intersubject error of clearance and its variance is ω^2_{Clj}.

In another mixed-effect model involving the analysis of lidocaine and maxiletine (Fig. 20-5), Vozeh and associates (1984) tested age, sex, time on drug therapy, and congestive heart failure (CHF) for effects on drug clearance. The effects of CHF and weight on V_D were also examined. The test statistic, DELS, or *difference extended least-squares,* was significant for CHF and moderately significant for weight on lidocaine clearance (Table 20.14).

Figure 20-5. The solid line and shaded area represent the average serum concentration and the interindividual variability (±SD) calculated from parameter estimates obtained from data for 58 patients. Squares and bars represent measured serum concentration (mean ± SD) in 26 of the 58 patients.
(From Vozeh et al, 1984, with permission.)

CLINICAL EXAMPLE

Fitting Warfarin Population Data

Population pharmacokinetics may be analyzed from various clinical sites. The population pharmacokinetics of racemic warfarin was evaluated using 613 measured warfarin plasma concentrations from 32 adult hospitalized patients and 131 adult outpatients (Mungall et al, 1985). Warfarin concentrations were measured in duplicate using a high-performance liquid chromatographic procedure. The pharmacokinetic model used was a one-compartment open model with first-order absorption and first-order elimination. The extent of availability was assumed to be 1. A linear regression model was used to evaluate the influence of various disease and demographic factors (Table 20.15) on warfarin drug clearance. Age appeared

TABLE 20.14   Testing for Factors Affecting Lidocaine Pharmacokinetics

HYPOTHESIS	ΔELS[a]
Cl influenced by:	
Age	0.1
Sex	2.4
Time on therapy	1.0
CHF $[Cl_{CHF} = Cl_{no}(1 - \theta_5)]$	52.7
V_1 influenced by CHF $[V_{1CHF} = V_{1no}(1 - \theta_6)]$	9.0
Cl and V_1 normalized for body weight	13.4

[a]ΔELS = change in extended least squares.

From Vozeh et al (1984).

TABLE 20.15   Population Pharmacokinetics of Warfarin Regression

PARAMETER	REGRESSION VALUE	EXPLANATION
P1	7.85 L/70 kg	Factor relating TBW to V_D
P2	0.460	exponential factor relating TBW to SIZECL
P3	3.31 L/day	Factor relating SIZECL to Cl
P4	0	Factors relating CHF to Cl
P5	0	Factor relating VAH site to Cl
P6	−0.0214 L/day/year of age	Factor relating age to Cl
P7	0	Factor relating gender to Cl
P8	0.367 L/day	Factor relating smoking to Cl
P9	0	Factor relating Caucasian vs Latin difference to Cl
P10	0	Factor relating Black vs Latin difference to Cl
P11	0	Factor relating drug inhibitor to Cl
P12	1.16 L/day	Factor relating drug inducer to Cl
P13	0	Factor relating drug displacer to Cl

From Mungall et al (1985).

to be an important determinant of warfarin clearance in this adult population. There was about a 1% per year decrease in oral clearance over the age range 20–70 years. Smoking appeared to result in a 10% increase in warfarin clearance, while co-administration of the inducer phenytoin or phenobarbital yielded about a 30% increase in clearance. Other factors such as race, gender, and hospital site did not significantly affect Cl_T based on this model. This study yielded a predictive model that, when combined with appropriate pharmacologic response data, may be useful in the design and adjustment of warfarin regimens.

$$SIZEVD = TBW/70$$

$$VD = SIZEVD \ (P1)$$

$$SIZECL = (TBW/70)^{P2}$$

$$Cl = SIZECL \ (P3 + P4 \ CHF + P5 \ VAH + P6 \ AGE + P7 \ GEN + P8 \ SKG + \\ P9 \ ANG + P10 \ BLK + P11 \ INH + P12 \ IND + P13 \ DIS)$$

The patient variables are the following: 1 = present; 0 = absent; CHF = congestive heart failure; VAH = VA hospital site; AGE = age in year; GEN = 1 for male and 0 for female; SKG = smoker; ANG = 1 if Caucasian; BLK = 1 if Black; INH = 1 if taking an inhibitor drug; IND = 1 if taking an inducer drug; DIS = 1 if taking a displacer (protein-binding) drug.

Thus, the information content is better when sampling is strategically designed. Proper sampling can yield valuable information about the distribution of pharmacokinetic parameters in a population. Pooled clinical drug concentrations taken from hospital patients are generally not well controlled and are much harder to analyze. This example shows that a mixed-effect model can yield valuable information about various demographic and pathophysiologic factors that may influence drug disposition in the patient population.

Model Selection Criteria

Data analysis in pharmacokinetics frequently selects either a monoexponential or polyexponential that will better describe the concentration–time relationship. The selection criteria for the better model is determined by the goodness-of-fit, taking into account the number of parameters involved. Three common model selection criteria are (1) the Akaike Information Criterion (AIC), (2) the Schwarz Criterion (SC), and (3) the F test (alpha = 0.05). The performance characteristics of these criteria were examined by Ludden et al (1994) using Monte Carlo (random or stochastic) simulations. The precision and bias of the estimated parameters were considered. The Akaike Information Criterion and the Schwarz Criterion lead to selection of the correct model more often than does the F test, which tends to choose the simpler model even when the more complex model is correct. The F test is also more sensitive to deficient sampling designs. Clearance was quite robust among the different methods and generally well estimated. Other pharmacokinetic parameters are more sensitive to model choice, particularly the apparent elimination rate constant. Prediction of concentrations is generally more precise when the correct model is chosen.

Decision Analysis Involving Diagnostic Tests

Diagnostic tests may be performed to determine the presence or absence of a disease. A scheme for the predictability of a disease by a diagnostic test is shown in Table 20.16. A true positive, represented by a indicates that the laboratory test correctly predicted the disease, whereas a false positive, represented by b, shows that the laboratory test incorrectly predicted that the patient had the disease when, in fact, the patient did not have the disease. In contrast, a true negative, represented by d, correctly gave a negative test in patients without the disease, whereas a false negative, represented by c, incorrectly gave a negative test when, in fact, the patient did have the disease.

CLINICAL EXAMPLE

A new diagnostic test for HIV$^+$/AIDS was developed and tested in 5772 intravenous drug users. The results of this study are tabulated in Table 20.17. From the results in

TABLE 20.16 Errors in Decision Predictability

	DIAGNOSTIC TEST RESULT		
DECISION	**Disease Present**	**Disease Absent**	**TOTALS**
Accept disease Present	Test positive (True positive) a	Test positive (False positive) b	$a + b$
Reject disease Present	Test negative (False negative) c	Test negative (True negative) d	$c + d$
Totals	$a + c$	$b + d$	$a + b + c + d$

TABLE 20.17   Results of HIV^+/AIDS Test

DECISION	DIAGNOSTIC TEST RESULT		TOTALS
	Disease Present	Disease Absent	
Accept HIV^+/AIDS Present	2756	107	2863
Reject HIV^+/AIDS Present	211	2698	2909
Totals	2967	2805	5772

Table 20.17, a total of 2863 subjects had a positive diagnostic test for HIV^+/AIDS and 2909 subjects had a negative diagnostic test for HIV^+/AIDS. Further tests on these subjects showed that 2967 subjects actually had HIV^+/AIDS, although 211 of these subjects had negative diagnostic test results. Moreover, 107 subjects who had a positive diagnostic test result did not, in fact, have HIV^+/AIDS after further tests were made.

1. The *positive predictability* of the test is the likelihood that the test will correctly predict the disease if the test is positive and is estimated as

$$\text{Positive predictability} = \frac{a}{a+b} = \frac{2756}{2863} = 0.963 \qquad (96.3\%)$$

2. The *negative predictability* of the test is the likelihood that the patient will not have the disease if the test is negative and is estimated as

$$\text{Negative predictability} = \frac{d}{c+d} = \frac{2698}{2909} = 0.927 \qquad (92.7\%)$$

3. The *total predictability* of the test is the likelihood that the patient will be predicted correctly and is estimated as

$$\text{Total predictability} = \frac{a+d}{a+b+c+d} = \frac{2756+2698}{5772} = 0.945 \qquad (94.5\%)$$

4. The *sensitivity* of the test is the likelihood that a test result will be positive in a patient with the disease and is estimated as

$$\text{Sensitivity} = \frac{a}{a+c} = \frac{2756}{2967} = 0.929 \qquad (92.9\%)$$

5. The *specificity* of the test is the likelihood that a test result will be negative in a patient without the disease and is estimated as

$$\text{Specificity} = \frac{d}{b+d} = \frac{2698}{2805} = 0.962 \qquad (96.2\%)$$

Analysis of the results in Table 20.17 shows that a positive result from the new test for HIV^+/AIDS will only predict the disease correctly 94.5% of the time. Therefore, the clinician must use other measures to predict whether the patient has the disease. These other measures may include physical diagnosis of the patient, other laboratory tests, normal incidence of the disease in the patient population (in this case, intravenous drug users), and the experience of the clinician. Each test has different predictive values.

REGIONAL PHARMACOKINETICS

Pharmacokinetics is the study of the time course of drug concentrations in the body. Pharmacokinetics is based generally on the time course of drug concentrations in systemic blood sampled from either a vein or an artery. This general approach is useful as long as the drug concentrations in the tissues of the body are well reflected by drug concentrations in the blood. Clinically, the blood drug concentration may not be proportional to the drug concentration in tissues. For example, after IV bolus administration, the distributive phase is attributed to temporally different changes in mixing and redistribution of drug in organs such as the lung, heart, and kidney (Upton, 1990). The time course for the pharmacodynamics of the drug may have no relationship to the time course for the drug concentrations in the blood. The pharmacodynamics of the drug may be related to local tissue drug levels and the status of homeostatic physiologic functions. After an IV bolus dose, Upton (1990) reported that lignocaine (lidocaine) rapidly accumulates in the spleen and kidney but is slowly sequestered into fat. More than 30 minutes were needed before the target-site (heart and brain) drug levels established equilibrium with drug concentrations in the blood. These *regional equilibrium factors* are often masked in conventional pharmacokinetic models that assume rapid drug equilibrium.

Regional pharmacokinetics is the study of pharmacokinetics within a given tissue region. The tissue region is defined as an anatomic area of the body between specified afferent and efferent blood vessels. For example, the myocardium includes the region perfused by the coronary arterial (afferent) and the coronary sinus (efferent) blood vessels. The selection of a region bounded by its network of blood vessel is based on the movement of drug between the blood vessels and the interstitial and intracellular spaces of the region. The conventional pharmacokinetic approach for calculating systemic clearance and volume of distribution tends to average various drug distributions together, such that the local perturbations are neglected. Regional pharmacokinetics (see Mather, 1991, chap. 10) supplement systemic pharmacokinetics when inadequate information is provided by conventional pharmacokinetics.

Various homeostatic physiologic functions may be responsible for the nonequilibrium of drug concentrations between local tissue regions and the blood. For example, most cells have an electrochemical difference across the cell membrane consisting of a membrane potential of negative 70 mV inside the membrane relative to the outside. Moreover, regional differences in pH normally exist within a cell. For example, the pH within the lysosome is between 4 and 5, which could allow a basic drug to accumulate within the lysosome with a concentration gradient of 400-fold to 160,000-fold over the blood. Other explanations for regional drug concentration differences have been reviewed by Upton (1990), who also considers that dynamic processes may be more important than equilibrium processes in affecting dynamic response. Thus, regional pharmacokinetics is another approach in applying pharmacokinetics to pharmacodynamics and clinical effect.

FREQUENTLY ASKED QUESTIONS

1. Can therapeutic drug monitoring be performed without taking blood samples?
2. What is meant by population pharmacokinetics? What advantages does population pharmacokinetics have over classical pharmacokinetics?
3. What are the major considerations in therapeutic drug monitoring?
4. Why is it possible to estimate individual pharmacokinetic parameters with just a few data points using the Bayesian method?
5. Why is pharmacokinetics important in studying drug interactions?

LEARNING QUESTIONS

1. Why is it harder to titrate patients with a drug whose elimination half-life is 36 hours compared to a drug whose elimination is 6 hours?
2. Penicillin G has a volume of distribution of 42 L/1.73 m^2 and an elimination rate constant of 1.034 hr^{-1}. Calculate the maximum peak concentration that would be produced if the drug were given intravenously at a rate of 250 mg every 6 hours for a week.
3. Dicloxacillin has an elimination half-life of 42 minutes and a volume of distribution of 20 L. Dicloxacillin is 97% protein bound. What would be the steady-state free concentration of dicloxacillin if the drug were given intravenously at a rate of 250 mg every 6 hours?
4. The normal elimination half-life of cefamandole is 1.49 hours and the apparent volume of distribution (V_D) is 39.2% of body weight. The elimination half-life for a patient with a creatinine clearance of 15 mL/min was reported by Czerwinski and Pederson (1979) to be 6.03 hour, and cefamandole's V_D is 23.75% of body weight. What doses of cefamandole should be given the normal and the uremic patient (respectively) if the drug is administered intravenously every 6 hours and the desired objective is to maintain an average steady concentration of 2 μg/mL?
5. The maintenance dose of digoxin was reported to be 0.5 mg/day for a 60-kg patient with normal renal function. The half-life of digoxin is 0.95 days and the volume of distribution is 306 L. The bioavailability of the digoxin tablet is 0.56.

   a. Calculate the steady-state concentration of digoxin.

   b. Determine whether the patient is adequately dosed (effective serum digoxin concentration is 1–2 ng/mL).

   c. What is the steady-state concentration if the patient is dosed with the elixir instead of the tablet? (Assume the elixir to be 100% bioavailable.)

  6. An antibiotic has an elimination half-life of 2 hours and an apparent volume of distribution of 200 mL/kg. The minimum effective serum concentration is 2 μg/mL and the minimum toxic serum concentration is 16 μg/mL. A physician ordered a dosage regimen of this antibiotic to be given at 250 mg every 8 hours by repetitive intravenous bolus injections.

   a. Comment on the appropriateness of this dosage regimen for an adult male patient (23 years, 80 kg) whose creatinine clearance is 122 mL/min.

   b. Would you suggest an alternative dosage regimen for this patient? Give your reasons and suggest an alternative dosage regimen.

  7. Gentamycin (Garamycin, Schering) is a highly water-soluble drug. The dosage of this drug in obese patients should be based on an estimate of the lean body mass or ideal body weight. Why?

  8. Why is the calculation for the loading dose (D_L) for a drug based on the apparent volume of distribution, whereas the calculation of the maintenance dose is based on the elimination rate constant?

  9. A potent drug with a narrow therapeutic index is ordered for a patient. After making rounds, the attending physician observes that the patient is not responding to drug therapy and orders a single plasma-level measurement. Comment briefly on the value of measuring the drug concentration in a single blood sample and on the usefulness of the information that may be gained.

 10. Calculate an oral dosage regimen for a cardiotonic drug for an adult male (63 years old, 68 kg) with normal renal function. The elimination half-life for this drug is 30 hours and its apparent volume of distribution is 4 L/kg. The drug is 80% bioavailable when given orally, and the suggested therapeutic serum concentrations for this drug range from 0.001 to 0.002 μg/mL.

   a. This cardiotonic drug is commercially supplied as 0.075-mg, 0.15-mg, and 0.30-mg white, scored, compressed tablets. Using these readily available tablets, what dose would you recommend for this patient?

   b. Are there any advantages for this patient to give smaller doses more frequently compared to a higher dosage less frequently? Any disadvantages?

   c. Would you suggest a loading dose for this drug? Why? What loading dose would you recommend?

   d. Is there a rationale for preparing a controlled-release product of this drug?

 11. The dose of sulfisoxazole (Gantrisin, Roche) recommended for an adult female patient (age 26, 63 kg) with a urinary tract infection was 1.5 g every 4 hours. The drug is 85% bound to serum proteins. The elimination half-life of this drug is 6 hours and the apparent volume of distribution is 1.3 L/kg. Sulfisoxazole is 100% bioavailable.

   a. Calculate the steady-state plasma concentration of sulfisoxazole in this patient.

   b. Calculate an appropriate loading dose of sulfisoxazole for this patient.

   c. Gantrisin (sulfisoxazole) is supplied in tablets containing 0.5 g of drug. How many tablets would you recommend for the loading dose?

d. If no loading dose was given, how long would it take to achieve 95–99% of steady state?

12. The desired plasma level for an antiarrhythmic agent is 5 $\mu g/mL$. The drug has an apparent volume of distribution of 173 mL/kg and an elimination half-life of 2.0 hours. The kinetics of the drug follow the kinetics of a one-compartment open model.

    a. An adult male patient (75 kg, 56 years of age) is to be given an IV injection of this drug. What loading dose (D_L) and infusion rate (R) would you suggest?

    b. The patient did not respond very well to drug therapy. Plasma levels of drug were measured and found to be 2 $\mu g/mL$. How would you readjust the infusion rate to increase the plasma drug level to the desired 5 $\mu g/mL$?

    c. How long would it take to achieve 95% of steady-state plasma drug levels in this patient assuming no loading dose was given and the apparent V_D was unaltered?

13. An antibiotic is to be given to an adult male patient (75 kg, 58 years of age) by intravenous infusion. The elimination half-life for this drug is 8 hours and the apparent volume of distribution is 1.5 L/kg. The drug is supplied in 30-mL ampules at a concentration of 15 mg/mL. The desired steady-state serum concentration for this antibiotic is 20 mg/mL.

    a. What infusion rate (R) would you suggest for this patient?

    b. What loading dose would you suggest for this patient?

    c. If the manufacturer suggests a starting infusion rate of 0.2 mL/hr per kilogram of body weight, what is the expected steady-state serum concentration in this patient?

    d. You would like to verify that this patient received the proper infusion rate. At what time after the start of the IV infusion would you take a blood sample to monitor the serum antibiotic concentration? Why?

    e. Assume that the serum antibiotic concentration was measured and found to be higher than anticipated. What reasons, based on sound pharmacokinetic principles, would account for this situation?

14. Nomograms are frequently used in lieu of pharmacokinetic calculations to determine an appropriate drug dosage regimen for a patient. Discuss the advantages and disadvantages for using nomograms to calculate a drug dosage regimen.

15. Based on the following pharmacokinetic data for drugs A, B, and C: **(a)** Which drug takes the longest time to reach steady state? **(b)** Which drug would achieve the highest steady-state drug concentration? **(c)** Which drug has the largest apparent volume of distribution?

	Drug A	Drug B	Drug C
Rate of infusion (mg/hr)	10	20	15
k (hr^{-1})	0.5	0.1	0.05
Cl (L/hr)	5	20	5

16. The effect of repetitive administration of phenytoin (PHT) on the single-dose pharmacokinetics of primidone (PRM) was investigated by Sato et al (1992) in three healthy male subjects. The peak concentration of unchanged PRM was achieved at 12 and 8 hours after the administration of PRM in the absence and the presence of PHT, respectively. The elimination half-life of PRM was decreased from 19.4 ± 2.2 (mean $\pm$ SE) to 10.2 ± 5.1 hours ($p < 0.05$) and the total body clearance was increased from 24.6 ± 3.1 to 45.1 ± 5.1 ml/hr/kg ($p < 0.01$) in the presence of PHT. No significant change was observed for the apparent volume of distribution between the two treatments. Based on pharmacokinetics of the two drugs, what are the possible reasons for phenytoin to reduce primidone elimination half-life and increase its renal clearance?

17. Traconazole (Sporanox, Janssen) is a lipophilic drug with extensive lipid distribution. The drug levels in fatty tissue and organs contains 2 to 20 times the drug levels in the plasma. Little or no drug was found in the saliva and in the cerebrospinal fluid and the half-life is 64 ± 32 hours. The drug is 99.8% bound. How does **(a)** plasma drug protein binding, **(b)** tissue drug distribution, and **(c)** lipid tissue partitioning contribute to the long elimination half-life for traconazole?

18. JL (29-year-old male, 180 kg) received oral ofloxacin 400 mg twice a day for presumed bronchitis due to *S. pneumoniae*. His other medications were the following: 400 mg cimetidine, orally, three times a day; 400 mg metronidazole, as directed. JL was still having a fever of 100.1°C a day after taking the quinolone antibiotic. Comment on any appropriate action.

19. CK (70-year-old male, 177 lb). Scr = 0.9 mg/dL. Allergy: PCN. Claudication, rhinitis: URI infection. His medication includes: Ilosone, 250 QID $\times$ 1 wk; Trental, 200 mg TID; Colace, 100 mg BID; Seldane, 1 TID PRN. Which of the following should the pharmacist conclude from this information?

a. There is an interaction between colace and seldane.

b. The dose of Trental is too high for this patient based on his renal function.

c. Seldane should be substituted with a therapeutic alternative because of an interaction.

REFERENCES

Abernethy DR: Drug therapy in the elderly. In Atkinson AJ, Daniels C, Dedrick R, et al (eds), *Principles of Clinical Pharmacology*. New York, Academic, 2001, chap 24

Abernethy DR, Greenblatt DJ: Pharmacokinetics of drugs in obesity. *Clin Pharmacokinet* **7**:108–124, 1982

Beal SL, Sheiner LB: The NONMEM system, AM. *Statistics* **34**:118–119, 1980

Beal SL, Sheiner LB: Methodology of population pharmacokinetics. In Garrett ER, Hirtz JL (eds), *Drug Fate and Metabolism: Methods and Techniques*, vol 5. New York, Marcel Dekker, 1985

Blouin RA, Warren GW: Pharmacokinetic considerations in obesity. *J Pharm Sci* **88**:1–7, 1999

Czerwinski AW, Pederson JA: Pharmacokinetics of cefamandole in patients with renal impairment. *Antimicrob Agents Chemother* **15**:161–164, 1979

D'Argenio DZ, Schumitzky A: A program package for simulation and parameter estimation in pharmacokinetic systems. *Comput Prog Biomed* **9**:115–134, 1979

DeHaan RM, Metzler CM, Schellenberg D, et al: Pharmacokinetic study of clindamycin hydrochloride in humans. *Int J Clin Pharmacol Biopharm* **6**:105–119, 1972

Erikson LO, Wahlin Boll-E, Odar Cederlof I, Lindholm L, Melander A: Influence of renal failure, rheumatoid arthritis and old age on the pharmacokinetics of diflunisal. *Eur J Clin Pharmacol* **36**(2):165–174, 1989

Evans WE, Schentag JJ, Jusko WJ: *Applied Pharmacokinetics. Principles of Therapeutic Drug Monitoring.* San Francisco, Applied Therapeutics, 1992

FDA Guidance for Industry: E11 Clinical investigation of medicinal products in the pediatric population. ICH, December, 2000.

Greenblatt DJ: Predicting steady state serum concentration of drugs. *Annu Rev Pharmacol Toxicol* **19**:347–356, 1979

Haverkos HW, Amsel Z, Drotman DP: Adverse virus–drug interactions. *Rev Infect Dis* **13**:697–704, 1991

Heden B, Ohlsson M, Rittner R, et al: Agreement between artificial neural networks and experienced electrocardiographer on electrocardiographic diagnosis of healed myocardial infarction. *J Am Coll Cardiol* **28**(4): 1012–1016, 1996

Hedman A, Angelin B, Arvidsson A, Beck O, Dahlqvist R, Nilsson B, Olsson M, Schenck-Gustafsson K: Digoxin–verapamil interaction: Reduction of biliary but not renal digoxin clearance in humans. *Clin Pharmacol Ther* **49**(3):256–262, 1991

Hendeles L, Weinberger M: Avoidance of adverse effects during chronic therapy with theophylline. *Drug Intell Clin Pharm* **14**:523, 1980

Hurley SF, McNeil JF: A comparison of the accuracy of a least-squares regression, a Bayesian, Chiou's and the steady state clearance method of individualizing theophylline dosage. *Clin Pharmacokinet* **14**:311–320, 1988

Iafrate RP, Glotz VP, Robinson JD, Lupkiewicz SM: Computer simulated conversion from intravenous to sustained-release oral theophylline drug. *Intell Clin Pharm* **16**:19–25, 1982

Landahl S, et al: Pharmacokinetics and blood pressure effects of felodipine in elderly hypertensive patients—A comparison with the young healthy subjects. *Clin Pharmacokinet* **14**:374–383, 1988

Lima DR, Santos RM, Werneck E, Andrade GN: Effect of orally administered misoprostol and cimetidine on the steady-state pharmacokinetics of diazepam and nordiazepam in human volunteers. *Eur J Drug Metab Pharmacokinet* **16**(3):61–70, 1991

Lindeman RD: Changes in renal function with aging. Implications for treatment. *Drugs Aging* **2**:423–431, 1992

Lindeman RD, Tobin J, Shock NW: Longitudinal studies on the rate of decline in renal function with age. *J Am Geriatr Soc* **33**:278–285, 1985

Ludden TM, Beal SL, Sheiner LB: Comparison of the Akaike Information Criterion, the Schwarz criterion and the F test as guides to model selection. *J Pharmacokinet Biopharm* **22**(5):431–445, 1994

Mawer GE: Computer assisted prescribing of drugs. *Clin Pharmacokinet* **1**:67–78, 1976

Mayersohn M: Pharmacokinetics in the elderly. *Environ Health Perspect Suppl* vol 102, suppl 11, 1994 (http://ehp.niehs.nih.gov/members/1994/Suppl-11/mayersohn-full.html)

Mentre F, Gomeni R: A two-step iterative algorithm for estimation in nonlinear mixed-effect models with an evaluation in population pharmacokinetics. *J Biopharm Stat* **5**(2):141–158, 1995

Mungall DR, Ludden TM, Marsh II J, Hawkin DW, Talbert RL, Crawford MH: Population pharmacokinetics of racemic warfarin in adult patients. *J Pharmacokinet Biopharm* **13**(3):213–227, 1985

National Institutes of Health, National Heart, Lung and Blood Institute: Clinical guidelines on the identification, evaluation and treatment of overweight and obesity in adults: The evidence report, 2003. (www.nhlb.nih.gov/obesity/ob-home.htm)

Okuno H, Takasu M, Kano H, Seki T, Shiozaki Y, Inoue K: Depression of drug metabolizing activity in the human liver by interferon-beta. *Hepatology* **17**(1):65–69, 1993

Perucca E, Gatti G, Cipolla G, Spina E, Barel S, Soback S, Gips M, Bialer M: Inhibition of diazepam metabolism by fluvoxamine: A pharmacokinetic study in normal volunteers. *Clin Pharmacol Ther* **56**(5):471–476, 1994

Regamey C, Gordon RC, Kirby WMM: Comparative pharmacokinetics of tobramycin and gentamicin. *Clin Pharmacol Ther* **14**:396–403, 1973

Sato J, Sekizawa Y, Yoshida A, Owada E, Sakuta N. Yoshihara M, Goto T, Kobayashi Y, Ito K: Single-dose kinetics of primidone in human subjects: Effect of phenytoin on formation and elimination of active metabolites of primidone, phenobarbital and phenylethylmalonamide. *J Pharmacobiodyn* **15**(9):467–472, 1992

Schellens JH, Ghabrial H, van-der-Wart HH, Bakker EN, Wilkinson GR, Breimer DD: Differential effects of quinidine on the disposition of nifedipine, sparteine, and mephenytoin in humans. *Clin Pharmacol Ther* **50**(5 pt 1):520–528, 1991

Schumucker DL: Aging and drug disposition: An update. *Pharmacol Rev* **37**:133–148, 1985a

Schumacher GE: Choosing optimal sampling times for therapeutic drug monitoring. *Clin Pharm* **4**:84–92, 1985b

Schumacker GE: *Therapeutic Drug Monitoring.* Norwalk, CT, Appleton & Lange, 1995

Sheiner LB, Beal SL: Bayesian individualization of pharmacokinetics. Simple implementation and comparison with nonBayesian methods. *J Pharm Sci* **71**:1344–1348, 1982

Sheiner LB, Ludden TM: Population pharmacokinetics/dynamics. *Annu Rev Pharmacol Toxicol* **32**:185–209, 1992

Smith BP, Brier ME: Statistical approach to neural network model building for gentamicin peak predictions. *J Pharm Sci* **85**(1):65–69, 1996

Spence JD: Drug interactions with grapefruit: Whose responsibility is it to warn the public? *Clin Pharmacol Ther* **61**:395–400, 1997

Stein GE, Haughey DB, Ross RJ, Vakoutis J: Conversion from intravenous to oral dosing using sustained release theophylline tablets. *Clin Pharm* **1**:772–773, 1982

Thomson AH, Whiting B: Bayesian parameter estimation and population pharmacokinetics. *Clin Pharmacokinet* **22**(6):447–467, 1992

Upton RN: Regional pharmacokinetics, I. Physiological and physicochemical basis. *Biopharm Drug Disp* **11**:647–662, 1990

Vozeh S, Wenk M, Follath F: Experience with NONMEM: Analysis of serum concentration data in patients treated with mexiletine and lidocaine. *Drug Metab Rev* **15**:305–315, 1984

West JR, Smith HW, Chasis H: Glomerular filtration rate, effective blood flow and maximal tubular excretory capacity in infancy. *J Pediatr* **32**:10, 1948

Whiting B, Kelman AW, Grevel J: Population pharmacokinetics: Theory and clinical application. *Clin Pharmacokin* **11**:387–401, 1986

Whiting B, Niven AA, Kelman AW, Thomson AH: A Bayesian kinetic control strategy for cyclosporin in renal transplantation. In D'Argenio DZ (ed), *Advanced Methods of Pharmacokinetic and Pharmacodynamic Systems Analysis.* New York, Plenum, 1991

BIBLIOGRAPHY

Abernethy DR, Azarnoff DL: Pharmacokinetic investigations in elderly patients. Clinical and ethical considerations. *Clin Pharmacokinet* **19**:89–93, 1990

Abernethy DR, Greenblatt DJ, Divoll M, et al: Alterations in drug distribution and clearance due to obesity. *J Pharmacol Exp Ther* **217**:681–685, 1981

Anderson KE: Influences of diet and nutrition on clinical pharmacokinetics. *Clin Pharmacokinet* **14**:325–346, 1988

Aranda JV, Stern L: Clinical aspects of developmental pharmacology and toxicology. *Pharmacol Ther* **20**:1–51, 1983

Atkinson AJ, Daniels CE, Dedrick RL, Grudzinskas CV, Markey SP: *Principles of Clinical Pharmacology.* New York, Academic, 2001

Beal SL: *NONMEM Users Guide VII: Conditional Estimation Methods.* San Francisco, NONMEM Project Group, University of California, San Francisco, 1992

Benet LZ (ed): *The Effect of Disease States on Drug Pharmacokinetics.* Washington, DC, American Pharmaceutical Association, 1976

Benowitz NL, Meister W: Pharmacokinetics in patients with cardiac failure. *Clin Pharmacokinet* **1**:389–405, 1976

Besunder JB, Reed MD, Blumer JL: Principles of drug biodisposition in the neonate: A critical evaluation of the pharmacokinetic–pharmacodynamic interface, Part I. *Clin Pharmacokinet* **14**:189–216, 1988

Chiou WL, Gadalla MAF, Pang GW: Method for the rapid estimation of total body clearance and adjustment of dosage regimens in patients during a constant-rate infusion. *J Pharmacokinet Biopharm* **6**:135–151, 1978

Chrystyn H, Ellis JW, Mulley BA, Peak MD: The accuracy and stability of Bayesian theophylline predictions. *Ther Drug Monit* **10**:299–303, 1988

Clinical Symposium on Drugs and the Unborn Child. *Clin Pharmacol Ther* **14**:621–770, 1973

Crooks J, O'Malley K, Stevenson IH: Pharmacokinetics in the elderly. *Clin Pharmacokinet* **1**:280–296, 1976

Crouthamel WG: The effect of congestive heart failure on quinidine pharmacokinetics. *Am Heart J* **90**:335, 1975

DeVane CL, Jusko WJ: Dosage regimen design. *Pharmacol Ther* **17**:143–163, 1982

Dimascio A, Shader RI: Drug administration schedules. *Am J Psychiatry* **126**:6, 1969

Friis-Hansen B: Body-water compartments in children: Changes during growth and related changes in body composition. *Pediatrics* **28**:169–181, 1961

Giacoia GP, Gorodisher R: Pharmacologic principles in neonatal drug therapy. *Clin Perinatol* **2**:125–138, 1975

Gillis AM, Kates R: Clinical pharmacokinetics of the newer antiarrhythmic agents. *Clin Pharmacokinet* **9**:375–403, 1984

Godley PJ, Black JT, Frohna PA, Garrelts JC: Comparison of a Bayesian program with three microcomputer programs for predicting gentamicin concentrations. *Ther Drug Monit* **10**:287–291, 1988

Gomeni R, Pineau G, Mentre F: Population kinetics and conditional assessment of the optimal dosage regimen using the P-pharm software package. *Cancer Res* **14**:2321–2326, 1994

Grasela TH, Sheiner LB: Population pharmacokinetics of procainamide from routine clinical data. *Clin Pharmacokinet* **9**:545, 1984

Gross G, Perrier CV: Intrahepatic portasystemic shunting in cirrhotic patients. *N Engl J Med* **293**:1046, 1975

Harnes HT, Shiu G, Shah VP: Validation of bioanalytical methods. *Pharm Res* **8**:421–426, 1991

Holloway DA: Drug problems in the geriatric patient. *Drug Intell Clin Pharm* **8**:632–642, 1974

Jaehde U, Sorgel F, Stephan U, Schunack W: Effect of an antacid containing magnesium and aluminum on absorption, metabolism, and mechanism of renal elimination of pefloxacin in humans. *Antimicrob Agents Chemother* **38**(5):1129–1133, 1994

Jensen EH: Current concepts for the validation of compendial assays. *Pharmacopoeial Forum* March–April: 1241–1245, 1986

Jusko WJ: Pharmacokinetic principles in pediatric pharmacology. *Pediatr Clin N Am* **19**:81–100, 1972

Kamimori GH, Somani SM, kawlton RG Perkins RM et al: The effects of obesity and exercise on the pharmacokinetics of caffeine in lean and obese volunteers. *Eur J Clin Pharmacol* **31**:595–600, 1987

Klotz U, Avant GR, Hoyumpa A, et al: The effects of age and liver disease on the disposition and elimination of diazepam in adult man. *J Clin Invest* **55**:347, 1975

Krasner J, Giacoia GP, Yaffe SJ: Drug–protein binding in the newborn infant. *Ann NY State Acad Sci* **226**:102–114, 1973

Kristensen M, Hansen JM, Kampmann J, et al: Drug elimination and renal function. *Int J Clin Pharmacol Biopharm* **14**:307–308, 1974

Latini R, Bonati M, Tognoni G: Clinical role of blood levels. *Ther Drug Monit* **2**:3–9, 1980

Latini R, Maggioni AP, Cavalli A: Therapeutic drug monitoring of antiarrhythmic drugs. Rationale and current status. *Clin Pharmacokinet* **18**:91–103, 1990

Lehmann K, Merten K: Die Elimination von Lithium in Abhangigkeit vom Lebensalten bei Gesunden und Niereninsuffizienten. *Int J Clin Pharmacol Biopharm* **10**:292–298, 1974

Levy G (ed): *Clinical Pharmacokinetics: A Symposium.* Washington, DC, American Pharmaceutical Association, 1974

Ludden TM: Population pharmacokinetics. *J Clin Pharmacol* **28**:1059–1063, 1988

Matzke GR, St Peter WL: Clinical pharmacokinetics 1990. *Clin Pharmacokinet* **18**:1–19, 1990

Maxwell GM: Paediatric drug dosing. Body weight versus surface area. *Drugs* **37**:113–115, 1989

Meister W, Benowitz NL, Melmon KL, Benet LZ: Influence of cardiac failure on the pharmacokinetics of digoxin. *Clin Pharmacol Ther* **23**:122, 1978

Mentre F, Pineau, Gomeni R: Population kinetics and conditional assessment of the optimal dosage regimen using the P-Pharm software package. *Anticancer Res* **14**:2321–2326, 1994

Morley PC, Strand LM: Critical reflections on therapeutic drug monitoring. *J Pharm Pract* **2**:327–334, 1989

Morselli PL: Clinical pharmacokinetics in neonates. *Clin Pharmacokinet* **1**:81–98, 1976

Mungall DR: *Applied Clinical Pharmacokinetics.* New York, Raven, 1983

Neal EA, Meffin PJ, Gregory PB, Blaschke TF: Enhanced bioavailability and decreased clearance of analgesics in patients with cirrhosis. *Gastroenterology* **77**:96, 1979

Niebergall PJ, Sugita ET, Schnaare RL: Potential dangers of common drug dosing regimens. *Am J Hosp Pharm* **31**:53–58, 1974

Rane A, Sjoquist F: Drug metabolism in the human fetus and newborn infant. *Pediatr Clin N Am* **19**:37–49, 1972

Rane A, Wilson JT: Clinical pharmacokinetics in infants and children. *Clin Pharmacokinet* **1**:2–24, 1976

Richey DP, Bender DA: Pharmacokinetic consequences of aging. *Annu Rev Pharmacol Toxicol* **17**:49–65, 1977

Roberts J, Tumer N: Age and diet effects on drug action. *Pharmacol Ther* **37**:111–149, 1988

Rowland M, Tozer TN: *Clinical Pharmacokinetics Concepts and Applications.* Philadelphia, Lea & Febiger, 1980

Schumacher GE, Barr JT: Pharmacokinetics in drug therapy. Bayesian approaches in pharmacokinetic decision making. *Clin Pharm* **3**:525–530, 1984

Schumacher GE, Barr JT: Applying decision analysis in therapeutic drug monitoring: Using decision trees to interpret serum theophylline concentrations. *Clin Pharm* **5**:325–333, 1986

Schumacher GE, Barr JT: Making serum drug levels more meaningful. *Ther Drug Monit* **11**:580–584, 1989

Schumacher GE, Griener JC: Using Pharmacokinetics in drug therapy II. Rapid estimates of dosage regimens and blood levels without knowledge of pharmacokinetic variables. *Am J Hosp Pharm* **35**:454–459, 1978

Sheiner LB, Benet LZ: Premarketing observational studies of population pharmacokinetics of new drugs. *Clin Pharmacol Ther* **35**:481–487, 1985

Sheiner LB, Rosenberg B, Marathe V: Estimation of population characteristics of pharmacokinetic parameters from routine clinical data. *J Pharmacokinet Biopharm* **9**:445–479, 1977

Shirkey HC: Dosage (dosology). In Shirkey HC (ed), *Pediatric Therapy.* St. Louis, Mosby, 1975, pp 19–33

Spector R, Park GD, Johnson GF, Vessell ES: Therapeutic drug monitoring. *Clin Pharmacol Ther* **43**:345–353, 1988

Thompson PD, Melmon KL, Richardson JA, et al: Lidocaine pharmacokinetics in advanced heart failure, liver disease, and renal failure in humans. *Ann Intern Med* **78**:499–508, 1973

Thomson AH: Bayesian feedback methods for optimizing therapy. *Clin Neuropharmacol* **15**(suppl 1, part A):245A–246A, 1992

Uematsu T, Hirayama H, Nagashima S, et al: Prediction of individual dosage requirements for lignocaine. A validation study for Bayesian forecasting in Japanese patients. *Ther Drug Monit* **11**:25–31, 1989

Vestel RE: Drug use in the elderly: A review of problems and special considerations. *Drugs* **16**:358–382, 1978

Vonesh EF, Carter RL: Mixed-effects nonlinear regression for unbalanced repeated measures. *Biometrics* **48**:1–17, 1992

Williams RW, Benet LZ: Drug pharmacokinetics in cardiac and hepatic disease. *Annu Rev Pharmacol Toxicol* **20**:289, 1980

Winter ME: *Basic Clinical Pharmacokinetics.* San Francisco, Applied Therapeutics, 1980

Yuen GJ, Beal SL, Peck CC: Predicting phenytoin dosages using Bayesian feedback. A comparison with other methods. *Ther Drug Monit* **5**:437–441, 1983

21

DOSE ADJUSTMENT IN RENAL AND HEPATIC DISEASE

RENAL IMPAIRMENT

The kidney is an important organ in regulating body fluids, electrolyte balance, removal of metabolic waste, and drug excretion from the body. Impairment or degeneration of kidney function affects the pharmacokinetics of drugs. Some of the more common causes of kidney failure include disease, injury, and drug intoxication. Table 21.1 lists some of the conditions that may lead to chronic or acute renal failure. Acute diseases or trauma to the kidney can cause *uremia*, in which glomerular filtration is impaired or reduced, leading to accumulation of excessive fluid and blood nitrogenous products in the body. Uremia generally reduces glomerular filtration and/or active secretion, which leads to a decrease in renal drug excretion resulting in a longer elimination half-life of the administered drug.

In addition to changing renal elimination directly, uremia can affect drug pharmacokinetics in unexpected ways. For example, declining renal function leads to disturbances in electrolyte and fluid balance, resulting in physiologic and metabolic changes that may alter the pharmacokinetics and pharmacodynamics of a drug. Pharmacokinetic processes such as drug distribution (including both the volume of distribution and protein binding) and elimination (including both biotransformation and renal excretion) may also be altered by renal impairment. Both therapeutic and toxic responses may be altered as a result of changes in drug sensitivity at the receptor site. Overall, uremic patients have special dosing considerations to account for such pharmacokinetic and pharmacodynamic alterations.

PHARMACOKINETIC CONSIDERATIONS

Uremic patients may exhibit pharmacokinetic changes in bioavailability, volume of distribution, and clearance. The oral bioavailability of a drug in severe uremia

673

TABLE 21.1 Common Causes of Kidney Failure

Pyelonephritis	Inflammation and deterioration of the pyelonephrons due to infection, antigens, or other idiopathic causes.
Hypertension	Chronic overloading of the kidney with fluid and electrolytes may lead to kidney insufficiency.
Diabetes mellitus	The disturbance of sugar metabolism and acid-base balance may lead to or predispose a patient to degenerative renal disease.
Nephrotoxic drugs/metals	Certain drugs taken chronically may cause irreversible kidney damage—eg, the aminoglycosides, phenacetin, and heavy metals, such as mercury and lead.
Hypovolemia	Any condition that causes a reduction in renal blood flow will eventually lead to renal ischemia and damage.
Neophroallergens	Certain compounds may produce an immune type of sensitivity reaction with nephritic syndrome—eg, quartan malaria nephrotoxic serum.

may be decreased as a result of disease-related changes in gastrointestinal motility and pH caused by nausea, vomiting, and diarrhea. Mesenteric blood flow may also be altered. However, the oral bioavailability of a drug such as propranolol (which has a high first-pass effect) may be increased in patients with renal impairment as a result of the decrease in first-pass hepatic metabolism (Bianchetti et al, 1978).

The apparent volume of distribution depends largely on drug protein binding in plasma or tissues and total body water. Renal impairment may alter the distribution of the drug as a result of changes in fluid balance, drug protein binding, or other factors that may cause changes in the apparent volume of distribution (see Chapter 10). The plasma protein binding of weak acidic drugs in uremic patients is decreased, whereas the protein binding of weak basic drugs is less affected. The decrease in drug protein binding results in a larger fraction of free drug and an increase in the volume of distribution. However, the net elimination half-life is generally increased as a result of the dominant effect of reduced glomerular filtration. Protein binding of the drug may be further compromised due to the accumulation of metabolites of the drug and accumulation of various biochemical metabolites, such as free fatty acids and urea, which may compete for the protein-binding sites for the active drug.

Total body clearance of drugs in uremic patients is also reduced by either a decrease in the glomerular filtration rate and possibly active tubular secretion or reduced hepatic clearance resulting from a decrease in intrinsic hepatic clearance.

In clinical practice, estimation of the appropriate drug dosage regimen in patients with impaired renal function is based on an estimate of the remaining renal function of the patient and a prediction of the total body clearance. A complete pharmacokinetic analysis of the drug in the uremic patient is not possible. Moreover, the patient's uremic condition may not be stable and may be changing too rapidly for pharmacokinetic analysis. Each of the approaches for the calculation of a dosage regimen have certain assumptions and limitations that must be carefully assessed by the clinician before any approach is taken. Dosing guidelines for individual drugs in patients with renal impairment may be found in various reference books, such as the *Physicians' Desk Reference,* and in the medical literature (Bennett 1988, 1990; St Peter et al, 1992).

GENERAL APPROACHES FOR DOSE ADJUSTMENT IN RENAL DISEASE

Several approaches are available for estimating the appropriate dosage regimen for a patient with renal impairment. Each of these approaches has similar assumptions, as listed in Table 21.2. Most of these methods assume that the required therapeutic plasma drug concentration in uremic patients is similar to that required in patients with normal renal function. Uremic patients are maintained on the same C_{av}^{∞} after multiple oral doses or multiple IV bolus injections. For IV infusions, the same C_{SS} is maintained. (C_{SS} is the same as C_{av}^{∞} after the plasma drug concentration reaches steady state.)

The design of dosage regimens for uremic patients is based on the pharmacokinetic changes that have occurred as a result of the uremic condition. Generally, drugs in patients with uremia or kidney impairment have prolonged elimination half-lives and a change in the apparent volume of distribution. In less severe uremic conditions there may be neither edema nor a significant change in the apparent volume of distribution. Consequently, the methods for dose adjustment in uremic patients are based on an accurate estimation of the drug clearance in these patients.

Several specific clinical approaches for the calculation of drug clearance based on monitoring kidney function are presented later in this chapter. Two general pharmacokinetic approaches for dose adjustment include methods based on drug clearance and methods based on the elimination half-life.

Dose Adjustment Based on Drug Clearance

Methods based on drug clearance try to maintain the desired C_{av}^{∞} after multiple oral doses or multiple IV bolus injections as total body clearance, Cl_T, changes. The calculation for C_{av}^{∞} is

$$C_{av}^{\infty} = \frac{FD_0}{Cl_T \tau} \qquad\qquad (21.1)$$

TABLE 21.2 Common Assumptions in Dosing Renal-Impaired Patients

ASUMPTION	COMMENT
Creatinine clearance accurately measures the degree of renal impairment	Creatinine clearance estimates may be biased. Renal impairment should also be verified by physical diagnosis and other clinical tests.
Drug follows dose-independent pharmacokinetics	Pharmacokinetics should not be dose-dependent (nonlinear).
Nonrenal drug elimination remains constant	Renal disease may also affect the liver and cause a change in nonrenal drug elimination (drug metabolism).
Drug absorption remains constant	Unchanged drug absorption from gastrointestinal tract.
Drug clearance, Cl_u, declines linearly with creatinine clearance, Cl_{Cr}	Normal drug clearance may include active secretion and passive filtration and may not decline linearly.
Unaltered drug protein binding	Drug protein binding may be altered due to accumulation of urea, nitrogenous wastes, and drug metabolites.
Target drug concentration remains constant	Changes in electrolyte composition such as potassium may affect sensitivity to the effect of digoxin. Accumulation of active metabolities may cause more intense pharmacodynamic response compared to parent drug alone.

For patients with a uremic condition or renal impairment, total body clearance of the uremic patient will change to a new value, Cl_T^u. Therefore, to maintain the same desired C_{av}^∞, the dose must be changed to a uremic dose, D_0^u or the dosage interval must be changed to τ^u, as shown in the following equation:

$$C_{av}^\infty = \underset{\text{(normal)}}{\frac{D_0^N}{Cl_T^N \tau^N}} = \underset{\text{(uremic)}}{\frac{D_0^u}{Cl_T^u \tau^u}} \tag{21.2}$$

where the superscripts N and u represent normal and uremic conditions, respectively. Rearranging Equation 21.2 and solving for D_0^u,

$$D_0^u = \frac{D_0^N Cl_T^u \tau^u}{Cl_T^N \tau^N} \tag{21.3}$$

If the dosage interval τ is kept constant, then the uremic dose D_0^u is equal to a fraction (Cl_T^u / Cl_T^N) of the normal dose, as shown in the equation

$$D_0^u = \frac{D_0^N Cl_T^u}{Cl_T^N} \tag{21.4}$$

For IV infusions the same desired C_{SS} is maintained both for patients with normal renal function and for patients with renal impairment. Therefore, the rate of infusion, R, must be changed to a new value, R^u, for the uremic patient, as described by the equation

$$C_{SS} = \underset{\text{(normal)}}{\frac{R}{Cl_T^N}} = \underset{\text{(uremic)}}{\frac{R^u}{Cl_T^u}} \tag{21.5}$$

Dose Adjustment Based on Changes in the Elimination Rate Constant

The overall elimination rate constant for many drugs is reduced in the uremic patient. A dosage regimen may be designed for the uremic patient either by reducing the normal dose of the drug and keeping the frequency of dosing (dosage interval) constant, or by decreasing the frequency of dosing (prolonging the dosage interval) and keeping the dose constant. Doses of drugs with a narrow therapeutic range should be reduced—particularly if the drug has accumulated in the patient prior to deterioration of kidney function.

The usual approach to estimating a multiple-dosage regimen in the normal patient is to maintain a desired C_{av}^∞, as shown in Equation 21.1. Assuming the V_D is the same in both normal and uremic patients and τ is constant, then the uremic dose D_0^u is a fraction (k^u / k^N) of the normal dose:

$$D_0^u = \frac{D_0^N k^u}{k^N} \tag{21.6}$$

When the elimination rate constant for a drug in the uremic patient cannot be determined directly, indirect methods are available to calculate the predicted elimination rate constant based on the renal function of the patient. The assumptions on which these dosage regimens are calculated include the following.

1. The renal elimination rate constant (k_R) decreases proportionately as renal function decreases. (Note that k_R is the same as k_e as used in previous chapters).

2. The nonrenal routes of elimination (primarily, the rate constant for metabolism) remain unchanged.

3. Changes in the renal clearance of the drug are reflected by changes in the creatinine clearance.

The overall elimination rate constant is the sum total of all the routes of elimination in the body, including the renal rate and the nonrenal rate constants:

$$k^u = k_{nr} + k_R^u \tag{21.7}$$

where k_{nr} is the nonrenal elimination rate constant and k_R is the renal excretion rate constant.

Renal clearance is the product of the apparent volume of distribution and the rate constant for renal excretion:

$$Cl_R^u = k_R^u V_D^u \tag{21.8}$$

Rearrangement of Equation 21.8 gives

$$k_R^u = Cl_R^u \frac{1}{V_D^u} \tag{21.9}$$

Assuming that the apparent volume of distribution and nonrenal routes of elimination do not change in uremia, then $k_{nr}^u = k_{nr}^N$ and $V_D^u = V_D^N$.

Substitution of Equation 21.9 into Equation 21.7 gives

$$k^u = k_{nr} + \frac{1}{V_D} Cl_R^u \tag{21.10}$$

From Equation 21.10, a change in the renal clearance, Cl_R^u, due to renal impairment will be reflected in a change in the overall elimination rate constant k_u. Because changes in the renal drug clearance cannot be assessed directly in the uremic patient, Cl_R^u is usually related to a measurement of kidney function by the glomerular filtration rate (GFR), which in turn is estimated by changes in the patient's creatinine clearance.

MEASUREMENT OF GLOMERULAR FILTRATION RATE

Several drugs and endogenous substances have been used as markers to measure GFR. These markers are carried to the kidney by the blood via the renal artery and are filtered at the glomerulus. Several criteria are necessary to use a drug to measure GFR:

1. The drug must be freely filtered at the glomerulus.
2. The drug must not be reabsorbed nor actively secreted by the renal tubules.
3. The drug should not be metabolized.
4. The drug should not bind significantly to plasma proteins.
5. The drug should not have an effect on the filtration rate nor alter renal function.
6. The drug should be nontoxic.
7. The drug may be infused in a sufficient dose to permit simple and accurate quantitation in plasma and in urine.

Therefore, the rate at which these drug markers are filtered from the blood into the urine per unit of time reflects the glomerular filtration rate of the kidney. Changes in GFR reflect changes in kidney function that may be diminished in uremic conditions.

Inulin, a fructose polysaccharide, fulfills most of the criteria listed above and is therefore used as a standard reference for the measurement of GFR. In practice, however, the use of inulin involves a time-consuming procedure in which inulin is given by intravenous infusion until a constant steady-state plasma level is obtained. Clearance of inulin may then be measured by the rate of infusion divided by the steady-state plasma inulin concentration. Although this procedure gives an accurate value for GFR, inulin clearance is not used frequently in clinical practice.

The clearance of creatinine is used most extensively as a measurement of GFR. *Creatinine* is an endogenous substance formed from creatine phosphate during muscle metabolism. Creatinine production varies with the age, weight, and gender of the individual. In humans, creatinine is filtered mainly at the glomerulus, with no tubular reabsorption. However, a small amount of creatinine may be actively secreted by the renal tubules, and the values of GFR obtained by the creatinine clearance tend to be higher than GFR measured by inulin clearance. Creatinine clearance tends to decrease in the elderly patient. As mentioned in Chapter 20, the physiologic changes due to aging may necessitate special considerations in administering drugs in the elderly.

Blood urea nitrogen (BUN) is a commonly used clinical diagnostic laboratory test for renal disease. Urea is the end product of protein catabolism and is excreted through the kidney. Normal BUN levels range from 10 to 20 mg/dL. Higher BUN levels generally indicate the presence of renal disease. However, other factors, such as excessive protein intake, reduced renal blood flow, hemorrhagic shock, or gastric bleeding, may affect increased BUN levels. The renal clearance of urea is by glomerular filtration and partial reabsorption in the renal tubules. Therefore, the renal clearance of urea is less than creatinine or inulin clearance and does not give a quantitative measure of kidney function.

SERUM CREATININE CONCENTRATION AND CREATININE CLEARANCE

Under normal circumstances, creatinine production is roughly equal to creatinine excretion, so the serum creatinine level remains constant. In a patient with reduced glomerular filtration, serum creatinine will accumulate in accordance with the degree of loss of glomerular filtration in the kidney. The serum creatinine concentration alone is frequently used to determine creatinine clearance, Cl_{Cr}. Creatinine clearance from the serum creatinine concentration is a rapid and convenient way to monitor kidney function.

Creatinine clearance may be defined as the rate of urinary excretion of creatinine/serum creatinine. Creatinine clearance can be calculated directly by determining the patient's serum creatinine concentration and the rate of urinary excretion of creatinine. The approach is similar to that used in the determination of drug clearance. In practice, the serum creatinine concentration is determined at the midpoint of the urinary collection period and the rate of urinary excretion of creatinine is measured for the entire day (24 hr) to obtain a reliable excretion rate. Creatinine clearance is expressed in mL/min and serum creatinine concentration in mg/dL or mg%. Other Cl_{Cr} methods based solely on serum creatinine are generally compared to the creatinine clearance obtained from the 24-hour urinary creatinine excretion.

The following equation is used to calculate creatinine clearance in mL/min when the serum creatinine concentration is known:

$$Cl_{Cr} = \frac{\text{rate of urinary excretion of creatinine}}{\text{serum concentration of creatinine}}$$

$$Cl_{Cr} = \frac{C_u V \times 100}{C_{Cr} \times 1440} \tag{21.11}$$

where C_{Cr} = creatinine concentration (mg/dL) of the serum taken at the 12th hour or at the midpoint of the urine-collection period, V = volume of urine excreted (mL) in 24 hours, C_u = concentration of creatinine in urine (mg/mL), and Cl_{Cr} = creatinine clearance in mL/min.

Creatinine is eliminated primarily by glomerular filtration. A small fraction of creatinine also is eliminated by active secretion and some nonrenal elimination. Therefore, Cl_{Cr} values obtained from creatinine measurements overestimate the actual glomerular filtration rate.

Creatinine clearance has been normalized both to body surface area, using 1.73 m^2 as the average, and to body weight for a 70-kg adult male. Creatinine distributes into total body water, and when clearance is normalized to a standard V_D, similar drug half-lives in adults and children correspond to identical clearances.

Creatinine clearance values must be considered carefully in special populations such as the elderly, obese, and emaciated patients. In elderly and emaciated patients, muscle mass may have declined, thus lowering the production of creatinine. However, serum creatinine concentration values may appear to be in the normal range, because of lower renal creatinine excretion. Thus, the calculation of creatinine clearance from serum creatinine may give an inaccurate estimation of the renal function. For obese patient, generally defined as patients more than 20% over *ideal body weight*, IBW, creatinine clearance should be based on ideal body weight. Estimation of creatinine clearance based on *total body weight*, TBW, would exaggerate the Cl_{Cr} values in the obese patient. Women with normal kidney function have smaller creatinine clearance values than men, approximately 80–85% of that in men with normal kidney function.

Several empirical equations have been used to estimate lean body weight, LBW, based on the patient's height and actual (total) body weight (see Chapter 20). The following equations have been used to estimate LBW in renally impaired patients:

LBW (males) = 50 kg + 2.3 kg for each inch over 5 ft

LBW (females) = 45.5 kg + 2.3 kg for each inch over 5 ft

For the purpose of dose adjustment in renal patients, normal creatinine clearance is generally assumed to be between 100 and 125 mL/min per 1.73 m^2 for a subject of ideal body weight: for a female adult, $Cl_{Cr} = 108.8 \pm 13.5$ mL/1.73 m^2, and for an average adult male, $Cl_{Cr} = 124.5 \pm 9.7$ mL/1.73 m^2 (*Scientific Table*, 1973). Creatinine clearance is affected by diet and salt intake. As a convenient approximation, the normal clearance has often been assumed by many clinicians to be approximately 100 mL/min.

Calculation of Creatinine Clearance from Serum Creatinine Concentration

The problems of obtaining a complete 24-hour urine collection from a patient, the time necessary for urine collection, and the analysis time preclude a direct estimation of creatinine clearance. *Serum creatinine concentration*, C_{Cr}, is related to creatinine clearance and is measured routinely in the clinical laboratory. Therefore, creatinine clearance, Cl_{Cr}, is most often estimated from the patient's C_{Cr}. Several methods are available for the calculation of creatinine clearance from the serum creatinine concentration. The more accurate methods are based on the patient's age, height, weight, and gender. These methods should be used only for patients with intact liver function and no abnormal muscle disease, such as hypertrophy or dystrophy. Moreover, most of the methods assume a stable creatinine clearance. The units for Cl_{Cr} are mL/min.

Adults

The method of Crockcroft and Gault (1976) shown in Equation 21.12 is used to estimate creatinine clearance from serum creatinine concentration. This method considers both the age and the weight of the patient. For males,

$$Cl_{Cr} = \frac{[140 - \text{age (yr)}] \times \text{body weight (kg)}}{72 \, (C_{Cr})} \tag{21.12}$$

For females, use 90% of the Cl_{Cr} value obtained in males.

The nomogram method of *Siersback-Nielsen* et al (1971) estimates creatinine clearance on the basis of age, weight, and serum creatinine concentration, as shown in Figure 21-1. Cockcroft and Gault (1976) compared their method with the nomogram method in adult males of various ages. Creatinine clearance estimated by both methods were comparable. Both methods also demonstrated an age-related linear decline in creatinine excretion (Figure 21-2), which may be due to the decrease in muscle mass with age.

Figure 21-1. Nomogram for evaluation of endogenous creatinine clearance. To use the nomogram, connect the patient's weight on the second line from the left with the patient's age on the fourth line with a ruler. Note the point of intersection on *R* and keep the ruler there. Turn the right part of the ruler to the appropriate serum creatinine value and the left side will indicate the clearance in mL/min.
(From Kampmann and Siersback-Nielsen, 1974, with permission.)

Children

There are a number of methods for calculation of creatinine clearance in children, based on body length and serum creatinine concentration. Equation 21.13 is a method developed by Schwartz and associates (1976):

$$Cl_{Cr} = \frac{0.55 \text{ body length (cm)}}{C_{Cr}} \tag{21.13}$$

where Cl_{Cr} is given in mL/min/1.73 m^2.

Another method of calculating creatinine clearance in children uses the nomogram of Traub and Johnson (1980), shown in Figure 21-3. This nomogram is based on observations of 81 children aged 6 to 12 years and requires the patient's height and serum creatinine concentration.

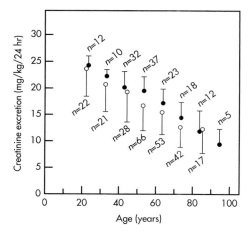

Figure 21-2. Creatinine excretion estimated by two different methods. ● = Kampmann and Siersback-Nielsen (1974), 149 males aged 20–99 years; O = Cockcroft and Gault (1976), 249 males aged 18–92 years.
(From Cockcroft and Gault, 1976, with permission.)

Figure 21-3. Nomogram for rapid evaluation of endogenous creatinine clearance (*Cl*Cr) in pediatric patients (aged 6–12 yr). To predict *Cl*Cr, connect the child's *S*Cr (serum creatinine) and Ht (height) with a ruler and read the *Cl*Cr where the ruler intersects the center line. (From Trub and Johnson, 1980, with permission.)

PRACTICE PROBLEMS

1. What is the creatinine clearance for a 25-year-old male patient with C_{Cr} of 1 mg/dL and a body weight of 80 kg?

   Solution

   Using the nomogram (Figure 21-1), join the points at 25 years (male) and 80 kg with a ruler—let the line intersect line R. Connect the intersection point at line R with the creatinine concentration point of 1 mg/dL, and extend the line to intersect the "clearance line." The extended line will intersect the clearance line at 110 mL/min, giving the creatinine clearance for the patient.

2. What is the creatinine clearance for a 25-year-old male patient with a C_{Cr} of 1 mg/dL? The patient is 5 ft, 4 inches in height and weighs 103 kg.

Solution

The patient is obese and the Cl_{Cr} calculation should be based on ideal body weight.

$$LBW \text{ (males)} = \frac{50 \text{ kg} + [2.3 \times 4]}{kg} = 59.2 \text{ kg}$$

Using the Cockcroft and Gault method (Eq. 21.12), the Cl_{Cr} can be calculated.

$$Cl_{Cr} = \frac{(140 - 25) \times (59.2 \text{ kg})}{72(1)} = 94.6 \text{ mL/min}$$

The serum creatinine methods for the estimation of the creatinine clearance assume stabilized kidney function and a steady-state serum creatinine concentration. In acute renal failure and in other situations in which kidney function is changing, the serum creatinine may not represent steady-state conditions. If C_{Cr} is measured daily and the C_{Cr} value is constant, then the serum creatinine concentration is probably at steady state. If the C_{Cr} values are changing daily, then kidney function is changing.

Although the Cockcroft and Gault method for estimating Cl_{Cr} has some biases, this method has gained general acceptance for the determination of renal impairment (Schneider et al, 2003; Hailemeskel et al, 1999; Spinler et al, 1998). A suggested representation of patients with various degrees of renal impairment based on creatinine clearance is shown in Table 21.3.

The practice problems show that, depending on the formula used, the calculated Cl_{Cr} can vary considerably. Consequently, unless a significant change in the creatinine clearance occurs, use of these methods will result in a rather large margin of error. According to St Peter et al (1992), dose adjustment of many antibiotic drugs is necessary only when the glomerular filtration rate as measured by Cl_{Cr} is less than 50 mL/min. For the aminoglycoside antibiotics and vancomycin, dose adjustment is individualized according to the wide range of Cl_{Cr}. Therefore, dose adjustment for all drugs on the basis of these Cl_{Cr} methods alone is not justified.

DOSE ADJUSTMENT FOR UREMIC PATIENTS

Dose adjustment for drugs in uremic or renally impaired patients should be made in accordance with changes in pharmacodynamics and pharmacokinetics of the

TABLE 21.3 *Renal Impairment Based on Creatinine Clearance*

GROUP	DESCRIPTION	ESTIMATED CREATININE CLEARANCE (mL/min)
1	Normal renal function	>80 mL/min
2	Mild renal impairment	50–80 mL/min
3	Moderate renal impairment	30–50 mL/min
4	Severe renal impairment	<30 mL/min
5	ESRD[a]	Requires dialysis

[a]ESRD = end-stage renal disease.

(Adapted from *FDA Guidance for Industry* (1988).

drug in the individual patient. Active metabolites of the drug may also be formed and must be considered for additional pharmacologic effects when adjusting dose. The following methods may be used to estimate an initial and maintenance dose regimen. After initiating the dosage, the clinician should continue to monitor the pharmacodynamics and pharmacokinetics of the drug. He or she should also evaluate the patient's renal function, which may be changing.

Basis for Dose Adjustment in Uremia

The loading drug dose is based on the apparent volume of distribution of the patient. It is generally assumed that the apparent volume of distribution is not altered significantly, and therefore that the loading dose of the drug is the same in uremic patients as in subjects with normal renal function.

The maintenance dose is based on clearance of the drug in the patient. In the uremic patient, the rate of renal drug excretion has decreased, leading to a decrease in total body clearance. Most methods for dose adjustment assume nonrenal drug clearance to be unchanged. The fraction of normal renal function remaining in the uremic patient is estimated from creatinine clearance.

After the remaining total body clearance in the uremic patient is estimated, a dosage regimen may be developed by (1) decreasing the maintenance dose, (2) increasing the dosage interval, or (3) changing both maintenance dose and dosage interval.

Although total body clearance is a more accurate index of drug dosing, the elimination half-life of the drug is more commonly used for dose adjustment because of its convenience. Clearance allows for the prediction of steady-state drug concentrations, while elimination half-life yields information on the time it takes to reach steady-state concentration.

Nomograms

Nomograms are charts available for use in estimating dosage regimens in uremic patients (Bjornsson, 1986; Chennavasin and Craig Brater, 1981; Tozer, 1974). The nomograms may be based on serum creatinine concentrations, patient data (height, weight, age, gender), and the pharmacokinetics of the drug. As discussed by Chennavasin and Craig Brater (1981), each nomogram has errors in its assumptions and drug database.

Most methods for dose adjustment in renal disease assume that nonrenal elimination of the drug is not affected by renal impairment and that the remaining renal excretion rate constant in the uremic patient is proportional to the product of a constant and the creatinine clearance, Cl_{Cr}:

$$k_u = k_{nr} + \alpha Cl_{Cr} \tag{21.14}$$

where k_{nr} is the nonrenal elimination rate constant and α is a constant. Equation 21.14 is similar to Equation 21.10, where $\alpha = 1/V_D$, and can be used for the construction of a nomogram. Figure 21-4 shows a graphical representation of Equation 21.14 for four different drugs, each with a different renal excretion rate constant. The fractions of drug excreted in the urine unchanged, *fe*, for drugs A, B, C, and D are 5%, 50%, 75%, and 90%, respectively. A creatinine clearance of

Figure 21-4.   Relationship between creatinine clearance and the drug elimination rate constant.

≥ 80 mL/min is considered an adequate glomerular filtration rate in subjects with normal renal function. The uremic elimination rate constant (k_u) is the sum of the nonrenal elimination rate constant and the renal elimination rate constant, which is decreased due to renal impairment. If the patient has complete renal shutdown (ie, creatinine clearance = 0 mL/min), then the intercept on the y axis represents the percent of drug elimination due to nonrenal drug elimination routes. Drug D, which is excreted 90% unchanged in the urine, has the steepest slope (equivalent to α in Eq. 21.14) and is most affected by small changes in creatinine clearance; whereas drug A, which is excreted only 5% unchanged in the urine (ie, 95% eliminated by nonrenal routes), is least affected by a decrease in creatinine clearance.

The nomogram method of Welling and Craig (1976) provides an estimate of the ratio of the uremic elimination rate constant (k_u) to the normal elimination rate constant (k_N) on the basis of creatinine clearance (Figure 21-5). For this

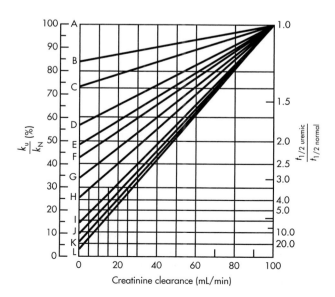

Figure 21-5.   This nomograph describes the changes in the percentage of normal elimination rate constant (left ordinate) and the consequent geometric increase in elimination half-life (right ordinate) as a function of creatinine clearance. The drugs associated with the individual slopes are given in Table 21.4.
(From Welling and Craig, 1976, with permission.)

method, Welling and Craig (1976) provided a list of drugs grouped according to the amount of drug excreted unchanged in the urine (Table 21.4). From the k_u/k_N ratio, the uremic dose can be estimated according to Equation 21.15:

$$\text{Uremic dose} = \frac{k_u}{k_N} \times \text{normal dose} \qquad (21.15)$$

TABLE 21.4   Elimination Rate Constants for Various Drugs[a]

GROUP	DRUG	k_N (hr^{-1})	k_{nr} (hr^{-1})	$k_{nr}/k_N\%$
A	Minocycline	0.04	0.04	100.0
	Rifampicin	0.25	0.25	100.0
	Lidocaine	0.39	0.36	92.3
	Digitoxin	0.114	0.10	87.7
B	Doxycycline	0.037	0.031	83.8
	Chlortetracycline	0.12	0.095	79.2
C	Clindamycin	0.16	0.12	75.0
	Chloramphenicol	0.26	0.19	73.1
	Propranolol	0.22	0.16	72.8
	Erythromycin	0.39	0.28	71.8
D	Trimethoprim	0.054	0.031	57.4
	Isoniazid (fast)	0.53	0.30	56.6
	Isoniazid (slow)	0.23	0.13	56.5
E	Dicloxacillin	1.20	0.60	50.0
	Sulfadiazine	0.069	0.032	46.4
	Sulfamethoxazole	0.084	0.037	44.0
F	Nafcillin	1.26	0.54	42.8
	Chlorpropamide	0.020	0.008	40.0
	Lincomycin	0.15	0.06	40.0
G	Colistimethate	0.154	0.054	35.1
	Oxacillin	1.73	0.58	33.6
	Digoxin	0.021	0.007	33.3
H	Tetracycline	0.120	0.033	27.5
	Cloxacillin	1.21	0.31	25.6
	Oxytetracycline	0.075	0.014	18.7
I	Amoxicillin	0.70	0.10	14.3
	Methicillin	1.40	0.19	13.6
J	Ticarcillin	0.58	0.066	11.4
	Penicillin G	1.24	0.13	10.5
	Ampicillin	0.53	0.05	9.4
	Carbenicillin	0.55	0.05	9.1
K	Cefazolin	0.32	0.02	6.2
	Cephaloridine	0.51	0.03	5.9
	Cephalothin	1.20	0.06	5.0
	Gentamicin	0.30	0.015	5.0
L	Flucytosine	0.18	0.007	3.9
	Kanamycin	0.28	0.01	3.6
	Vancomycin	0.12	0.004	3.3
	Tobramycin	0.32	0.010	3.1
	Cephalexin	1.54	0.032	2.1

[a]k_N is for patients with normal renal function, k_{nr} is for patients with severe renal impairment, and $k_{nr}/k_N\%$ = percent of normal elimination in severe renal impairment.

From Welling and Craig (1976), with permission.

When the dosage interval τ is kept constant, the uremic dose is always a smaller fraction of the normal dose. Instead of reducing the dose for a uremic patient, the usual dose is kept constant and the dosage interval τ is prolonged according to the following equation:

$$\text{Dosage interval in uremia, } \tau_u = \frac{k_N}{k_u} \times \tau_N \tag{21.16}$$

where τ_u is the dosage interval for the dose in uremic patients and τ_N is the dosage interval for the dose in patients with normal renal function.

PRACTICE PROBLEM

Lincomycin is given at 500 mg every 6 hours to a 75-kg normal patient. What doses would be used **(a)** in complete renal shutdown ($Cl_{Cr} = 0$) and **(b)** when $Cl_{Cr} = 10$ mL/min?

Solution

To use the nomogram method, follow the steps below:

1. Locate the group to which the drug belongs in Table 21.4.

2. Find k_u/k_N at the point corresponding to the Cl_{Cr} of the patient (Figure 21-5).

3. Determine k_u for the patient.

4. Make the dose adjustment in accordance with pharmacokinetic principles.

    a. When $Cl_{Cr} = 0$,

$$k_u = k_{nr} + k_R$$

In complete renal shutdown ($k_R = 0$),

$$k_u = k_{nr} = 0.06 \text{ hr}^{-1} \qquad \text{(Table 21.4, group F)}$$

or find k_u/k_N in Figure 21-5, group F, at $Cl_{Cr} = 0$ mL/min:

$$\frac{k_u}{k_N} = 0.425$$

$$k_u = 0.425 \, (0.15) = 0.0638 \text{ hr}^{-1}$$

$$\text{Uremic dose} = 500 \text{ mg} \times \frac{0.0638}{0.15} = 212 \text{ mg every 6 hr}$$

    b. At $Cl_{Cr} = 10$ mL/min,

$$\frac{k_u}{k_N} = 0.48$$

$$k_{\mathrm{N}} = 0.15 \ \mathrm{hr}^{-1}$$

$$k_{\mathrm{u}} = (0.48)(0.15) = 0.072 \ \mathrm{hr}^{-1}$$

$$\mathrm{Dose} = 500 \ \mathrm{mg} \times \frac{0.072}{0.15} = 240 \ \mathrm{mg}$$

Alternatively,

$$\mathrm{Dose} = (0.48)(500) = 240 \ \mathrm{mg}$$

Fraction of Drug Excreted Unchanged (*fe*) Methods

For many drugs, the fraction of drug excreted unchanged (*fe*) is available in the literature. Table 21.5 lists various drugs with their *fe* value and elimination half-life. The *fe* method for estimating a dosage regimen in the uremic patient is a general method that may be applied to any drug whose *fe* is known.

TABLE 21.5   Fraction of Drug Excreted Unchanged (*fe*) and Elimination Half-Life Values

DRUG	fe	$t_{1/2}$ normal (hr)[a]	DRUG	fe	$t_{1/2}$ normal (hr)[a]
Acebutolol	0.44 ± 0.11	2.7 ± 0.4	Chlorphentermine	0.2	120
Acetaminophen	0.03 ± 0.01	2.0 ± 0.4	Chlorpropamide	0.2	36
Acetohexamide	0.4	1.3	Chlorthalidone	0.65 ± 0.09	44 ± 10
Allopurinol	0.1	2–8	Cimetidine	0.77 ± 0.06	2.1 ± 1.1
Active metabolite		16–30	Clindamycin	0.09–0.14	2.7 ± 0.4
Alprenolol	0.005	3.1 ± 1.2	Clofibrate	0.11–0.32	13 ± 3
Amantadine	0.85	10	Clonidine	0.62 ± 0.11	8.5 ± 2.0
Amikacin	0.98	2.3 ± 0.4	Colistin	0.9	3
Amiloride	0.5	8 ± 2	Cytarabine	0.1	2
Amoxicillin	0.52 ± 0.15	1.0 ± 0.1	Cyclophosphamide	0.3	5
Amphetamine	0.4–0.45	12	Dapsone	0.1	20
Amphotericin B	0.03	360	Dicloxacillin	0.60 ± 0.07	0.7 ± 0.07
Ampicillin	0.90 ± 0.08	1.3 ± 0.2	Digitoxin	0.33 ± 0.15	166 ± 65
Atenolol	0.85	6.3 ± 1.8	Digoxin	0.72 ± 0.09	42 ± 19
Azlocillin	0.6	1.0	Disopyramide	0.55 ± 0.06	7.8 ± 1.6
Bacampicillin	0.88	0.9	Doxycycline	0.40 ± 0.04	20 ± 4
Baclofen	0.75	3–4	Erythromycin	0.15	1.1–3.5
Bleomycin	0.55	1.5–8.9	Ethambutol	0.79 ± 0.03	3.1 ± 0.4
Bretylium	0.8 ± 0.1	4–17	Ethosuximide	0.19	33 ± 6
Bumetanide	0.33	3.5	Flucytosine	0.63–0.84	5.3 ± 0.7
Carbenicillin	0.82 ± 0.09	1.1 ± 0.2	Flunitrazepam	0.01	15 ± 5
Cefalothin	0.52	0.6 ± 0.3	Furosemide	0.74 ± 0.07	0.85 ± 0.17
Cefamandole	0.96 ± 0.03	0.77	Gentamicin	0.98	2–3
Cefazolin	0.80 ± 0.13	1.8 ± 0.4	Griseofulvin	0	15
Cefoperazone	0.2–0.3	2.0	Hydralazine	0.12–0.14	2.2–2.6
Cefotaxime	0.5–0.6	1–1.5	Hydrochlorothiazide	0.95	2.5 ± 0.2
Cefoxitin	0.88 ± 0.08	0.7 ± 0.13	Indomethacin	0.15 ± 0.08	2.6–11.2
Cefuroxime	0.92	1.1	Isoniazid		
Cephalexin	0.96	0.9 ± 0.18	Rapid acetylators	0.07 ± 0.02	1.1 ± 0.2
Chloramphenicol	0.05	2.7 ± 0.8	Slow acetylators	0.29 ± 0.05	3.0 ± 0.8

TABLE 21.5 Fraction of Drug Excreted Unchanged (fe) and Elimination Half-Life Values (continued)

DRUG	fe	$t_{1/2}$ normal (hr)[a]	DRUG	fe	$t_{1/2}$ normal (hr)[a]
Isosorbide dinitrate	0.05	0.5	Pivampicillin	0.9	0.9
Kanamycin	0.9	2.1 ± 0.2	Polymyxin B	0.88	4.5
Lidocaine	0.02 ± 0.01	1.8 ± 0.4	Prazosin	0.01	2.9 ± 0.8
Lincomycin	0.6	5	Primidone	0.42 ± 0.15	8.0 ± 4.8
Lithium	0.95 ± 0.15	22 ± 8	Procainamide	0.67 ± 0.08	2.9 ± 0.6
Lorazepam	0.01	14 ± 5	Propranolol	0.005	3.9 ± 0.4
Meperidine	0.04–0.22	3.2 ± 0.8	Quinidine	0.18 ± 0.05	6.2 ± 1.8
Methadone	0.2	22	Rifampin	0.16 ± 0.04	2.1 ± 0.3
Methicillin	0.88 ± 0.17	0.85 ± 0.23	Salicylic acid	0.2	3
Methotrexate	0.94	8.4	Sisomicin	0.98	2.8
Methyldopa	0.63 ± 0.10	1.8 ± 0.2	Sotalol	0.6	6.5–13
Metronidazole	0.25	8.2	Streptomycin	0.96	2.8
Mexiletine	0.1	12	Sulfisoxazole	0.53 ± 0.09	5.9 ± 0.9
Mezlocillin	0.75	0.8	Sulfinpyrazone	0.45	2.3
Minocycline	0.1 ± 0.02	18 ± 4	Tetracycline	0.48	9.9 ± 1.5
Minoxidil	0.1	4	Thiamphenicol	0.9	3
Moxalactam	0.82–0.96	2.5–3.0	Thiazinamium	0.41	
Nadolol	0.73 ± 0.04	16 ± 2	Theophylline	0.08	9 ± 2.1
Nafcillin	0.27 ± 0.05	0.9–1.0	Ticarcillin	0.86	1.2
Nalidixic acid	0.2	1.0	Timolol	0.2	3–5
Netilmicin	0.98	2.2	Tobramycin	0.98	2.2 ± 0.1
Neostigmine	0.67	1.3 ± 0.8	Tocainide	0.20-0.70	1.6–3
Nitrazepam	0.01	29 ± 7		(0.40 mean)	
Nitrofuraniton	0.5	0.3	Tolbutamide	0	5.9 ± 1.4
Nomifensine	0.15–0.22	3.0 ± 1.0	Triamterene	0.04 ± 0.01	2.8 ± 0.9
Oxacillin	0.75	0.5	Trimethoprim	0.53 ± 0.02	11 ± 1.4
Oxprenolol	0.05	1.5	Tubocurarine	0.43 ± 0.08	2 ± 1.1
Pancuronium	0.5	3.0	Valproic acid	0.02 ± 0.02	16 ± 3
Pentazocine	0.2	2.5	Vancomycin	0.97	5–6
Phenobarbital	0.2 ± 0.05	86 ± 7	Warfarin	0	37 ± 15
Pindolol	0.41	3.4 ± 0.2			

[a]Half-life is a derived parameter that changes as a function of both clearance and volume of distribution. It is independent of body size, because it is a function of these two parameters (Cl, V_D), each of which is proportional to body size. It is important to consider that half-life is the time to eliminate 50% of the "drug" from the body (plasma), not the time in which 50% of the effect is lost.

From Benet et al (1984), with permission.

The *Giusti–Hayton* (1973) method assumes that the effect of reduced kidney function on the renal portion of the elimination constant can be estimated from the ratio of the uremic creatinine clearance, Cl^u_{Cr}, to the normal creatinine clearance, Cl^N_{Cr}:

$$\frac{k^u_r}{k^N} = \frac{Cl^u_{Cr}}{Cl^N_{Cr}} \qquad (21.17)$$

where k^u_r is the uremic renal excretion rate constant and k^N_r is the normal renal excretion rate constant.

$$k^u_r = k^N_r \frac{Cl^u_{Cr}}{Cl^N_{Cr}} \qquad (21.18)$$

Because the overall uremic elimination rate constant, k_u, is the sum of renal and nonrenal elimination,

$$k_u = k_{nr}^u + k_r^u \tag{21.19}$$

$$k_u = k_{nr}^u + k_r^N \left(\frac{Cl_{Cr}^u}{Cl_{Cr}^N} \right)$$

Dividing Equation 21.19 by k_N on both sides yields

$$\frac{k_u}{k_N} = \frac{k_{nr}^u}{k_N} + \frac{k_r^N}{k_N} \left(\frac{Cl_{Cr}^u}{Cl_{Cr}^N} \right) \tag{21.20}$$

Let $fe = k_r^N / k_N$ = fraction of drug excreted unchanged in the urine and $1 - fe = k_{nr}^u / k_N$ = fraction of drug excreted by nonrenal routes. Substitution into Equation 21.20 yields the Giusti–Hayton equation, where G is the Giusti–Hayton factor, which can be calculated from the fe and the ratio of uremic to normal clearance:

$$\frac{k_u}{k_N} = (1 - fe) + fe \left(\frac{Cl_{Cr}^u}{Cl_{Cr}^N} \right)$$

or

$$\frac{k_u}{k_N} = 1 - fe \left(1 - \frac{Cl_{Cr}^u}{Cl_{Cr}^N} \right) = G \tag{21.21}$$

The Giusti–Hayton equation is useful for most drugs for which the fraction of drug excreted by renal routes has been reported in the literature. The ratio k_u / k_N can be calculated from the fraction of drug excreted by the kidney, normal creatinine clearance, and the creatinine clearance in the uremic patient.

PRACTICE PROBLEM

The maintenance dose of gentamicin is 80 mg every 6 hours for a patient with normal renal function. Calculate the maintenance dose for a uremic patient with creatinine clearance of 20 mL/min. Assume a normal creatinine clearance of 100 mL/min.

Solution

From the literature, gentamicin is reported to be 100% excreted by the kidney (ie, $fe = 1$). Using Equation 21.21,

$$\frac{k_u}{k_N} = 1 - 1 \left(1 - \frac{20}{100} \right) = 0.2$$

Because

$$\frac{D_u}{D_N} = \frac{k_u}{k_N} \qquad \text{or} \qquad D_u = D_N \times \frac{k_u}{k_N}$$

where D_u = uremic dose and D_N = normal dose,

$$D_u = 80 \text{ mg} \times 0.2 = 16 \text{ mg}$$

The maintenance dose is 16 mg every 6 hours. Alternatively, the dosing interval can be adjusted without changing the dose:

$$\frac{\tau_u}{\tau_N} = \frac{k_N}{k_u} \qquad \text{or} \qquad \tau_u = \tau_N \times \frac{k_N}{k_u}$$

$$\tau_u = 6 \text{ hr} \times \frac{1}{0.2} = 30 \text{ hr}$$

where t_u and t_N are dosing intervals for uremic and normal patients, respectively. The patient may be given 80 mg every 30 hours.

Other approaches for using fraction of drug excreted unchanged have been developed by Tozer (1974) and Bjornsson (1986). These methods use *fe* for dosing regimen design and the following equation:

$$Q = 1 - fe\,(1 - k_f) \qquad\qquad (21.22)$$

where Q is the dosage adjustment factor, $k_f = Cl^u_{Cr}/Cl^N_{Cr}$, and *fe* is the fraction of unchanged drug excreted renally. Actually Q is exactly the same as G in Eq. 21.21, the Giusti-Hayton approach developed in 1973.

The value of Q in Equation 21.22 is multipled by the normal dose, D_N, to give the uremic dose, D_u:

$$D_u = Q \times D_N \qquad\qquad (21.23)$$

All the methods discussed so far assume that nonrenal elimination, k_{nr}, is unchanged, thereby ignoring potential side effects resulting from an increase in the half-life of metabolism of the parent drug and/or an accumulation of active metabolites of the drug.

Bodenham and associates (1988) have shown that although lorazepam pharmacokinetics were not significantly altered in patients with chronic renal failure, the clearance of lorazepam glucuronide, a major metabolite, was reduced significantly. Therefore, there are potential sedative side effects in the renally impaired patient as a result of the longer metabolite half-life. Bodenham and co-workers (1988) also cited literature references to potentiation of sedative and analgesic drug effects in renal, liver, and other multisystem disease states.

In addition to pharmacokinetic changes, possible changes in pharmacodynamic effects in patients with renal and other diseases must be considered. Neuromuscular-blocking drugs may be potentiated or antagonized by changes in potassium, phosphate, and hydrogen ion concentration brought about by uremic states. Morphine potentiation has been reported in hypocalcemic states. In many patients, plasma creatinine concentration may not rise for some time, until creatinine clearance has fallen significantly, thereby adding to the uncertainty of any method that depends on plasma C_{Cr} for dose adjustment.

Comparison of the Various Methods for Dose Adjustment in Uremic Patients

All of the methods mentioned previously have similar limitations (see Table 21.2). For example, the drug must follow dose-independent kinetics and the volume of distribution of the drug must remain relatively constant in the uremic patient. As mentioned, it is usually assumed that the nonrenal routes of elimination, such as hepatic clearance, do not change. Because no correction for metabolites is made, any drug having an active pharmacologic metabolite must be additionally modified. Another assumption in the use of these methods is that pharmacologic response is unchanged in the uremic patient. This assumption may be unrealistic for drugs that act differently in the disease state. For example, the pharmacologic response with digoxin is dependent on the potassium level in the body, and the potassium level in the uremic patient may be rather different from that of the normal individual. In a patient undergoing dialysis, loss of potassium may increase the potential of toxic effect of the drug digoxin. For many drugs, studies have shown that the incidence of adverse effects is increased in uremic patients. It is often impossible to distinguish whether the increase in adverse effect is due to a pharmacokinetic change or to a pharmacodynamic change in the receptor sensitivity to the drug. In any event, these observations point out the fact that dose adjustment must be regarded as a preliminary estimation to be followed with further adjustments in accordance with the observed clinical response.

PRACTICE PROBLEMS

1. An adult male patient (52 years old, 75 kg) whose serum creatinine is 2.4 mg/dL is to be given gentamicin sulfate for a confirmed Gram-negative infection. The usual dose of gentamicin in adult patients with normal renal function is 1 mg/kg every 8 hours by multiple IV bolus injections. Gentamicin sulfate (Garamycin) is available in 2-mL vials containing 40 mg of gentamicin sulfate per milliliter. Calculate (a) the creatinine clearance in this patient by the Cockcroft and Gault method and (b) the appropriate dosage regimen of gentamicin sulfate for this patient in mg and mL.

Solution

a. The creatinine clearance is calculated by the Cockcroft and Gault method using Equation 21.13:

$$Cl_{Cr} = \frac{(140 - 52)\,(75)}{72\,(2.4)} = 38.19 \text{ mL/min}$$

b. The initial dose of gentamicin sulfate in this patient may be estimated using Equation 21.21. Normal creatinine clearance is assumed to equal 100 mL/min. The fraction of dose excreted unchanged in the urine, $fe = 0.98$ for gentamicin sulfate (Table 21.5).

$$\frac{k_u}{k_N} = Q = 1 - 0.98 \left(1 - \frac{38.19}{100}\right) = 0.39$$

The usual dose of gentamicin sulfate = 1 mg/kg every 8 hours. Therefore, for a 75-kg adult, the usual dose is 75 mg every 8 hours. The uremic dose may be estimated by:

(1) Reducing the maintenance dose and keeping the dosing interval constant:

$$\text{Uremic dose} = \frac{k_u}{k_N} \times \text{normal dose}$$

Uremic dose = $0.39 \times 75 = 29.25$ mg

Give 29.25 mg (about 30 mg) every 8 hours. Because the concentration of gentamicin sulfate solution is 40 mg/mL, then 30 mg gentamicin sulfate is equivalent to 0.75 mL.

(2) Increasing the dosing interval and keeping the maintenance dose constant:

$$\text{Dosage interval in uremia}, \tau_u = \frac{k_N}{k_u} \times \tau_N$$

$\tau_u = 2.564 \times 8 = 20.5$ hr (2.564 is the reciprocal of 0.39)

Give 75 mg every 20.5 hours.

(3) Change both the maintenance dose and dosing interval. Using the dosing rate $D_\tau = 29.25$ mg/8 hr $= 3.66$ mg/hr, a dose of 21.9 mg every 6 hours or 43.8 mg every 12 hours will produce the same average steady-state plasma drug concentration.

Although each estimated dosage regimen shown above produces the same average steady-state plasma drug concentration, the peak drug concentration, trough drug concentration, and duration of time in which the drug concentration will be above or below the minimum effective plasma drug concentration will be different. Choice of an appropriate dosage regimen requires consideration of these issues, the patient, and the safety and efficacy of the drug.

2. Calculate the dose adjustment needed for uremic patients with **(a)** 75% of normal kidney function (ie, $Cl_{Cr}^u / Cl_{Cr}^N = 75\%$); **(b)** 50% of normal kidney function; and **(c)** 25% of normal kidney function. Make calculations for **(1)** a drug that is 50% excreted by the kidney, and **(2)** a drug that is 75% excreted by the kidney.

Solution

The values for percent of normal creatinine clearance in uremic patients with various renal functions are listed in Table 21.6. The percent of dose adjustment in a given uremic state is obtained using the procedure detailed below. The important facts to remember are (1) although the elimination rate constant is usually composed of two components, only the renal component is reduced in a uremic patient, and (2) the kidney function of the uremic patient may be expressed as a percent of uremic Cl_{Cr}^u/normal Cl_{Cr}^N. The reduction in the renal elimination rate constant can be estimated from the percent of kidney function remaining in the patient. The steps involved in making the calculations are as follows:

a. Determine fe, or the fraction of drug excreted by the kidney.

b. Determine k_f by dividing Cl_{Cr}^u of the uremic patient by Cl_{Cr}^N.

c. Calculate Q (Eq. 21.22).

d. Multiply Q by the normal dose to give the fraction of normal dose required for a uremic patient.

3. What is the dose for a drug that is 75% excreted unchanged through the kidney in a uremic patient with a creatinine clearance of 10 mL/min?

Solution

$fe = 75\%$

Renal function of uremic patient $= \dfrac{10}{100} = 10\%$ normal

Percent of uremic patient's renal elimination constant $= 75\% \times 10\%$
$= 7.5\%$ normal

Percent of uremic patient's overall elimination constant $= 7.5\% + (100\% - 75\%)$
$= 7.5\% + 25\% = 32.5\%$

Therefore, the uremic patient's dose should be 32.5% of that of normal patient. Table 21.6 provides some calculated dose adjustments for drugs eliminated to various degrees by renal excretion in different stages of renal failure.

General Clearance Method

The general clearance method is based on the methods discussed above. This method is popular in clinical settings because of its simplicity. The method assumes

TABLE 21.6 *Dosage Adjustment in Uremic Patients*

FRACTION OF DRUG EXCRETED UNCHANGED (k_r/k_N) or fe	PERCENT OF NORMAL DOSE			
	50% Normal Cl_{Cr}	25% Normal Cl_{Cr}	10% Normal Cl_{Cr}	0% Normal Cl_{Cr}
0.25	87	81	77	75
0.50	75	62	55	50
0.75	62	44	32	25
0.90	55	32	19	10

that creatinine clearance, Cl_{Cr}, is a good indicator of renal function and that the renal clearance of a drug, Cl_R, is proportional to Cl_{Cr}. Therefore, renal drug clearance, Cl_R^u, in the uremic patient is

$$Cl_R^u = \frac{Cl_{Cr}^u}{Cl_{Cr}^N} \times Cl_R \tag{21.24}$$

$$Cl_u = Cl_{nr} + Cl_R \frac{Cl_{Cr}^u}{Cl_{Cr}^N} \tag{21.25}$$

where Cl_u is the total body clearance in the uremic patient.

If the ratio Cl_{Cr}^u / Cl_{Cr}^N, Cl_{nr}, and Cl_R are known, the total body clearance in the uremic patient may be estimated using Equation 21.25. Alternatively, if the normal total body clearance, Cl, and fe are known, Equation 21.26 may be obtained by substitution in Equation 21.25:

$$Cl_u = Cl(1 - fe) + fe\, Cl \frac{Cl_{Cr}^u}{Cl_{Cr}^N} \tag{21.26}$$

Equation 21.26 calculates drug clearance in the uremic patient using the fraction of drug excreted unchanged (fe), total body clearance of the drug (Cl) in the normal subject, and the ratio of creatinine clearance of the uremic to that of the normal patient.

Dividing Equation 21.26 on both sides by Cl yields the ratio Cl_u/Cl, reflecting the fraction of the uremic/normal drug dose.

$$\frac{Cl_u}{Cl} = (1 - fe) + fe \frac{Cl_{Cr}^u}{Cl_{Cr}^N} \tag{21.27}$$

PRACTICE PROBLEM

M.S., a 34-year-old, 110-lb female patient, is to be given tobramycin for sepsis. The usual dose of tobramycin is 150 mg twice a day by intravenous injection. The creatinine clearance in this patient has decreased to a stable level of 50 mL/min. Calculate the appropriate dose of tobramycin for this patient.

Solution

Obtain $fe = 0.9$ from the literature (Appendix D) and apply Equation 21.27:

$$\frac{Cl_u}{Cl} = (1 - fe) + fe \frac{Cl_{Cr}^u}{Cl_{Cr}^N}$$

$$\frac{Cl_u}{Cl} = 1 - 0.9 + 0.9 \left(\frac{50}{100} \right) = 0.55$$

Therefore, the dose for the uremic patient = 150 mg $\times$ 0.55 = 82.5 mg (given twice a day).

The Wagner Method

The methods for renal dose adjustment discussed in the previous sections all assume that the volume of distribution and the fraction of drug excreted by nonrenal routes are unchanged. These assumptions are convenient and hold true for many drugs. However, in the absence of reliable information assuring the validity of these assumptions, the equations should be demonstrated as statistically reliable in practice. A statistical approach was used by Wagner (1975), who established a linear relationship between creatinine concentration and the first-order elimination constant of the drug in patients. The Wagner method is described in greater detail in the previous edition.

This method takes advantage of the fact that the elimination constant for a patient can be obtained from the creatinine clearance, as follows:

$$k\% = a + bCl_{Cr} \tag{21.28}$$

The values of a and b are determined statistically for each drug from pooled data on uremic patients. The method is simple to use and should provide accurate determination of elimination constants for patients when a good linear relationship exists between elimination constant and creatinine concentration. The theoretical derivation of this approach is as follows:

$k\%$ = total elimination rate constant

k_{nr} = nonrenal elimination rate constant ($\%$)

k_R = renal excretion rate constant

Cl = Total body clearance of drug

$$R = \frac{Cl}{Cl_{Cr}} \tag{21.29}$$

$$Cl = R\,Cl_{Cr}$$

$$k = k_{nr} + \frac{R}{V_D}Cl_{Cr}$$

$$100k = 100k_{nr} + \frac{100R}{V_D}Cl_{Cr}$$

$$k\% = a + bCl_{Cr} \tag{21.30}$$

Equation 21.30 can also be used with drugs that follow the two-compartment model. In such cases the terminal half-life is used and b, the terminal slope of elimination curve, is substituted for the elimination rate constant, k. Since the equation assumes a constant nonrenal elimination constant (k_{nr}) and volume of distribution, any change in these two parameters will result in an error in the estimated elimination constant.

EXTRACORPOREAL REMOVAL OF DRUGS

Patients with *end-stage renal disease* (ESRD) and patients who have become intoxicated with a drug as a result of a drug overdose require supportive treatment to remove the accumulated drug and its metabolites. Several methods are available for the extracorporeal removal of drugs, including hemoperfusion, hemofiltration, and dialysis.

The objective of these methods is to rapidly remove the undesirable drugs and metabolites from the body without disturbing the fluid and electrolyte balance in the patient.

Patients with impaired renal function may be taking other medication concurrently. For these patients, dosage adjustment may be needed to replace drug loss during extracorporeal drug and metabolite removal.

Dialysis

Dialysis is an artificial process in which the accumulation of drugs or waste metabolites is removed by diffusion from the body into the dialysis fluid. Two common dialysis treatments are *peritoneal dialysis* and *hemodialysis*. Both processes work on the principle that as the uremic blood or fluid is equilibrated with the dialysis fluid across a dialysis membrane, waste metabolites from the patient's blood or fluid diffuse into the dialysis fluid and are removed. The dialysate contains water, dextrose, electrolytes (potassium, sodium, chloride, bicarbonate, acetate, calcium, etc), and other elements similar to normal body fluids without the toxins.

Peritoneal Dialysis

Peritoneal dialysis uses the peritoneal membrane in the abdomen as the filter. The peritoneum consists of visceral and parietal components. The peritoneum membrane provides a large natural surface area for diffusion of approximately 1–2 m² in adults; the membrane is permeable to solutes of molecular weights $\leq$ 30,000 Da (Merck Manual, 1996–1997). Total splanchnic flow is 1200 mL/min at rest, but only a small portion, approximately 70 mL/min, comes into contact with the peritoneum. Placement of a peritoneal catheter is surgically simpler than hemodialysis and does not require vascular surgery and heparinization. The dialysis fluid is pumped into the peritoneal cavity, where waste metabolites in the body fluid are discharged rapidly. The dialysate is drained and fresh dialysate is reinstilled and then drained periodically. Peritoneal dialysis is also more amenable to self-treatment. However, slower drug clearance rates are obtained with peritoneal dialysis compared to hemodialysis, and thus longer dialysis time is required.

Continuous ambulatory peritoneal dialysis (CAPD) is the most common form of peritoneal dialysis. Many diabetic patients become uremic as a result of lack of control of their diabetes. About 2 L of dialysis fluid is instilled into the peritoneal cavity of the patient through a surgically placed resident catheter. The objective is to remove accumulated urea and other metabolic waste in the body. The catheter is sealed and the patient is able to continue in an ambulatory mode. Every 4–6 hours, the fluid is emptied from the peritoneal cavity and replaced with fresh dialysis fluid. The technique uses about 2 L of dialysis fluid; it does not require a dialysis machine and can be performed at home.

Hemodialysis

Hemodialysis uses a dialysis machine and filters blood through an artificial membrane. Hemodialysis requires access to the blood vessels to allow the blood to flow to the dialysis machine and back to the body. For temporary access, a shunt is created in the arm, with one tube inserted into an artery and another tube inserted in a vein. The tubes are joined above the skin. For permanent access to the blood vessels, an arteriovenous fistula or graft is created by a surgical procedure to allow access to the artery and vein. Patients who are on chronic hemodialysis treatment need to be aware of the need for infection control of the surgical site of the fistula. At the start of the hemodialysis procedure, an arterial needle allows the blood to flow to the dialysis machine, and blood is returned to the patient to the venous side. Heparin is used to prevent blood clotting during the dialysis period.

During hemodialysis, the blood flows through the dialysis machine, where the waste material is removed from the blood by diffusion through an artificial membrane before the blood is returned to the body. Hemodialysis is a much more effective method of drug removal and is preferred in situations when rapid removal of the drug from the body is important, as in overdose or poisoning. In practice, hemodialysis is most often used for patients with end-stage renal failure. Early dialysis is appropriate for patients with acute renal failure in whom resumption of renal function can be expected and in patients who are to be renally transplanted. Other patients may be placed on dialysis according to clinical judgment concerning the patient's quality of life and risk/benefit ratio (Carpenter and Lazarus, 1994).

Dialysis may be required from once every 2 days to 3 times a week, with each treatment period lasting 2 to 4 hours. The time required for dialysis depends on the amount of residual renal function in the patient, any complicating illness (eg, diabetes mellitus), the size and weight of the patient, including muscle mass, and the efficiency of the dialysis process. Dosing of drugs in patients receiving hemodialysis is affected greatly by the frequency and type of dialysis machine used and by the physicochemical and pharmacokinetic properties of the drug. Factors that affect drug removal in hemodialysis are listed in Table 21.7. These factors are carefully considered before hemodialysis is used for drug removal.

In hemodialysis, blood is pumped to the dialyzer by a roller pump at a rate of 300–450 mL/min. The drug and metabolites diffuse from the blood through the semipermeable membrane. In addition, hydrostatic pressure also forces the drug

TABLE 21.7 *Factors Affecting Dialyzability of Drugs*

PHYSICOCHEMICAL AND PHARMACOKINETIC PROPERTIES OF THE DRUG	
Water solubility	Insoluble or fat-soluble drugs are not dialyzed—eg, glutethimide, which is very water insoluble.
Protein binding	Tightly bound drugs are not dialyzed because dialysis is a passive process of diffusion—eg, propranolol is 94% bound.
Molecular weight	Only molecules with molecular weights of less than 500 are easily dialyzed—eg, vancomycin is poorly dialyzed and has a molecular weight of 1800.
Drugs with large volumes of distribution	Drugs widely distributed are dialyzed more slowly because the rate-limiting factor is the volume of blood entering the machine—eg, for digoxin, V_D = 250–300 L. Drugs concentrated in the tissues are usually difficult to remove by dialysis.

CHARACTERISTICS OF THE DIALYSIS MACHINE	
Blood flow rate	Higher blood flows give higher clearance rates.
Dialysate	Composition of the dialysate and flow rate.
Dialysis membrane	Permeability characteristics and surface area.
Transmembrane pressure	Ultrafiltration increases with increase in transmembrane pressure.
Duration and frequency of dialysis	

molecules into the dialysate by ultrafiltration. The composition of the dialysate is similar to plasma but may be altered according to the needs of the patient. Many dialysis machines use a hollow fiber or capillary dialyzer in which the semipermeable membrane is made into fine capillaries, of which thousands are packed into bundles with blood flowing through the capillaries and the dialysate is circulated outside the capillaries. The permeability characteristics of the membrane and the membrane surface area are determinants of drug diffusion and ultrafiltration.

The efficacy of hemodialysis membranes for the removal of vancomycin by hemodialysis has been reviewed by De Hart (1996). Vancomycin is an antibiotic effective against most Gram-positive organisms such as *Staphylococcus aureus,* which may be responsible for vascular access infections in patients undergoing dialysis. In De Hart's study, vancomycin hemodialysis in patients was compared using a cuprophan membrane or a cellulose acetate and polyacrylonitrile membrane. The cellulose acetate and polyacrylonitrile membrane is considered a "high-flux" filter. Serum vancomycin concentrations decreased only 6.3% after dialysis when using the cuprophan membrane, whereas the serum drug concentration decreased 13.6–19.4% after dialysis with the cellulose acetate and polyacrylonitrile membrane.

In dialysis involving uremic patients receiving drugs for therapy, the rate at which a given drug is removed depends on the flow rate of blood to the dialysis machine and the performance of the dialysis machine. The term *dialysance* is used to describe the process of drug removal from the dialysis machine. Dialysance is a clearance term similar in meaning to renal clearance, and it describes the amount of blood completely cleared of drugs (in mL/min). Dialysance is defined by the equation

$$Cl_D = \frac{Q(C_a - C_v)}{C_a} \tag{21.31}$$

where C_a = drug concentrations in arterial blood (blood entering kidney machine), C_v = drug concentration in venous blood (blood leaving kidney machine), Q = rate of blood flow to the kidney machine, and Cl_D = dialysance. Dialysance is sometimes referred to as *dialysis clearance.*

PRACTICE PROBLEM

Assume the flow rate of blood to the dialysis machine is 350 mL/min. By chemical analysis, the concentrations of drug entering and leaving the machine are 30 and 12 μg/mL, respectively. What is the dialysis clearance?

Solution

The rate of drug removal is equal to the volume of blood passed through the machine divided by the arterial difference in blood drug concentrations before and after dialysis. Thus,

Rate of drug removal = 350 mL/min × (30 − 12) μg/mL = 6300 μg/min

Since clearance is equal to the rate of drug removal divided by the arterial concentration of drug,

$$Cl_D = \frac{6300 \ \mu g/min}{30 \ \mu g/mL} = 210 \ mL/min$$

Alternatively, using Equation 21.31,

$$Cl_D = 350 \ mL/min \times \frac{(30 - 12)}{30} = 210 \ mL/min$$

These calculations show that the two terms are the same. In practice, dialysance has to be measured experimentally by determining C_a, C_v, and Q. In dosing of drugs for patients on dialysis, the average plasma drug concentration of a patient is given by

$$C_{av}^{\infty} = \frac{FD_0}{(Cl_T + Cl_D) \tau} \tag{21.32}$$

where F represents fraction of dose absorbed, Cl_T is total body drug clearance of the patient, C_{av}^{∞} is average steady-state plasma drug concentration, and τ is the dosing interval.

In practice, if Cl_D is 30% or more of Cl_T, adjustment is usually made for the amount of drug lost in dialysis.

The elimination half-life, $t_{1/2}$, for the drug in the patient off dialysis is related to the remaining total body clearance Cl_T and the volume of distribution V_D, as shown below.

$$t_{1/2} = \frac{0.693 V_D}{Cl_T} \tag{21.33}$$

Drugs that are easily dialyzed will have a high dialysis clearance Cl_D, and the elimination half-life $t_{1/2}$ is shorter in a patient on dialysis.

$$t_{1/2} = \frac{0.693 V_D}{Cl_T + Cl_D} \tag{21.34}$$

$$k_{ON} = \frac{Cl_T + Cl_D}{V_D} \tag{21.35}$$

where k_{ON} is the first-order elimination half-life of the drug in the patient on dialysis.

The *fraction of drug lost* due to elimination and dialysis may be estimated from Equation 21.36.

Fraction of drug lost $= 1 - e^{-(Cl_T + Cl_D) \ t/V_D}$ \hfill (21.36)

Equation 21.36 is based on first-order drug elimination and the substitution of t hours for the dialysis period.

TABLE 21.8 Predicted Effects of Hemodialysis on Drug Half-Life and Removal in the Overdose Setting

DRUG	V_D (L)	Cl (mL/min)	Cl_D (mL/min)	$t_{1/2 \text{ off}}$ (hr)	$t_{1/2 \text{ on}}$ (hr)	FL[a]
Digoxin[b]	560	150	20	43	38	0.07
Digoxin[c]	300	40	20	86	58	0.05
Ethchlorvynol	300	35	60	99	36	0.07
Phenobarbital	50	5	70	115	8	0.30
Phenytoin	100	5	10	231	77	0.04
Salicylic acid	40	20	100	23	4	0.51

[a]FL = fraction lost during a dialysis period of 4 hours.
[b]Parameters for a patient with normal renal function.
[c]Parameters for a patient with no renal function.

From Gambertoglio (1984), with permission.

Several hypothetical examples illustrating the use of Equation 21.36 have been developed by Gambertoglio (1984). These are given in Table 21.8.

Equation 21.36 shows that as V_D increases, the fraction of drug lost decreases. The fraction of drug lost during a 4-hour dialysis period for phenobarbital and salicylic acid was 0.30 and 0.50, respectively, whereas for digoxin and phenytoin, the fraction of drug lost was only 0.07 and 0.04, respectively. Both phenobarbital and salicylic acid are easily dialyzed because of their smaller volumes of distribution, small molecular weights, and aqueous solubility. In contrast, digoxin has a large volume of distribution and phenytoin is highly bound to plasma proteins, making these drugs difficult to dialyze. Thus, dialysis is not very useful for treating digoxin intoxication, but is useful for salicylate overdose.

An example of the effect of hemodialysis on drug elimination is shown in Figure 21-6. During the interdialysis period, the patient's total body clearance is very low and the drug concentration declines slowly. In this example, the drug has an elimination $t_{1/2}$ of 48 hours during the interdialysis period. When the patient is placed on dialysis, the drug clearance (sum of the total body clearance and the dialysis clearance) removes the drug more rapidly.

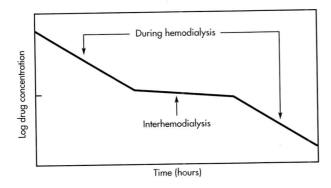

Figure 21-6. Effect of dialysis on drug elimination.

CLINICAL EXAMPLES

1. The aminoglycoside antibiotics, such as gentamicin and tobramycin, are eliminated primarily by the renal route. Dosing of these aminoglycosides is adjusted according to the residual renal function in the patient as estimated by creatinine clearance. During hemodialysis or peritoneal dialysis, the elimination half-lives for these antibiotics are significantly decreased, as shown in Table 21.8. After dialysis, the aminoglycoside concentrations are below the therapeutic range, and the patient needs to be given another dose of the aminoglycoside antibiotic. The data in Table 21.9 also show that hemodialysis is more efficient in removing the aminoglycoside antibiotic, as shown by a smaller half-life during the dialysis period compared to peritoneal dialysis.

2. An adult male (73 years old, 65 kg) with diabetes mellitus is placed on hemodialysis. His residual creatinine clearance is <5 mL/min. The patient is given tobramycin, an aminoglycoside antibiotic, at a dose of 1 mg/kg by IV bolus injection. Tobramycin is 90% excreted unchanged in the urine, is less than 10% bound to plasma proteins, and has an elimination half-life of approximately 2.2 hours in patients with normal renal function. In this patient, tobramycin has an elimination $t_{1/2}$ of 50 hours during the interdialysis period and an elimination $t_{1/2}$ of 8 hours during hemodialysis. The apparent volume of distribution for tobramycin is about 0.33 L/kg. For this patient, calculate (a) the initial plasma antibiotic concentration after the first dose of tobramycin; (b) the plasma drug concentration just before the start of hemodialysis (48 hours after the initial tobramycin dose); (c) the plasma drug concentration at the end of 4 hours of hemodialysis; (d) the amount of drug lost from the body after dialysis; and (e) the tobramycin dose (replenishment dose) needed to be given to the patient after hemodialysis.

Solution

a. Initial plasma antibiotic concentration after the first dose of tobramycin:

$$\text{Patient dose} = \frac{1\,\text{mg}}{\text{kg}} \times 65\ \text{kg} = 65\ \text{mg}$$

$$V_\text{D} = \frac{0.33\ \text{L}}{\text{kg}} \times 65\ \text{kg} = 21.45\ \text{L}$$

$$\text{Plasma drug concentration,}\ C_\text{p}^0 = \frac{D_0}{V_\text{D}} = \frac{65\ \text{mg}}{21.45\ \text{L}} = 3.03\ \text{mg/L}$$

b. Plasma drug concentration just before the start of hemodialysis (48 hours after the initial tobramycin dose): After 48 hours, the plasma drug concentration declines according to first-order kinetics:

$$C_\text{p} = 3.03\, e^{-(0.693/50)(48)} = 1.58\ \text{mg/L}$$

c. Plasma drug concentration at the end of a 4-hour hemodialysis:

$$C_\text{p} = 1.58\, e^{-(0.693/8)(4)} = 0.547\ \text{mg/L}$$

d. Amount of drug lost from the body after dialysis:

Amt of drug lost after dialysis = Amt of drug in the body before dialysis
− Amt of drug in the body after dialysis =

$$\frac{1.58\text{ mg}}{L}(21.45\text{ L}) - \frac{5.47\text{ mg}}{L}(21.45\text{ L}) = 22.16\text{ mg}$$

e. Tobramycin dose (replenishment dose) needed to be given to the patient after hemodialysis: The recommended ranges of peak and trough concentrations of tobramycin (Mathews, 1995) are 5 to 10 mg/L (peak) and 0.5 to <2 mg/L (trough). The usual replenishment dose of tobramycin after hemodialysis is 1 to 1.5 mg/kg.

If a replenishment dose of 65 mg (ie, 1 mg/kg) is given to the patient, then the estimated plasma drug concentration is estimated as

Plasma drug conc. after 65 mg
given by IV bolus injection
after hemodialysis
$$= \frac{65\text{ mg}}{21.45\text{ L}} + 0.547\text{ mg/L} = 3.58\text{ mg/L}$$

The patient is given 65 mg of tobramycin by IV bolus injection after completion of hemodialysis to produce a tobramycin plasma concentration of 3.58 mg/L.

Hemoperfusion

Hemoperfusion is the process of removing drug by passing the blood from the patient through an adsorbent material and back to the patient. Hemoperfusion is a useful procedure for rapid drug removal in accidental poisoning and drug overdosage. Because the drug molecules in the blood are in direct contact with the adsorbent material, any molecule that has great affinity for the adsorbent material will be removed. The two main adsorbents used in hemoperfusion include **(1)** activated charcoal, which adsorbs both polar and nonpolar drugs, and **(2)** Amberlite resins. Amberlite resins, such as Amberlite XAD-2 and Amberlite XAD-4, are available as insoluble polymeric beads, each bead containing an agglomerate of cross-linked polystyrene microspheres. The Amberlite resins have a greater affinity for

TABLE 21.9 Range of Aminoglycoside Half-Lives (Hours) during Dialysis[a]

AMINOGLYCOSIDE	INTERDIALYSIS[b]	HEMODIALYSIS	PERITONEAL DIALYSIS
Kanamycin	40–96	5	12
Gentamicin	21–59	6–11	5–29
Tobramycin	27–70	3–10	10–37
Amikacin	28–87	4–7	18–29
Netlimicin	24–52	5	—

[a]Patient renal function creatinine clearance ≤5 mL/min.
[b]Interdialysis, period in between dialysis treatment.

From *Facts and Comparisons* (1992), with permission.

nonpolar organic molecules than does activated charcoal. The important factors for drug removal by hemoperfusion include affinity of the drug for the adsorbent, surface area of the adsorbent, absorptive capacity of the adsorbent, rate of blood flow through the adsorbent, and the equilibration rate of the drug from the peripheral tissue into the blood.

Hemofiltration

An alternative to hemodialysis and hemoperfusion is hemofiltration. *Hemofiltration* is a process by which fluids, electrolytes, and small-molecular-weight substances are removed from the blood by means of low-pressure flow through hollow artificial fibers or flat-plate membranes (Bickley, 1988). Because fluid is also filtered out of the plasma during hemofiltration, replacement fluid is administered to the patient for volume replacement. Hemofiltration is a slow, continuous filtration process that removes nonprotein bound, small molecules (<10,000 Da) from the blood by convective mass transport. The clearance of the drug depends on the sieving coefficient and ultrafiltration rate. Hemofiltration provides a creatinine clearance of approximately 10 mL/min (Bickley, 1988) and may have limited use for drugs that are widely distributed in the body, such as aminoglycosides, cephalosporins, and acyclovir. A major problem with this method is the formation of blood clots within the hollow filter fibers.

Continuous Renal Replacement Therapy (CRRT)

Because of the initial loss of fluid that results during hemofiltration, intermittent hemofiltration results in concentration of red blood cells in the resulting reduced plasma volume. Therefore, viscous blood with a high hematocrit and high colloid oncotic pressure results at the distal end of the hemofilter. *Predilution* may be used to circumvent this problem, but this method is rarely used because of cost and inefficiency.

Continuous replacement therapy allows ongoing removal of fluid and toxins by relying on a patient's own blood pressure to pump blood through a filter. The continuous filtration is better tolerated by patients than intermittent therapy, provides optimal control of circulating volumes, and provides ongoing toxin removal. Because continuous replacement therapies are hemofiltration methods, replacement fluid must be administered to the patient to replace fluid lost to the hemofiltrate, though the volume of fluid removed can be easily controlled compared to intermittent hemofiltration. Heparin infusions are also provided for anticoagulation.

Continuous renal replacement therapy (CRRT) includes *continuous veno-venous hemofiltration* (CVVH) and *continuous arteriovenous hemofiltration* (CAVH). In CAVH, blood passes through a hemofilter that is placed between a cannulated femoral artery and vein. A dialysis filter may be added to CAVH to improve small-molecule clearance. Circulating dialysate on the outside of the filters allows more efficient toxin removal. However, this method is inefficient (10–15 mL filtered per minute) and complex, and is not widely used in comparison to CVVH.

CVVH provides a hemofilter that is placed between cannulated femoral, subclavian, or internal jugular veins. Rather than relying on arterial pressure to filter blood, a pump can be used to provide filtration rates greater than 100 mL/min. Like CAVH, a dialysis filter may be added to CVVH to improve clearance of small molecules.

As with other extracorporeal removal systems, hemofiltration methods can alter drug pharmacokinetics. A study by Hansen et al. (2001) showed that acute renal failure patients on CVVH demonstrated a 50% decrease in clearance of levofloxacin. However, because of the high volume and moderate renal clearance of fluoroquinolones, levofloxacin did not require dosing adjustment.

Drug Removal during Continuous Renal Replacement Therapy

During CAVH, solutes are removed by convection, in which a *sieving coefficient, S,* reflects the solute removal ability during hemofiltration and is equal to the ratio of solute concentration in the ultrafiltrate to the solute concentration in the retentate. When $S = 1$, solute passes freely through the membrane, whereas when $S = 0$, the solute is retained in the plasma. S is constant and independent of blood flow; therefore,

$$Cl = S \times \text{rate}_{uf} \tag{21.37}$$

where rate_{uf} if the ultrafiltration rate. The concentration of drug in the ultrafiltrate is also equal to the unbound drug concentration in the plasma, and so the amount of drug removed during CAVH is

$$\text{Amount removed} = C_p + \alpha \times \text{rate}_{uf} \tag{21.38}$$

where α = the unbound fraction.

EFFECT OF HEPATIC DISEASE ON PHARMACOKINETICS

Drugs are often metabolized by one or more enzymes located in cellular membranes in different parts of the liver. Drugs and metabolites may also be excreted by biliary secretion. Hepatic disease may lead to drug accumulation, failure to form an active or inactive metabolite, increased bioavailability after oral administration, and other effects including possible alteration in drug protein binding, and kidney function.

The major difficulty in estimating hepatic clearance in patients with hepatic disease is the complexity and stratification of the liver enzyme systems. In contrast, creatinine clearance has been used successfully to measure kidney function and renal clearance of drugs. Clinical laboratory tests measure only a limited number of liver functions. Some clinical laboratory tests, such as the aspartate aminotransferase (AST) and alanine aminotransferases (ALT), are common serum enzyme tests that detect liver cell damage rather than liver function. Other laboratory tests, such as serum bilirubin, are used to measure biliary obstruction or interference with bile flow. Presently, no single test accurately assesses the total liver function. Usually, a series of clinical laboratory tests are used in clinical practice to detect the presence of liver disease, distinguish among different types of liver disorders, gauge the extent of known liver damage, and follow the response to treatment. A few tests have been used to relate the severity of hepatic impairment to predicted changes in the pharmacokinetic profile of the drug (*FDA Guidance for Industry,* 2003). Examples of these tests include the ability of the liver to eliminate marker drugs such as antipyrine, indocyanine green, monoethylglycine-xylidide, and galactose. Furthermore, endogenous substrates such as albumin or bilirubin, or a functional measure such as prothrombin time, have been used for the evaluation of liver impairment.

Dosage Considerations in Hepatic Disease

Several physiologic and pharmacokinetic factors are relevant in considering dosage of a drug in patients with hepatic disease (Table 21.10). Chronic disease or tissue injury may change the accessibility of some enzymes as a result of redirection or detour of hepatic blood circulation. Liver disease affects the quantitative and qualitative synthesis of albumin, globulins, and other circulating plasma proteins that subsequently affect drug plasma protein binding and distribution (Chapter 11). As mentioned, most liver function tests indicate only that the liver has been damaged; they do not assess the function of the cytochrome P-450 enzymes or intrinsic clearance by the liver.

Because there is no readily available measure of hepatic function that can be applied to calculate appropriate doses, enzyme-dependent drugs are usually given to patients with hepatic failure in half-doses, or less. Response or plasma levels then must be monitored. Drugs with flow-dependent clearance are avoided if possible in patients with liver failure. When necessary, doses of these drugs may need to be reduced to as low as one-tenth of the conventional dose, for an orally administered agent. Starting therapy with low doses and monitoring response or plasma levels provides the best opportunity for safe, efficacious treatment.

Fraction of Drug Metabolized

Drug elimination in the body may be divided into: (1) fraction of drug excretion unchanged, fe, and (2) fraction of drug metabolized. The latter is usually estimated

TABLE 21.10 Considerations in Dosing Patients with Hepatic Impairment

ITEM	COMMENTS
Nature and severity of liver disease	Not all liver diseases affect the pharmacokinetics of the drugs to the same extent
Drug elimination	Drugs eliminated by the liver >20% are less likely to be affected by liver disease. Drugs that are eliminated mainly via renal route will be least affected by liver disease
Route of drug administration	Oral drug bioavailability may be increased by liver disease due to decrease first-pass effects
Protein binding	Drug protein binding may be altered due to alteration in hepatic synthesis of albumin
Hepatic blood flow	Drugs with flow dependent hepatic clearance will be more affected by change in hepatic blood flow
Intrinsic clearance	Metabolism of drugs with high intrinsic clearance may be impaired
Biliary obstruction	Biliary excretion of some drugs and metabolites, particularly glucuronide metabolites, may be impaired
Pharmacodynamic changes	Tissue sensitivity to drug may be altered
Therapeutic range	Drugs with a wide therapeutic range will be less affected by moderate hepatic impairment

from $1 - fe$; alternatively, the fraction of drug metabolized may be estimated from the ratio of Cl_h/Cl, where Cl_h is hepatic clearance and Cl is total body clearance. Knowing the fraction of drug eliminated by the liver allows estimation of total body clearance when hepatic clearance is reduced. Drugs with low fe values (or, conversely, drugs with a higher fraction of metabolized drug) are more affected by a change in liver function due to hepatic disease.

$$Cl_h = Cl(1 - fe) \tag{21.39}$$

Equation 21.39 assumes that all metabolism occurs in the liver, and all the unchanged drug is excreted in the urine. Assuming linear kinetics are applicable (after determining that there is no enzyme saturation), dosing adjustment may be based on residual hepatic function in patients with hepatic disease, as shown in the following example.

PRACTICE PROBLEM

The hepatic clearance of a drug in a patient is reduced by 50% due to chronic viral hepatitis. How is the total body clearance of the drug affected? What should be the new dose of the drug in the patient? Assume that renal drug clearance ($fe = 0.4$) and plasma drug protein binding are not altered.

Solution

RL = residual liver function, estimated by $\dfrac{[Cl_h]_{hepatitis}}{[Cl_h]_{normal}}$

$[Cl_h]_{normal}$ = hepatic clearance of drug in normal subject
$[Cl_h]_{hepatitis}$ = hepatic clearance of drug in patient with hepatitis
Cl_{normal} = total clearance of drug in normal subject
$Cl_{hepatitis}$ = total clearance of drug in patient with hepatitis
fe = fraction of drug excreted unchanged
$1 - fe$ = fraction of drug metabolized
$[Cl_h]_{hepatitis} = RL\,[Cl_h]_{normal}$

Substituting for $[Cl_h]_{normal}$ with $Cl_{normal}(1 - fe)$,

$$[Cl_h]_{hepatitis} = RL\,Cl_{normal}(1 - fe) \tag{21.40}$$

Assuming no renal clearance deterioration due to hepatitis,

$$Cl_{hepatitis} = [Cl_h]_{hepatitis} + [Cl_R]_{normal} \tag{21.41}$$

Substituting Equation 21.40 with Equation 21.41 in terms of total body clearance

$$Cl_{hepatitis} = RL\,Cl_{normal}(1 - fe) + Cl_{normal}\,fe \tag{21.42}$$

$$Cl_{\text{hepatitis}} = Cl_{\text{normal}}[RL\,(1 - fe) + fe] \qquad\qquad \text{(21.43)}$$

$$\frac{D_{\text{hepatitis}}}{D_{\text{normal}}} = \frac{Cl_{\text{hepatitis}}}{Cl_{\text{normal}}} = \frac{RL\,(1 - fe) + fe}{1} \qquad\qquad \text{(21.44)}$$

where $D_{\text{hepatitis}}$ and D_{normal} are the doses in a hepatitis patient and in a normal liver function patient, respectively. Substituting in Equation 21.44 with $RL = 0.5$ and $fe = 0.4$,

$$\frac{D_{\text{hepatitis}}}{D_{\text{normal}}} = 0.5(1 - 0.4) + 0.4 = 0.3 + 0.4 = 0.7 \qquad (\text{or } 70\%)$$

The adjusted dose of the drug for the hepatic patient is 70% of that for the normal subject as a result of the 50% decrease in hepatic function in the above case ($fe = 0.4$).

An example of a correlation established between actual residual liver function (measured by marker) and hepatic clearance was reported for cefoperazone (Hu et al, 1995) and other drugs in patients with cirrhosis. The method should be applied only to drugs that have linear pharmacokinetics, low protein binding, or that are non-restrictively bound.

Many variables can complicate dose correction when binding profoundly affects distribution, elimination, and penetration of the drug to the active site. For drugs with restrictive binding, the fraction of free drug must be used to correct the change in free drug concentration and the change in free drug clearance. In some cases, the increase in free drug is partly offset by a larger volume of distribution resulting from the decrease in protein binding. Since there are many variables that complicate dose correction for patients with hepatic disease, dose correction is limited to drugs whose hepatic metabolism is approximated by linear pharmacokinetics.

Active Drug and the Metabolite

For many drugs, both the drug and the metabolite contribute to the overall therapeutic response of the patient to the drug. The concentration of both the drug and the metabolite in the body should be known. When the pharmacokinetic parameters of the metabolite and the drug are similar, the overall activity of the drug can become more or less potent as a result of a change in liver function; that is, **(1)** when the drug is more potent than the metabolite, the overall pharmacologic activity will increase in the hepatic-impaired patient because the parent drug concentration will be higher; **(2)** when the drug is less potent than the metabolite, the overall pharmacologic activity in the hepatic patient will decrease because less of the active metabolite is formed.

Changes in pharmacologic activity due to hepatic disease (Table 21.11) may be much more complex when both the pharmacokinetic parameters as well as the pharmacodynamics of the drug change as a result of the disease process. In such cases, the overall pharmacodynamic response may be greatly modified, making it necessary to monitor the response change with the aid of a pharmacodynamic model (see Chapter 19).

TABLE 21.11   Pugh's Modification of Child's Classification[a]

	1 POINT	2 POINTS	3 POINTS
Encephalopathy (grade)	None	1 or 2	3 or 4
Ascites	Absent	Slight	Moderate
Bilirubin (mg/dL)	1–2	2–3	>3
Albumin (gm/dL)	>3.5	2.8–3.5	<2.8
Prothrombin time (sec > control)	1–4	4–10	>10

[a]Total points: 5–6 = mild dysfunction; 7–9 = moderate dysfunction; >9 = severe dysfunction.

From Brouwer et al (1992).

Hepatic Blood Flow and Intrinsic Clearance

Blood flow changes can occur in patients with chronic liver disease (often due to viral hepatitis or chronic alcohol use). In some patients with severe liver cirrhosis, fibrosis of liver tissue may occur, resulting in intra- or extrahepatic shunt. Hepatic arterial-venous shunts may lead to reduced drug fraction of drug extracted (see Chapter 11) and an increase in the bioavailability of drug. In other patients, resistance to blood flow may be increased as a result of tissue damage and fibrosis, causing a reduction in intrisic hepatic clearance.

The following equation may be applied to estimate hepatic clearance of a drug after assessing changes in blood flow and intrinsic clearance (Cl_{int}):

$$Cl_h = \frac{Q\,Cl_{int}}{Q + Cl_{int}} \tag{21.45}$$

Alternatively, when both Q and the extraction ratio, ER, are known in the patient, Cl may also be estimated:

$$Cl = Q\,(ER) \tag{21.46}$$

Unlike changes in renal disease, in which serum creatinine concentration may be used to monitor changes in renal function such as glomerular filtration (GFR), the above physiologic model equation may not be adequate to account for accurate prediction of changes in hepatic clearance. Calculations based on model equations must be corroborated by clinical assessment.

Pathophysiologic Assessment

In practice, patient information about changes in hepatic blood flow may not be available, because special electromagnetic (Nuxmalo et al, 1978) or ultrasound techniques are required to measure blood flow and are not routinely available. The clinician/pharmacist may have to make an empirical estimate of the blood flow change after examining the patient and reviewing the available liver function tests (Table 21.12).

While chronic hepatic disease is more likely to change the metabolism of a drug (Howden et al, 1989), acute hepatitis due to hepatotoxin or viral inflammation is often associated with marginal or less severe changes in metabolic drug clearance

TABLE 21.12   Severity Classification Schemes for Liver Disease

	CHILD–TURCOTTE CLASSIFICATION		
	Grade A	Grade B	Grade C
Bilirubin (mg/dL)	<2.0	2.0–3.0	>3.0
Albumin (gm/dL)	>3.5	3.0–3.5	<3.0
Ascites	None	Easily controlled	Poorly controlled
Neurological disorder	None	Minimal	Advanced
Nutrition	Excellent	Good	Poor

From Brouwer et al (1992).

(Farrel et al, 1978). The clinician may make an assessment based on acceptable risk criteria on a case-by-case basis. Brouwer et al (1992) list useful endpoints for assessing the extent of hepatic dysfunction (Table 21.12).

In general, basic pharmacokinetics treats the body globally and more readily applies to dosing estimation. However, drug clearance based on individual eliminating organs is more informative and provides more insight into the pharmacokinetic changes in the disease process. A practical method for dosing hepatic-impaired patients is still in its early stages of development. While the hepatic blood flow model (Chapter 11) is useful for predicting changes in hepatic clearance resulting from alterations in hepatic blood flow, Q_a, and Q_v, extrahepatic changes can also influence pharmacokinetics in hepatic-impaired patients. Global changes in distribution may occur outside the liver. Extrahepatic metabolism and other hemodynamic changes may also occur and can be accounted for more completely by monitoring total body clearance of the drug using basic pharmacokinetics. For example, lack of local change in hepatic drug clearance should not be prematurely interpreted as "no change" in overall drug clearance. Reduced albumin and α acid glycoprotein (AAG), for example, may change the volume of distribution of the drug and therefore alter total body clearance on a global basis.

Hormonal Influence

Hormones can also affect the rate of metabolism. In hyperthyroid patients, the rate of metabolism of many drugs is increased, as are, for example, the rates for theophylline, digoxin, and propranolol. In hypothyroid disease, the rate of metabolism

TABLE 21.13   Drugs with Significantly Decreased Metabolism in Chronic Liver Disease

Antipyrine	Caffeine
Cefoperazone	Chlordiazepoxide
Chloramphenicol	Diazepam
Erythromycin	Hexobarbital
Metronidazole	Lidocaine
Meperidine	Metoprolol
Pentazocine	Propranolol
Tocainide	Theophylline
Verapamil	Promazine

Sources: Howden et al (1989), Williams (1983), Hu et al (1995).

of these drugs may be decreased (Table 21.13). In children with human growth hormone (HGH) deficiency, administration of HGH decreases the half-life of theophylline.

EXAMPLE

After IV bolus administration of 1 g of cefoperazone to normal and chronic hepatitis patients, urinary excretion of cefoperazone was significantly increased in cirrhosis patients, from 23.95 ± 5.06% for normal patients to 51.09 ± 11.50% in cirrhosis patients (Hu et al, 1995). Explain (**a**) why there is a change in the percent of unchanged cefoperazone excreted in the urine of patients with cirrhosis, and (**b**) suggest a quantitative test to monitor the hepatic elimination of cefoperazone. (*Hint:* consult Hu et al, 1994.)

Liver Function Tests and Hepatic Metabolic Markers

Drug markers used to measure residual hepatic function may correlate well with hepatic clearance of one drug but correlate poorly with substrate metabolized by a different enzyme within the same cytochrome P-450 subfamily. Some useful marker compounds are listed below.

1. *Aminotransferase* (normal ALT, male, 10–55 U/L; female, 7–30 U/L; normal AST, male, 10–40, U/L; female, 9–25 U/L). Aminotransferases are enzymes found in many tissues that include serum glutamic oxaloacetic transaminase (AST, formerly SGOT) and alanine aminotransferase (ALT, formerly SGPT). ALT is liver-specific, but AST is found in liver and many other tissues, including cardiac and skeletal muscle. Leakage of aminotransferases into the plasma is used as an indicator of many types of hepatic disease and hepatitis. The AST/ALT ratio is used in differential diagnosis. In acute liver injury, AST/ALT is ≤ 1, whereas in alcoholic hepatitis the AST/ALT > 2.

2. *Alkaline phosphatase* (male, 45–115 U/L; female, 30–100 U/L). Like amino-transferase, alkaline phosphatase (AP) is normally present in many tissues, and is present on the canalicular domain of the hepatocyte plasma membrane. Plasma AP may be elevated in hepatic disease because of increased AP production and released into the serum. In cholestasis, or bile flow obstruction, AP release is facilitated by bile acid solubilization of the membranes. Marked AP elevations may indicate hepatic tumors or biliary obstruction in the liver, or disease in other tissues such as bone, placenta, or intestine.

3. *Bilirubin* (normal total = 0–1.0 mg/dL, direct = 0–0.4 mg/dL). Bilirubin consists of both a water-soluble, conjugated, "direct" fraction and a lipid-soluble, uncon-jugated, "indirect" fraction. The unconjugated form is bound to albumin and is

therefore not filtered by the kidney. Since impaired biliary excretion results in increases in conjugated (filtered) bilirubin, hepatobiliary disease can result in increases in urinary bilirubin. Unconjugated hyperbilirubinemia results from either increased bilirubin production or defects in hepatic uptake or conjugation. Conjugated hyperbilirubinemia results from defects in hepatic excretion.

4. *Prothrombin time* (PT; normal, 11.2–13.2 sec). With the exception of Factor VIII, all coagulation factors are synthesized by the liver. Therefore, hepatic disease can alter coagulation. Decreases in PT (the rate of conversion of prothrombin to thrombin) therefore is suggestive of acute or chronic liver failure or biliary obstruction. Vitamin K is also important in coagulation, so vitamin K deficiency can also decrease PT.

EXAMPLE

Paclitaxel, an anticancer agent for solid tumors and leukemia, has extensive tissue distribution, high plasma protein binding (approximately 90–95%), and variable systemic clearance. Average paclitaxel clearance ranges from 87 to 503 mL/min/m^2 (5.2–30.2 L/h/m^2) with minimal renal excretion of parent drug, 10% (Sonnichsen and Relling, 1994). Paclitaxel is extensively metabolized by the liver to three primary metabolites. Cytochrome P-450 enzymes of the CYP3A and CYP2C subfamilies appear to be involved in hepatic metabolism of paclitaxel. What are the precautions in administering paclitaxel to patients with liver disease?

Solution

Although paclitaxel has first-order pharmacokinetics at normal doses, its elimination may be saturable in some patients with genetically reduced intrinsic clearance due to CYP3A or CYP2C. The clinical importance of saturable elimination will be greatest when large dosages are infused over a shorter period of time. In these situations, achievable plasma concentrations are likely to cause saturation of binding. Thus, small changes in dosage or infusion duration may result in disproportionately large alterations in paclitaxel systemic exposure, potentially influencing patient response and toxicity.

FREQUENTLY ASKED QUESTIONS

1. What are the main factors that influence drug dosing in renal disease?

2. Name and contrast the two methods for adjusting drug dose in renal disease.

3. What are the pharmacokinetic considerations in designing a dosing regimen? Why is dosing once a day for aminoglycosides recommended by many clinicians?

4. Protein binding of drugs is often affected by renal and hepatic disease. How are those changes accounted for in dose adjustment?

5. Drug clearance is often decreased 20–50% in many patients with congestive heart failure (CHF). Explain how it may affect drug disposition.

LEARNING QUESTIONS

1. The normal dosing schedule for a patient on tetracycline is 250 mg PO (peroral) every 6 hours. Suggest a dosage regimen for this patient when laboratory analysis shows his renal function to have deteriorated from a Cl_{Cr} of 90 to 20 mL/min.

2. A patient receiving antibiotic treatment is on dialysis. The flow rate of serum into the kidney machine is 50 mL/min. Assays shows that the concentration of drug entering the machine is 5 μg/mL and the concentration of drug in the serum leaving the machine is 2.4 μg/mL. The drug clearance for this patient is 10 mL/min. To what extent should the dose be increased if the average concentration of the antibiotic is to be maintained?

3. Glomerular filtration rate may be measured by either insulin clearance or creatinine clearance.

   a. Why is creatinine or insulin clearance used to measure GFR?

   b. Which clearance method, insulin or creatinine, gives a more accurate estimate of GFR? Why?

4. A uremic patient has a urine output of 1.8 L/24 hours and an average creatinine concentration of 2.2 mg/dL. What is the creatinine clearance? How would you adjust the dose of a drug normally given at 20 mg/kg every 6 hours in this patient (assume the urine creatinine concentration is 0.1 mg/mL and creatinine clearance is 100 mL/min)?

5. A patient on lincomycin at 600 mg every 12 hours intramuscular was found to have a creatinine clearance of 5 mL/min. Should the dose be adjusted? If so, **(a)** adjust the dose by keeping the dosing interval constant; **(b)** adjust the dosing interval and give the same dose; and **(c)** adjust both dosing interval and dose. What are the significant differences in the adjustment methods?

6. Using the method of Cockcroft and Gault, calculate the creatinine clearance for a woman (38 years old, 62 kg) whose serum creatinine is 1.8 mg/dL.

7. Would you adjust the dose of cephamandole, an antibiotic which is 98% excreted unchanged in the urine, for the patient in Question 6? Why?

8. What assumptions are usually made when adjusting a dosage regimen according to the creatinine clearance in a patient with renal failure?

9. The usual dose of gentamicin in patients with normal renal function is 1.0 mg/kg every 8 hours by multiple IV bolus injections. Using the nomogram method (Figure 21-5), what dose of gentamicin would you recommend for a 55-year-old male patient weighing 72 kg with a creatinine clearance of 20 mL/min?

10. A single intravenous bolus injection (1 g) of an antibiotic was given to a male anephric patient (age 68, 75 kg). During the next 48 hours, the elimination half-life of the antibiotic was 16 hours. The patient was then placed on hemodialysis for 8 hours and the elimination half-life was reduced to 4 hours.

   a. How much drug was eliminated by the end of the dialysis period?

   b. Assuming the apparent volume of distribution of this antibiotic is 0.5 L/kg, what was the plasma drug concentration just before and just after dialysis?

11. There are several pharmacokinetic methods for adjustment of a drug dosage regimen for patients with uremic disease based on the serum creatinine concentration in that patient. From your knowledge of clinical pharmacokinetics, discuss the following questions.

   a. What is the basis of these methods for the calculation of drug dosage regimens in uremic patients?

   b. What is the validity of the assumptions on which these calculations are made?

12. After assessment of the uremic condition of the patient, the drug dosage regimen may be adjusted by one of two methods: **(a)** by keeping the dose constant and prolonging the dosage interval, τ, or **(b)** by decreasing the dose and maintaining the dosage interval constant. Discuss the advantages and disadvantages of adjusting the dosage regimen using either method.

REFERENCES

Benet LZ, Massoud N, Gambertoglio JG (eds): *Pharmacokinetic Basis for Drug Treatment.* New York, Raven, 1984

Bennett WM: Guide to Drug Dosage in Renal Failure. *Clin Pharmacokinet* **15:**326–354, 1988

Bennett WM: Guide to Drug Dosage in Renal Failure. In *Clinical Pharmacokinetics Drug Data Handbook.* New York, Adis, 1990

Bianchetti G, Graziani G, Brancaccio D, et al: Pharmacokinetics and effects of propranolol in terminal uremic patients and in patients undergoing regular dialysis treatment. *Clin Pharmacokinet* **1:**373–384, 1978

Bickley SK: Drug dosing during continuous arteriovenous hemofiltration. *Clin Pharm* **7:**198–206, 1988

Bjornsson TD: Nomogram for drug dosage adjustment in patients with renal failure. *Clin Pharmacokinet* **11:**164–170, 1986

Bodenham A, Shelly MP, Park GR: The altered pharmacokinetics and pharmacodynamics of drugs commonly used in critically ill patients. *Clin Pharmacokinet* **14:**347–373, 1988

Brouwer KBR, Dukes GE, Powell JR: Influence of liver function on drug disposition. In Evans WE, Schewtag, J and Jusko, J (eds): *Applied Pharmacokinetics—Principles of Therapeutic Drug Monitoring.* Lippincott Williams & Wilkins, Baltimore, MD, 1992, chap 6

Carpenter CB, Lazarus JM: Dialysis and transplantation in the treatment of renal failure. In Isselbacher KJ, et al (eds): *Harrison's Principles of Internal Medicine.* New York, McGraw-Hill, 1994, chap 238

Chennavasin P, Craig Brater D: Nomograms for drug use in renal disease. *Clin Pharmacokinet* **6:**193–215, 1981

Cockcroft DW, Gault MH: Prediction of creatinine clearance from serum creatinine. *Nephron* **16:**31–41, 1976

De Hart RM: Vancomycin removal via newer hemodialysis membranes. *Hosp Pharm* **31:**1467–1477, 1996

Farrel GC, et al: Drug metabolism in liver disease. Identification of patients with impaired hepatic drug metabolism. *Gastroenterology* **75:**580, 1978

FDA Guidance for Industry: Pharmacokinetics in patients with impaired renal function—Study design, data analysis and impact on dosing and labeling, 1998. www.fda.gov/cder/guidance/index.htm

FDA Guidance for Industry: Pharmacokinetics in patients with impaired hepatic function: Study design, data analysis, and impact on dosing and labeling, 2003. www.fda.gov/cder/guidance/index.htm

Gambertoglio JG: Effects of renal disease: Altered pharmacokinetics. In Benet LZ, Massoud N, Gambertoglio JG (eds): *Pharmacokinetic Basis of Drug Treatment.* New York, Raven, 1984

Giusti DL, Hayton WL: Dosage regimen adjustments in renal impairment. *Drug Intell Clin Pharm* **7:**382–387, 1973

Hailmeskel B, Lakew D, Yohannes L, Wutoh AK, Namanny M: Creatinine clearance estimation in elderly patients using the Cockcroft and Gault equation with ideal, actual, adjusted or no body weight. *Consultant Pharmacist* **14:**72–75, 1999

Hansen E, Bucher M, Jakob W, Lemberger P: Pharmacokinetics of levofloxacin during continuous venovenous hemofiltration. *Intensive Care Med* **27:**371–375, 2001

Howden CW, Birnie GG, Brodie MJ: Drug metabolism in liver disease. *Pharmacol Ther* **40:**439, 1989

Hu OY, Tang HS, Chang CL: The influence of chronic lobular hepatitis on pharmacokinetics of cefoperazone—A novel galactose single-point method as a measure of residual liver function. *Biopharm Drug Dispos* **15**(7):563–576, 1994

Hu OY, Tang HS, Chang CL: Novel galactose single point method as a measure of residual liver function: Example of cefoperazone kinetics in patients with liver cirrhosis. *J Clin Pharmacol* **35**(3):250–258, 1995

Mathews SJ: Aminoglycosides. In Schumacher GE (ed), *Therapeutic Drug Monitoring.* Norwalk, CT, Appleton & Lange, 1995, chap 9

Merck Manual. Whitehouse Station, NJ, Merck, 1996–1997

Nuxmalo JL, Teranaka M, Schenk WG JR: Hepatic blood flow measurement. *Arch Surg* **113:**169, 1978

Physicians' Desk Reference. Montvale, NJ, Medical Economics (published annually).

Schneider V, Henschel V, Tadjalli-Mehr K, Mansmann U, Haefeli WE: Impact of serum creatinine measurement error on dose adjustment in renal failure. *Clin Pharmacol Ther* **74:**458–467, 2003

Schwartz GV, Haycock GB, Edelmann CM, Spitzer A: A simple estimate of glomerular filtration rate in children derived from body length and plasma creatinine. *Pediatrics* **58:**259–263, 1976

Scientific Tables, 7th ed. Ciba Geigy, 1973

Siersback-Nielson K, Hansen JM, Kampmann J, Kirstensen M: Rapid evaluation of creatinine clearance. *Lancet* **i:**1133–1134, 1971

Sonnichsen DS, Relling MV: Clinical pharmacokinetics of paclitaxel. *Clin Pharmacokinet* **27**(4):256–269, 1994

Spinler SA, Nawarskas JJ, Boyce EG, Connors Je, Charland SL, Goldfarb S: Predictive performance of ten equations for estimating creatinine clearance in cardiac patients. *Ann Pharmacother* **32:**1275–1283, 1998

St Peter WL, Redic-Kill KA, Halstenson CE: Clinical pharmacokinetics of antibiotics in patients with impaired renal function. *Clin Pharmacokinet* **22:**169–210, 1992

Tozer TN: Nomogram for modification of dosage regimen in patients with chronic renal function impairment. *J Pharmacokinet Biopharm* **2:**13–28, 1974

Traub SL, Johnson CE: Comparison methods of estimating creatinine clearance in children. *Am J Hosp Pharm* **37:**195–201, 1980

Wagner JG: *Fundamentals of Clinical Pharmacokinetics.* Hamilton, IL, Drug Intelligence, 1975, p 161

Welling PG, Craig WA: Pharmacokinetics in disease states modifying renal function. In Benet LZ (ed): *The Effects of Disease States on Drug Pharmacokinetics.* Washington, DC, American Pharmaceutical Association, 1976

Williams RL: Drug administration in hepatic disease. *N Engl J Med* **309:**1616, 1983

BIBLIOGRAPHY

Benet L: *The Effect of Disease States on Drug Pharmacokinetics.* Washington, DC, American Pharmaceutical Association, 1976

Bennett WM, Singer I: Drug prescribing in renal failure: Dosing guidelines for adults—An update. *Am J Kidney Dis* **3:**155–193, 1983

Bjornsson TD: Use of serum creatinine concentration to determine renal function. *Clin Pharmacokinet* **4:**200–222, 1979

Bjornsson TD, Cocchetto DM, McGowan FX, et al: Nomogram for estimating creatinine clearance. *Clin Pharmacokinet* **8:**365–399, 1983

Brater DC: *Drug Use in Renal Disease.* Boston, AIDS Health Science Press, 1983

Brater DC: Treatment of renal disorders and the influence of renal function on drug disposition. In Melmon KL, Morrelli HF, Hoffman BB, Nierenberg DW (eds): *Clinical Pharmacology—Basis Principles in Therapeutics,* 3rd ed. New York, McGraw-Hill, 1992, chap 11

Brenner and Rector, *The Kidney,* 6th ed. Philadelphia, Saunders, 2000, pp 2610–2614

Chennavasin P, Brater DC: Nomograms for drug use in renal disease. *Clin Pharmacokinet* **6**:193–214, 1981

Craig Brater D, Chennavasin P: Effects of renal disease: Pharmacokinetic considerations. In Benet LZ (eds): *Pharmacokinetic Basis of Drug Treatment.* New York, Raven, 1984

Cutler RE, Forland SC, St. John PG, et al: Extracorporeal removal of drugs and poisons by hemodialysis and hemoperfusion. *Annu Rev Pharmacol Toxicol* **27**:169–191, 1987

Dettli L: Elimination kinetics and dosage adjustment of drugs in patients with kidney disease. In Grobecker H, et al (eds): *Progress in Pharmacology,* vol 1. New York, Gustav Fischer Verlag, 1977

Fabre J, Balant L: Renal failure, drug pharmacokinetics and drug action. *Clin Pharmacokinet* **1**:99–120, 1976

Facts and Comparisons, Walter Kluwer Health. St. Louis, MO. (updated monthly), 1992

Feldman: Biochemical liver tests. In Sleisenger, Fordtran (eds): *Gastrointestinal and Liver Diseases,* 7th ed. Elsevier, 2002, pp 1227–1231

Ford, *Clinical Toxicology.* Philadelphia: Saunders, 2001, pp 43–48

Gibaldi M: Drug distribution in renal failure. *Am J Med* **62**:471–474, 1977

Gibson TP, Nelson HA: Drug kinetics and artificial kidneys. *Clin Pharmacokinet* **2**:403–426, 1977

Giusti DL, Hayton WL: Dosage regimen adjustments in renal impairment. *Drug Intell Clin Pharm* **7**:382–387, 1973

Hallynck TH, Soeph HH, Thomis VA, et al: Should clearance be normalized to body surface or lean body mass? *Br J Clin Pharm* **11**:523–526, 1981

Jellife RW: Estimation of creatinine clearance when urine cannot be collected. *Lancet* **1**:975–976, 1971

Jellife RW: Estimation of creatinine clearance in patients with unstable renal function, without a urine specimen. *Am J Nephrol* **22**:320–324, 2002.

Jellife RW, Jellife SM: A computer program for estimation of creatinine clearance from unstable serum creatinine concentration. *Math Biosci* **14**:17–24, 1972

Kampmann JP, Hansen JM: Glomerular filtration rate and creatinine clearance. *Br J Clin Pharmacol* **12**:7–14, 1981

Lee CC, Marbury TC: Drug therapy in patients undergoing haemodialysis. Clinical pharmacokinetic considerations. *Clin Pharmacokinet* **9**:42–66, 1984

LeSher DA: Considerations in the use of drugs in patients with renal failure. *J Clin Pharmacol* **16**:570, 1976

Levy G: Pharmacokinetics in renal disease. *Am J Med* **62**:461–465, 1977

Lott RS, Hayton WL: Estimation of creatinine clearance from serum creatinine concentration—A review. *Drug Intell Clin Pharm* **12**:140–150, 1978

Maher JF: Principle of dialysis and dialysis of drugs. *Am J Med* **62**:475–481, 1977

Parker PR, Parker WA: Pharmacokinetic considerations in the haemodialysis of drugs. *J Clin Hosp Pharm* **7**:87–99, 1982

Paton TW, Cornish WR, Manuel MA, Hardy BG: Drug therapy in patients undergoing peritoneal dialysis. Clinical pharmacokinetic considerations. *Clin Pharmacokinet* **10**:404–426, 1985

Ratz A, Ewandrowski K: Normal reference laboratory values. *N Engl J Med* **339**:1063–1071, 1998

Rhodes PJ, Rhodes RS, McClelland GH, et al: Evaluation of eight methods for estimating creatinine clearance in man. *Clin Pharm* **6**:399–406, 1987

Rosenberg J, Benowitz NL, Pond S: Pharmacokinetics of drug overdosage. *Clin Pharmacokinet* **6**:161–192, 1981

Schumacher GE: Practical pharmacokinetic techniques for drug consultation and evaluation, II: A perspective on the renal impaired patient. *Am J Hosp Pharm* **30**:824–830, 1973

Traub SL: Creatinine and creatinine clearance. *Hosp Pharm* **13**:715–722, 1978

Watanabe AS: Pharmacokinetic aspects of the dialysis of drugs. *Drug Intell Clin Pharm* **11**:407–416, 1977

Watkins PB, Hamilton TA, Annesley TM, Ellis CN, Kolars JC, Voorhees JJ: The erythromycin breath test as a predictor of cyclosporine blood levels. *Clin Pharmacol Ther* **48**:120–129, 1990

22

PHYSIOLOGIC PHARMACOKINETIC MODELS, MEAN RESIDENCE TIME, AND STATISTICAL MOMENT THEORY

The study of pharmacokinetics describes the absorption, distribution, and elimination of the active drug and metabolites in quantitative terms (Chapter 1). Ideally, a pharmacokinetic model uses the observed time course for drug concentration in the body and, from this data, obtains various pharmacokinetic parameters to predict drug dosing outcomes, pharmacodynamics, and toxicity.

In developing a model, certain underlying assumptions are made by the pharmacokineticist as to the type of pharmacokinetic model, the order of the rate process, the blood flow to a tissue, the method for the estimation of the plasma or tissue volume, and other factors. Even with a more general approach such as model-independent analysis, first-order drug elimination is often assumed in the calculation of AUC_0^∞. In selecting a model for data analysis, the pharmacokineticist may choose more than one method of modeling, depending on the many factors including experimental condition, study design, and completeness of data. The goodness-of-fit to the model and the desired pharmacokinetic parameters are other considerations. Each estimated pharmacokinetic parameter has an inherent variability because of the variability of the biologic system and of the observed data. Moreover, because pharmacokinetic studies are performed on a limited number of subjects, the estimated pharmacokinetic parameters may not be representative of the entire population.

Figure 22-1. In describing drug transfer, the physiologic pharmacokinetic model divides a body organ into three parts: capillary vessels, extracellular space, and intracellular space.

In spite of difficulties in the construction of these pharmacokinetic models, such models have been extremely useful in describing the time course of drug action, improving drug therapy by enhancing drug efficacy, and minimizing adverse reactions through more accurate dose regimens. Pharmacokinetic models are also applied to the development of new drug delivery systems. Three main types of pharmacokinetic models—physiologic, compartment, and statistical moment approach models—are discussed in this chapter.

The human body is composed of organ systems containing living cells bathed in an extracellular aqueous fluid (Chapter 10). Both drugs and endogenous substances, such as hormones, nutrients, and oxygen, are transported to the organs by the same network of blood vessels (arteries). The drug concentration within a target organ depends on plasma drug concentration, the rate of blood flow to an organ and the rate of drug uptake into the tissue. Physiologically, uptake (accumulation) of drug by organ tissues occurs from the extracellular fluid, which equilibrates rapidly with the capillary blood in the organ. Some drugs cross the plasma membrane into the interior fluid (intracellular water) of the cell (Fig. 22-1).

In addition to drug accumulation, some organs of the body are involved in drug elimination, either by excretion (eg, kidney) or by metabolism (eg, liver). The elimination of drug by an organ may be described by drug clearance in the organ (Chapters 6 and 11). The liver is an example of an organ with drug metabolism and drug uptake (accumulation). Physiologic pharmacokinetic models consider all processes of drug uptake and elimination.

PHYSIOLOGIC PHARMACOKINETIC MODELS

Drugs are carried by blood flow from the administration (input) site to various body organs, where the drug rapidly equilibrates with the interstitial water in the organ. Physiologic pharmacokinetic models are mathematical models describing drug movement and disposition in the body based on organ blood flow and the organ spaces penetrated by the drug. In its simplest form, a physiologic pharmacokinetic model considers the drug to be blood flow limited. Drugs are carried to organs by arterial blood and leave organs by venous blood (Fig. 22-2). In such a model, transmembrane movement of drug is rapid, and the capillary membrane does not offer any resistance to drug permeation. Uptake of drug into the tissues is rapid, and a constant ratio of drug concentrations between the organ and the venous blood is quickly established. This ratio is the tissue/blood partition coefficient:

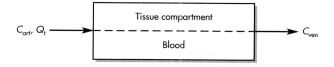

Figure 22-2. Noneliminating tissue organ. The extracellular water is merged with the plasma water in the blood

$$P_{\text{tissue}} = \frac{C_{\text{tissue}}}{C_{\text{blood}}} \tag{22.1}$$

where P is the partition coefficient.

The magnitude of the partition coefficient can vary depending on the drug and on the type of tissue. Adipose tissue, for example, has a high partition for lipophilic drugs. The rate of drug carried to a tissue organ and tissue drug uptake depend on the rate of blood flow to the organ and the tissue/blood partition coefficient, respectively.

The rate of blood flow to the tissue is expressed as Q_t (mL/min), and the rate of change in the drug concentration with respect to time within a given tissue organ is expressed as

$$\frac{d(V_{\text{tissue}} C_{\text{tissue}})}{dt} = Q_t(C_{\text{in}} - C_{\text{out}}) \tag{22.2}$$

$$\frac{d(V_{\text{tissue}} C_{\text{tissue}})}{dt} = Q_t(C_{\text{art}} - C_{\text{ven}}) \tag{22.3}$$

where C_{art} is the arterial blood drug concentration and C_{ven} is the venous blood drug concentration. Q_t is blood flow and represents the volume of blood flowing through a typical tissue organ per unit of time.

If drug uptake occurs in the tissue, the incoming concentration, C_{art}, is higher than the outgoing venous concentration, C_{ven}. The rate of change in the tissue drug concentration is equal to the rate of blood flow multiplied by the difference between the blood drug concentrations entering and leaving the tissue organ. In the *blood flow-limited model*, drug concentration in the blood leaving the tissue and the drug concentration within the tissue are in equilibrium, and C_{ven} may be estimated from the tissue/blood partition coefficient in Equation 22.1. Substituting in Equation 22.3 with $C_{\text{ven}} = C_{\text{tissue}}/P_{\text{tissue}}$ yields

$$\frac{d(V_{\text{tissue}} C_{\text{tissue}})}{dt} = Q_t\left(C_{\text{art}} - \frac{C_{\text{tissue}}}{P_{\text{tissue}}}\right) \tag{22.4}$$

Equation 22.4 describes drug distribution in a noneliminating organ or tissue group. For example, drug distribution to muscle, adipose tissue, and skin is represented in a similar manner by Equations 22.5, 22.6, and 22.7, respectively, as shown below. For tissue organs in which drug is eliminated (Fig. 22-3), parmeters representing drug elimination from the liver (k_{LIV}) and kidney (k_{KID}) are added to account for drug removal through metabolism or excretion. Equations 22.8 and 22.9 are derived similarly to those for the noneliminating organs above.

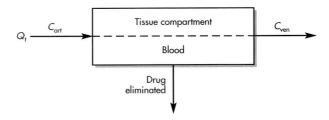

Figure 22-3. A typical eliminating tissue organ.

Removal of drug from any organ is described by drug clearance (Cl) from the organ. The rate of drug elimination is the product of the drug concentration in the organ and the organ clearance.

$$\text{Rate of drug elimination} = \frac{V_{\text{tiss}}\, dC_{\text{tiss}}}{dt} = C_{\text{tiss}} \times Cl_{\text{tiss}}$$

The rate of drug elimination may be described for each organ or tissue (Fig. 22-4).

$$\textit{Muscle:}\ \frac{d(V_{\text{MUS}} C_{\text{MUS}})}{dt} = Q_{\text{MUS}}\left(C_{\text{MUS}} - \frac{C_{\text{MUS}}}{P_{\text{MUS}}}\right) \tag{22.5}$$

$$\textit{Adipose tissue:}\ \frac{d(V_{\text{FAT}} C_{\text{FAT}})}{dt} = Q_{\text{FAT}}\left(C_{\text{FAT}} - \frac{C_{\text{FAT}}}{P_{\text{FAT}}}\right) \tag{22.6}$$

$$\textit{Skin:}\ \frac{d(V_{\text{SKIN}} C_{\text{SKIN}})}{dt} = Q_{\text{SKIN}}\left(C_{\text{SKIN}} - \frac{C_{\text{SKIN}}}{P_{\text{SKIN}}}\right) \tag{22.7}$$

$$\textit{Liver:}\ \frac{d(V_{\text{LIV}} C_{\text{LIV}})}{dt} = C_{\text{LIV}}(Q_{\text{LIV}} - Q_{\text{GI}} - Q_{\text{SP}}) + Q_{\text{GI}}\left(\frac{C_{\text{GI}}}{P_{\text{GI}}}\right)$$

$$+ Q_{\text{SP}}\left(\frac{C_{\text{SP}}}{P_{\text{SP}}}\right) - Q_{\text{LIV}}\left(\frac{C_{\text{LIV}}}{P_{\text{LIV}}}\right) - C_{\text{LIV}}\left(\frac{Cl_{\text{int}}}{P_{\text{LIV}}}\right) \tag{22.8}$$

$$\textit{Kidney:}\ \frac{d(V_{\text{KID}} C_{\text{KID}})}{dt} = Q_{\text{KID}}\left(C_{\text{KID}} - \frac{C_{\text{KID}}}{P_{\text{KID}}}\right) - C_{\text{KID}}\left(\frac{Cl_{\text{KID}}}{P_{\text{KID}}}\right) \tag{22.9}$$

$$\textit{Lung:}\ \frac{d(V_{\text{LU}} C_{\text{LU}})}{dt} = Q_{\text{LU}}\left(\frac{C_{\text{LU}}}{P_{\text{LU}}}\right) \tag{22.10}$$

where LIV = liver, SP = spleen, GI = gastrointestinal tract, KID = kidney, LU = lung, FAT = adipose, SKIN = skin, and MUS = muscle.

The mass balance for the rate of change in drug concentration in the blood pool is

$$\frac{d(V_{\text{b}} C_{\text{b}})}{dt} = Q_{\text{MUS}}\left(\frac{C_{\text{MUS}}}{P_{\text{MUS}}}\right) + Q_{\text{LIV}}\left(\frac{C_{\text{LIV}}}{P_{\text{LIV}}}\right) + Q_{\text{KID}}\left(\frac{C_{\text{KID}}}{P_{\text{KID}}}\right)$$
$$\text{(muscle)}\qquad\quad \text{(liver)}\qquad\quad \text{(kidney)}$$

$$+ Q_{\text{SKIN}}\left(\frac{C_{\text{SKIN}}}{P_{\text{SKIN}}}\right) + Q_{\text{FAT}}\left(\frac{C_{\text{FAT}}}{P_{\text{FAT}}}\right) + Q_{\text{LU}}\left(\frac{C_{\text{LU}}}{P_{\text{LU}}}\right) - Q_{\text{b}} C_{\text{b}} \tag{22.11}$$
$$\text{(skin)}\qquad\quad \text{(adipose)}\qquad\quad \text{(lung)}\qquad \text{(blood)}$$

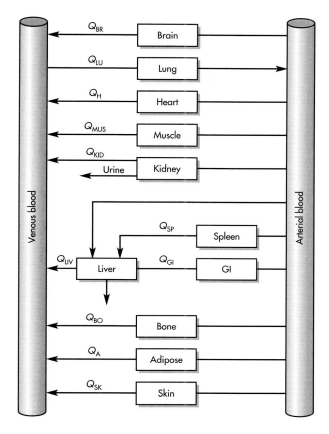

Figure 22-4. Example of blood flow to organs in a physiologic pharmacokinetic model.

Lung perfusion is unique because the pulmonary artery returns venous blood flow to the lung, where carbon dioxide is exchanged for oxygen and the blood becomes oxygenated. The blood from the lungs flows back to the heart (into the left atrium) through the pulmonary vein, and the quantity of blood that perfuses the pulmonary system ultimately passes through the remainder of the body. In describing drug clearance through the lung, perfusion from the heart (right ventricle) to the lung is considered as venous blood (Fig. 22-4). Therefore, the terms in Equation 22.11 describing lung perfusion are reversed compared to those for the perfusion of other tissues. With some drugs, the lung is a clearing organ besides serving as a merging pool for venous blood. In those case, a lung clearance term could be included in the general model.

After intravenous drug administration, drug uptake in the lungs may be very significant if the drug has high affinity for lung tissue. If actual drug clearance is at a much higher rate than the drug clearance accounted for by renal and hepatic clearance, then lung clearance of the drug should be suspected, and a lung clearance term should be included in the equation in addition to lung tissue distribution.

The system of differential equations used to describe the blood flow-limited model is usually solved through computer programs. The *Runge–Kutta method* is often used in computer methods for series of differential equations. Because of the large number of parameters involved in the mass balance, more than one set of parameters may fit the experimental data. This is especially true with human data, in which many of the organ tissue data items are not available. The lack of sufficient tissue data sometimes leads to unconstrained models. As additional data become available, new or refined models are adopted. For example, methotrexate was initially described by a flow-limited model, but later work described the model as a *diffusion-limited model.*

Because invasive methods are available for animals, tissue/blood ratios or partition coefficients can be determined accurately by direct measurement. Using experimental pharmacokinetic data from animals, physiologic pharmacokinetic models may yield more reliable predictions.

Physiologic Pharmacokinetic Model with Binding

The physiologic pharmacokinetic model assumes flow-limited drug distribution without drug binding to either plasma or tissues. In reality, many drugs are bound to a variable extent in either plasma or tissues. With most physiologic models, drug binding is assumed to be linear (not saturable or concentration dependent). Moreover, bound and free drug in both tissue and plasma are in equilibrium. Further, the free drug in the plasma and in the tissue equilibrates rapidly. Therefore, the free drug concentration in the tissue and the free drug concentration in the emerging blood are equal:

$$[C_b]_f = [C_t]_f \tag{22.12}$$
$$[C_b]_f = f_b[C_b] \tag{22.13}$$
$$[C_t]_f = f_t[C_t] \tag{22.14}$$

where f_b is the blood free drug fraction, f_t is the tissue free drug fraction, C_t is the total drug concentration in tissue, and C_b is the total drug concentration in blood.

Therefore, the partition ratio, P_t, of the tissue drug concentration to that of the plasma drug concentration is

$$\frac{f_b}{f_t} = \frac{[C_t]}{[C_b]} = P_t \tag{22.15}$$

By assuming linear drug binding and rapid drug equilibration, the free drug fraction in tissue and blood may be incorporated into the partition ratio and the differential equations. These equations are similar to those above except that free drug concentrations are substituted for C_b. Drug clearance in the liver is assumed to occur only with the free drug. The inherent capacity for drug metabolism (and elimination) is described by the term Cl_{int} (Chapter 11). General mass balance of various tissues is described by Equation 22.16:

$$\frac{d(V_{tissue} C_{tissue})}{dt} = Q_t(C_{art} - C_{ven})$$

$$\frac{d(V_{tissue} C_{tissue})}{dt} = Q_t\left(C_{art} - \frac{C_t}{P_t}\right) \tag{22.16}$$

or

$$\frac{d(V_{\text{tissue}} C_{\text{tissue}})}{dt} = Q_t\left(C_{\text{art}} - \frac{C_t f_t}{f_b}\right)$$

For liver metabolism,

$$\frac{d(V_{\text{LIV}} C_{\text{LIV}})}{dt} = C_b (Q_{\text{LIV}} - Q_{\text{GI}} - Q_{\text{SP}}) - Q_{\text{LIV}}\left(\frac{C_{\text{LIV}}}{P_{\text{LIV}}}\right)$$

$$\text{(hepatic drug elimination)}$$

$$+ Q_{\text{GI}}\left(\frac{C_{\text{GI}}}{P_{\text{GI}}}\right) + Q_{\text{SP}}\left(\frac{C_{\text{SP}}}{P_{\text{SP}}}\right) \tag{22.17}$$

The mass balance for the drug in the blood pool is

$$\frac{d(V_b C_b)}{dt} = Q_{\text{MUS}} C_{\text{MUS}} + Q_{\text{LIV}}\left(\frac{C_{\text{LIV}}}{P_{\text{LIV}}}\right) + Q_{\text{KID}}\left(\frac{C_{\text{KID}}}{P_{\text{KID}}}\right) + Q_{\text{SKIN}}\left(\frac{C_{\text{SKIN}}}{P_{\text{SKIN}}}\right)$$

$$\text{(muscle)} \qquad \text{(liver)} \qquad \text{(kidney)} \qquad \text{(skin)}$$

$$+ Q_{\text{FAT}}\left(\frac{C_{\text{FAT}}}{P_{\text{FAT}}}\right) + Q_{\text{LU}}\left(\frac{C_{\text{LU}}}{P_{\text{LU}}}\right) - Q_b C_b \tag{22.18}$$

$$\text{(adipose)} \qquad \text{(lung)} \qquad \text{(blood)}$$

The influence of binding on drug distribution is an important factor in inter-species differences in pharmacokinetics. In some instances, animal data may predict drug distribution in humans by taking into account the differences in drug binding. For the most part, extrapolations from animals to humans or between species are rough estimates only, and there are many instances in which species differences are not entirely attributable to drug binding and metabolism.

Blood Flow-Limited versus Diffusion-Limited Model

Most physiologic pharmacokinetic models assume rapid drug distribution between tissue and venous blood. Rapid drug equilibrium assumes that drug diffusion is extremely fast and that the cell membrane offers no barrier to drug permeation. If no drug binding is involved, the tissue drug concentration is the same as that of the venous blood leaving the tissue. This assumption greatly simplifies the mathematics involved. Table 22.1 lists some of the drugs that have been described by a flow-limited model. This model is also referred to as the *perfusion model*. A more complex type of physiologic pharmacokinetic model is called the *diffusion-limited model* or the *membrane-limited model*. In the diffusion-limited model, the cell membrane acts as a barrier for the drug, which gradually permeates by diffusion. Because blood flow is very rapid and drug permeation is slow, a drug concentration gradient is established between the tissue and the venous blood (Lutz and Dedrick, 1985). The rate-limiting step of drug diffusion into the tissue depends on the permeation across the cell membrane rather than blood flow. Because of the time lag

TABLE 22.1 Drugs Described by Physiologic Pharmacokinetic Model

DRUG	CATEGORY	COMMENT	REFERENCE
Thiopental	Anesthetic	Blood, flow limited	Chen and Andrade (1976)
BSP	Diagnostic	Plasma, flow limited	Luecke and Thomason (1980)
Nicotine	Stimulant	Blood, flow limited	Gabrielsson and Bondesson (1987)
Lidocaine	Antiarrhythmic	Blood, flow limited	Benowitz et al (1974)
Methotrexate	Antineoplastic	Plasma, flow limited	Bischoff et al (1970)
Biperiden	Anticholinergic	Blood, flow limited	Nakashima and Benet (1988)
Cisplatin	Antineoplastic	Plasma, multiple metabolite, binding	King et al (1986)

in equilibration between blood and tissue, the pharmacokinetic equation for the diffusion-limited model is very complicated.

Application and Limitations of Physiologic Pharmacokinetic Models

The physiologic pharmacokinetic model is related to drug concentration and tissue distribution using physiologic and anatomic information. For example, the effect of a change in blood flow on the drug concentration in a given tissue may be estimated once the model is characterized. Similarly, the effect of a change in mass size of different tissue organs on the redistribution of drug may also be evaluated using the system of physiologic model differential equations generated. When several species are involved, the physiologic model may predict the pharmacokinetics of a drug in humans when only animal data are available. Changes in drug–protein binding, tissue organ drug partition ratios, and intrinsic hepatic clearance may be inserted into the physiologic pharmacokinetic model.

Most pharmacokinetic studies are modeled based on blood samples drawn from various venous sites after either IV or oral dosing. Physiologists have long recognized the unique difference between arterial and venous blood. For example, arterial tension (pressure) of oxygen drives the distribution of oxygen to vital organs. Chiou (1989) and Mather (2001) have discussed the pharmacokinetic issues when differences in drug concentrations in arterial and venous are considered (Chapter 10). The implication of venous versus arterial sampling is hard to estimate and may be more drug dependent. Most pharmacokinetic models are based on sampling of venous data. In theory, mixing occurs quickly when venous blood returns to the heart and becomes reoxygenated again in the lung. Chiou (1989) has estimated that for drugs that are highly extracted, the discrepancies may be substantial between actual concentration and concentration estimated from well-stirred pharmacokinetic models.

Interspecies Scaling

Various approaches have been used to compare the toxicity and pharmacokinetics of a drug among different species. *Interspecies scaling* is a method used in toxicokinetics and the extrapolation of therapeutic drug doses in humans from nonclinical animal

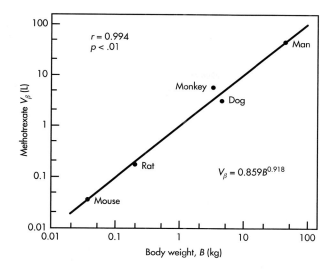

Figure 22-5. Interspecies correlation between methotrexate volume of distribution V_β and body weight. Linear regression analysis was performed on logarithmically transformed data.

(From Boxenbaum, 1982, with permission.)

drug studies. *Toxicokinetics* is the application of pharmacokinetics to toxicology and pharmacokinetics for interpolation and extrapolation based on anatomic, physiologic, and biochemical similarities (Mordenti and Chappell, 1989; Bonate and Howard 2000; Mahmood, 2000; Hu and Hayton, 2001).

The basic assumption in interspecies scaling is that physiologic variables, such as clearance, heart rate, organ weight, and biochemical processes, are related to the weight or body surface area of the animal species (including humans). It is commonly assumed that all mammals use the same energy source (oxygen) and energy transport systems across animal species (Hu and Hayton, 2001). Interspecies scaling uses a physiologic variable, *y*, that is graphed against the body weight of the species on log–log axes to transform the data into a linear relationship (Fig. 22-5). The general allometric equation obtained by this method is

$$y = bW^a \tag{22.19}$$

where *y* is the pharmacokinetic or physiologic property of interest, *b* is an allometric coefficient, *W* is the weight or surface area of the animal species, and *a* is the allometric exponent. *Allometry* is the study of size.

Both *a* and *b* vary with the drug. Examples of various pharmacokinetic or physiologic properties that demonstrate allometric relationships are listed in Table 22.2. In the example shown in Figure 22-5, methotrexate volume of distribution is related to body weight *B* of five animal species by the equation $V_\beta = 0.859B^{0.918}$.

The allometric method gives an empirical relationship that allows for approximate interspecies scaling based on the size of the species. Not considered in the method are certain specific interspecies differences such as gender, nutrition, pathophysiology, route of drug administration, and polymorphisms. Some of these more specific cases, such as the pathophysiologic condition of the animal or human, may preclude pharmacokinetic or allometric predictions.

TABLE 22.2   Examples of Allometric Relationship for Interspecies Parameters

PHYSIOLOGIC OR PHARMACOKINETIC PROPERTY	ALLOMETRIC EXPONENT a	ALLOMETRIC COEFFICIENT b
Basal O_2 consumption (mL/hr)	0.734	3.8
Endogenous N output (g/hr)	0.72	0.000042
O_2 consumption by liver slices (mL/hr)	0.77	3.3
Clearance		
Creatinine (mL/hr)	0.69	8.72
Inulin (mL/hr)	0.77	5.36
PAH (mL/hr)	0.80	22.6
Antipyrine (mL/hr)	0.89	8.16
Methotrexate (mL/hr)	0.69	10.9
Phenytoin (mL/hr)	0.92	47.1
Aztreonam (mL/hr)	0.66	4.45
Ara-C and Ara-U (mL/hr)	0.79	3.93
Volume of distribution (V_D)		
Methotrexate (L/kg)	0.92	0.859
Cyclophosphamide (L/kg)	0.99	0.883
Antipyrine (L/kg)	0.96	0.756
Aztreonam (L/kg)	0.91	0.234
Kidney weight (g)	0.85	0.0212
Liver weight (g)	0.87	0.082
Heart weight (g)	0.98	0.0066
Stomach and intestines weight (g)	0.94	0.112
Blood weight (g)	0.99	0.055
Tidal volume (mL)	1.01	0.0062
Elimination half-life:		
Methotrexate (min)	0.23	54.6
Cyclophosphamide (min)	0.24	36.6
Digoxin (min)	0.23	98.3
Hexobarbital (min)	0.35	80.0
Antipyrine (min)	0.07	74.5
Turnover times:		
Serum albumin (1/day)	0.30	5.68
Total body water (1/day)	0.16	6.01
RBC (1/day)	0.10	68.4
Cardiac circulation (min)	0.21	0.44

From Ritschel and Banerjee (1986), with permission.

Interspecies scaling has been refined by considering the aging rate and life span of the species. In terms of physiologic time, each species has a characteristic life span, its *maximum life-span potential* (MLP), which is controlled genetically (Boxenbaum, 1982). Because many energy-consuming biochemical processes, including drug metabolism, vary inversely with the aging rate or life span of the animal, the allometric approach has been used for drugs that are eliminated mainly by hepatic intrinsic clearance.

Through the study of various species in handling several drugs that are metabolized predominantly by the liver, some empirical relationships regarding drug clearance of several drugs have been related mathematically in a single equation. For example, drug hepatic intrinsic clearance of biperiden in rat, rabbit, and dog was extrapolated to humans (Nakashima et al, 1987). Equation 22.20 describes the relationship between biperiden intrinsic clearance with body weight and MLP:

$$Cl_{int} \times MLP = 1.36 \times 10^7 \times B^{0.892} \tag{22.20}$$

where MLP is the maximum life-span potential of the species, B is the body weight of the species, and Cl_{int} is the hepatic intrinsic clearance of the free drug.

Although further model improvements are needed before accurate prediction of pharmacokinetic parameters can be made from animal data, some interesting results were obtained by Sawada et al (1985) on nine acid and six basic drugs. When interspecies differences in protein–drug binding are properly considered, the volume of distribution of many drugs may be predicted with 50% deviation from experimental values (Table 22.3).

The application of MLP to pharmacokinetics has been described by Boxenbaum (1982). Initially, hepatic intrinsic clearance was considered to be related to volume or body weight. Indeed, a plot of the log drug clearance versus body weight for various animal species resulted in an approximately linear correlation (ie, a straight line). However, after correcting intrinsic clearance by MLP, an improved log–linear relationship was achieved between free drug Cl_{int} and body weight for many drugs. A possible explanation for this relationship is that the biochemical processes, including Cl_{int}, in each animal species are related to the animal's normal life expectancy (estimated by MLP) through the evolutionary process. Animals with a shorter MLP have higher basal metabolic rates and tend to have higher intrinsic hepatic clearance and thus metabolize drugs faster. Boxenbaum (1982, 1983) postulated a constant "life stuff" in each species, such that the faster the life stuff is consumed, the more quickly the life stuff is used up. In the fourth-dimension scale (after correcting for MLP), all species share the same intrinsic clearance for the free drug.

$$\frac{(MLP)(Cl_{int})}{B} = constant \tag{22.21}$$

$$Cl_{int} = aB^{\times} \tag{22.22}$$

Extensive work with caffeine in five species (mouse, rat, rabbit, monkey, and humans) by Bonati and associates (1985) verified this approach. Caffeine is a drug that is metabolized predominantly by the liver. For caffeine,

$$Q = 0.0554 \times B^{0.894}$$

$$L = 0.0370 \times B^{0.849}$$

where B is body weight, L is liver weight, and Q is blood flow.

Hepatic clearance for the unbound drug did not show a direct correlation among the five species (Fig. 22-6). After intrinsic clearance was corrected for MLP (calculation based on brain weight), an excellent relationship was obtained among the five species (Fig. 22-7).

More recently, the subject of interspecies scaling was investigated using Cl values for 91 substances for several species by Hu and Hayton (2001). These investigators used $Y = a\,(BW)^b$ in their analysis, similar to Equation 22.19 above but with

TABLE 22.3 Relationship between Predicted and Observed Values of Various Pharmacokinetic Parameters in Humans for 15 Drugs

DRUG	V (L/kg)			Cl_m (mL/min per kg)			$t_{1/2,z}$ (min)		
	Observed	Predicted	Percent[a]	Observed	Predicted	Percent[a]	Observed	Predicted	Percent[a]
Phenytoin	0.640	0.573	10.5	0.574	0.483	15.9	792	822	3.79
Quinidine	3.20	3.69	22.2	2.91	3.25	11.7	470	785	67.0
Hexobarbital	1.27	0.735	42.1	3.57	4.25	19.0	261	120	54.0
Pentobarbital	0.999	1.57	57.2	0.524	0.964	84.0	1340	1126	16.0
Phenylbutazone	0.122[b]	0.0839[c]	31.2	0.0205	0.0162	21.0	4110	3590	12.7
Warfarin	0.108	0.109	0.926	0.0367	0.0165	55.0	2040	4560	124
Tolbutamide	0.112	0.116	3.57	0.180	0.0589	67.3	434	1360	214
Chlorpromazine	11.2[b]	9.05[c]	19.2	4.29	4.63	7.93	1810	1350	25.2
Propranolol	3.62	3.77	4.14	11.2	15.56	38.9	167	135	19.2
Pentazocine	5.56	7.19	29.3	18.3	11.6	36.6	203	408	101
Valproate	0.151	0.482	219	0.110	0.159	44.5	954	2110	121
Diazepam	0.950	1.44	51.6	0.350	2.13	509	1970	469	76.2
Antipyrine	0.869	0.878	1.04	0.662	0.664	3.02	654	917	40.2
Phenobarbital	0.649	0.817	25.9	0.0530	0.0825	55.7	6600	5870	11.0
Amobarbital	1.04	1.21	16.3	0.556	1.01	81.7	1360	827	39.2

[a]Absolute percent of error.
[b]The value of V_{SS}.
[c]Predicted from the value of V_{SS} in the rat.

From Sawada et al (1985), with permission.

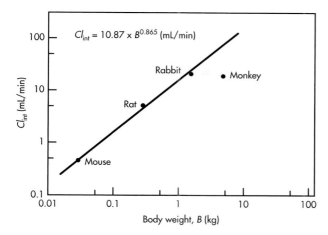

Figure 22-6. Caffeine Cl_{int} (free drug) in mammalian species as a function of body weight. Line does not utilize man and monkey points.
(From Bonati et al, 1985, with permission.)

different symbols: Y = biological variable dependent on the body weight of the species, a = allometric coefficient, b = allometric exponent, BW = body weight of the species. One issue discussed by Hu and Hayton is the uncertainty in the allometric exponent (b) of xenobiotic clearance (CL). Published literature has focused on whether the basal metabolic rate scale is a 2/3 or 3/4 power of the body mass (BW). When the uncertainty in the determination of a b value is relatively large, a fixed-exponent approach might be feasible according to Hu and Hayton. In this regard, 0.75 might be used for substances that are eliminated mainly by metabolism or by metabolism and excretion combined, whereas 0.67 might apply for drugs that are eliminated mainly by renal excretion. The researchers pointed out that genetic (intersubject) difference may be a limitation for using a single universal constant.

Physiologic versus Compartment Approach

Compartmental models represent a simplified kinetic approach to describe drug absorption, distribution, and elimination (Chapters 3 and 4). The major

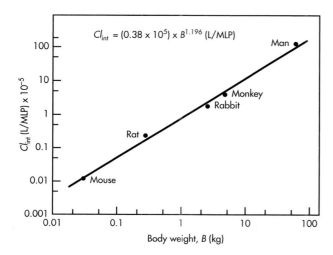

Figure 22-7. Caffeine (free drug) Cl_{int} per maximum life-span potential (MLP) in mammalian species as a function of body weight. MLP values were calculated for monkeys, rabbits, rats, and mice employing the following numeric values: MLP = $10.389 \times$ (brain weight)$^{0.636} \times$ (body weight)$^{0.225}$.
(From Bonati et al, 1985, with permission.)

advantage of compartment models is that the time course of drug in the body may be monitored quantitatively with a limited amount of data. Generally, only plasma drug concentrations and limited urinary drug excretion data are available. Compartmental models have been applied successfully to prediction of the pharmacokinetics of the drug and the development of dosage regimens. Moreover, compartmental models are very useful in relating plasma drug levels to pharmacodynamic and toxic effects in the body.

The simplicity and flexibility of the compartment model is the principal reason for its wide application. For many applications, the compartmental model may be used to extract some information about the underlying physiologic mechanism through model testing of the data. Thus, compartment analysis may lead to a more accurate description of the underlying physiologic processes and the kinetics involved. In this regard, compartmental models are sometimes misunderstood, overstretched, and even abused. For example, the tissue drug levels predicted by a compartment model represent only a composite pool for drug equilibration between all tissue and the circulatory system (plasma compartment). However, extrapolation to a specific tissue drug concentration is inaccurate and analogous to making predictions without experimental data. Although specific tissue drug concentration data are missing, many investigators may make general predictions about average tissue drug levels.

Compartment models account accurately for the mass balance of the drug in the body and the amount of drug eliminated. Mass balance includes the drug in the plasma, the drug in the tissue pool, and the amount of drug eliminated after dosage administration. The compartment model is particularly useful for comparing the pharmacokinetics of related therapeutic agents. In the clinical pharmacokinetic literature, drug data comparisons are based on compartment models. Though alternative pharmacokinetic models have been available for approximately 20 years, the simplicity of the compartment model allows easy tabulation of parameters such as V_{DSS}, alpha $t_{1/2}$, and beta $t_{1/2}$. The alternative pharmacokinetic models, including the physiologic and statistical moment (mean residence time) approaches, are used much less frequently, even though a substantial body of data has been generated using both of these models.

In spite of these advantages, the compartmental model is generally regarded as somewhat empirical and lacking physiologic relevance. Many disease-related changes in pharmacokinetics are the result of physiologic changes, such as impairment of blood flow or a change in organ mass. These pathophysiologic changes are better evaluated using a physiologic-based pharmacokinetic model.

Because of its simplicity, the compartment model often serves as a "first model" that requires further refinement in order to describe the physiologic and drug distribution processes in the body accurately. The physiologic pharmacokinetic model—which accounts for processes of drug distribution, drug binding, metabolism, and drug flow to the body organs—is much more realistic. Disease-related changes in physiologic processes are more readily related to changes in the pharmacokinetics of the drug. Furthermore, organ mass, volumes, and blood perfusion rates are often scalable, based on size, among different individuals and even among different species. This allows a perturbation in one parameter and the prediction of changing physiology on drug distribution and elimination.

The physiologic pharmacokinetic model may also be modified to include a specific feature of a drug. For example, for an antitumor agent that penetrates into the cell, both the drug level in the interstitial water and the intracellular water may be considered in the model. Blood flow and tumor size may even be included in the model to study any change in the drug uptake at that site.

The physiologic pharmacokinetic model can calculate the amount of drug in the blood and in any tissues for any time period if the initial amount of drug in the blood is known and the dose is given by IV bolus. In contrast, the tissue compartment in the compartmental model is not related to any actual anatomic tissue groups. The tissue compartment is needed when the plasma drug concentration data are fitted to a multicompartment model. In theory, when tissue drug concentration data are available, the multiple-compartment models may be used to fit both tissue and plasma drug data together, including the drug concentration in a specific tissue. In such a case, the compartment model would mimic the system of equations used in the physiologic model, except that in place of blood flows, transfer constants would be used to describe the mass transfer in the model. The latter approach would probably, at best, yield less useful information than that obtained from the physiologic model.

MEAN RESIDENCE TIME

After an intravenous bolus drug dose (D_0), the drug molecules distribute throughout the body. These molecules stay (reside) in the body for various time periods. Some drug molecules leave the body almost immediately after entering, whereas other drug molecules leave the body at later time periods. The term *mean residence time* (MRT) describes the average time for all the drug molecules to reside in the body. MRT may be considered also as the mean transit time or mean sojourn time. The residence time for the drug molecules in the dose may be sorted into groups i ($i = 1, 2, 3, \ldots, m$) according to their residing time. The total residence time is the summation of the number of molecules in each group i multiplied by the residence time, t_i, for each group. The summation of n_i (number of molecules in each group) is the total number of molecules, N. Thus, MRT is the total residence time for all molecules in the body divided by the total number of molecules in the body, as shown in Equation 22.23:

$$\text{MRT} = \frac{\text{total residence time for all drug molecules in body}}{\text{total number of drug molecules}}$$

$$\text{MRT} = \frac{\sum_{i=1}^{m} n_i t_i}{N} \tag{22.23}$$

where n_i is the number of molecules and t_i is the residence time of the ith group of molecules.

The drug dose (mg) may be converted to the number of molecules by dividing the dose (mg) by 1000 and the molecular weight of the drug to obtain the number of moles of drug, and then multiplying the number of moles of drug by

6.023×10^{23} (Avogadro's number) to obtain the number of drug molecules. For convenience, Equation 22.23 may be written in terms of milligrams (instead of molecules) by substitution of n_i with $De_i \times f$, where De_i is the number of drug molecules (as mg) leaving the body with residence time t_i ($i = 1, 2, 3, \ldots, m$). The f is a conversion factor. The number of molecules or milligrams of drug cancels out in Equation 22.24, showing that MRT is independent of mass:

$$\text{MRT} = \frac{\sum_{i=1}^{m} De_i f t_i}{\sum_{i=1}^{m} De_i f} = \frac{\sum_{i=1}^{m} De_i t_i}{\sum_{i=1}^{m} De_i} \tag{22.24}$$

where De_i ($i = 1, 2, 3, \ldots, m$) is the amount of drug (mg) in the ith group with residence time t_i.

Drug molecules may have a residence time ranging from values near zero (eg, 0.1, 0.2) to very large values (100, 1000, 10,000). The number of i groups may be large and the summation approach to calculate MRT will be only an approximation. Also, for the summation process to be accurate, data must be collected continuously in order not to miss any groups. Integration is an accurate method that replaces summation when the data or function needs to be continuously summed over time.

Mean Residence Time—IV Bolus Dose

The drug concentration in the body after an IV bolus injection for a drug that follows the pharmacokinetics of a one-compartment model is given by

$$C_p = \left(\frac{D_0}{V_D}\right) e^{-kt} \tag{22.25}$$

$$D_p = D_0 e^{-kt} \tag{22.26}$$

where V_D is the apparent volume of distribution, k is the first-order elimination rate constant, and t is the time after the injection of the drug. The drug exit rate was generated in Table 22.4 with a numerical example until most drug was eliminated.

The rate of change in the amount of drug in the body with respect to time (dD_p/dt) reflects the rate at which the drug molecules leave the body at any time t. Although all drug molecules enter the body at the same time, the exit time, or the residing time, for each molecule is different. Equation 22.27 is obtained by taking the derivative of Equation 22.26, with all the drug molecules exiting the body from $t = 0$ to ∞ (Table 22.4):

$$\frac{dD_p}{dt} = -kD_0 e^{-kt} \tag{22.27}$$

Alternatively, the rate of drug molecules exiting at any time t is given by

$$\frac{dDe}{dt} = \frac{-dD_p}{dt} = kD_0 e^{-kt} \tag{22.28}$$

TABLE 22.4 Simulated Plasma Data after an IV Bolus Dose, Illustrating Calculation of MRT[a]

TIME (hr)	RATE ELIMINATED dDe/dt (mg/hr)	RATE ELIMINATED Time $(t) \times dt$ (mg/hr)	C_p (mg/L)
0	231.000	0	100
1	183.354	183.354	79.374
2	145.535	291.070	63.002
3	115.517	346.551	50.007
4	91.690	366.762	39.693
5	72.778	363.891	31.506
6	57.767	346.602	25.007
7	45.852	320.964	19.849
8	36.395	291.156	15.755
9	28.888	259.990	12.506
10	22.929	229.293	9.926
42	0.014	0.593	0.006
43	0.011	0.482	0.005
44	0.009	0.392	0.004
45	0.007	0.318	0.003
46	0.006	0.258	0.002
47	0.004	0.209	0.002
48	0.004	0.170	0.002
49	0.003	0.137	0.001
Total drug exited = 1004.43[b]		Total drug residence time = 4310[c]	

[a]Drug exiting (first-order rate) tank or body compartment after IV bolus injection. Data generated with Equation 22.25. Dose = 1000 mg, volume = 10 L, $k = 0.231$ hr^{-1}.
[b]Total drug exited = average rate $\times$ dt and sum total.
[c]Total drug residence time (expressed as mg hr) = rate $\times$ $t \times$ dt and sum total.

Rearranging yields

$$dDe = kD_0 e^{-kt}\, dt \tag{22.29}$$

At any time t, dDe molecules exit. Therefore, multiplying Equation 22.29 by t on both sides yields the residence for each molecule exiting with a residence time t. Summation of the residence time for each drug molecule, and division by the total number of molecules, estimates the mean residence time (Eq. 22.30):

$$\frac{\int_0^\infty dD_0 e^{-kt} t}{D_0} = \frac{\int_0^\infty kD_0 e^{-kt} t\, dt}{D_0} \tag{22.30}$$

$$\mathrm{MRT} = \int_0^\infty ke^{-kt} t\, dt \tag{22.31}$$

As shown in Equation 22.30, the MRT is related to the product of the elimination rate constant k and the function describing drug elimination in the body. MRT is the integrated normalized form of the differential function representing drug amount (or concentration) in the body. The term *differential probability* is used to reflect that the function is a *probability density function* (PDF), which represents the residence time probability of a molecule in the population. The mean residence time is the normalized (divided by D_0) differential of the function governing drug elimination in the body. When a function is normalized, it becomes dimensionless, without units.

Equation 22.30 was derived in terms of amount of drug. Because $D_0 = C_p^0 V_D$, substituting for D_0 with $C_p^0 V_D$ into the right side of Equation 22.30 yields

$$\frac{\int_0^\infty dD_e t}{D_0} = \frac{\int_0^\infty kC_p^0 t \, dt}{C_p^0} \tag{22.32}$$

Equation 22.32 may be used to determine MRT directly or may be rearranged to Equation 22.33 by dividing the numerator and denominator by k to yield a moment equation.

$$\text{MRT} = \frac{\int_0^\infty d\,\mathrm{D}_e\, t}{D_0} = \frac{\int_0^\infty C_p^0 e^{-kt} t \, dt}{C_p^0/k} \tag{22.33}$$

The plasma concentration equation [function $f(t)$] multiplied by time and integrated from $0 = \infty$ gives a term called the *first moment* of the plasma drug curve. The denominator is the area under the curve, AUC_0^∞. The AUC_0^∞ is equal to $\int_0^\infty C_p \, dt$ or $D_0/V_D k$. Because $C_p^0 = D_0/V_D$, the denominator of Equation 22.33 is the AUC_0^∞ of the time–concentration curve ($\text{AUC}_0^\infty = D_0/kV_D$); see Chapter 6. Equation 22.33 is used in pharmacokinetics to determine MRT; the equation is abbreviated in the literature as shown in Equation 22.34:

$$\text{MRT} = \frac{\text{AUMC}}{\text{AUC}} \tag{22.34}$$

where AUMC is the area under the (first) moment-versus-time curve from $t = 0$ to infinity. AUC is the area under plasma time-versus-concentration curve from $t = 0$ to infinity. AUC is also known as the *zero moment curve*. Table 22.5 shows how

TABLE 22.5 Equations and Parameters Used in Generating Data for Figure 22.8. Summation Method Was Used to Mimic Actual Calculation of MRT by the Moment Method[a]

Parameters	
$i = 0, \ldots, 50$	Number of groups summed
$t_i = 1 \times i$	Residence time t_i
$k = 0.231$	
Dose $= 1000$ mg	
Volume $= 10$ L	
$Db_i = 1000 \times \exp(-kt_i)$	Equation showing drug in body at t_i
$De_i = 1000k \times \exp(-kt_i)$	Equation showing drug exiting at t_i
$rt_i = De_i \times t_i$	
$\sum_i rt_i = 4.31 \times 10^3$	Total residence time found by summation, $\text{MRT} = \dfrac{4310}{1004.43}$ $= 4.29$ hr
$\dfrac{1}{0.231} = 4.329$	MRT by calculation from $1/k$

[a]MATHCAD was used for calculation. Complete data generated are listed in Table 22.4.

summation may be used to calculate MRT from generated data when the function is known.

 # EXAMPLE

A drug that follows the kinetics of a one-compartment model is given by IV bolus injection at a dose of 1000 mg. The drug has an elimination rate constant of $0.231\ hr^{-1}$ and a volume of distribution of 10 L. The body is considered as a single compartment with no drug permanently bound in the body. (Use Table 22.4 for this problem; 50 data points were generated with Equation 22.25 for C_p and Equation 22.28 for dDe/dt.)

1. Calculate the MRT of the drug molecules in the body using the moment method. Assume AUC is 432.9 (mg/L) hr and AUMC is 1865.465 (mg/L)hr².

2. Calculate MRT using the total residence times of all molecules exited and divide by the total dose. Compare the answer to part 1.

Solution

1. Using the equation MRT = AUMC/AUC,

$$MRT = \frac{1865.465\ (mg/L)\ hr^2}{432.9\ (mg/L)\ hr} = 4.309\ hr$$

2. The residence time for most of the drug molecules exiting from the body ($t = 0$ to ∞) is approximated by the first 50 points (only few drug molecules remained in the body after 50 hours). Total residence time is the sum of the number of molecules at each exit time point multiplied by the time. The mean residence time is the sum of all the residence times for all drug molecules divided by the total number of molecules (Eq. 22.23). Multiplying columns 1 and 2 yields column 3:

> Total drug molecule residence time = 4310 mg hr
>
> Sum of drug exited = 1004.43 mg

(The sum of drug exited was obtained by averaging the rate of drug exited for each time point and multiplied by the time interval, 1 hour in this case; then sum up to obtain the total drug excreted. See Table 22.4.)

$$MRT = \frac{4310}{1004.43\ hr} = 4.29\ hr$$

The example is basically a verification of Equation 22.30. The approximation shows that when the function is not known, MRT may be estimated from the rate of drug excreted or from the plasma drug concentration–time curve. In practice, unless the entire dose is known, there is no assurance that all drug molecules are excreted through the plasma compartment if multiple compartments are involved.

MRT may also be calculated using the compartmental approach by considering the MRT for a drug after IV bolus injection as the reciprocal of the elimination rate constant, k. In this case, MRT is inversely related to the elimination constant, and MRT $= 1/k$. Therefore, MRT $= 1/0.231$ hr$^{-1} = 4.329$ hr. MRT was estimated earlier as 4.309 hr using the moment method. The slightly smaller value for the MRT here is due to approximation in the summation of the moment area and AUC.

Using the method of MRT $=$ AUMC/AUC, MRT may be estimated using the AUC calculated from the C_p–t curve (Table 22.4). Alternatively, the MRT can be estimated accurately using integration when the function that describes plasma drug concentrations is known (Table 22.5). A plot of De and C_p versus time, and the moment curve De $\times$ t versus t, are shown in Figure 22-8. For drugs that follow the kinetics of a one-compartment model with drug elimination only from the plasma, MRT may be calculated by either the area method or from the first moment curve. In data analysis, the function that governs drug disposition is generally not known, and the MRT is generally calculated from the plasma drug concentration–time curve.

STATISTICAL MOMENT THEORY

Statistical moment theory provides a unique way to study time-related changes in *macroscopic events*. A macroscopic event is considered as the overall event brought about by the constitutive elements involved. For example, in chemical processing, a dose of tracer molecules may be injected into a reactor tank to track the transit

Figure 22-8. Plot of **(A)** drug eliminated versus time; **(B)** C_p versus time; and **(C)** De versus time. The data generated for these plots are tabulated in Table 22.4. The actual equations and parameters used are listed in Table 22.5.

A. Tracer concentration in tank

$\int_0^{50} f(t)\, dt = 432.896$

B. Tracer in tank after normalization

$\int_0^{50} g(t)\, dt = 4.329$

C. Tracer exit rate after normalization

$\int_0^{50} h(t) \cdot t\, dt = 4.328$

$\int_0^{50} h(t)\, dt = 1$

Parameters

$t = 0, \ldots, 50$		Variable of time from 0 to 50 hr
$k = 0.231$		Elimination constant k
A	$f(t) = 100 \exp(-kt)$	Equation showing first-order exit of tracer
B	$g(t) = \exp(-kt)$	Equation after $f(t)$ divided by C_0, or 100. This normalizes the function.
C	$h(t) = k \exp(-kt)$	Multiplying $g(t)$ with k converts it to a PDF

Figure 22-9. Simulated tracer concentration in a tank over time. The three plots were generated by MATHCAD. The AUC under each curve is evaluated by integration. In **C,** the tracer concentration exit rate plot is a PDF and the AUC is 1. The mean of this function is simply the first moment and equal to the mean residence time of 4.328.

time (residence time) of materials that stay in the tank. The constitutive elements in this example are the tracer molecules, and the macroscopic events are the residence times shared by groups of tracer molecules. Each tracer molecule is well mixed and distributes noninteractively and randomly in the tank. In the case of all the molecules ($\int_0^{D_0} d\mathrm{De} = D_0$) that exit from the tank, the rate of exit of tracer molecules ($-d\mathrm{De}/dt$) divided by D_0 yields the probability of a molecule having a given residence time t (Fig. 22-9C). A mathematical formula describing the probability of a tracer molecule exited at any time is a probability density function. MRT is merely the expected value or mean of the distribution.

MRT provides a fundamentally different approach than classical pharmacokinetic models, which involve the concept of dose, half-life, volume, and concentration. The classical approach is macroscopic and does not account for the observation that molecules in a cluster move individually through space and are more appropriately tracked as statistical distribution based on residence-time considerations. Consistent with the concept of mass and the dynamic movement of molecules within a region or "space," MRT is an alternative concept to describe how drug molecules move in and out of a system. The concept is well established in chemical kinetics, where the relationships between MRT and rate constants for different systems are known.

In the last two decades, MRT has been well characterized for various pharmacokinetic models, although MRT application is less developed in pharmacodynamics. In the future, the residence-time concept will probably be applied further in pharmacodynamics if a useful model can be developed relating MRT to the intensity and duration of drug action that yields more insight than a conventional pharmacokinetic model. Empirically, it has been observed that changing from a slow rate of IV injection of a fast-acting drug may result in quite different response in a subject compared to rapid injection of the same drug solution. This observation has been attributed to a transient change in concentration at the site. Alternatively, the response may be explained by modeling the MRT change of the drug at the site.

EXAMPLE

Assume the tracer molecules are eliminated according to a kinetic function, $f(t) = C_0 e^{-kt}$. The tank volume V_D and k are similar to the previous one-compartment-model example ($k = 0.231$ hr^{-1}, $D_0 = 1000$ mg, $V_D = 10$). What is the MRT? What is the probability density function?

Because $f(t)$ describes drug elimination in terms of concentration units, $f(t)$ is divided by C_0 for normalization (Fig. 22-9B). The function is then differentiated to obtain $h(t)$. Next, $h(t) = ke^{-kt}$ is plotted in Figure 22-9C. This is the PDF (probability density function), also obtained by $k \times C$. Integration of $h(t)$ t dt yields MRT (4.329 hours) directly. Integration of $f(t)$ yields the AUC of 432.896 (mg/L) hr. All integration in Figure 22-9 were computed using MATHCAD software.

In the one-compartment model, AUC divided by C_0 also yields MRT (432.896/100 = 4.33 hr). This example is another way to calculate MRT, as will be demonstrated later. MRT may also be computed by integrating $f(t)/C_0$ (Fig. 22-9B). However, if $f(t)$ represents a two- or multicompartment function, the computed MRT using this method is only for the central compartment, whereas using the AUMC/AUC approach leads to an MRT for the body (a larger value). The latter method treats the molecules as a single population within the body, tracking them only as they exit and without supposing any knowledge of molecular exchanges between the plasma and tissue compartments.

In the previous discussion, Equation 22.34 was derived to estimate MRT without applying the concept of probability density functions. However, the equation may be rearranged in the form of a PDF, as in Equation 22.31. This result is plotted in Figure 22-9C for comparison. The moment theory facilitates calculation of MRT and related parameters from the kinetic function, as discussed below.

A probability density function $f(t)$ multiplied by t^m and integrated over time yields the moment curve (Eq. 22.35). The moment curve shows the characteristics of the distribution.

$$\mu_m \text{ or } m\text{th moment} = \int_0^\infty t^m f(t) \ dt \qquad (22.35)$$

where $f(t)$ is the probability density function, t is time, and m is the mth moment.

For example, when $m = 0$, substituting for $m = 0$ yields Equation 22.36, called the *zero moment*, μ_0:

$$\mu_0 = \int_0^\infty f(t) \ dt \qquad (22.36)$$

If the distribution is a true probability function, the area under the zero moment curve is 1.

Substituting into Equation 22.35 with $m = 1$, Equation 22.37 gives the first moment μ_1

$$\mu_1 = \int_0^\infty t^1 f(t)\ dt \tag{22.37}$$

The area under the curve $f(t)$ times t is called the AUMC, or the *area under the first moment curve*. The *first moment, μ_1*, defines the *mean* of the distribution.

Similarly, when $m = 2$, Equation 22.35 becomes the *second moment, μ_2*:

$$\mu_2 = \int_0^\infty t^2 f(t)\ dt \tag{22.38}$$

where μ_2 defines the variance of the distribution. Higher moments, such as μ_3 or μ_4, represent skewness and kurtosis of the distribution. Equation 22.35 is therefore useful in characterizing family of moment curves of a distribution.

The principal use of the moment curve is the calculation of the MRT of a drug in the body. The elements of the distribution curve describe the distribution of drug molecules after administration and the residence time of the drug molecules in the body.

In Equation 22.31, the plasma equation, $f(t) = C_p^0 e^{-kt}$, was converted to a PDF [ie, $f(t) = ke^{-kt}$]. It can be shown that μ_0 for this function = 1 (total probability adds up to 1 by summing zero moment), and the mean of the function is the area under the first moment curve (the mean is the MRT).

By comparison, Equation 22.25 is not a true PDF, because its mean is not given by the AUMC, and its AUC is not 1. Nonetheless, Equation 22.34 may be used to calculate MRT independent of the PDF concept, although some confusion over its application appears in the literature.

EXAMPLE

An antibiotic was given to two subjects by an IV bolus dose of 1000 mg. The drug has a volume of distribution of 10 L and follows a one-compartment model with an elimination constant of (1) 0.1 hr^{-1} and (2) 0.2 hr^{-1} in the two subjects. Determine the MRT from each C_p–time curve (Table 22.6) and compare your values with the MRT determined by taking the reciprocal of k.

Solution

Noncompartmental Approach (MRT = AUMC/AUC)

1. From Table 22.6, multiply each time point with the corresponding plasma C_p to obtain points for the moment curve. Use the trapezoid rule and sum the area

TABLE 22.6 Simulated Data for a Drug Administered by IV Bolus[a]

				SUBJECTS 1 AND 2	
	C_p1	C_p2	t	AUMC1	AUMC2
0	100.000	100.000	0	0.000	0.000
1	90.484	81.873	1	90.484	81.873
2	81.873	67.032	2	163.746	134.064
3	74.082	54.881	3	222.245	164.643
4	67.032	44.933	4	268.128	179.732
5	60.653	36.788	5	303.265	183.940
6	54.881	30.119	6	329.287	180.717
7	49.659	24.660	7	347.610	172.618
8	44.933	20.190	8	359.463	161.517
9	40.657	16.530	9	365.913	148.769
10	36.788	13.534	10	367.879	135.335
11	33.287	11.080	11	366.158	121.883
12	30.119	9.072	12	361.433	108.862
13	27.253	7.427	13	354.291	96.556
14	24.660	6.081	14	345.236	85.134
15	22.313	4.979	15	334.695	74.681
16	20.190	4.076	16	323.034	65.220
17	18.268	3.337	17	310.562	56.735
18	16.530	2.732	18	297.538	49.183
19	14.957	2.237	19	284.180	42.504
20	13.534	1.832	20	270.671	36.631
21	12.246	1.500	21	257.158	31.491
22	11.080	1.228	22	243.767	27.010
23	10.026	1.005	23	230.595	23.119
24	9.072	0.823	24	217.723	19.751
25	8.208	0.674	25	205.212	16.845
26	7.427	0.552	26	193.111	14.343
27	6.721	0.452	27	181.455	12.195
28	6.081	0.370	28	170.268	10.354
29	5.502	0.303	29	159.567	8.780
30	4.979	0.248	30	149.361	7.436
91	0.011167	0.00000125	91	1.0162	0.0001135
92	0.010104	0.00000102	92	0.9296	0.0000939
93	0.009142	0.00000084	93	0.8502	0.0000777
94	0.008272	0.00000068	94	0.7776	0.0000643
95	0.007485	0.00000056	95	0.7111	0.0000532
96	0.006773	0.00000046	96	0.6502	0.0000440
97	0.006128	0.00000038	97	0.5944	0.0000364
98	0.005545	0.00000031	98	0.5434	0.0000301
99	0.005017	0.00000025	99	0.4967	0.0000249
100	0.004540	0.00000021	100	0.4540	0.0000206

[a](1) $k = 0.1$ hr^{-1}, (2) $k = 0.2$ hr^{-1}.

Note the corresponding AUMC for the two subjects in the last two columns.

to obtain area under the moment curve (AUMC$_1$) for subject 1. Also, determine the area under the plasma curve using the trapezoid rule.

2. The steps are as follows.

    a. Multiply each C_p by t as in column 5 of Table 22.6.

b. Sum all $C_p \times t$ values, and find the area under the moment curve (AUMC)—that is, 9986.45 $(\mu g/mL)$ hr^2.

c. Estimate tail area of the moment curve (beyond the last data point) using the equation

$$\text{AUMC} = \frac{C_p t}{k} + \frac{C_p}{k^2} \qquad (22.39)$$

Substituting the last data point, $C_p = 0.00454\ \mu g/mL$, the last time point, 100 hours, and the last moment curve point, 0.454 $(\mu g/mL)$ hr^2:

$$\text{Tail AUMC} = \frac{0.454}{0.1} + \frac{0.00454}{0.1^2} = 4.99\ (\mu g/mL)\ hr^2$$

$$\text{Total AUMC} = 9986.46 + 4.99 = 9991.45\ (\mu g/mL)\ hr^2$$

(Note that k is determined from the slope to be 0.1 hr^{-1}.)

d. Estimate AUC using the trapezoid rule from columns 1 and 2 (AUC = 1000.79 $\mu g/mL/hr$).

e. $\text{MRT} = \dfrac{\text{AUMC}}{\text{AUC}} = \dfrac{9991.45\ (\mu g/mL)\ hr^2}{1000.79\ (\mu g/mL)\ hr} = 9.98\ hr$

When data are available for a long period, 6 to 7 half-lives and beyond, the last C_p will be very small and no extrapolation will be needed. If a model-independent approach is needed, no extrapolation beyond the data should be used (in this example, extrapolation was used only for illustration). Instead, additional data should be collected, or the assay sensitivity improved so that more data at later time periods may be obtained. All data extrapolation, linear or log-linear, will be subject to error, because the real rate process is determined from the experimental data and is not assumed.

Note that without the extrapolation to infinity, MRT = 9986.45/1000.79 = 9.978 hours, because extensive plasma drug concentration data are available. This value is fairly close to the value of 9.98 hours when the plasma drug concentration data are extrapolated to infinity.

2. From the tabulated results, summing up column 6, $\text{AUMC}_2 = 2491.68\ (\mu g/mL)$ hr^2. AUC for patient 2 = 500 $(\mu g/mL)$ hr (calculated from the trapezoid rule using the time–plasma concentration data for subject 2).

(*Note:* In this case, the AUMC tail area was not extrapolated because the drug concentration was already very low at the last data point.)

$$\text{MRT} = \frac{2491.68\ (\mu g/mL)\ hr^2}{500\ (\mu g/mL)\ hr} = 4.98\ hr$$

Compartment Approach

1. If a one-compartment model is assumed and k is determined from the slope, MRT is simply $1/k = 1/0.1 = 10$ hours.

2. As determined from the slope of a C_p–t curve, $k = 0.2$ hr^{-1}, and MRT = $1/0.2$ = 5 hours.

In a one-compartment model IV bolus, MRT is inversely proportional to the elimination constant and directly proportional to the half-life of the drug in the patient. The elimination half-lives of the drug in the two patients are 6.93 and 3.47 hours, respectively.

The plasma drug concentration–time curves for the two cases above were plotted with the moment curves. The use of moment ($C_p \times t$) changes the typical monoexponential plasma–time curve into a profile very similar to that of a nonsymmetric bell-shaped curve (Fig. 22.10) similar to a statistical distribution (see Appendix A). Furthermore, in the one-compartment IV bolus case, the mean of the distribution may be seen as 10 and 5 hours, respectively, from the curve. A smaller k widens the distribution and increases the total residence times of all the drug molecules in the body. The shape of the moment curve depends on the function describing the plasma drug concentration, and may be skewed.

MRT for Multicompartment Model with Elimination from the Central Compartment

The moment theory provides a means for calculating MRT for the body from plasma drug concentration data obtained for drugs that follow one-compartment models. In this section, the MRT is determined for a drug that has a plasma (central) compartment and one or more tissue or peripheral compartments. The assumptions

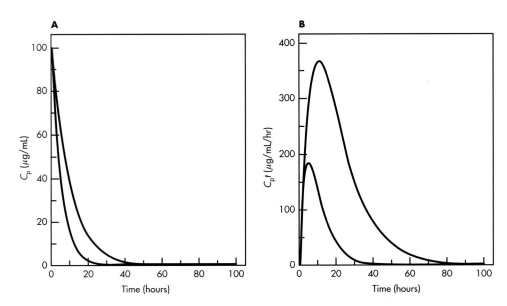

Figure 22-10. Simulated plasma drug concentration curves (left) and the corresponding AUMC curves (right). Dose = 1000 mg, V_D = 10 L, k = 0.1, and 0.2 hr^{-1}, by IV bolus administration.

are (1) that the drug is eliminated only from the central compartment and (2) that all drug is eliminated by a linear process (constant clearance). The MRT for a multicompartment model drug is the summation of the residence time of the drug in each compartment,

$$\text{MRT}_{\text{body}} = \text{MRT}_{\text{c}} + \text{MRT}_{\text{p1}} + \text{MRT}_{\text{p2}} + \cdots + \text{MRT}_{\text{pn}} \tag{22.40}$$

where MRT_{pi} represents MRT in the ith peripheral or tissue compartments and $\text{MRT}_{c} = $ MRT for the central compartment.

MRT for the body may be calculated from the plasma concentration curve using AUMC/AUC as discussed earlier, because the body (including all compartments) may be treated as a single compartment.

MRT_{c} is known as the mean residence time or mean transit time for the central compartment. This is calculated by AUC/C_{p}^{0}, where AUC is the area under the plasma drug concentration curve and C_{p}^{0} is the initial plasma drug concentration curve.

Derivation of MRT$_c$

Let

    De = amount of drug eliminated at time t

    D_0 = does or drug at time zero

    D_{p} = amount of drug in the plasma compartment from which drug is eliminated at time t

    C_{p} = drug concentration in the plasma compartment (volume, V_{D})

At time t, dDe units of drug are eliminated, the residence time is $t\, d$De, and integrating from 0 to D_{e}^{∞} yields the total residence time (see the numerator of Eq. 22.41). Integrating De will yield the total units of drug eliminated (see the denominator of Eq. 22.41), and MRT is obtained by dividing the total residence time by the total unit of drugs. If elimination occurs only from the central compartment, then at any instant dt, dDe $= -dD_{p}$.

$$\text{MRT}_{\text{c}} = \frac{\displaystyle\int_{0}^{\text{De}^{0}} t\, d\text{De}}{\displaystyle\int_{0}^{\text{De}^{0}} d\text{De}} = \frac{\displaystyle\int_{0}^{D_{0}} t\, d\text{D}_{\text{p}}}{\displaystyle\int_{0}^{D_{0}} d\text{D}_{\text{p}}} \tag{22.41}$$

$$\text{MRT}_{\text{C}} = \frac{\displaystyle\int_{0}^{C_{\text{p}}^{0}} t V_{\text{D}}\, dC_{\text{p}}}{\displaystyle\int_{0}^{C_{\text{p}}^{0}} V_{\text{D}}\, dC_{\text{p}}} = \frac{\displaystyle\int_{0}^{C_{\text{p}}^{0}} t\, dC_{\text{p}}}{\displaystyle\int_{0}^{C_{\text{p}}^{0}} dC_{\text{p}}} \tag{22.42}$$

Since

$$t\, dC_p = -C_p\, dt \quad \text{and} \quad \int_0^0 dC_p = C_p^0$$

$$\text{MRT}_c = \frac{\displaystyle\int_0^\infty C_p\, dt}{C_p^0} = \frac{\text{AUC}_0^\infty}{C_p^0} \tag{22.43}$$

When a drug is distributed between a central and one or more peripheral compartments, the peripheral compartment is not available for sampling. Therefore, both the drug and tissue MRT have to be determined from the plasma data. If a two-compartment model is involved, the peripheral MRT is given by

$$\text{MRT}_p = \frac{\text{AUMC}}{\text{AUC}} - \frac{\text{AUC}}{C_p^0} \tag{22.44}$$

EXAMPLE

The plasma drug concentrations of a drug that follows a two-compartment model after IV bolus were simulated with the following parameters (Nagashima and Benet, 1988) and the plasma concentration equation for the two-compartment model. Determine MRT for the plasma and tissue compartments and verify Equation 22.43. Use these parameters: $a = 2.2346$, $b = 0.4654$, $k = 0.946$ (overall elimination constant from the central compartment), $k_{12} = 0.655$, $k_{21} = 1.1$ (all rate constants in hr^{-1}). Also, $V_p = 10$ L, $D_0 = 1000$ mg, $C_0 = 100$ μg/mL.

Using the above parameters, the plasma drug concentrations, C_p, at any point is given by Equation 22.45 (Table 22.7) and is plotted in Figure 22-11.

$$C_p = 100\left[\left(\frac{k_{21} - a}{b - a}\right)e^{-at} - \left(\frac{k_{21} - b}{a - b}\right)e^{-bt}\right] \tag{22.45}$$

The AUMC is found by determining the $C_p \times t$ at each point and summing up for the entire curve (Table 22.7). The AUMC = 177.915 and the AUC = 106.6. The MRT of the drug in the body is 1.67 hours. MRT of the drug in the plasma is $\text{AUC}/C_0 = 106.6/100 = 1.066$ hours. The MRT for the tissue compartment is $1.67 - 1.066 = 0.604$ hour.

From statistical moment theory, MRT is the mean of the statistical distribution, $k \times C_p \times dt$, where k is the elimination constant and each C_p has been normalized by dividing by C_0 (to give a PDF). MRT for the body is then simply the first moment of the distribution:

$$\text{MRT} = \int_0^\infty \frac{100}{C_0}\left[\left(\frac{k_{21} - a}{b - a}\right)e^{-at} - \left(\frac{k_{21} - b}{a - b}\right)e^{-bt}\right]k\, dt \tag{22.46}$$

MRT = 1.687 hr

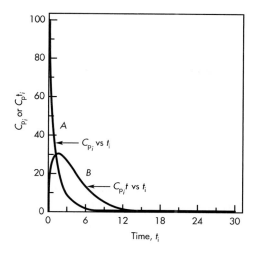

Figure 22-11. Plot of (A) C_p and (B) C_p versus time $C_p\,dt$ after a bolus dose IV.

The answer should agree with that given above, by AUMC/AUC. The second method illustrates the relationship of the plasma concentration data and the PDF. Because k (the elimination constant from the central compartment) is not known from plasma data, the second approach is not applied directly. The PDF approach may also be used to determine MRT_c, or mean residence time from the central compartment. Taking the derivative of the two-compartment equation for plasma drug concentration yields a PDF; this function may be calculated directly using software such as MATHCAD. Integration of the result yields $MRT = 1.066$ hours

TABLE 22.7   Simulated Data Showing How to Calculate MRT from AUMC/AUC; 50 Points Were Generated Using Two-Compartment Equation after IV Bolus

t	C_p	AUC	$C_p t$	AUMC
0	100	21.076	0	2.144
0.25	68.611	14.752	17.153	5.232
0.5	49.404	10.838	24.702	6.585
0.75	37.302	8.336	27.976	7.170
1	29.386	6.670	29.386	7.419
1.25	23.974	5.508	29.968	7.513
1.5	20.092	4.658	30.138	7.523
1.75	17.170	4.006	30.048	7.475
2	14.876	3.485	29.752	7.377
10	0.342	0.081	3.416	0.817
10.25	0.304	0.072	3.117	0.745
10.5	0.271	0.064	2.842	0.679
10.75	0.241	0.057	2.590	0.619
11	0.214	0.051	2.359	0.563
11.25	0.191	0.045	2.148	0.513
11.5	0.17	0.040	1.954	0.467
11.75	0.151	0.036	1.778	0.424
12	0.135	0.032	1.616	0.386
12.25	0.12	0.028	1.469	0.35
Total sum of column		106.6		177.915

(the mean of the PDF), the same as that calculated using $\mathrm{AUC}/C_\mathrm{p}^0$. AUMC/AUC of the differential function also yields an MRT of 1.066 hours.

In contrast, when AUMC/AUC is applied to the plasma drug concentration equation directly, $\mathrm{AUC}/C_\mathrm{p}^0$ yields 1.066 hours, while AUMC/AUC yields 1.687 hours. The latter approach has caused some controversy in the literature because two different definitions were independently derived that apply independently during calculation. When the PDF approach is applied, this confusion is avoided. When the PDF is applied to the equation describing the drug in the body, an MRT of 1.687 hours is obtained, which is the sum of MRT in the tissue and the plasma compartment. In each case, MRT is simply the mean of the distribution that has a definite variance. The MRT may still be calculated without any knowledge of the distribution function, in which case the MRT is the ratio of two area-under-the-curve terms used in calculating V_SS or Cl. The two approaches are contrasted below.

Analysis Based on $f(t)$, the Function Describing Plasma Drug Concentration

$$f(t) = \frac{(k_{21} - a)e^{-at}}{b - a} + \frac{(k_{21} - b)e^{-bt}}{a - b}$$

$$\int_0^{50} f(t)\, t\, dt = \mathrm{AUC}_0^\infty = 1.058$$

$$\int_0^{50} f(t)\, t\, dt = \mathrm{AUMC}_0^\infty = 1.784$$

$$\frac{\mathrm{AUMC}}{\mathrm{AUC}} = \frac{1.784}{1.058} = 1.688$$

$$\mathrm{MRT} = \frac{\mathrm{AUC}}{C_\mathrm{p}^0} = \frac{1.058}{1} = 1.058$$

Analysis Based on Differential Function, $f'(t)$, the Derivative of $f(t)$

$$g(t) = \frac{(k_{21} - a)e^{-at}}{b - a}(a) + \frac{(k_{21} - b)e^{-bt}}{a - b}(b)$$

$$\int_0^{50} g(t)\, t\, dt = \mathrm{AUMC}_0^\infty = 1.058 \qquad \text{(MRT from PDF)}$$

$$\int_0^{50} g(t)\, dt = \mathrm{AUC}_0^\infty = 1$$

$$\frac{\mathrm{AUMC}}{\mathrm{AUC}} = \frac{1.058}{1} = 1.058 \qquad \text{(MRT using AUMC/AUC)}$$

The first approach depends on C_p^0 evaluation. The second approach allows two ways to evaluate MRT. The two approaches agree with each other.

The Model-Independent and Model-Dependent Nature of MRT

MRT evaluated from AUMC/AUC assumes that most drugs are excreted through the central compartment or that they are metabolized in highly vascular tissues that kinetically are considered part of the central compartment. For drugs eliminated through tissues that are not part of the central compartment, the MRT calculated by AUMC/AUC is smaller than that calculated by considering both peripheral and central compartment elimination.

Compare models A and B generated by Nakashima and Benet (1988) in Figure 22-12 and Table 22.8. Both models A and B have identical rate constants except that model B has an elimination rate constant, k_{20}, from the peripheral compartment. MRT calculated using the new approach, referred to as MRT (new), is 1.687 hours for model A and 2.212 hours for model B. The new equation for MRT (new) of model B is

$$\text{MRT (new)} = \frac{\text{AUMC}}{\text{AUC}} + \frac{k_{20} V_2}{E_2 \, Cl} \tag{22.47}$$

where k_{20} = elimination rate for drug eliminated in compartment 2; V_2 = the distribution volume of compartment 2; E_2 = the sum of rate constants exiting from compartment 2 (in model B, $E_2 = k_{20} + k_{21}$); Cl = total body clearance; MRT_c = MRT from the central compartment; MRT_p = MRT from the peripheral or tissue compartment, also referred to as MRT_t; MRT = AUMC/AUC; and MRT (new) = MRT as calculated with correction for peripheral elimination.

The equation also applies for other multicompartment models. For a three-compartment model, Figure 22-12 (model E), a third term is added to Equation 22.47 to reflect drug exiting in compartment 3, as in Equation 22.48.

$$\text{MRT (new)} = \frac{\text{AUMC}}{\text{AUC}} + \frac{k_{20} V_2}{E_2 \, Cl} + \frac{k_{30} V_3}{E_3 \, Cl} \tag{22.48}$$

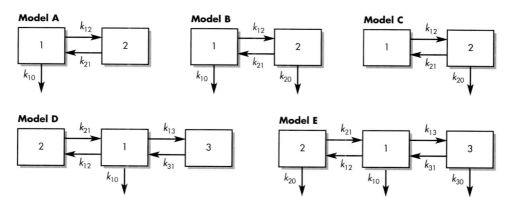

Figure 22-12. The three possible linear two-compartment open models and two possible three-compartment models. In each case, the concentration in compartment 1 (the central compartment) represents the measurable concentration of drug.
(From Nagashima and Benet, 1988, with permission.)

TABLE 22.8   Parameter Values for Models Depicted in Figure 22-12 Consistent with the Following Equations: $C_p = 64.131e^{-2.2346t} + 35.869e^{-0.4654t}$ for Models A, B, and C; and $C_p = 53.55e^{-0.1212t} + 18.4e^{-0.0361t} + 28.013e^{-0.01049t}$ for Models D and E

PARAMETER	TWO-COMPARTMENT MODELS			THREE-COMPARTMENT MODELS	
	Model A	Model B	Model C	Model D	Model E
Dose (D_0)	1000	1000	1000	1000	1000
V_1	10	10	10	10	10
V_{SS}	15.95	20.91	24.55	20.73	25.83
V_{area}	20.32	28.91	35.21	26.31	34.80
Cl	9.455	9.455	9.455	0.276	0.276
k_{12}	0.655	1.2	1.6	0.0323	0.0379
k_{21}	1.1	0.6	0.45	0.0693	0.0593
k_{10}	0.946	0.4	0	0.0276	0.0118
k_{20}	0	0.5	0.65	0	0.01
K_{13}	—	—	—	0.0146	0.0249
k_{31}	—	—	—	0.024	0.0141
k_{30}	—	—	—	0	0.01
f_1	1.0	0.423	0	1.0	0.4265
f_2	0	0.577	1	0	0.1983
f_3	—	—	—	0	0.3752
MRTC	1.058	1.058	1.058	36.23	36.23
$MRTP_2$	0.629	1.154	1.538	16.89	19.83
$MRTP_3$	—	—	—	22.07	37.52
MRT from Eq. 22.48	1.687	2.212	2.596	75.19	93.57
AUMC	178.4	178.4	178.4	272335	272335
AUC	105.8	105.8	105.8	3622	3622
AUMC/AUC	1.687	1.687	1.687	75.19	75.19
MRT from urine	1.687	1.687	ND[a]	75.19	75.19

[a]Intact drug will not be measured in urine.

From Nakashima and Benet (1988), with permission.

From Table 22.8, MRT (new) calculated using Equations 22.47 and 22.48 is model dependent. The original MRT calculated using AUMC/AUC yields the same MRT value of 1.687 hours for models A, B, and C. The original method, frequently quoted as a model-independent method for calculating MRT from plasma data, in effect, treats the body as a single unit from which drugs are eliminated from the plasma pool regardless of the true nature of the model. Unfortunately, it is not possible to know, from plasma data alone, whether drug elimination occurs in the peripheral compartment. Therefore, it is not possible to interpret unambiguously the calculated MRT parameters without making some assumptions. Benet and Galeazzi (1979) and Nakashima and Benet (1988) showed that MRT is related to V_{SS} and clearance (Eq. 22.49), as illustrated in Table 22.8. The clearances among models A, B, and C are identical, showing that clearance is site independent and may be calculated through MRT. However, the three-compartment model clearances were clearly different.

$$\text{MRT} = \frac{Cl}{V_{SS}} \tag{22.49}$$

MRT is useful in calculating the steady-state volume of distribution and additional parameters in compartmental and other models. In the compartmental

TABLE 22.9   Mean Residence Time for Different Pharmacokinetic Models

MODEL	MRT
One-compartment bolus IV	$1/k$
One-compartment oral bolus	$1/k_a + 1/k$
Two-compartment bolus IV	$(k_{12} + k_{21})/kk_{21}$ [a]
Two-compartment oral bolus	$1/k_a + (k_{12} + k_{21})/kk_{21}$
One-compartment infusion (for period τ)	$1/k + \tau/2$
Two-compartment IV bolus	$AUMC = A_1/a^2 + A_2/b^2$

[a] Alternatively, this may be calculated as $1/a + 1/b - 1/k_{21}$.

Compiled from Riegelman and Collier (1980) and Yamoaka et al (1978).

models, MRT may give some idea of how long the drug molecules stay in the peripheral compartment. For example, for the drug digoxin, MRT for the body is 49.5 hours; for the central and peripheral compartments, MRT is 3.68 hours and 45.8 hours as calculated (Veng-Pedersen, 1989). The peripheral MRT is the mean total time the drug molecules spend in the peripheral tissue, considering the first entry as well as possibly subsequent entries into the peripheral tissue from the central, general systemic circulation. An overview of MRT values for various pharmacokinetic models is given in Table 22.9.

Mean Absorption Time (MAT) and Mean Dissolution Time (MDT)

After IV bolus injecton, the rate of systemic drug absorption is zero, because the drug is placed directly into the bloodstream. The MRT calculated for a drug after IV bolus injection basically reflects the elimination rate processes in the body. After oral drug administration, the MRT is the result of both drug absorption and elimination. The relationship between the *mean absorption time*, MAT, and MRT is given by

$$\text{MRT}_{oral} = \text{MAT} + \text{MRT}_{IV} \tag{22.50}$$

$$\text{MAT} = \text{MRT}_{oral} - \text{MRT}_{IV} \tag{22.51}$$

For a one-compartment model, $\text{MRT}_{IV} = 1/k$:

$$\text{MAT} = \text{MRT}_{oral} - \frac{1}{k}$$

In some cases, IV data are not available and an MRT for a solution may be calculated. The *mean dissolution time* (MDT), or *in-vivo* mean dissolution time, for a solid drug product is

$$\text{MDT}_{solid} = \text{MRT}_{solid} - \text{MRT}_{solution} \tag{22.52}$$

MDT reflects the time for the drug to dissolve *in vivo*. Equation 22.52 calculates the *in-vivo* dissolution time for a solid drug product (tablet, capsule) given orally. MDT has been evaluated for a number of drug products. MDT is most readily estimated for the drugs that follow the kinetics of a one-compartment model. MDT is considered model independent because MRT is model independent. MDT has been used to compare the *in-vitro* dissolution versus *in-vivo* bioavailability for immediate-release and extended-release drug products (Chapters 14 and 17). Even with complete experimental data, the parameters obtained are quite dependent on the method of computation method employed.

EXAMPLE

Data for ibuprofen (Gillespie et al, 1982) are shown in Table 22.10. Serum concentrations for ibuprofen after a capsule and a solution are tabulated as a function of time in Tables 22.10 and 22.11.

The MRT was determined using the trapezoid method and Equation 22.43. The MRT for the solution was 2.63 hours and for the product was 4.48 hours. Therefore, MDT for the product is $4.48 - 2.63 = 1.85$ hours.

$$\text{MAT}_{\text{solution}} = \text{MRT}_{\text{solution}} - \frac{1}{k} = 2.63 - \frac{1}{0.455} = 2.2 \text{ hr}$$

$$\text{MAT}_{\text{product}} = \text{MRT}_{\text{product}} - \frac{1}{k} = 4.48 - \frac{1}{0.347} = 4.48 - 2.88 = 1.6 \text{ hr}$$

TABLE 22.10 Serum Concentrations for Capsule Ibuprofen

TIME (hr)	C_p	$C_p t$	$tC_p \Delta t$
0	0	0	
0.167	0.06	0.01002	0.000836
0.333	3.59	1.195	0.1000
0.50	7.79	3.895	0.425
1	13.3	13.300	4.298
1.5	14.5	21.750	8.762
2	16.9	33.80	63.887
3	16.6	49.80	41.80
4	11.9	47.60	48.70
6	6.31	37.86	85.46
8	3.54	28.32	66.18
10	1.36	13.60	41.92
12	0.63	7.56	21.16
			Total AUMC = 382.695

$k = 0.347 \text{ hr}^{-1}$, $\text{AUC}_0^\infty = 91.5$

$$\text{AUMC of tail piece} = \frac{C_p' t}{k} + \frac{C_p}{k^2} = \frac{(0.63)(12)}{0.347} + \frac{0.63}{0.347^2}$$

(extrapolation to ∞) $\quad = 21.79 + 5.23 = 27.02$

$\text{AUMC}_0^\infty = 382.695 + 27.02 = 409.72$

$$\text{MRT}_{\text{product}} = \frac{409.72}{91.5} = 4.48 \text{ hr}$$

Data adapted from Gillespie et al (1982), with permission.

TABLE 22.11 Serum Concentrations for Solution Ibuprofen

TIME (hr)	C_p	$C_p t$	$t C_p \Delta t$
0	0	0	
0.167	17.8	2.973	0.248
0.333	29.0	9.657	1.048
0.5	29.7	14.85	2.046
1	25.7	25.7	10.14
1.5	19.7	29.55	13.81
2	17.0	34.0	15.88
3	11.0	33.0	33.50
4	7.1	28.4	30.70
6	3.82	22.92	51.33
8	1.44	11.52	34.45
10	0.57	5.70	17.22
12	0.38	4.56	10.26
			Total AUMC = 220.64

$k = 0.455 \ \text{hr}^{-1}$, $\text{AUC}_0^\infty = 88.5$

$$\text{AUMC (tailpiece, extrapolation to } \infty) = \frac{C_p t}{k} = \frac{C_p}{k^2} = \frac{(0.38)(12)}{0.455} + \frac{0.38}{0.455^2}$$

$$= 10.02 + 1.84 = 11.86$$

$\text{AUMC}_0^\infty = 220.64 + 11.86 = 232.50 \ (\mu g/mL) \ \text{hr}^2$

$\text{MRT}_{\text{solution}} = \dfrac{232.50}{88.5} = 2.63 \ \text{hr}$

Data adapted from Gillespie et al (1982), with permission.

Applying Equation 22.52 directly (Riegelman and Collier, 1980),

$$\text{MDT} = 4.48 - 2.63 = 1.85 \ \text{hr}$$

Alternatively,

$$\text{MDT} = \text{MAT}_{\text{product}} - \text{MAT}_{\text{solution}} = 2.69 - 2.2 = 0.49 \ \text{hr}$$

The MDT obtained for the product differs according to the method of calculation. Therefore, the errors in calculating the elimination constant, k, may greatly affect the values for MAT and MDT. Equation 22.52 is recommended because it is less affected by k. When the above data are fitted to an oral one-compartment model and the AUMC and AUC are calculated using Equation 22.34, the results in Table 22.12 are obtained.

SELECTION OF PHARMACOKINETIC MODELS

Several objectives should be considered when using mathematical models to study rate processes (eg, pharmacokinetics of a drug). The primary objective in developing a model is to conceptualize the kinetic process in a quantitative manner that can be tested experimentally (Chapter 1). A model that cannot be tested is weak

TABLE 22.12 Parameters for Capsule and Solution Ibuprofen

PARAMETER	UNITS	CAPSULE	SOLUTION
AUC	$(\mu g/mL)$ hr	92.55	85.50
AUMC	$(\mu g/mL)$ hr^2	396.1	210.5
k_a	hr^{-1}	0.46	4.90
k	hr^{-1}	0.47	0.437
MRT	hr	4.28	2.49

Parameters were calculated from data of Gillespie et al (1982).

and will not improve or yield new knowledge about the process. In contrast, a wrong model that can be tested may be useful if the proposed hypotheses and its subsequent rejection leads to the correct model. To be statistically vigorous, a hypothesis or model is tested with the *null hypothesis* (H_0) (Appendix A). Only after rejection of the null hypothesis (tested beyond chance probability) is the hypothesis accepted. When the null hypothesis is rejected, the probability (eg, $p < 0.05$) means that the chance of error is less than 5% and the hypothesis or model is accepted. In fitting data using linear regression, the correlation of coefficient, r^2, is calculated, where r^2 is an indication of how well the data are predicted by the model. For example, $r = 0.9$ or $r^2 = 0.81$ indicates that 81% of the data agree with the model. The r^2 is not always a very good criterion. The sum of the squared differences (between the observed and predicted data) is a better criterion.

Adequate experimental design and the availability of valid data are important considerations in model selection and testing. For example, the experimental design should determine whether a drug is being eliminated by saturable (dose-dependent) or simple linear kinetics. A plot of metabolic rate versus drug concentration can be used to determine dose dependence, as in Figure 22-13. Metabolic rate can be measured at various drug concentrations using an *in-vitro* system (Chapter 11). In Figure 22-13, curve *B*, saturation occurs at higher drug concentration.

For illustration, consider the drug concentration–time profile for a drug given by IV bolus. The combined metabolic and distribution processes may result in profiles like those in Figure 22-14. Curve *A* represents a slow initial decline due to saturation and a faster terminal decline as drug concentration decreases. Curve *C* represents a dominating distributive phase masking the effect of nonlinear metabolism. Finally, a combination of *A* and *C* may approximate a rough overall linear decline (curve *B*). Notice that the drug concentration–time profile is shared by many different processes and that the goodness-of-fit is not an adequate criterion for adopting a model. For example, concluding linear metabolism based

Figure 22-13. Metabolic rate versus drug concentration. Drug *A* follows first-order pharmacokinetics, whereas drug *B* follows nonlinear pharmacokinetics and saturation occurs at higher drug concentrations.

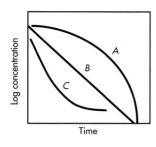

Figure 22-14. Plasma drug concentration profiles due to distribution and metabolic process. (See text for description of *A, B,* and *C.*)

only on curve *B* would be incorrect. Contrary to common belief, complex models tend to mask opposing variables that must be isolated and tested through better experimental designs. In this case, a constant infusion until steady-state experiment would yield information on saturation without the influence of initial drug distribution.

The use of pharmacokinetic models has been critically reviewed by Rescigno and Beck (1987) and by Riggs (1963). These authors emphasize the difference between model building and simulation. A model is a secondary system designed to test the primary system (real and unknown). The assumptions in a model must be realistic and consistent with physical observations. On the other hand, a simulation may emulate the phenomenon without resembling the true physical process. A simulation without identifiable support of the physical system does little to aid understanding of the basic mechanism. The computation has only hypothetical meaning.

For example, the data in Figure 22-15 may be described by three different equations: a straight line, a hyperbola, and an equation with trigonometric functions. Without physical support, the model gives little understanding of the mechanisms involved. Regression or data fitting (computation of parameters of a given equation so that divergence of the data from the equation is minimized) is considered to be modulation. All forms of modulation represent data manipulation and, as such, decrease information. Information comes from observations and observations only. If more points were available in this example, we could distinguish different processes if the data represent a straight line. Simulations within the realm of data allow for the determination of a quantitative relationship that is useful but does not actually increase understanding of the underlying physiologic processes governing the sojourn of the drug in the body.

Data dredging, such as manipulating the data to influence a stated study objective or model, is considered statistically undesirable because it may lead to a biased or a nonobjective analysis of the study. Ideally, statisticians prefer that details such as inclusion and exclusion criteria, the number of subjects per group, and the

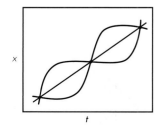

Figure 22-15. Data described by a straight line, a hyperbola, and an equation with trigonometric functions.
(From Rescigno and Beck, 1987, with permission.)

method of analysis or modeling be designed with sufficient power written into the protocols in advance. Pharmacokineticists are interested in understanding underlying kinetic processes that yield the results (data); statisticians are more interested in knowing that the conclusions drawn are real and not the result of random distribution.

It is perhaps refreshing to reexamine the basic paradigm of pharmacokinetics, or kinetics, which may be described as "observing how a given process changes over time." For example, by monitoring a change in the drug concentration in a patient over time, drug absorption and elimination from the patient may be modeled. If a statistician wishes to extrapolate the conclusion to a larger population, he or she may choose to enroll a sufficient number of subjects, and consider inclusion or exclusion criteria such as age, sex, other diseases, and genetics.

Basic pharmacokinetic concepts should be simple with few assumptions are made. The clinician may choose to weigh the risk of extrapolating the data and conclusions from a study with a few patients to a larger patient population. With recent advances in genetics, there are thousands of known genomic and environmental factors that may potentially influence disease and pharmacotherapy. The combination of genetic and environmental factors is very large and may make it very difficult to apply average information to an individual subject (see Chapter 12). However, the concept of adjusting dosing based on individual pharmacokinetic/pharmacodynamic information is still the most reliable approach to optimize dosing and drug efficacy and avoid toxicity. Ultimately, individual pharmacokinetic information will be combined with pharmacogenetic information obtained from the patient to allow the development of even better models to improve drug therapy.

FREQUENTLY ASKED QUESTIONS

1. Why are differential equations used to describe physiologic models?
2. Why do we assume that drug concentrations in venous and arterial blood are the same in pharmacokinetics?
3. Why is statistical moment used in pharmacokinetics?
4. Why is MRT used in pharmacokinetics?

LEARNING QUESTIONS

1. After an intravenous dose (500 mg) of an antibiotic, plasma–time concentration data were collected and the area under the curve was computed to be 20 mg/L hr. The $AUMC_0^\infty$ area was found to be 100 mg/L hr^2.

    a. What is the mean residence time of this drug?

b. What is the clearance of this drug?

c. What is the steady-state volume of distribution of this drug?

2. Why is MRT calculated from moment and AUC curves (ie $[\text{AUMC}]_0^\infty/[\text{AUC}]_0^\infty$) rather than $[\text{AUC}]_0^\infty/C_0$ directly, as the term was defined in Equation 22.43?

3. If the data in Question 1 above are fit to a one-compartment model with an elimination k that is found to be 0.25 hour, MRT may be calculated simply as $1/k$. What different assumptions are used in here versus Question 1?

4. What are the principal considerations in interspecies scaling?

5. What are the key considerations in fitting plasma drug data to a pharmacokinetic model?

REFERENCES

Benet LZ, Galeazzi RL: Noncompartmental determination of the steady-state volume of distribution. *J Pharm Sci* **68:**1071–1073, 1979

Benowitz N, Forsyth RP, Melmon KL, Rowland M: Lidocaine disposition kinetics in monkey and man, 1. Prediction by a perfusion model. *Clin Pharmacol Ther* **16:**87–98, 1974

Bischoff KB, Dedrick RL, Zaharko DS: Preliminary model for methotrexate pharmacokinetics. *J Pharm Sci* **59:**149–154, 1970

Bonate PL, Howard D: Prospective allometric scaling: Does the emperor have clothes? *J Clin Pharmacol* **40:**665–670, 2000

Bonati M, Latini R, Tognoni G, et al: Interspecies comparison of in vivo caffeine pharmacokinetics in man, monkey, rabbit, rat, and mouse. *Drug Metab Rev* **15:**1355–1383, 1985

Boxenbaum H: Interspecies scaling, allometry, physiological time, and the ground plan of pharmacokinetics. *J Pharmacokinet Biopharm* **10:**201–227, 1982

Boxenbaum H: Evolution biology, animal behavior, fourth-dimensional space, and the raison d'etre of drug metabolism and pharmacokinetics. *Drug Metab Rev* **14:**1057–1097, 1983

Chen CN, Andrade JD: Pharmacokinetic model for simultaneous determination of drug levels in organs and tissues. *J Pharm Sci* **65:**717–724, 1976

Chiou WL: The phenomenon and rationale of marked dependence of drug concentration on blood sampling site: Implication in pharmacokinetics, pharmacodynamics, toxicology and therapeutics. Part I, *Clin Pharmacokinet* **17**(3):175–199, 1989; Part II, *Clin Pharmacokinet* **17**(3):275–290, 1989.

Gabrielsson J, Bondesson U: Constant-rate infusion of nicotine and cotinine, I. A physiological pharmacokinetic analysis of the cotinine disposition, and effects on clearance and distribution in the rat. *J Pharmacokinet Biopharm* **15:**583–599, 1987

Gillespie WR, Disanto AR, Monovich RE, Albert DS: Relative bioavailability of commercially available ibuprofen oral dosage forms in humans. *J Pharm Sci* **71:**1034–1038, 1982

Hu Teh-Min, Hayton WL: Allometric scaling of xenobiotic clearance: Uncertainty versus universality. *AAPS PharmSci* **3**(4), article 29, 2001 (www.pharmsci.org).

King FG, Dedrick RL, Farris FF: Physiological pharmacokinetic modeling of *cis*-dichlorodiammineplatinum(II) (DDP) in several species. *J Pharmacokinet Biopharm* **14:**131–157, 1986

Luecke RH, Thomason LE: Physiological flow model for drug elimination interactions in the rat. *Comput Prog Biomed* **11:**88–89, 1980

Lutz RJ, Dedrick RL: Physiological pharmacokinetics: Relevance to human risk assessment. In Li AP (ed), *New Approaches in Toxicity Testing and Their Application in Human Risk Assessment.* New York, Raven, 1985, pp 129–149

Mahmood I. Critique of prospective allometric scaling: Does the emperor have clothes? *J Clin Pharmacol* **40:**671–674, 2000

Mordenti J, Chappell W: The use of interspecies scaling in toxicology. In Yacobi A, Skelly JP, Batra VK (eds), *Toxicokinetic and Drug Development.* New York, Pergamon, 1989

Nakashima E, Benet LZ: General treatment of mean residence time, clearance, and volume parameters in linear mammillary models with elimination from any compartment. *J Pharmacokinet Biopharm* **16:**475–492, 1988

Nakashima E, Yokogawa K, Ichimura F, et al: A physiologically based pharmacokinetic model for biperiden in animals and its extrapolation to humans. *Chem Pharm Bull* **35:**718–725, 1987

Rescigno A, Beck JS: Perspective in pharmacokinetics and the use and abuses of models. *J Pharmacokinet Biopharm* **15:**327–344, 1987

Riegelman S, Collier P: The application of statistical moment theory to the evaluation of in vivo dissolution time and absorption. *J Pharmacokinet Biopharm* **8:**509–534, 1980

Riggs DS: *A Mathematical Approach to Physiological Problems*. Baltimore, Williams & Wilkins, 1963

Ritschel WA, Banerjee PS: Physiological pharmacokinetic models: Principles, applications, limitations and outlook. *Meth Find Exp Clin Pharmacol* **8:**603–614, 1986

Sawada Y, Hanano M, Sugiyama Y, Iga T: Prediction of the disposition of nine weakly acidic and six weakly basic drugs in humans from pharmacokinetic parameters in rats. *J Pharmacokinet Biopharm* **13:**477–492, 1985

Veng-Pedersen P: Mean time parameters in pharmacokinetics: Definition, computation and clinical implications, I. *Clin Pharmacol* **17:**345–366, 1989

Yamaoka K, Nakagawa T, Uno T: Statistical moments in pharmacokinetics. *J Pharmacokinet Biopharm* **6:**547–558, 1978

BIBLIOGRAPHY

Banakar UV, Block LH: Beyond bioavailability testing. *Pharm Technol* **7:**107–117, 1983

Benet LZ: Mean residence time in the body versus mean residence time in the central compartment. *J Pharmacokinet Biopharm* **13:**555–558, 1985

Bischoff KB, Dedrick RL, Zaharko DS, Longstreth JA: Methotrexate pharmacokinetics. *J Pharm Sci* **60:**1128–1133, 1971

Boxenbaum H, D'Souza RW: Interspecies pharmacokinetics scaling, biological design and neoteny. In Testa B, D'Souza WD (eds), *Advances in Drug Research*. New York, Academic, 1990, vol 19, pp 139–196

Chanter DO: The determination of mean residence time using statistical moments: Is it correct? *J Pharmacokinet Biopharm* **13:**93–100, 1985

Coburn WA, Sheiner LB: Perspective in pharmacokinetics: Pharmacokinetic/pharmacodynamic model: What is it! *J Pharmacokinet Biopharm* **15:**545–555, 1987

Himmelstein KJ, Lutz RJ: A review of the applications of physiologically based pharmacokinetic modeling. *J Pharmacokinet Biopharm* **7:**127–145, 1979

Kasuya Y, Hirayama H, Kubota N, Pang KS: Interpretation and estimation of mean residence time with statistical moment theory. *Biopharm Drug Disp* **8:**223–234, 1987

Sawada Y, Hanano M, Sugiyama Y, Iga T: Prediction of the disposition of nine weakly acidic and six weakly basic drugs in humans from pharmacokinetic parameters in rats. *J Pharmacokinet Biopharm* **13:**477–492, 1985

Veng-Pedersen P, Gillespie W: The mean residence time of drugs in the systemic circulation. *J Pharm Sci* **74:**791–792, 1985

Wagner JG: Do you need a pharmacokinetic model, and, if so, which one? *J Pharmacokinet Biopharm* **3:**457–478, 1975

Wagner JG: Dosage intervals based on mean residence times. *J Pharm Sci* **76:**35–38, 1987

Wagner JG: Types of mean residence times. *Biopharm Drug Disp* **9:**41–57, 1988

West GB. The origin of universal scaling laws in biology. *Physica A* **263:**104–113, 1999

APPENDIX A

STATISTICS

PROBABILITY

Probability is widely applied to measure risk associated with disease and drug therapy. *Risk factor* is a condition or behavior that increases the chance of developing disease in a healthy subject over a period of time. An example could be the risk of developing lung cancer over time with tobacco smoking. Another example of risk factor is the possibility of developing hearing loss after receiving an aminoglycoside antibiotic for a period of time.

The term *relative risk* (RR) or *risk ratio* is the most frequently used probability term to measure association of risk with exposure (to a drug or a behavior). Risk factors may be genetic, environmental, or behavioral. They have important implications in both pharmacokinetics and drug therapy (see Chapter 12). Risk factors may be casual or merely a marker that increases the probability of a disease.

$$RR = \frac{risk_{(exposed)}}{risk_{(unexposed)}}$$

$$RR = relative\ risk = \frac{disease\ probability\ of\ exposed}{disease\ probability\ of\ unexposed}$$

Often risk information is collected in a controlled manner over a period of time by survey, either from the past or forward in time. In a *prospective cohort study* (also known as a *cohort study, prospective, follow-up,* or *longitudinal study*), a cohort of healthy subjects exposed to different levels of a suspected risk is followed forward in time to determine the incidence of risk in each group. For example, in a hypothetical study, the risk of thrombophlebitis was studied in a group of randomly selected women: 500 women taking and 500 matched women not taking a birth control pill for 10 years. The RR of 10 for thrombophlebitis was calculated from a risk of thrombophlebitis in women exposed to the birth control pill versus women not exposed to the drug using a dichotomous 2×2 table as shown in Table A.1, where A and B are the number of subjects who developed thrombophlebitis. The probability of *exposed* in this case is $A/(A + B)$ and that of *not exposed* is $C/(C + D)$. In this case, assume the exposed risk is 0.025 and the not-exposed risk is 0.0025. Then RR = 0.025/0.0025 = 10. Thus, the relative risk

TABLE A.1 Tabulation from a Hypothetical Cohort Study of Female Subjects on the Pill—with and without Developing Thrombophlebitis for 10 Years

	POSITIVE OUTCOME (+THROMBOPHLEBITIS)	NEGATIVE OUTCOME (−THROMBOPHLEBITIS)	SUBTOTAL
Risk factor present (eg, taking the pill—exposed)	A	B	A + B
Risk factor absent (eg, not taking the pill—not exposed)	C	D	C + D
Subtotal	A + C	B + D	

of thrombophlebitis in women on the birth control pill for 10 years is 10 for this group of women studied.

A second method of studying risk is the *historical* or *retrospective cohort study,* which looks backward in time to determine the present risk. The cohort of exposed and unexposed subjects is retrieved from past records to determine risk outcome. In the next section relative risks are described in terms of *odds,* a similar concept that is also widely applied.

ODDS

The probability of drawing an ace from a deck of cards is 4/52, or 1/13 for a deck of cards containing 4 aces in 52 cards. The odds of drawing an ace is the number of times an ace will be drawn divided by the number of times it will not be drawn. The odds are

$$\text{ODDS} = \frac{4/52}{48/52} = \frac{4}{48} = \frac{1}{12}$$

This can be read as a 1:12 odds of drawing an ace. The absence of four aces in the denominator makes the difference in the odds outcome. Odds are numerically not equal to probability as defined.

The point may be illustrated by considering the opening of a standard deck of cards, one card at a time. For example, we may encounter 4 aces after 40 cards are opened, before the entire deck is open. We can see that the number of cards opened (we stopped at 40 cards) becomes a factor in the odds obtained. In this case, after opening the first 40 cards, 4 cards were aces and 36 cards were not aces. The odds are 4/36 = 1/9 instead of 1/12 as calculated for 52 cards. Using this analogy, it is inappropriate to pick sample sizes that do not reflect the natural risk course of the disease or drug treatment involved. If we decide to sample only 40 cards, stop sampling, and then calculate the odds (or RR in observing a disease), the results will be in error. In statistics, the sample size and how samples represent the population at large are important considerations for accurate determination of the RR of a disease or drug treatment.

A common approach to studying risk outcome is the *case-control study* (also known as the *retrospective study*). In the case-control study, the exposure histories of two groups of subjects are selected on the basis of whether or not they develop a particular disease (eg, thrombophlebitis), in order to evaluate disease frequency resulting from drug (eg, the pill) exposure. The investigator selects the size of the subject population that has the disease or is disease free to determine exposure to the risk factor. The number of subjects who do and do not have the disease may not necessarily reflect the natural frequency of the disease. It is therefore improper to compute a "relative risk (RR)" from the odds ratio (OR) for a case-control study, because the investigator can manipulate the size of the relative risk.

$$OR = \frac{\text{odds of case exposure}}{\text{odds of case unexposed}}$$

If the disease is rare, then OR ≈ RR. When the sample size is large, the difference between OR and RR diminishes.

In statistical analysis, it is important to guard against *selection error* or *bias*. Investigators may look harder for cancer, for example, in smokers than in a control group of healthy subjects. The resultant disparity is often called *surveillance bias*. In a case-control group there may also be *recall bias;* for example, medical history taken on surgical lung cancer (case) may be more likely to contain information on smoking than other type of surgical controls (Knapp and Miller, 1992).

EXPERIMENTAL DESIGN AND COLLECTION OF DATA

Statistics have important applications in scientific studies, whether in studies involving hypothesis testing or in finding ways to improve a product. Statistical design is widely used at the experimental planning stage. Later, when data are collected, statistical methods are applied for data analysis and to help draw conclusions from the studies.

Experimental design may be simple or may involve an elaborate model. The method may be applied to optimize a drug or drug product based on a set of criteria (Deming and Morgan, 1987). Experimental design may be used to optimize an analytical method to separate a drug from impurities, such as a HPLC method. In pharmacokinetics, experimental design is used to design better sampling time for drawing blood samples for drug analysis in pharmacokinetic parameter estimation. A common approach to optimizing a drug product is the *factorial design*. For example, we may be interested in determining whether 0, 0.25, 0.5, 0.75 or 1% of magnesium stearate should be formulated into a tablet granulation to allow adequate flow of the tablet granulation mixture during manufacturing. This problem may be viewed as a simple one-factorial-design experiment to determine the amount of lubricant needed to provide best powder flow (1 factor × 5 lubricant levels). The object of the experimental design is to try to pick the tablet lubricant level that will result in the optimal powder flow from the hopper to the die cavity during tablet compression.

In practice, tablet granulation flow is more complex. Moisture level, particle size, and tackiness (of the drug substance) are other factors that influence flow. We may decide to reduce the increment level and select the lubricant levels to 0, 0.5, and 1% only. This provides three lubricant levels—high, medium, and low—for each factor. We then can apply a factorial design of 4 factors at 3 levels, which involves $4^3 = 64$

trials in the above case to generate a geometric response space that represents all the factors involved. The full factorial design is tedious, so a reduced design, the *fractional factorial* design, is often used. How to reach the optimal point efficiently when several factors are involved is a problem for many optimization experiments.

The identical concept for optimizing flow can be applied to optimizing the media composition supporting antibiotic production by fermentation using *Streptomyces* or a new microbe engineered by recombinant DNA. The factorial design may be employed to find the optimum composition for the growth medium. Factorial design yields knowledge about the system but is tedious. An alternative approach to carry out the optimization is the *sequential simplex method,* which optimizes the factors through sequentially planned experiments. This method is often applied in parameter estimation from data using computerized iteration algorithms. In designing experiments, it is important to know the factors involved and the range of each factor. How much change in drug concentration is occurring in plasma samples over an hour or in a minute? How much difference in drug concentrations can the analytical method detect? Good design requires some knowledge of the system and a strategy to obtain data for analysis that saves time and resources.

The same principle applies to human clinical studies. In clinical trials, studies are often done with a limited number of subjects, due to either cost or the availability of subjects who meet the study requirements. Based on good clinical practices, the study subjects are selected according to exclusion and inclusion criteria that are written into the protocol. All subjects must give informed consent to be in the study. Since most studies are done over a period of time, it is important to ensure that both the treatment and control groups are balanced and to avoid any temporal influence. For example, in bioequivalency trials, adequate time (*wash-out time*) between study dosing periods is allowed for the drug to be eliminated from the subject and to avoid residual effects due to carryover of the drug from the first dosing period to the next dosing period.

All scientific studies must be designed properly to obtain valid conclusions that may be applied to the population intended. The experimental design of a study includes the following:

1. A clearly stated hypothesis for the study
2. Assurance that the samples have been randomly selected
3. Control of all experimental variables
4. Collection of adequate data to allow experimental testing of the hypothesis

For example, we may wish to test the hypothesis that the average weight of young males is greater than the average weight of females in the United States. First, we may decide that young male and female subjects aged 18 to 24 will be selected and other ages excluded. The subjects are randomly selected from a pool of subjects who are not interrelated in a way that might affect their body weights. We may want to exclude subjects with certain diseases (exclusion criteria). A sufficient number of subjects must be selected (sampled) randomly so that the total number of subjects (sample size) represents the general population in the United States. The need for randomization is easily understood but often poorly met because of the difficulties in recruiting subjects, or in the methods used for recruiting. For example, if all the subjects in this example are randomly recruited from one health club in a given city, the samples will not be typical of the population intended even though the subjects are randomly selected. Are we too ambitious to include the population of the entire United States? Second, many of the subjects exercise at the health club to lose weight, and this may not be representative of the general population. A true sample is one selected randomly from the population of the entire country without connection by any variable that affects their weights.

The identification of all covariates in a study is generally difficult and requires thorough consideration. The subject of sample size, inclusion criteria, and exclusion criteria are major considerations in experimental design that will affect the statistical outcome. After careful consideration, we may realize that there are many variables to be considered and may wish to modify the scope to tailor the study objectives more efficiently.

Age, gender, genetic background, and health of the subjects are important variables in clinical drug testing. The statistical design of a study is based on the study objectives. Each study should have clearly stated objectives and an appropriate study design indicating how the study is to be performed. Often, the population may be subdivided according to the objectives of the study. For example, a new drug for the treatment of Alzheimer's disease in the elderly may initially be tested in male subjects aged 55 and above. Later, clinical studies might test the drug in other patient populations. Many different statistical designs are possible. Some of these designs control experimental variables better than others. Specific statistical designs are given in other chapters and in standard statistical texts.

The quality of the data is very important and may be controlled by the researcher and the method of measurement. For example, if the weights of the young males and females in the example above are obtained using different scales, the investigator must ascertain that each scale weighs the subject accurately. *Accuracy* refers to the closeness of the observation (ie, observed weight) to the actual or true value. *Reproducibility* or *precision* refers to the closeness of repeated measurements.

ANALYSIS AND INTERPRETATION OF DATA

The objective of data analysis is to obtain as much information about the population as possible based on the sample data collected. A common method for analyzing data of a sample population is to classify the data and then plot the frequency of occurrence of all the samples. For example, the frequency of weight distribution of a class of students may be plotted in the form of a histogram that relates frequency to weight (Fig. A-1).

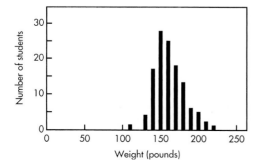

Figure A-1. *Weight distribution of 120 students.*

An important observation in this example is that the weight of most students lies in the middle of the weight distribution. There is a common tendency for most sample values to occur around the mean. This is described in the *central limit theorem,* which states that the frequency of the values of measurements drawn randomly from a population tends to approximate a *bell-shaped curve* or *normal distribution.* Extensive data collection is needed to determine the distributional nature of a sample population. Once the parameters of a distribution are determined, the probability of a given sample's occurrence in the population may be calculated.

DESCRIPTIVE TERMS

Descriptive terms are used in statistics to generalize the nature of the data and provide a measure of central tendency. The *mean or average* is the sum of the observations divided by the number, *n,* of observations (Table A.2). The *median* is the middle value of the observation between the highest and lowest value. The *mode* is the most frequently occurring value. The term *range* is used to describe the *dispersion* of the observations and is the difference between the highest and lowest values. For data that are distributed as a normal distribution (discussed below), the mean, median, and mode have the same value.

THE NORMAL DISTRIBUTION

If data are plotted according to the frequency of occurrence, a pattern for the distribution of the data is observed. Most data approximate a normal or *Gaussian distribution.* The *normal distribution* is a bell-shaped curve that is symmetric on both sides of the mean. Statistical tests that assume the data follow normal distribution patterns are known as *parametric tests. Nonparametric tests* do not make any assumption about the central tendency of the data and may be used to analyze data without assuming normal distribution. Nonparametric tests require no

TABLE A.2   Descriptive Statistics for a Set of Data[a]

DATA		DESCRIPTIVE TERMS
21	63	Sum = 1274
25	67	Mean = 57.9
29	67	Mode = 67
35	67	Median = 62
37	67	n = 22
42	67	Range = 21–91
45	72	SD = 20.3
49	73	RSD = 35.1%
56	75	
57	88	
61	91	

[a] The data represent a set of measurements (observations) in study. The descriptive terms are often used to describe the data. Each term is defined in the text.

SD, standard deviation; RSD, relative standard deviation.

assumption of normality and are less powerful. Examples are the Wilcoxan test and the side test.

The shape of the normal distribution is determined by only two parameters, the population mean and the variance, both of which may be estimated from the samples. The *variance* is a measure of the spread or variability of the sample. Many biologic and physical random variables are described by the normal distribution (or may be transformed to a normal distribution). These may include the weight and height of humans and animal species, the elimination half-lives of many drugs in a population of patients, the duration of a telephone call, and other variables. In statistics, the item investigated is termed the *random variable.* For convenience, the standardized normal distribution is introduced to allow easy probability calculation when the standard deviation is known (Fig. A-2). The probability of a sample value occurring from 1 *standard deviation* (SD) above to 1 SD below the mean is 68% (z of -1 to $+1$). This value is calculated by finding the probability corresponding to $z = -1$ and $z = 1$ from curve B in Figure A-2 as follows:

- Probability between z of -4 to -1 is 0.16.
- Probability between z of -4 to $+1$ is 0.84.
- Therefore, the probability between z of -1 to $+1$ is $0.84 - 0.16 = 0.68$ or 68%.

The area representing probability between any two points on the normal distribution is calculated from this graph. In practice, a cumulative standardized normal distribution table is used to allow better accuracy.

Standard deviation measures the variability of a group of data. SD for n number of measurements is calculated according to the following equation:

$$\text{SD} = \sqrt{\frac{\sum_{i}^{n} (x_i - \bar{x})^2}{n - 1}} \tag{A.1}$$

where $\bar{x}$ is the mean, x_i is the observed value, and n is the number of observations (data). The standard deviation is often calculated by computer or calculator and gives an indication of the spread of data (Fig. A-2). A larger standard deviation indicates that the spread of data about the mean is larger compared to data with the same mean but with a smaller standard deviation.

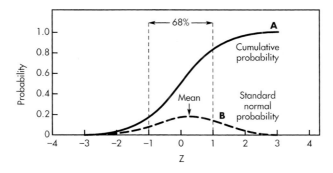

Figure A-2.   Probability of a normal distribution. (A = cumulative probability, B = standard normal probability.)

Relative standard deviation or *coefficient of variation* allows comparison of the variance of measurements. The standard deviation is divided by the mean to give the relative standard deviation (RSD) or coefficient of variation (CV):

$$RSD = \frac{SD}{\bar{x}} \qquad (A.2)$$

The RSD may be expressed as a percent or %CV by multiplying the RSD by 100. This is commonly known as *percent standard deviation* or *percent variation.*

The difference between the mean, $\bar{x}$, and each observed datum, x_i, is the deviation from the mean. Because the deviation from the mean can be either negative or positive, the deviations are squared and summed to give an estimation of the total spread or deviation of the data from the mean. The term $\sum_i^n (x_i - \bar{x})^2$ is the *sum of the squares.* This term incorporates measurement error as well as inherent variance of the samples. If a single sample is measured several times, the sum of the squares should be very small if the method of measurement is reproducible. The concept of least squares for minimizing error due to model fitting is fundamental in many statistical methods.

CONFIDENCE LIMIT

If normal distribution of the data is assumed, the probability of a random variable in the population can be calculated. For example, data that falls within 1 SD above and below the mean ($\bar{x} \pm 1$ SD) represents approximately 68% of the data, whereas data that falls within 2 SD above and below the mean ($\bar{x} \pm 2$ SD) represents approximately 95% of the data. In the examples below, the random variable in which we are interested is the diameters of drug particles measured from a powdered drug sample lot.

 EXAMPLE

The particle size of a powdered drug sample was measured. The average (mean) particle size was 130 μm with a standard deviation of 20 μm.

1. Determine the range of particle sizes that represents the middle 68% of the powdered drug.

Solution

From a normal distribution table or Figure A-2, 68% of the middle particles represent 34% above and below the mean, corresponding to the mean ± 1 SD.

Small particle size = mean − SD = 130 − 20 = 110 μm
Large particle size = mean + SD = 130 + 20 = 150 μm

Therefore, 68% of the particles will have a particle size ranging from 110 to 150 μm.

2. Determine the range of particle sizes that represents the middle 95% of the powdered drug.

Solution

95% ÷ 2 or 47.5% on each side of the mean, corresponding to ±2 SD (Fig. A-2)

Smallest particle size = 130 − (2 × 20) = 90 μm
Largest particle size = 130 + (2 × 20) = 170 μm

Therefore, 95% of the particles will have a particle size ranging from 90 to 170 μm.

In the above example, the calculation shows that most of the particles lie around the mean. To be 95% certain, simply extend from the mean ±2 SD. This approach estimates the 95% confidence limit. A 95% confidence limit implies that if an experiment is performed 100 times, 95% of the data will be in this range above and below the mean.

This example shows how to reconstruct a population based on the two parameters, mean and variance (approximated by the SD). A more common application is the estimation of experimental data such as assay measurements. Such 95% confidence limits are often calculated from the standard deviation to estimate the reliability of the assay measurement.

In the example above, the mean for the particle size was 130 μm and the SD was 20 mm. Therefore, from equation A.2, the RSD = 20/130 or 0.15. The RSD may be expressed as a percent or %CV by multiplying the RSD by 100.

As mentioned, *accuracy* refers to the agreement with the observed value or measurement in a group of data and the actual or true value of the population. Unfortunately, the true value is unknown in many studies. The term *precision* refers to the reproducibility of the data or the variation within a set of measurements. Data that are less precise will demonstrate a larger variance or a larger relative standard deviation, whereas more precise data will have a smaller variance.

 # EXAMPLE

A lot of 10-mg tablets was assayed five times by three students (Fig. A-3). Which student assayed the tablets most accurately?

Solution

The mean and SD of assays by each student were determined. Because the same lot was assayed, the difference in SD among the students is attributed to assay variations. Student A is closest to the target—that is, the labeled claimed dose (LCD) of 10 mg. Student C is most precise (with the smallest %SD), but is consistently off target.

The data obtained by Student C is considered biased because all the observed data are above 10 mg. Data are also considered biased if all the observed data are below the true value of 10 mg.

Bias refers to a systematic error when the measurement is consistently not on target. Repeated measurements may be very reproducible (precise) but miss the target. In the example above, Student C was most precise, but Student A was most accurate. In determining accuracy and precision, a standard (known sample) is usually prepared and assayed several times to determine the variation due to assay errors. In the example above, we assumed that the students used known 10-mg standard tablets. If the tablets were unknown samples, it would not be possible to conclude which student was more accurate, because the true value would be unknown. In practice, assay methods are validated for precision and accuracy based on known standards before unknown samples (eg, plasma samples) are assayed.

In the analysis and interpretation of data, statistics makes inferences about a population using experimental data gathered in a sample. After analysis of data, the statistician calculates the likelihood or probability that a given result would happen. *Probability* (P) is the fraction of the population indicating that a given result or event would occur by random sampling or chance. For example, if $P <0.05$, then the likelihood that a result occurs by random sampling is 5/100, 1/20, or 5%. By convention, if the statistical inference produces a P value of 0.05 or less, it is considered atypical or uncommon of the population. As shown in Figure A-1, the probability of finding a student weighing above 250 lb is small ($P <0.05$), and we may conclude (somewhat erroneously) that a student who weighs 250 lb is significantly different from the rest. This concept for determining the probability of how typical a given sample value occurs in a population may be extended to hypothesis

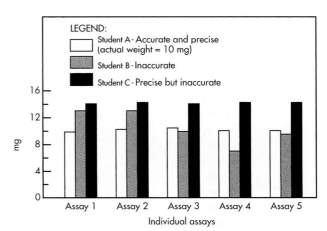

Figure A-3. Comparison of assays (5 each) of 10-mg tablet by three students.

testing. Hypothesis testing estimates the probability of whether a given value is typical of the control group or of the treated group.

STATISTICAL DISTRIBUTIONS AND APPLICATION

The frequency distribution of some data does not appear to be symmetrically shaped. The term *skewness* relates to the asymmetry of the data. The data distribution may be skewed to the left or right of the mean. In many pharmacologic studies, the sample size in the study is small, and the investigator cannot always be certain that the data obtained from the study are normally distributed. An incorrect assumption of a normal distribution may lead to a biased conclusion. In such cases, a nonparametric test may be used, because it does not make any assumption about the underlying test except that it may be continuous.

During data analysis, a value or observation may be observed that is several standard deviations above or below the mean; such a value is called an *outlier*. A value that is an outlier is difficult to use statistically. An observed value that deviates far from the majority of the data may indicate non-normal distribution, an error in measurement, or an error in data entry. If an error is found during checking, it should be corrected. In general, outlier values should not be excluded from the statistical analysis. Some investigators use log transformation of the data to make the distribution of the data appear to be more normally distributed. A geometric mean is obtained after log transformation of the data. In some cases, with sufficient data collection, a bimodal distribution may be observed. For example, the acetylation of isoniazid in humans follows a bimodal distribution, indicating two populations consisting of fast acetylators and slow acetylators. In this study, if the data were obtained from subjects of whom all but one were fast acetylators, then the single datum for the slow acetylator might be considered an outlier (and possibly be discarded from the data analysis).

When a specific distribution is not known, it may be possible to use the bootstrap/jackknife method. A *bootstrap* is a paradoxical means of getting started on something when you need some of that something in order to get started. The concept derives from the phrase "to pull oneself up by one's bootstraps." Rather than attributing an assumption to the distribution, the actual data collected will be used to extrapolate further about the larger population it represents. Instead of collecting more samples by actual experiment, one simply puts all the data into a "virtual bag" and randomly samples (not actually taking the original data out) from the bag until the desired number of samples is collected to yield a glimpse of what the population will be like. The method was a great innovation by Bradley Efron and is easily adapted to many applications with computer technology. The basic bootstrap method is essentially the same. The method has worked well and has been modified for many practical applications where assumption of specific distribution failed (Efron, Bradley, Tibshirani, 1993). It should be appreciated that the nature of the data from an original study is new and unknown. The greatest difficulty facing the investigator is characterizing the distribution and applying it to a proper model. The bootstrap method avoids the problem of assuming the wrong distribution. In Chapter 22, statistical distribution is discussed with further application to pharmacokinetics.

The normal, binomial, Poisson, chi-square distributions are frequently applied in statistics and engineering. Some distributions are related mathematically. References for further information are listed at the end of this appendix.

Statistical analysis is referred to as a statistical *test* when the data are formulated for hypothesis testing. The most common test involves the *Student's t-test,* which is a test of means of two groups assuming the same variance. If the variances are different, the Student's *t*-test will be a *t*-test with unequal variance. When the sample size increases to very large, the *t*-distribution approaches the normal distribution. The *t*-test becomes more powerful if the subjects meet the criteria for a paired *t*-test. The *F*-test is a simple test of variance of two groups. When more groups are involved, analysis of variance may be applied.

Statistics are broadly applied in pharmacokinetics. Special statistical methods have been developed to provide a platform for rational argument or decision making in accepting or rejecting a theory. The information generated in many controlled clinical studies is often sparse due to limited sample size (eg, few subjects) and limited sampling (eg, few blood samples). For this reason, all drugs under development in clinical studies are monitored for side effects and rare events. After FDA approval and marketing, pharmacovigilance is needed to assure safety in the larger population of patients who will be using the drug.

In testing the effect of a drug across different groups, the term *interaction* is often heard. An *effect* is a difference in treatment response, and an *interaction* is a difference in differences. Examples might be treatment-by-center interactions, or treatment-by-gender interactions. When large interactions are noted, it is not appropriate to combine groups and make an overall assessment of the treatment effect statistically. Clinical trials often involve pivotal and supporting studies. An analysis that combines multiple studies to obtain an overall result, such as an overall estimate of the size of the treatment effect of a drug, is termed *meta-analysis.*

HYPOTHESIS TESTING

Hypothesis testing is an objective way of analyzing data and determining whether the data support or reject the hypothesis postulated. For example, we might want to test the hypothesis that a given steroid causes a weight increase. We want to test this hypothesis using two groups of healthy volunteers, one group (treated) that took the given steroid and another (control) that took no drug. The two hypotheses generated are as follows:

H_0: There is no difference in weight between the treated and control groups (null hypothesis).

H_1: There is a difference in weight between the treated and control groups (alternative hypothesis).

The null hypothesis H_0, states that there is no difference between the treatments. The experimental data will either reject or fail to reject (accept) the null hypothesis. If the null hypothesis is rejected, then the alternative hypothesis is accepted, since there are only two possibilities. A simple hypothesis testing data from two groups is the two-sample Student's *t*-test involving a control group and a treated group (the *t*-distribution approximates the normal distribution and is commonly used).

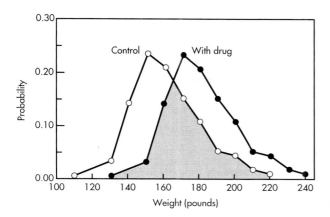

Figure A-4. Hypothesis testing example.

The data for the study (simulated) is shown in Figure A-4 using 120 students in the control and treated groups. The mean weight of the treated group is about 175 lb, whereas the mean weight for the control group is about 155 lb. There is a shift to the right in the weight distribution of the treated group. However, a considerable overlapping (shaded area) in weights is observed, making it difficult to reject the null hypothesis. In practice, H_0 is rejected at a known level of uncertainty called the *level of significance*. A level of 5% ($\alpha = 0.05$) is considered statistically significant, and a level of 1% ($\alpha = 0.01$) is considered highly significant. Commonly, this level of significance is reported as $P < 0.05$ or $P < 0.01$, respectively, to indicate the different levels of significance. Because uncertainty is involved, whenever the null hypothesis is rejected or accepted, the level of significance is stated. A significance level of 25% ($P < 0.25$) in the above example suggests that there is a 25% probability that the weight change is not due to drug treatment. A 25% probability is a level far too large to reject the H_0 with certainty. The level of significance is therefore related to the probability of incorrectly rejecting H_0 when it should have been accepted. This level of error is called *Type I error*. Whenever a decision is made, there is the possibility of making the wrong decision. Four possible decisions for a statistical test may be made (Table A.3). A *Type II error* is committed when H_0 is accepted as being true when it should have been rejected. In contrast, a Type I error is committed when H_0 is rejected when it should have been accepted.

The probability of committing a Type I error is defined as the significance level of the statistical test, and is denoted as P or α (alpha). The probability of a Type II error, denoted as β (beta), can also be computed.

The *power test* determines the probability that the statistical test results in the rejection of the null hypothesis if H_0 is really false. The larger the power, the more

TABLE A.3 *Decisions Based on a Statistical Test*

	ACCEPT NULL HYPOTHESIS (H_0)	REJECT NULL HYPOTHESIS (H_0)
H_0 true	Correct decision	Type I error
H_1 true	Type II error	Correct decision

sensitive are the tests. Because power is defined as $1 - \beta$, the larger the β-error (Type II error), the weaker is the power. The power of the test would equal $1 - \beta$ for a particular power.

To reduce Type I or Type II errors, the sample sizes need to be increased or the assay method improved. Because time, expense, and ethical concerns for performing a study are important issues, the investigator generally tries to keep the sample size (usually the number of subjects in a clinical study) to a minimum. The variability within the samples, number of samples (sample size), and desired level of significance will affect the power of the statistical test. Usually, the greater the variability within the samples, the larger will be the sample size needed to obtain sufficient power.

ANALYSIS OF VARIANCE (ONE-WAY)

When more than two data sets are compared, analysis of variance (ANOVA) is used to determine the probability of the data sets being identical or different among groups. *One-way* analysis of variance is a method for testing the differences between the population means of k treatment groups, where each group i ($i = 1, 2, \ldots, k$) consists of n_i observations X_{ij} ($j = 1, 2, \ldots, n_i$). For example, we may want to test whether there is a difference in the peak plasma level of a drug resulting from the administration of three different dosage forms—solution, capsule, and tablet. If we decide to have three groups of 20 patients per group, $i = 1, 2, 3, j = 1, 2, \ldots, 20$, and the observation in each group will be X_{ij}. The formulas for calculation are as follows:

$$\text{Sum of observation in group} = \sum_{j}^{n_j} x_{ij}$$

$$\text{Total sum of squares SS} = \sum_{i}^{k} \sum_{j}^{n_j} x_{ij}^2 - \frac{\left(\sum_{i}^{k} \sum_{j}^{n} x_{ij}^2 \right)}{\sum_{i}^{k} n_i}$$

$$\text{Total sum of squares TSS} = \sum_{i}^{k} \sum_{j}^{n_j} x_{ij}^2 - \frac{\left(\sum_{i}^{k} \sum_{j}^{n_j} x_{ij}^2 \right)}{\sum_{i}^{k} n_i}$$

$$\text{Error sum squares (ESS)} = \text{SS} - \text{TSS} = \text{total sum of squares} - \text{treatment sum of squares}$$

The value of the F-statistic is

$$F = \frac{\text{DF}_2 \times \text{TSS}}{\text{DF}_1 \times \text{ESS}} = \frac{\text{TSS}/\text{DF}_1}{\text{ESS}/\text{DF}_2}$$

Alteratively, F is expressed as the ratio of treatment mean squares (TMS)/error mean squares (EMS):

$$F = \frac{\text{TSS}/\text{DF}_1}{\text{ESS}/\text{DF}_2} = \frac{\text{TMS}}{\text{EMS}}$$

Error degrees of freedom $\text{DF}_1 = k - 1$

Error degrees of freedom $\text{DF}_2 = \sum_{j=1}^{k} n_i - k$

The ANOVA employed depends on the objectives and design of the study. ANOVA methods can estimate the variance among different subjects (intersubject variability), groups, or treatments. Using ANOVA, the statistician determines whether to accept or reject the null hypothesis (H_0), deciding whether there is no significant difference (accept H_0) or there is a significant difference (reject H_0) between the data groups.

ANOVA is a test for a difference in means between two or more groups. It is very similar to the t-test, which tests for a difference between two groups. It is applicable when several groups are involved. An ANOVA on two groups is analogous to as a two-sample t-test. ANOVA assumes that the groups have equal variances and that the outcome is normally distributed within each group. These assumptions are less important when one has large samples and equal sample sizes for each group (as with the t-test). If one rejects the null hypothesis in the ANOVA, one can conclude that the groups are not all equal, but the test does not yield any information on each pair of comparisons.

After completion of the study and statistical analysis of the data, the investigator must decide whether any statistically significant differences in the data groups have clinical relevance. For example, it may be possible to demonstrate that a new antihypertensive agent lowers the systolic blood pressure in patients by 10 mm Hg and that this effect is statistically significant ($P < 0.05$) using the appropriate statistical test. From these results and statistical treatment of the data, the principal investigator must decide whether the study is clinically relevant and whether the drug will be efficacious for its intended use. An example of ANOVA appears in Chapter 15, Table 15.5.

In clinical tests involving a comparison of a drug to a control, it is important to establish some criteria in advance with the clinicians. What is the size of the difference (Δ) that is considered clinically meaningful? How large should the sample size be in order to have adequate statistical power? If the variance is large, a large sample may be needed. On the other hand, "Over-powering" may occur if the study sample size is so large that an extremely small treatment effect could be found statistically significant but not clinically useful. When two similar studies testing the treatment effect of a drug found different results and conclusions, as is sometimes reported in the literature, it is important to look for study flaws and biases. If an estimate is biased, it means that it is not accurately estimating the true value (true mean, true median, true standard deviation, etc). It may be due to a flaw in the study design, conduct, or analysis. Any of these can shift the results in favor of either the new drug or the control. Is the drug tested in one of the studies using an old standard of care? A new drug believed by most physicians to be superior can influence the result. Bias includes not blinding the study or having many dropouts, especially if the dropouts are due to the study drug. The consequence of the study bias may lead to a drug that may be found statistically better than the control but not clinically important. Clinical judgment should be used to evaluate the magnitude of the treatment and eliminate over-powering. This is especially important for superiority trials of new drugs. Most clinical trials for regulatory purposes are quality checked or audited to assure accuracy. On the other hand, the literature or information published, although useful, may not be adequately reviewed or does not always meet statistical design requirements. It is important for the pharmacist to check the source of information and determine whether test methods are validated.

POWER TEST

A Type I error may be observed when the result of an ANOVA rejects the null hypothesis when it should have been accepted. The power of a statistical hypothesis test provides a high level of certainty that the correct decision was made—that is, to reject the null hypothesis when it is actually false. The power of a hypothesis test is the probability of not committing a Type II error. It is calculated by subtracting the probability of a Type II error from 1, usually expressed as

$$\text{Power} = 1 - \text{P (Type II error)} = 1 - \beta$$

The values for the power test range from 0 to 1. Ideally, the values for the power test should have a high power or value close to 1. To calculate the power of a given test, it is necessary to specify α (the probability that the test will lead to the rejection of the hypothesis tested when that hypothesis is true) and to specify a specific alternative hypothesis. Usually, α is set at 0.05. The power test is influenced by sample size and by intrasubject variability. For drugs whose bioavailability demonstrates high intrasubject variability ($>30\%$ CV), a larger number of subjects (larger sample size) is required to obtain a high power (>0.95).

BIOEQUIVALENCE STUDIES

Statistics have wide application in bioequivalence studies for the comparison of drug bioavailability for two or more drug products (see Chapter 15). The FDA has published two Guidance for Industry for the statistical determination of bioequivalence (2001, 1992) that describe the comparison between a test (T) and reference (R) drug product. These trials are needed for approval of new or generic drugs. If the drug formulation changes, bioequivalence studies may be needed to compare the new drug formulation to the previous drug formulation. For new drugs, several investigational formulations may be used at various stages, or one formulation with several strengths must show equivalency by extent and rate (eg, 2×250-mg tablet versus 1×500-mg tablet, suspension versus capsule, immediate-release versus extended-release product). The blood levels of the drug are measured for both the new and the reference formulation. The derived pharmacokinetic parameters, such as maximum concentration (C_{max}) and area under the curve (AUC), must meet accepted statistical criteria for the two drugs to be considered bioequivalent. In bioequivalence trials, a 90% confidence interval of the ratio of the mean of the new formulation to the mean of the old formulation

(Test/Reference) is calculated. That confidence interval needs to be completely within 0.80 to 1.25 for the drugs to be considered bioequivalent. Adequate power should be built into the design and validated methods used for analysis of the samples. Typically, both the rate (reflected by C_{max}) and extent (AUC) are tested. The ANOVA may also reveal any sequence effects, period effects, treatment effects, or inter- and intrasubject variability. Because of the small subject population usually employed in bioequivalence studies, the ANOVA uses log-transformed data to make an inference about the difference of the two groups.

PHARMACOKINETIC MODELS

In data analysis involving a model, the number of data points should exceed the number of parameters in the model with a sufficient degree of freedom. Otherwise, the model is unconstrained and the parameters estimated are not valid.

REFERENCES

Deming SN, Morgan SL: *Experimental Design: A Chemometric Approach.* Elsevier, 1987

Efron, Bradley, Tibshirani RJ: *An Introduction to the Bootstrap.* New York, London, Chapman & Hall, 1993

FDA Guidance for Industry—Statistical Approaches to Establishing Bioequivalence. www.fda.gov/cder/guidance, 2001

FDA Guidance for Industry—Statistical Procedures for Bioequivalence Studies Using a Standard Two-Treatment Crossover Design. www.fda.gov/cder/guidance, 1992

Knapp RG, Miller MC III: *Clinical Epidemiology and Biostatistics.* Lippincott Williams & Wilkins, 1992

APPENDIX B

APPLICATIONS OF COMPUTERS IN PHARMACOKINETICS

The availability of computers and improvements in bioanalytical chemistry have greatly accelerated the development of pharmacokinetics. Computer software programs now allow for the rapid solution of complicated pharmacokinetic equations and rapid modeling of pharmacokinetic processes. Computers simplify tedious calculations and allow more time for the development of new approaches to data analysis and pharmacokinetics modeling. In addition, computer software is used for the development of experimental study designs, statistical data treatment, data manipulation, graphical representation of data, pharmacokinetic model simulation, and projection or prediction of drug action. Furthermore, computers are used frequently for written reports, documentation, and archiving.

A variety of computers are now available. Personal computers (PCs) may be used independently or linked together into local networks (LANs) that share many application software packages. Each type of computer has an operating system (OS), which is a collection of programs that allocates resources and enables algorithms (well-defined rules or processes for solving a problem in a finite number of steps) to be processed. UNIX, Windows, and more recently, LINUX, are examples of commonly used operating systems. Windows NT is used mostly in network systems that link many PCs. Most PCs today are equipped with a modem to allow access to remote information. Netscape and Microsoft Internet Explorer are browsers that allow PCs to access remote information at various sites on the Internet referred to as Websites.

A program of instructions known as a computer package or software is written in a computer language. This software is needed to run the computer. The computer operating system must support the computer language of the software. In the past, computer users needed to be competent in computer programming and usually had knowledge of at least one computer language such as Pascal, C, or Basic. As a result of the availability of various commercial and noncommercial

775

pharmacokinetic applications and spreadsheets, such as Excel, very little computer programming is required for many applications in pharmacokinetics. Some examples are given below.

PHARMACOKINETIC SOFTWARE

Pharmacokinetic software consists of computer programs designed for computation and easy solution of pharmacokinetic problems. Not all computer programs satisfy the user's full requirements, but many provide the following.

1. Fitting drug concentration-versus-time data to a series of pharmacokinetic models, and choosing the one that best describes the data statistically

   Typically, a least-squares program is employed, in which the sum of squared differences between observed data points and theoretic prediction is minimized. Usually, a mathematical procedure is used iteratively (repetitively) to achieve a minimum in the sum of squares (convergence). Some data may allow easier convergence with one procedure rather than another. The mathematical method employed should be reviewed before use.

2. Fitting data into a pharmacokinetic or pharmacodynamic model defined by the user

   This method is by far the most useful, because any list of prepared models is often limited. The flexibility of user-defined models allows continuous refinement of the model as new experimental information becomes available. Some software merely provides a utility program for fitting the data to a series of polynomials. This utility program provides a simple, quantitative way of relating the variables, but offers little insight into the underlying pharmacokinetic processes.

3. Simulation

   Some software programs generate data based on a model with parameter input by the user. When the parameters are varied, new data are generated based on the model chosen. The user is able to observe how the simulated model data matches the experimental observed data. Because pharmacokinetic processes are conveniently described by systems of differential equations, the simulation process involves a numerical solution of the equation with predefined precision.

4. Experimental design

   To estimate the parameters of any model, the experimental design of the study must have points appropriately spaced to allow curve description and modeling. Although statisticians stress the need for proper experimental design, little information is generally available for experimental design in pharmacokinetics when a study is performed for the first time. For the first pharmacokinetic study, an empirical or a statistical experiment design is necessarily based on assumptions that may later prove to be wrong.

5. Clinical pharmacokinetic applications

   Some software programs are available for the clinical monitoring of narrow-therapeutic-index drugs (ie, critical-dose drugs) such as the aminoglycosides, other antibiotics, theophylline, or antiarrythmics. These programs may include calculations for creatinine clearance using the Cockcroft–Gault equation (see

Chapter 21), dosage estimation, pharmacokinetic parameter estimation for the individual patient, and pharmacokinetic simulations.

6. **Computer programs for teaching**

Software applications for teaching have been reviewed by Charles and Duffull (2001). These authors taught a course in which students used (download free ware). Pharmacalc and PharmaSim may be used for pharmacokinetic computations. SAAM II or Stella and ModelMaker may be used for "system dynamics." The latter takes into account stochastic processes in the simulation and may be more suitable when variability is considered to be an important factor in a clinical situation. Other software reviewed includes ADAPT for use in parameter estimation, simulation, and experimental (sample schedule) design.

VALIDATION OF SOFTWARE PACKAGES

Software used for data analysis such as statistical and pharmacokinetic calculations should be validated with respect to the accuracy, quality, integrity, and security of the data. One approach for determining the accuracy of the data analysis is to compare the results obtained from two different software packages using the same set of data (Heatherington et al, 1998). Because software packages may have different functionalities, different results (eg, pharmacokinetic parameter estimates) may be obtained.

PHARMACOKINETIC SOFTWARE

Various pharmacokinetic programs (software) are available on the Internet. These programs may not have been validated by the programmer. Thus, the user is responsible for validating the program. Other programs are available from commercial suppliers. Dr. David Bourne of the University of Oklahoma has compiled a listing of pharmacokinetic programs, general references in pharmacokinetics, pharmacodynamics, and other information, available at www.boomer.org. The Website www.cpb.uokhsc.edu/pkin/soft.html lists numerous pharmacokinetic software packages with user comments. Students should consult the site for updated information.

Popular Programs

Some popular commercially available computer software programs are listed below. The descriptions may not represent the latest versions. New features are often added or old features improved. The user should contact the program vendor directly for more information. See below for information about Internet resources, including user evaluations of software packages.

PCNonlin

PCNonlin is a powerful least-squares program for parameter estimation. Both a user-defined model and a library of over 20 compartmental models are available. The program accepts both differential and regular (analytical) equations. Users may select the Hartley-modified or Levenberg-type Gauss–Newton algorithm or the (Nelder and Mead) simplex algorithm for minimizing the sum of squared residuals. Some training is needed. Until its commercial release, Nonlin was installed mostly on mainframe computers. PCNonlin includes additional features and was designed to run on PCs. PCGRAPH (Version 4) was bundled to improve the quality of the plots from previous versions of Nonlin. Compartmental models, curve fitting, and simulations are specially designed for pharmacokinetics.

WinNonlin

Pharsight Corporation Main
800 W. El Camino Real, Suite 200
Mountain View, CA 94040
(650) 314-3800
www.pharsight.com/products/winnonlin

WinNonlin is Windows-based software for pharmacokinetic, pharmacodynamic, and noncompartmental analysis. It is designed for easy interfacing and secure data management with PkS Suite. WinNonlin can calculate individual bioequivalences for all of the common replicated crossover designs. WinNonMix is associated software for population pharmacokinetic analysis. WinNonlin has an improved user interface that makes it easier to use and to interface with other Windows applications. WinNonlin is relatively easy to use for modeling or noncompartmental analysis of data files and handles large numbers of subjects or profiles. WinNonlin's input and output data may be managed via Excel (Microsoft)-compatible spreadsheet files. The Noncompartmental Analysis module computes derived pharmacokinetic parameters ($AUC_{t \to 0}$, $AUC_{0 \to \infty}$, C_{max}, cumulative excretion, etc). PCNonlin's extensive library of models for nonlinear regression and parameter estimation are included in this software. Standard descriptive statistics and confidence intervals are determined from datasets.

SAS

SAS Institute, Inc.
Cary, NC 27511
(919) 677-8000
www.sas.com

An all-purpose data analysis system with a flexible application-development language, SAS Graph allows for multidimension plots, for bar, pie, and contour charts, and for all sorts of other graphs. Over 5000 SAS products are reported to be available. Various "procs" (subroutines) are available for statistics as well as general linear and nonlinear regression models. There are over 80 procedures for univariate descriptive statistics; t-test, chi-square, correlation, autoregression, multidimensional scaling, nonparametric test, factor analysis, and discriminant and stepwise analysis. SAS runs in many user environments, including PCSAS for personal computers. A special startup interface, ASSIST, facilitates beginners who are unfamiliar with the default batch data entry.

The U.S. Code of Federal Regulations, 21CFR Part 11, requires all datasets to be provided in special format for review and inspection. SAS Institute published the SAS XPORT format (Version 5) for electron data submission for regulatory purposes.

Details about SAS EXPORT can be found at www.sas.com/fda-esub. *Guidance for Industry: Providing regulatory submissions in electronic format—General considerations 1999.*

RSTRIP

> MicroMath Research
> 1710 South Brentwood Blvd.
> Saint Louis, MO 63144
> www.micromath.com

RSTRIP is menu-driven and very suitable for student use; it fits data to models, mono-, bi-, and tri-exponentials based on model selection criteria (Akaike Information Criteria). A good statistics menu is available for AUC, C_{max}, T_{max}, and mean residence time. The program gives initial parameter estimates and final parameters after iteration. However, the program does not handle differential equations or user-defined models. Plot outputs are available, as are pharmacokinetic curve stripping, and least-squares parameter optimization. The original software was written for PC DOS but has now been replaced by a Windows version with additional features.

Scientist for Windows

Scientist for Windows V2.01 is a general mathematical modeling application from MicroMath, www.micromath.com. It can perform nonlinear least-squares minimization and simulation. Models can consist of both analytic and differential equations. The software has many functions with pharmacokinetic applications.

PKAnalyst for Windows

> MicroMath Scientific Software
> PO Box 21550
> Salt Lake City, UT 84121

PKAnalyst is a bundled pharmacokinetic software incorporating many features of RSTRIP but with more statistics and mathematical functions. The program operates under Windows and is generally easy to use. It is very user-friendly for routine data analysis in pharmacokinetics.

DIFFEQ and DIFFEQ Pharmacokinetics Library

> MicroMath Scientific Software
> PO Box 21550
> Salt Lake City, UT 84121

DIFFEQ is a nonlinear least-squares program for PCs. Model entry uses a generic language with syntax similar to Basic; it may be used with DIFFEQ Pharmacokinetic Library, which includes many models used in pharmacokinetics. The original version was updated under a different name.

P-STAT

> P-Stat Inc.
> Princeton, NJ 08540
> (609) 924-9100

This program supplies statistical data handling for mainframe computers.

STELLA

High Performance Systems
Lyme, NH 03755
(603) 643-9636

STELLA is a structural thinking experimental learning laboratory with animation, available for Windows-based PCs. The program was developed on the MAC. STELLA solves differential equations and simulates pharmacokinetic models and other physiologic systems. The software is particularly suitable for teaching because of its animation and learning simulation by drawing the model.

NONMEM

NONMEM Project Group, C255
University of California
San Francisco, CA 94143

NONMEM (Nonlinear Mixed Effects Model), developed by S. L. Beal and L. B. Sheiner, is a statistical program used for fitting parameters in population pharmacokinetics. The NONMEM program first appeared in 1979. It is useful in evaluating relationships between pharmacokinetic parameters and demographic data such as age, weight, and disease state. Average population parameters and intersubject variance are estimated. The program fits the data of all the subjects simultaneously and estimates the parameters and their variances. The parameters are useful in estimating doses for individuals based on population pharmacokinetics with calculated risks. A regression program is written in ANSI (American National Standards Institute) Fortran 77 for mainframe computers.

The current version of NONMEM (Version IV) consists of several parts. The NONMEM program itself is a general (noninteractive) regression program which can be used to fit many different types of data. PREDPP consists of subroutines that can be used by NONMEM to compute predictions for population pharmacokinetics. NM-TRAN is a preprocessor, allowing control and other needed inputs and error messages to NONMEM/PREDPP.

MKMODEL

Biosoft
PO Box 10398
Ferguson, MO

MKMODEL, by N. Holford, is a pharmacokinetic program from the National Institutes of Health-supported PROPHET system. The program, available for the PC, performs nonlinear least-squares regression and includes both pharmacokinetic and pharmacodynamic models (effect compartment).

ADAPT II

D. Z. D'Argenio and A. Schumitzky
Biomedical Simulation Resource
University of Southern California
Los Angeles, CA

Supplied as Fortran code for various operating systems, this program performs simulations, nonlinear regression, and optimal sampling, and includes extended least-squares and Bayesian optimization. Models can be expressed as integrated or differential equations (D'Argenio and Schumitzky, 1992).

USC*PACK PC PROGRAMS

USC Laboratory of Applied Pharmacokinetics
2250 Alcazar St, CSC 134B
Los Angeles, CA 90033
www.usc.edu/hsc/lab_apk

This software package consists of various pharmacokinetic programs bundled for clinical pharmacokinetic applications and model parameter estimation. The program NPEM2 (Version 3) is an improved version of the nonparametric expectation maximization algorithm that is well adapted for population pharmacokinetics. The program is now available for a three-compartment model with various routes of dosing. Lahey Fortran F77EM32 and its associated package is used in this program.

Clinical programs include related routines in which past therapy data for individual patients are entered into files along with parameter and dose-prediction programs for various drugs (eg, aminoglycosides, other antibiotics, and drugs of special interest). Bayesian fitting procedures are included to fit a selected drug population model to a patient's data of doses and serum concentrations and to adaptive control of the individual dose regimen. Some program selections include:

- Amikacin (Amik)
- Gentamicin (Gent)
- Netilmicin (Net)
- Tobramycin (Tob)
- Bayesian General Modeling (MB)
- Least-Squares General Modeling (MLS)

Many patient-oriented programs for adaptive dosing based on pharmacokinetics and pharmacodynamic are featured in the package. Maximum Aposteriori Probability (MAP) Bayesian fitting is useful in individual dosing; an example is shown in Figure B-1 for gentamicin dose prediction. This method yields better prediction than conventional clinical methods even in patients with unstable renal function.

S-Plus

S-plus is a versatile package that can be used for analyzing data using the included software, and also includes its own programming language, which can be used to write your own routines. S is a statistical package developed at AT&T's Bell Laboratories. S-Plus is an extension of this statistical language produced by the StatSci Division of MathSoft in Seattle. The software is used extensively by many pharmacokinetics and statisticians for model analysis.

MathCAD

www.mathcad.com

MathCAD 11 has many general mathematical and statistical functions which can be easily adaptable for data analysis or fitting data to probability distribution models.

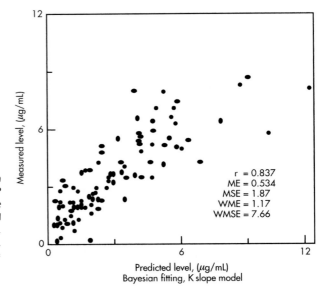

Figure B-1. An example of gentamicin dosing prediction in patients using MAP Bayesian fitting and K slope method (one compartment): Predicted versus measured serum gentamicin. (r = correlation coefficient, ME = mean error, MSE = mean squared error, WME = mean weighted error. WMSE = weighted mean squared error.)
(From Jelliffe et al, 1995, with permission.)

Differential equation solvers support ordinary differential equations, systems of differential equations, and boundary-value problems both at the command line and in Solve blocks that use natural notation to specify the differential equations and constraints.

Cyber Patient

Cyber Patient is a Windows-based multimedia pharmacokinetic simulation program that can be used for development and presentation of problem-solving case studies from Michael B. Bolger, USC School of Pharmacy. This program is suitable for simulations in pharmacy courses and research in development of pharmacokinetic drug models.

GastroPLUS

GastroPlus is a computer simulation program that predicts the rate and extent of drug absorption from the gastrointestinal tract. This innovative program was developed by a team of scientist-programmers under the direction of Dr. Michael B. Bolger at Simulations Plus, Inc., in collaboration with Dr. Gordon L. Amidon.

Instructional Programs

The **Modern Biopharmaceutics Version 6** Computer Based Training Software provides a complete information base for both university biopharmaceutics courses and continuing education courses. The program teaches both basic principles and important applications. Course material is available in modules on CD for individualized learning. For more information see www.tsrlinc.com/mbindex.htm or www.simulations-plus.com.

Other Pharmacokinetic Programs

ACSL BioMed Software based on the ACSL language that is used to simulate clinical trials of drugs. Pharsight Corporation, www.pharsight.com.

BIOPAK A pharmacokinetic program for bioavailability/bioequivalence studies, available from SCI Software.

BOOMER/MULTI-FORTE A simulation program by D. W. A. Bourne, College of Pharmacy, University of Oklahoma.

PCDCON A convolution/deconvolution program by W. R. Gillespie (see Karol et al, 1991).

FUNFIT A parameter estimation regression program.

Kinetica 4.0 A pharmacokinetic/pharmacodynamic analysis and simulation program that supports nonlinear mixed-effect model fitting. Available at www.innaphase.com.

LAGRAN A parameter estimation regression program.

MATLAB A powerful program that handles complex models, mostly in chemical engineering but found useful in pharmacokinetics.

NCOMP An Excel-based program for noncompartmental analysis of pharmacokinetic data, by Paul B. Laub. For integration of AUC and other uses, with choice of splines obtained from Lagrange polynomials or the hybrid method recommended by Purves (1996). J Pharm Sci 85:393–395, 1996.

NPEM A nonparametric expectation maximization program by A. Schumitzky (1991). It is part of the USC*PACK collection (see above).

Pharsight Trial Simulator A comprehensive computer-assisted trial simulation software system by Pharsight Corporation, www.pharsight.com/products/trial _simulator.

PDx-Pop Integrates with NONMEM and other software to expedite population modeling and analysis. UNIX version published by GloboMax LLC.

SAAM A program for pharmacokinetics and other biological models that was developed at the National Institutes of Health (NIH).

SAAM/CONSAM Performs nonlinear regression in batch (SAAM) or conversational mode (CONSAM). The SAAM/CONSAM programs are provided by the NIH. Available from L. A. Zech and P. C. Greif, Laboratory of Mathematical Biology, NIH, zech@ncifcrf.gov.

P-PHARM A population pharmacokinetic-dynamic data modeling program from InnaPhase, science@innaphase.com.

PK-Sim A whole-body physiology-based pharmacokinetic (PBPK) simulation software by Bayer Technology Services GmbH, www.pk-sim.com.

PopKinetics A population pharmacokinetics analysis program. It is a companion application to SAAM II that uses parametric algorithms, Standard Two-Stage and Iterated Two-Stage, to compute population parameters. Available from the SAAM Institute, info@saam.com.

TOPFIT A PC-based pharmacokinetic program with both data fitting and clinical application, available from Gustav Fischer (VCH Publishers, Transwell and Koup, 1993).

WinNonMix A program for nonlinear mixed-effects modeling provided in an interactive and easy-to-use Windows application. By Pharsight Corporation, www.pharsight.com.

WinSAAM   A Windows version of the original interactive biological modeling program, CONSAAM, developed in 1980 at the NIH. WinSAAM adds Windows features and enhances application environment and is maintained by Peter C. Grief.

ELECTRONIC SPREADSHEETS

For general computation, many programs, such as electronic spreadsheets, are very adaptable to calculation and pharmacokinetic curve plotting. Spreadsheet software

	A	B	C	D	E	F
1	D	100000		0	0.00	
2	KA	2		0.1	1.78	
3	K	0.4		0.2	3.16	
4	V	10000		0.3	4.23	
5	TAU	4		0.4	5.04	
6	F	1		0.5	5.64	
7	N	1		0.6	6.07	
8	EXP(-KA*TAU)	0.00033546		0.7	6.36	
9	EXP(-K*TAU)	0.20189652		0.8	6.55	
10	FKAD	200000		0.9	6.65	
11	V(K-KA)	-16000		1	6.69	
12	AA	1		1.1	6.67	
13	BB	1		1.2	6.60	
14				1.3	6.50	
15	FD/VK	25	AUC	1.4	6.38	
16				1.5	6.24	
17	FD/V...	8.86435343	Cmax-ss	1.6	6.08	
18				1.7	5.92	
19				1.8	5.74	
20	TMAX	1.0058987	tmax-1	1.9	5.57	
21				2	5.39	
22				2.1	5.21	
23	TMAX-SS	0.86516026	tmax-ss	2.2	5.03	
24				2.3	4.86	
25				2.4	4.68	
26				2.5	4.51	
27				2.6	4.35	
28				2.7	4.19	
29				2.8	4.03	
30				2.9	3.88	
31				3	3.73	
32				3.1	3.59	
33				3.2	3.45	
34				3.3	3.32	
35				3.4	3.19	
36				3.5	3.07	
37				3.6	2.95	
38				3.7	2.84	
39				3.8	2.73	
40				3.9	2.62	
41			tmin	4	2.52	Cmin
42						
43						
44						
45						
46						
47	PARAMETER	PARAM. VAL	PHARM-TERM	TIME (HRS)	CONC (MCG/ML)	

Figure B-2.   Example of a Microsoft Excel spreadsheet used to calculate time–concentration data according to an oral one-compartment model after *n* doses.

programs such as Quattro and Microsoft Excel are easy to use. Data are entered in columns (referred to alphabetically as A, B, C, . . .) and rows (referred to numerically as 1, 2, 3, . . .). Manuals are generally displayed on screen and can be selected by moving the arrow keys followed by pressing the Return or Enter key. An example of a Microsoft Excel worksheet used to generate time-versus-concentration data after n doses of a drug given orally according to a one-compartment model is given in Figure B-2. The parameter inputs are in column B, time is in column D, and concentration is in column E.

EXAMPLE 1

From a series of time–concentration data (Fig. B-3, rows A and B), determine the elimination rate constant using the regression feature of MS Excel.

Solution

a. Type in the time and concentration data shown in columns A and B (Fig. B-3).
b. Convert in column C all concentration data to ln concentration. Data point #1 may be omitted because ln of zero cannot be determined.
c. From the main menu, select Insert:

Select function
SLOPE
Y data range (select last 4 value)
X data range (select last 4 value)

The slope, given in Fig. B-3 is −0.1. In this case, the ln concentration is plotted versus time, and the slope is simply the elimination rate constant.

Note: To check this result, students may be interested in simulating the data with dose = 10,000 μg/kg, V_D = 1000 mL/kg, k_a = 0.8 hr^{-1}, and k = 0.1 hr^{-1}.

	A	B	C		
1	Time	Conc	Ln		
2	(hr)		(conc)		
3	0	0.00			
4	2	7049.53	8.86		
5	4	7194.95	8.88		
6	6	6178.08	8.73		
7	8	5116.20	8.54		
8	10	4200.50	8.34		
9	12	3441.45	8.14	Slope	−0.1
10	14	2818.09	7.94		
11	16	2307.36	7.74		

Figure B-3. A sample spreadsheet showing a set of time–concentration data (Time and Conc) being analyzed to obtain the slope or the elimination constant. Note: Only four points from the terminal part of the curve were regressed [t versus ln (conc)].

EXAMPLE 2

Generate some data for a two-compartment model using two differential equations. Initial conditions are dose $= 1$, $V = 1$, and $k_{12} = 0$, $k_{21} = 1$, and $k = 3$.

Solution

The data may be generated with MathCAD (Fig. B-4). Note that k_{12} is abbreviated as k_1, k_{21} is abbreviated as k_2, and k is abbreviated at k_3 in the program for simplicity. Also, $dC_p/dt = F(t, x, y)$; $x = C_p$; $y = C_t$; $t = $ time; and $dC_t/dt = G(t, x, y)$.

Model Fitting

An example of a set of oral plasma data was fitted to a one-compartment model by RSTRIP (Fig. B-5). The software makes an initial estimate as well as a final parameter after several iterations. An example of some oral plasma data was generated with PCNonlin (Figs. B-6A, B, C).

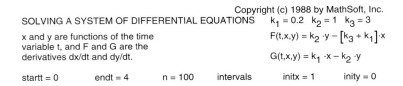

SOLVING A SYSTEM OF DIFFERENTIAL EQUATIONS

Copyright (c) 1988 by MathSoft, Inc. $k_1 = 0.2$ $k_2 = 1$ $k_3 = 3$

x and y are functions of the time variable t, and F and G are the derivatives dx/dt and dy/dt.

$F(t,x,y) = k_2 \cdot y - [k_3 + k_1] \cdot x$

$G(t,x,y) = k_1 \cdot x - k_2 \cdot y$

startt = 0   endt = 4   n = 100   intervals   initx = 1   inity = 0

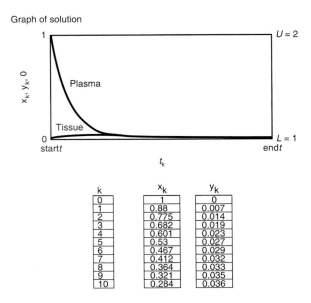

k	x_k	y_k
0	1	0
1	0.88	0.007
2	0.775	0.014
3	0.682	0.019
4	0.601	0.023
5	0.53	0.027
6	0.467	0.029
7	0.412	0.032
8	0.364	0.033
9	0.321	0.035
10	0.284	0.036

Figure B-4. A sample of the MathCAD application program used to solve the two-differential equation for a two-compartment model after IV bolus dose. (The first 10 data points are shown.)

```
                Summary of Least Squares for dataset oral absorption

          computation time:     1.04 secs   A[1]=  12.801      k[1]=  0.40724
         calculated lag time:   0.00000     k[2]= -12.800      k[2]=  1.9428
    sum of squared residuals:   0.0048572
    Model Selection Criterion:  8.1157
         Weighting Factor:      0.00000

     time           y-obs          y-calc          resid          wt*res-sq

    0.00000        0.00000        0.00051906     -0.00051906     2.694E-007
    0.40000        5.0000         4.9919          0.0080675      6.509E-005
    0.80000        6.5000         6.5363         -0.036276       0.0013160
    1.2000         6.6600         6.6087          0.051306       0.0026323
    2.0000         5.3900         5.4062         -0.016228       0.00026334
    2.4000         4.6800         4.6961         -0.016060       0.00025791
    2.8000         4.0300         4.0373         -0.0072648      5.278E-005
    3.2000         3.4500         3.4520         -0.0020411      4.166E-006
    3.6000         2.9500         2.9431          0.0069157      4.783E-005
    4.0000         2.5200         2.5053          0.014746       0.00021745
                        press any key to continue
```

Figure B-5. *Sample output from RSTRIP pharmacokinetic software showing a good fit of the theoretical data to actual data (columns 2 and 3). The parameters estimated are given in the top right-hand corner.*

 # EXAMPLE 3

After a drug is administered orally, a series of plasma drug concentration–time data may be fitted to a one-compartment model, to estimate the absorption rate constant, elimination rate constant, and volume of distribution. Other pharmacokinetic parameters of interest may also be calculated using the NONLIN program, as shown in Figure B-6. Three parameters were estimated—V, k_{01}, and k_{10}—representing volume of distribution, k_a, and k (see model). Initial estimates were derived from either curve stripping or feathering. Dose is CON (1). In this case, NOBS = 9, showing that there are 9 data points. There is only one function that describes the model FUNC 1. S(1) represents the calculation of AUC, S(2) the calculation of absorption, and S(3) the calculation of elimination half-life.

```
LISTING OF INPUT COMMANDS

MODEL 3, 'ONE'
MODEL 3
REMARK    ONE COMPARTMENT MODEL - FIRST ORDER INPUT AND OUTPUT
REMA
REMA    NO.    PARAMETER         CONSTANT         SECONDARY PARM.
REMA    ---    ---------         --------         ---------------
REMA     1     VOLUME            DOSE             AUC
REMA     2     K01                                K01 HALF LIFE
REMA     3     K10                                K10 HALF LIFE
REMA     4                                        TMAX
REMA     5                                        CMAX
REMA****************************************************************
REMA              I---------------------I
REMA              I                     I
REMA    K01  --> I     COMPARTMENT 1    I    ---> K10
REMA              I                     I
REMA              I---------------------I
REMA****************************************************************
COMM
NPARM 3
NCON 1
MSEC 5
PNAMES 'VOLUME', 'K01', 'K10'
SNAMES 'AUC', 'K01-HL', K10-HL', 'TMAX', 'CMAX'
END
TEMP
D=CON(1)
V=P(1)
K01=P(2)
K10=P(3)
T=X
END
FUNC1
COEF=D*K01/(V*(K01-K10))
F=COEF*(DEXP(-K10*T)-DEXP(-K01*T))
END
SECO
S(1)=D/V/K10
S(2)=-DLOG(.5)/K01
S(3)=-DLOG(.5)/K10
TMAX=(DLOG(K01/K10)/(K01-K10))
S(4)=TMAX
S(5)=(D/V)*DEXP(-K10*TMAX)
END
EOM
CONS 250
INIT 100.7, 1.03, .13
NOBS 9
DATA
BEGIN


PCNONLIN NONLINEAR ESTIMATION PROGRAM

ITERATION WEIGHTED SS      VOLUME       K01          K10
    0        1.34180        100.7       1.030        .1300
                   TAU  = .1583E-04   RANK = 3   COND = 1049.
    1         .136818       100.7        .5689       .1706
                   TAU  = .1108E-04   RANK = 3   COND = 1701.
    2        .358976E-01    100.7        .4396       .1788
                   TAU  = .1008E-04   RANK = 3   COND = 2489.
    3        .357194E-01    100.7        .4439       .1795
                   TAU  = .1005E-04   RANK = 3   COND = 2451.
    4        .357049E-01    100.7        .4442       .1791
                   TAU  = .1008E-04   RANK = 3   COND = 2447.
    5        .356635E-01     99.63       .4392       .1816
                   TAU  = .9998E-05   RANK = 3   COND = 2473.
    6        .356553E-01     99.63       .4383       .1815
                   TAU  = .1000E-04   RANK = 3   COND = 2481.


CONVERGENCE ACHIEVED
RELATIVE CHANGE IN WEIGHTED SUM OF SQUARES LESS THAN        .000100
    6        .356553E-01     99.57       .4377       .1817
```

Figure B-6A.   Sample output from PCNONLIN showing data fitted to Model 3, a one-compartment model with first-order absorption and first-order elimination.

PARAMETER	ESTIMATE	STANDARD ERROR	95% CONFIDENCE LIMITS		
VOLUME	99.568030	19.182331	52.630524	146.505537	UNIVARIATE
			24.795837	174.340224	PLANAR
K01	.437738	.117793	.149508	.725969	UNIVARIATE
			-.021417	.896894	PLANAR
K10	.181749	.043746	.074706	.288792	UNIVARIATE
			.011228	.352271	PLANAR

*** SUMMARY OF NONLINEAR ESTIMATION ***

    FUNCTION   1

X	OBSERVED Y	CALCULATED Y	RESIDUAL	WEIGHT	SD-YHAT	STANDARDIZED RESIDUAL
1.000	.7000	.8085	-.1085	1.000	.4987E-01	-1.847
2.000	1.200	1.196	.3927E-02	1.000	.4740E-01	.6460E-01
3.000	1.400	1.334	.6581E-01	1.000	.4034E-01	1.002
4.000	1.400	1.330	.7008E-01	1.000	.4253E-01	1.090
6.000	1.100	1.132	-.3226E-01	1.000	.4620E-01	-.5228
8.000	.8000	.8737	-.7371E-01	1.000	.4000E-01	-1.119
10.00	.6000	.6435	-.4349E-01	1.000	.3919E-01	-.6552
12.00	.5000	.4624	.3760E-01	1.000	.4469E-01	.5986
16.00	.3000	.2305	.6954E-01	1.000	.4888E-01	1.167

CORRECTED SUM OF SQUARED OBSERVATIONS = 1.28889
WEIGHTED CORRECTED SUM OF SQUARED OBSERVATIONS = 1.28889
SUM OF SQUARED RESIDUALS = .356533E-01
SUM OF WEIGHTED SQUARED RESIDUALS = .356533E-01
S = .770857E-01 WITH 6 DEGREES OF FREEDOM

SUMMARY OF ESTIMATED SECONDARY PARAMETERS

PARAMETER	ESTIMATE	STANDARD ERROR
AUC	13.814898	.847009
KO1-HL	1.583474	.425680
K10-HL	3.813757	.917038
TMAX	3.433715	.217994
CMAX	1.345203	.040455

Figure B-6B. Sample output from PCNONLIN.

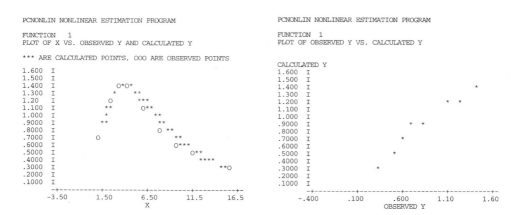

Figure B-6C. Sample output from PCNONLIN.

REFERENCES

Charles BG, Duffull SB: Pharmacokinetic software for the health sciences: Choosing the right package for teaching purposes. *Clin Pharmacokinet* **40**(6):395–403, 2001

D'Argenio DZ, Schumitzky A: *ADAPT II User's Guide.* Los Angeles, Biomedical Simulation Resource, University of Southern California, 1992

Heatherington AC, Vicini P, Golde H: A pharmacokinetic/pharmacodynamic comparison of SAAM II and PC/WIN Nonlin Modeling software. *J Pharm Sci* **87**:1255–1263, 1998

Jelliffe RW, Schumitzky A, Van Guilder M, Jiang F: *User Manual for Version 10.7 USC*PACK Collection of PC Programs.* USC Laboratory of Applied Pharmacokinetics, University of Southern California, 1995

Karol M, Gillespie WR, Veng-Pederson P: *AAPS Short Course: Convolution, Deconvolution and Linear Systems,* Washington, DC, AAPS (1991)

Schumitzky A: Nonparametric EM algorithms for estimating prior distributions. *Appl Math Comput* **45**:143–157, 1991

Tanswell P, Koup J: *Int J Clin Pharmacol Ther Toxicol* **31**(10):514–420, 1993

BIBLIOGRAPHY

Bourne DWA: Mathematical modeling of pharmaceutical data. In Swarbrick J, Boylan JC (eds), *Encyclopedia of Pharmaceutical Technology,* Vol 9. New York, Marcel Dekker, 1994

Gabrielsson J, Wiener D: *Pharmacokinetics and Pharmacodynamic Data Analysis: Concepts and Applications,* 2nd ed. Swedish Pharmaceutical Press, 1998

Gex-Fabry M, Balant LP: Consideration on data analysis using computer methods and currently available software for personal computers. In Welling PG, Balant LP (eds), *Handbook of Experimental Pharmacology, Vol 110, Pharmacokinetics of Drugs,* Berlin, Springer-Verlag, 1994

Maronda R (ed): Clinical applications of pharmacokinetics and control theory: Planning, monitoring, and adjusting dosage regiments of aminoglycosides, lidocaine, digoxitin, and digoxin. In Jelliffe RW (ed), *Selected Topics in Clinical Pharmacology.* New York, Springer-Verlag, 1986, chap 3

The NONMEM Project Group: *NONMEM User Manuals I–VI.* San Francisco, University of California, San Francisco, www.micromath.com/http://www.micromath.com, 1995

APPENDIX C

SOLUTIONS TO FREQUENTLY ASKED QUESTIONS (FAQ) AND LEARNING QUESTIONS

CHAPTER 1

FREQUENTLY ASKED QUESTIONS

1. Blood is composed of plasma and red blood cells (RBCs). Serum is the fluid obtained from blood after it is allowed to clot. Serum and plasma do not contain identical proteins. RBCs may be considered a cellular component of the body in which the drug concentration in the serum or plasma is in equilibrium, in the same way as with the other tissues in the body. Whole blood samples are generally harder to process and assay than serum or plasma samples.

2. Physiologic models are complex, and require more information for accurate prediction compared to compartment models. Missing information in the physiologic model will lead to bias or error in the model. Compartment models are more simplistic in that they assume that both arterial and venous drug concentrations are similar. The compartment model accounts for a rapid distribution phase and a slower elimination phase. Physiologic clearance models postulate that arterial blood drug levels are higher than venous blood drug levels. In practice, only venous blood samples are usually sampled. Organ drug clearance is useful in the treatment of cancers and in diagnosis of certain diseases involving arterial perfusion. Physiologic models are difficult to use for general application.

3. The exact site of drug action is generally unknown for most drugs. The time needed for the drug to reach the site of action, produce a pharmacodynamic effect, and reach equilibrium are deduced from studies on the relationship of the time course for the drug concentration and the pharmacodynamic effect. Often, the drug concentration is sampled during the elimination phase after the drug has been distributed and reached equilibrium. For multiple-dose studies, both the peak and trough drug concentrations are frequently taken.

LEARNING QUESTIONS

1. The plasma drug level–time curve describes the pharmacokinetics of the systemically absorbed drug. Once a suitable pharmacokinetic model is obtained, plasma drug concentrations may be predicted following various dosage regimens such as single oral and IV bolus doses, multiple-dose regimens, IV infusion, etc. If the pharmacokinetics of the drug relate to its pharmacodynamic activity (or

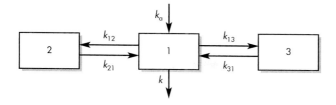

Figure C-1

any adverse drug response or toxicity), then a drug regimen based on the drug's pharmacokinetics may be designed to provide optimum drug efficacy. In lieu of a direct pharmacokinetic–pharmacodynamic relationship, the drug's pharmacokinetics describe the bioavailability of the drug including inter- and intrasubject variability; this information allows for the development of drug products that consistently deliver the drug in a predictable manner.

2. The purpose of pharmacokinetic models is to relate the time course of the drug in the body to its pharmacodynamic and/or toxic effects. The pharmacokinetic model also provides a basis for drug product design, the design of dosage regimens, and a better understanding of the action of the body on the drug.

3. (Figure C-1)

4. a. Nine parameters: V_1, V_2, V_3, k_{12}, k_{21}, k_e, k_b, k_m, k_u

b. Compartment 1 and compartment 3 may be sampled.

c. $k = k_b + k_m + k_e$

d. $\dfrac{dC_1}{dt} = k_{21} C_2 - (k_{12} + k_m + k_e + k_b) C_1$

6.

Compartment 1	Compartment 2
C_1	C_2

a. C_1 and C_2 are the *total* drug concentration in each compartment respectively. $C_1 > C_2$ may occur if the drug concentrates in compartment 1 due to protein binding (compartment 1 contains a high amount of protein or special protein binding), due to partitioning (compartment 1 has a high lipid content and the drug is poorly water soluble), if the pH is different in each compartment and the drug is a weak electrolyte (the drug may be more ionized in compartment 1), or if there is an active transport mechanism for the drug to be taken up into the cell (eg, purine drug). Other explanations for $C_1 > C_2$ may be possible.

b. Several different experimental conditions are needed to prove which of the above hypotheses is the most likely cause for $C_1 > C_2$. These experiments may use *in-vivo* or *in-vitro* methods, including intracellular electrodes to measure pH *in vivo*, protein binding studies *in vitro*, and partitioning of drug in chloroform/water *in vitro*, among others.

c. In the case of protein binding, the total concentration of drug in each compartment may be different (eg, $C_1 > C_2$) and, at the same time, the free (non-protein bound) drug concentration may be equal in each compart-ment—assuming that the free or unbound drug is easily diffusable. Similarly, if $C_1 > C_2$ is due to differences in pH and the nonionized drug is easily diffusable, then the nonionized drug concentration may be the same in each compartment. The total drug concentrations will be $C_1 = C_2$ when there is similar affinity for the drug and similar conditions in each compartment.

d. The total amount of drug, A, in each compartment depends on the volume, V, of the compartment and the concentration, C, of the drug in the compartment. Since the amount of drug (A) = concentration (C) times volume (V), any condition that causes the product, $C_1 V_1 \neq C_2 V_2$, will result in $A_1 \neq A_2$. Thus, if $C_1 = C_2$ and $V_1 \neq V_2$, then $A_1 \neq A_2$.

CHAPTER 2

 FREQUENTLY ASKED QUESTIONS

1. A semilog plot spaces the data at logarithmic intervals on the y axis and rectangular (evenly spaced) intervals on the x axis. The paper comes in one or more cycles. Two-cycle semilog paper covers two logarithmic intervals (eg, 1 to 100). The semilog scale does not start with zero.

2. A common error in using logs is failing to remember that $\ln x = 2.3 \log x$. For the slope formula using a semilog plot,

$$\text{Slope} = \frac{\log y_2 - \log y_1}{x_2 - x_1} = \frac{-k}{2.3}$$

$$k = -\text{slope} \times 2.3 \qquad \text{(Did you forget the 2.3 factor?)}$$

Alternatively, if you determine the slope with natural logs,

$$\text{slope} = \frac{\ln y_2 - \ln y_1}{x_2 - x_1} = -k$$

$$k = -\text{slope} \qquad \text{(You should not use the 2.3 factor in this case)}$$

3. Use the natural antilog of the intercept, or the inverse of ln.

LEARNING QUESTIONS

1. a. Zero-order process (Fig. C-2).

   b. Rate constant, k_0:

   Method 1

   Values obtained from the graph (Fig. C-2):

t (min)	A (mg)
40	71
80	41

   $$-k_0 = \text{slope} = \frac{\Delta Y}{\Delta X} = \frac{y_2 - y_1}{x_2 - x_1}$$

   $$-k_0 = \frac{41 - 71}{80 - 40} \qquad k_0 = 0.75 \text{ mg/min}$$

   Notice that the negative sign shows that the slope is declining.

   Method 2

   By extrapolation:

   $A_0 = 103.5$ at $t = 0$; $A = 71$ at $t = 40$ min
   $A = k_0 t + A_0$
   $71 = -40 k_0 + 103.5$
   $k_0 = 0.81 \text{ mg/min}$

   Notice that the answer differs in accordance with the method used.

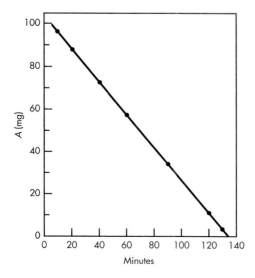

Figure C-2

c. $t_{1/2}$

For zero-order kinetics, the larger the initial amount of drug A_0, the longer the $t_{1/2}$.

Method 1

$$t_{1/2} = \frac{0.5\ A_0}{k_0}$$

$$t_{1/2} = \frac{0.5\,(103.5)}{0.78} = 66 \text{ min}$$

Method 2

The zero-order $t_{1/2}$ may be read directly from the graph (Fig. C-2):

At $t = 0$, $A_0 = 103.5$ mg.

At $t_{1/2}$, $A = 51.8$ mg.

Therefore, $t_{1/2} = 66$ min.

d. The amount of drug A does extrapolate to zero on the x axis.

e. The equation of the line is

$$A = -k_0 t + A_0$$
$$A = -0.78t + 103.5$$

2. a. First-order process (Fig. C-3).

   b. Rate constant, k:

Method 1

Obtain the first-order $t_{1/2}$ from the semilog graph (Fig. C-3):

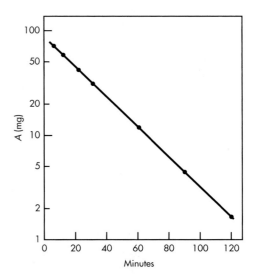

Figure C-3

t (min)	A (mg)
30	30
53	15

$t_{1/2} = 23$ min

$$k = \frac{0.693}{t_{1/2}} = \frac{0.693}{23} = 0.03 \text{ min}^{-1}$$

Method 2

$$\text{Slope} = \frac{-k}{2.3} = \frac{\log Y_2 - \log Y_1}{X_2 - X_1}$$

$$k = \frac{-2.3(\log 15 - \log 30)}{53 - 30} = 0.03 \text{ min}^{-1}$$

c. $t_{1/2} = 23$ min (see Method 1 above).

d. The amount of drug A does not extrapolate to zero on the x axis.

e. The equation of the line is

$$\log A = -\frac{kt}{2.3} + \log A_0$$

$$\log A = -\frac{0.03t}{2.3} + \log 78$$

$$A = 78e^{-0.03t}$$

On a rectangular plot, the same data shows a curve (not plotted).

3. a. Zero-order process (Fig. C-4).

b. $k_0 = \text{slope} = \dfrac{\Delta Y}{\Delta X}$

Values obtained from the graph (Fig. C-4):

t (hr)	C (μg/mL)
1.2	80
4.2	60

It is always best to plot the data. Obtain a regression line (ie, the line of best fit), then use points C and t from that line.

$$-k_0 = \frac{60 - 80}{4.2 - 1.2}$$

$$k_0 = 6.67 \ \mu\text{g/mL hr}$$

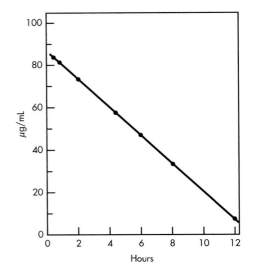

Figure C-4

c. By extrapolation:

At t_0, $C_0 = 87.5$ μg/mL.

d. The equation (using a ruler only) is

$$A = -k_0 t + A_0 = -6.67t + 87.5$$

4. Given:

C (mg/mL)	t (days)
300	0
75	30

a. $\log C = \dfrac{-kt}{2.3} + \log C_0$

$\log 75 = \dfrac{-30k}{2.3} + \log 300$

$k = 0.046$ days^{-1}

$t_{1/2} = \dfrac{0.693}{k} = \dfrac{0.693}{0.046} = 15$ days

b. Method 1

300 mg/mL = C_0 at $t = 0$

75 mg/mL = C at $t = 30$ days

225 mg/mL = difference between initial and final drug concentration

$$k_0 = \frac{225 \text{ mg/mL}}{30 \text{ days}} = 7.5 \text{ mg/mL/day}$$

The time, $t_{1/2}$, for the drug to decompose to $\frac{1}{2}$ C_0 (from 300 to 150 mg/mL) is calculated by (assuming zero order)

$$t_{1/2} = \frac{150 \text{ mg/mL}}{7.5 \text{ mg/mL day}} = 20 \text{ days}$$

Method 2

$$C = -k_0 t + C_0$$
$$75 = -30 k_0 + 300$$
$$k_0 = 7.5 \text{ mg/mL/day}$$
$$\text{At } t_{1/2}, C = 150 \text{ mg/mL}$$
$$150 = -7.5 t_{1/2} + 300$$
$$t_{1/2} = 20 \text{ days}$$

Method 3

A $t_{1/2}$ value of 20 days may be obtained directly from the graph by plotting C against t on rectangular coordinates.

5. Assume the original concentration of drug to be 1000 mg/mL.

Method 1

mg/mL	No. of Half-Lives	mg/mL	No. of Half-Lives
1000	0	15.6	6
500	1	7.81	7
250	2	3.91	8
125	3	1.95	9
62.5	4	0.98	10
31.3	5		

99.9% of 1000 = 999

Concentration of drug remaining = 0.1% of 1000

1000 − 999 = 1 mg/mL

It takes approximately 10 half-lives to eliminate all but 0.1% of the original concentration of drug.

Method 2

Assume any $t_{1/2}$ value:

$$t_{1/2} = \frac{0.693}{k}$$

Then

$$k = \frac{0.693}{t_{1/2}}$$

$$\log C = \frac{-kt}{2.3} + \log C_0$$

$$\log 1.0 = \frac{-kt}{2.3} + \log 1000$$

$$t = 9.96 t_{1/2}$$

Substituting $0.693/t_{1/2}$ for k:

$$\log 1.0 = \frac{-0.693t}{2.3 \times t_{1/2}} + \log 1000$$

$$t = 9.96 \ t_{1/2}$$

6. $t_{1/2} = 12$ hr

$$k = \frac{0.693}{t_{1/2}} = \frac{0.693}{12} = 0.058 \ \text{hr}^{-1}$$

If 30% of the drug decomposes, 70% is left.

$$70\% \text{ of } 125 \text{ mg} = (0.70)(125) = 87.5 \text{ mg}$$
$$A_0 = 125 \text{ mg}$$
$$A = 87.5 \text{ mg}$$
$$k = 0.058 \ \text{hr}^{-1}$$
$$\log A = -\frac{kt}{2.3} + \log A_0$$
$$\log 87.5 = -\frac{0.058t}{2.3} + \log 125$$
$$t = 6.1 \text{ hr}$$

7. Immediately after the drug dissolves, the drug degrades at a constant, or zero-order, rate. Since concentration is equal to mass divided by volume, it is necessary to calculate the initial drug concentration (at $t = 0$) to determine the original volume in which the drug was dissolved. From the data, calculate the zero-order rate constant, k_0:

$$-k_0 = \text{slope} = \frac{\Delta Y}{\Delta X} = \frac{0.45 - 0.3}{2.0 - 0.5} \qquad k_0 = 0.1 \text{ mg/mL hr}$$

Then calculate the initial drug concentration, C_0, using the following equation:

$$C = -k_0 t + C_0$$

At $t = 2$ hours,

$$0.3 = -0.1(2) + C_0$$
$$C_0 = 0.5 \text{ mg/mL}$$

Alternatively, at $t = 0.5$ hour,

$$0.45 = -0.1(0.5) - C_0$$
$$C_0 = 0.5 \text{ mg/mL}$$

Since the initial mass of drug D_0 dissolved is 300 mg and the initial drug concentration C_0 is 0.5 mg/mL, the original volume may be calculated from the following relationship:

$$C_0 = \frac{D_0}{V}$$

$$0.5 \text{ mg/mL} = \frac{300 \text{ mg}}{V(\text{mL})}$$

$$V = 600 \text{ mL}$$

8. First order.

9. The volume of the culture tube is not important. In 8 hours (480 minutes), the culture tube is completely full. Because the doubling time for the cells is 2 minutes (ie, one $t_{1/2}$), then in 480 minutes less 2 minutes (478 minutes) the culture tube is half full of cells.

10. Data is often reported as the mean $\pm$ standard deviation or SD (see Fig. A-2, Appendix A). One SD above and below the mean represents 95% of the population, assuming a normal distribution of the data. In this example,

Mean + 2SD = 9.8 L + 8.4 L = 18.2 L
Mean − 2SD = 9.8 L − 8.4 L = 1.4 L

Thus, 95% of the population would have a volume of distribution approximately ranging from 1.4 to 18.2 L.

11. The answer is **A.** Each of the equations are in the form of $y = Ae^{kt}$, where k is the slope of the line connecting the data points. A positive slope indicates that the direction of the line is slanted upward from left to right, whereas a negative slope indicates that the line slants downward (declines) from left to right. Answer **C** would have a rising slope.

12. The answer is **C.** Recall that $e^{-kt} = 1/e^{kt}$, and that, as k or t gets larger, the fraction, $1/e^{kt}$ gets smaller (for both A and B). (Note: You may check the values using your calculator.)

13. The answer is **D.** You cannot obtain a log from a negative number.

14. The answer is **B.** Substitute the same value for t in each example and notice your answers.

CHAPTER 3

 FREQUENTLY ASKED QUESTIONS

1. A rate represents the change in amount or concentration of drug in the body per time unit. For example, a rate equal to -5 mg/hr means the amount of drug is decreasing at 5 mg per hour. A *positive* or *negative* sign indicates that the rate is increasing or decreasing, respectively. Rates may be zero order, first order, or higher orders. For a first-order rate, the rate of change of drug in the body is determined by the *product of the elimination rate constant, k*, and by the *amount of drug* remaining in the body, ie, rate $= -kD_B$, where k represents "the fraction" of the amount of drug in the body that is eliminated per hour. If $k = 0.1 \text{ hr}^{-1}$ and $D_B = 10$ mg, then the rate $= 0.1 \text{ hr}^{-1} \times 10 \text{ mg} = 1$ mg/hr. The rate constant in this example shows that one-tenth of the drug is eliminated per hour, whatever amount of drug is present in the body. For a first-order rate, the rate states the absolute amount eliminated per unit time (which changes with the amount of drug in the body), whereas the first-order rate constant, k, gives a constant fraction of drug that is eliminated per unit time (which does not change with the amount of drug in the body).

2. The first-order rate constant k has no concentration or mass units. In the calculation of the slope, k, the unit for mass or concentration is canceled when taking the log of the number:

$$\text{Slope} = \frac{\ln y_2 - \ln y_1}{x_2 - x_1} = \frac{\ln(y_2/y_1)}{x_2 - x_1}$$

3. The one-compartment model uses a single homogeneous compartment to represent the fluid and the vascular tissues. This model ignores the heterogeneity of the tissues in the body, so there is no merit in predicting precise tissue–drug levels. However, the model provides useful insight into the mass balance of drug distribution in and out of the plasma fluid in the body. If V_D is larger than the physiologic vascular volume, the conclusion is that there is some drug outside the vascular pool, ie, in the tissues. If V_D is small, then there is little extravascular tissue drug storage, except perhaps in the lung, liver, kidney, and heart. With some knowledge about the lipophilicity of the drug and an understanding of blood flow and perfusion within the body, a postulation may be made as to which organs are involved in storing the extravascular drug. The concentration of a biopsy sample may support or refute the postulation.

4. Clearance is the volume of plasma fluid that is cleared of drug per unit time. Clearance may also be derived for the physiologic model as the fraction of drug that is eliminated by an organ as blood flows through it. The former definition

is equivalent to $Cl = kV_D$ and is readily adapted to dosing since V_D is the volume of distribution. If the drug is eliminated solely by metabolism in the liver, then $Cl_H = Cl$. Cl_H is usually estimated by the difference between $Cl - Cl_R$. Cl_H is directly estimated by the product of the hepatic blood flow and the extraction ratio.

5. Since mass balance (ie, relating dose to plasma drug concentration) is based on volume of distribution rather than blood volume, the compartment model is used in determining dose. Generally, the total blood concentrations of most drugs are not known, since only the plasma or serum concentration is assayed. Some drugs have a RBC/plasma drug ratio much greater than 1, making the application of the physiologic model difficult without knowing the apparent volume of distribution.

LEARNING QUESTIONS

1. The C_p decreased from 1.2 to 0.3 $\mu g/mL$ in 3 hours.

t (hr)	C_P ($\mu g/mL$)
2	1.2
5	0.3

$$\log C_p = -\frac{kt}{2.3} + \log C_p^0$$

$$\log 0.3 = -\frac{k(3)}{2.3} + \log 1.2$$

$$k = 0.462 \text{ hr}^{-1}$$

$$t_{1/2} = \frac{0.693}{k} = \frac{0.693}{0.462}$$

$$t_{1/2} = 1.5 \text{ hr}$$

These data may also be plotted on a semilog graph and $t_{1/2}$ obtained from the graph.

2. Dose (IV bolus) = 6 mg/kg × 50 kg = 300 mg

a. $V_D = \dfrac{\text{dose}}{C_p^0} = \dfrac{300 \text{ mg}}{8.4 \text{ } \mu g/mL} = \dfrac{300 \text{ mg}}{8.4 \text{ mg/L}} = 35.7 \text{ L}$

(1) Plot the data on semilog graph paper and use two points from the line of best fit.

t (hr)	C_p (μg/mL)
2	6
6	3

(2) $t_{1/2}$ (from graph) $= 4$ hr $k = \dfrac{0.693}{4} = 0.173 \text{ hr}^{-1}$

b. $C_p^0 = 8.4 \ \mu\text{g/mL}$ $C_p = 2 \ \mu\text{g/mL}$ $k = 0.173 \text{ hr}^{-1}$

$$\log C_p = -\frac{kt}{2.3} + \log C_p^0$$

$$\log 2 = -\frac{0.173t}{2.3} + \log 8.4$$

$$t = 8.29 \text{ hr}$$

Alternatively, time t may be found from a graph of C_p versus t.

c. Time required for 99.9% of the drug to be eliminated:

(1) Approximately $10t_{1/2}$

$$t = 10(4) = 40 \text{ hr}$$

(2) $C_p^0 = 8.4 \ \mu\text{g/mL}$

With 0.1% of drug remaining,

$$C_p = 0.001\,(8.4 \ \mu\text{g/mL}) = 0.0084 \ \mu\text{g/mL}$$

$$k = 0.173 \text{ hr}^{-1}$$

$$\log 0.0084 = \frac{-0.173t}{2.3} + \log 8.4$$

$$t = 39.9 \text{ hr}$$

d. If the dose is doubled, then C_p^0 will also double. However, the elimination half-life or first-order rate constant will remain the same. Therefore,

$$C_p^0 = 16.8 \ \mu\text{g/mL}   C_p = 2 \ \mu\text{g/mL}   k = 0.173 \text{ hr}^{-1}$$

$$\log 2 = \frac{0.173t}{2.3} + \log 16.8$$

$$t = 12.3 \text{ hr}$$

Notice that doubling the dose does not double the duration of activity.

3. $D_0 = 200$ mg

$V_D = 10\%$ of body weight $= 0.1 \ (80 \text{ kg}) = 8000 \text{ mL} = 8 \text{ L}$

At 6 hours:

$$C_p = 1.5 \text{ mg}/100 \text{ mL}$$

$$V_D = \frac{\text{drug in body } (D_B)}{C_p}$$

$$D_B = C_p V_D = \frac{1.5 \text{ mg}}{100 \text{ mL}} (8000 \text{ mL}) = 120 \text{ mg}$$

$$\log D_B = -\frac{kt}{2.3} + \log D_B^0$$

$$\log 120 = -\frac{k(6)}{2.3} + \log 200$$

$$k = 0.085 \text{ hr}^{-1}$$

$$t_{1/2} = \frac{0.693}{k} = \frac{0.693}{0.085} = 8.1 \text{ hr}$$

4. $C_p = 78e^{-0.46t}$ (the equation is in the form $C_p = C_p^0 e^{-kt}$)

$$\ln C_p = \ln 78 - 0.46t$$

$$\log C_p = -\frac{0.46t}{2.3} + \log 78$$

Thus, $k = 0.46 \text{ hr}^{-1}$, $C_p^0 = 78 \ \mu g/mL$.

a. $t_{1/2} = \dfrac{0.693}{k} = \dfrac{0.693}{0.46} = 1.5 \text{ hr}$

b. $V_D = \dfrac{\text{dose}}{C_p^0} = \dfrac{300{,}000 \ \mu g}{78 \ \mu g/mL} = 3846 \text{ mL}$

Dose $= 4 \text{ mg/kg} \times 75 \text{ kg} = 300 \text{ mg}$

c. (1) $\log C_p = -\dfrac{0.46(4)}{2.3} + \log 78 = 1.092$

$$C_p = 12.4 \ \mu g/mL$$

(2) $C_p = 78e^{-0.46(4)} = 78e^{-1.84} = 78(0.165)$

$$C_p = 12.9 \ \mu g/mL$$

d. At 4 hours:

$$D_B = C_p V_D = 12.4 \ \mu g/mL \times 3846 \text{ mL} = 47.69 \text{ mg}$$

e. $V_D = 3846 \text{ mL}$

Average weight $= 75 \text{ kg}$

Percent body wt $= (3.846 \text{ kg}/75 \text{ kg}) \times 100 = 5.1\%$

The apparent V_D approximates the plasma volume.

f. $C_p = 2 \ \mu g/mL$.

Find t.

$$\log 2 = -\frac{0.46t}{2.3} + \log 78$$

$$t = -\frac{2.3(\log 2 - \log 78)}{0.46}$$

$$t = 7.96 \text{ hr} \approx 8 \text{ hr}$$

Alternate Method

$$2 = 78e^{-0.46t}$$

$$\frac{2}{78} = 0.0256 = e^{-0.46t}$$

$$-3.7 = -0.46t$$

$$t = \frac{3.7}{0.46} = 8 \text{ hr}$$

6. For first-order elimination kinetics, one-half of the initial quantity is lost each $t_{1/2}$. The following table may be developed:

Time (hr)	Number of $t_{1/2}$	Amount of Drug in Body (mg)	Percent of Drug in Body	Percent of Drug Lost
0	0	200	100	0
6	1	100	50	50
12	2	50	25	75
18	3	25	12.5	87.5
24	4	12.5	6.25	93.75

Method 1

From the above table the percent of drug remaining in the body after each $t_{1/2}$ is equal to 100% times $(1/2)^n$, where n is the number of half-lives, as shown below:

Number of $t_{1/2}$	Percent of Drug in Body	Percent of Drug Remaining in Body after n $t_{1/2}$
0	100	
1	50	$100 \times 1/2$
2	25	$100 \times 1/2 \times 1/2$
3	12.5	$100 \times 1/2 \times 1/2 \times 1/2$
n		$100 \times (1/2)^n$

$$\text{Percent of drug remaining} = \frac{100}{2^n}, \text{ where } n = \text{number of } t_{1/2}$$

$$\text{Percent of drug excreted} = 100 - \frac{100}{2^n}$$

At 24 hours, $n = 4$, since $t_{1/2} = 6$ hours.

$$\text{Percent of drug lost} = 100 - \frac{100}{16} = 93.75\%$$

Method 2

The equation for a first-order elimination after IV bolus injection is

$$\log D_B = \frac{-kt}{2.3} + \log D_0$$

where

$$D_B = \text{amount of drug remaining in the body}$$

$$D_0 = \text{dose} = 200 \text{ mg}$$

$$k = \text{elimination rate constant} = \frac{0.693}{t_{1/2}} = 0.1155 \text{ hr}^{-1}$$

$$t = 24 \text{ hr}$$

$$\log D_B = \frac{-0.1155(24)}{2.3} + \log 200$$

$$D_B = 12.47 \text{ mg} \approx 12.5 \text{ mg}$$

$$\% \text{ of drug lost} = \frac{200 - 12.5}{12.5} \times 100 = 93.75\%$$

7. The zero-order rate constant for alcohol is 10 mL/hr. Since the specific gravity for alcohol is 0.8,

$$0.8 \text{ g/mL} = \frac{x(\text{g})}{10 \text{ mL}}$$

$$x = 8 \text{ g}$$

Therefore, the zero-order rate constant, k_0, is 8 g/hr.

Drug in body at $t = 0$:

$$D_B^0 = C_p V_D = \frac{210 \text{ mg}}{0.100 \text{ L}} \times (0.60)(75 \text{ L}) = 94.5 \text{ g}$$

Drug in body at time t:

$$D_B = C_p V_D = \frac{100 \text{ mg}}{0.100 \text{ L}} \times (0.60)(75 \text{ L}) = 45.0 \text{ g}$$

For a zero-order reaction:

$$D_B = -k_0 t + D_B^0$$

$$45 = -8t + 94.5$$

$$t = 6.19 \text{ hr}$$

8. a. $C_p^0 = \dfrac{\text{dose}}{V_D} = \dfrac{500 \text{ mg}}{(0.1 \text{ L/kg})(55 \text{ kg})} = 90.9 \text{ mg/L}$

b. $\log D_B = \dfrac{-kt}{2.3} + \log D_B^0$

$\log D_B = \dfrac{(0.693/0.75)\,(4)}{2.3} + \log 500$

$D_B = 12.3$ mg

c. $\log 0.5 = \dfrac{-(0.693/0.75)\,t}{2.3} + \log 90.0$

$t = 5.62$ hr

9. $\log D_B = \dfrac{-kt}{2.3} + \log D_B^0$

$\log 25 = \dfrac{-k(8)}{2.3} + \log 100$

$k = 0.173$ hr^{-1}

$t_{1/2} = \dfrac{0.693}{0.173} = 4$ hr

10.

$\log D_B = \dfrac{-kt}{2.3} + \log D_B^0$

$= \dfrac{(-0.693/8)\,(24)}{2.3} + \log 600$

$D_B = 74.9$ mg

Percent drug lost $= \dfrac{600 - 74.9}{600} \times 100 = 87.5\%$

C_p at $t = 24$ hours:

$C_p = \dfrac{74.9 \text{ mg}}{(0.4 \text{ L/kg})\,(62 \text{ kg})} = 3.02$ mg/L

11. The total drug concentration in the plasma is not usually equal to the total drug concentration in the tissues. A one-compartment model implies that the drug is rapidly equilibrated in the body (in plasma and tissues). At equilibrium, the drug concentration in the tissues may differ from the drug concentration in the body because of drug protein binding, partitioning of drug into fat, differences in pH in different regions of the body causing a different degree of ionization for a weakly dissociated electrolyte drug, an active tissue uptake process, etc.

12. Set up the following table:

Time (hr)	D_u (mg)	D_u/t	mg/hr	t^*
0	0			
4	100	100/4	25	2
8	26	26/4	6.5	6

The elimination half-life may be obtained graphically after plotting mg/hr versus t^*. The $t_{1/2}$ obtained graphically is approximately 2 hours.

$$\log \frac{dD_u}{dt} = \frac{-kt}{2.3} + \log k_e D_B^0$$

$$\text{Slope} = \frac{-k}{2.3} = \frac{\log Y_2 - \log Y_1}{X_2 - X_1} = \frac{\log 6.5 - \log 25}{6 - 2}$$

$$k = 0.336 \text{ hr}^{-1}$$

$$t_{1/2} = \frac{0.693}{k} = \frac{0.693}{0.336} = 2.06 \text{ hr}$$

CHAPTER 4

FREQUENTLY ASKED QUESTIONS

1. *Mathematical* and *hypothetical* are indeed vague and uninformative terms. Mathematical equations are developed to calculate how much drug is in the vascular fluid, as well as outside the vascular fluid (ie, extravascular or in the tissue pool). *Hypothetical* refers to an unproven model. The assumptions in the compartmental models simply imply that the model simulates the mass transfer of drug between the circulatory system and the tissue pool. The mass balance of drug moving out of the plasma fluid is described even though we know the tissue pool is not real (the tissue pool represents the virtual tissue mass that receives drug from the blood). While the model is a less than perfect representation, we can interpret it, knowing its limitations. All pharmacokinetic models need interpretation. We use a model when there are no simple ways to obtain needed information. As long as we know the model limitations (ie, that the tissue compartment is not the brain, nor the muscle!) and stay within the bounds of the model, we can extract useful information from it. For example, we may determine the amount of drug that is stored outside the plasma compartment at any desired time point. After an IV bolus drug injection, the drug distributes rapidly throughout the plasma fluid and more slowly into the fluid-filled tissue spaces. Drug distribution is initially rapid and confines to a fixed fluid volume known as the V_p or the initial volume. As drug distribution expands into other tissue regions, the volume of the penetrated spaces increases, until a critical point (steady state) is obtained when all penetrable tissue regions are equilibrated with the drug. Knowing that there is heterogenous drug distribution within and between tissues, the

tissues are grouped into compartments to determine the amount of drugs in them. Mass balance, including drug inside and outside the vascular pool, accounts for all body drug storage ($D_B = D_t + D_p$). Assuming steady state, the tissue drug concentration equal to the plasma drug concentration, C_{PSS}, and one may determine size of the tissue volume using D_t/C_{PSS}. This volume is really a "numerical factor" that is used to describe the relationship of the tissue storage drug relative to the drug in the blood pool. The sum of the two volumes is the steady-state volume of distribution. The product of the steady-state concentration, C_{PSS}, and the $(V_D)ss$ yields the amount of drug in the body at steady state. The amount of drug in the body at steady state is considered vital information in dosing drugs clinically. Students should realize that tissue drug concentrations are not predicted by the model. However, plasma drug concentration is fully predictable after any given dose once the parameters become known. Initial pharmacokinetic parameter estimation may be obtained from the literature using comparable age and weight for a specific individual.

2. Apparent volumes of distribution are not real tissue volumes, but rather reflect the volume in which the drug is contained. For example,

   V_p = initial or plasma volume

   V_t = tissue volume

   $(V_D)_{ss}$ = steady-state volume of distribution (most often listed in the literature)

The steady-state drug concentration multiplied by $(V_D)_{ss}$ yields the amount of drug in the body. $(V_D)_\beta$ is a volume usually determined from area under the curve (AUC), and differs from $(V_D)_{ss}$ somewhat in magnitude. $(V_D)_\beta$ multiplied by b gives clearance of the drug.

3. A physiologic model is a detailed representation of drug disposition in the body. The model requires blood flow, extraction ratio, and specific tissue and organ size. This information is not often available for the individual. Thus, the less sophisticated compartment models are used more often.

4. Clearance is used to calculate the steady-state drug concentration and to calculate the maintenance dose. However, clearance alone is not useful in determining the maximum and minimum drug concentrations in a multiple-dosing regimen.

5. If the two-compartment model is ignored and the data are treated as a one-compartment model, the estimated values for the pharmacokinetic parameters are distorted. For example, during the distributive phase, the drug declines rapidly according to distribution α half-life, while in the elimination (terminal) part of the curve, the drug declines according to a β elimination half-life.

6. Compartment models have been used to develop dosage regimens and for the development of pharmacodynamic models. Compartment models have improved the dosing of drugs such as digoxin, gentamicin, lidocaine, and many others. The principal use of compartment models in dosing is to simulate a plasma drug concentration profile based on pharmacokinetic (PK) parameters. This information allows comparison of PK parameters in patients with only two or three points to a patient with full profiles using generated PK parameters.

LEARNING QUESTIONS

1. Equation for the curve:

$$C_p = 52e^{-1.39t} + 18e^{-0.135t}$$

$$k = 0.41 \text{ hr}^{-1} \qquad k_{12} = 0.657 \text{ hr}^{-1} \qquad k_{21} = 0.458 \text{ hr}^{-1}$$

2. Equation for the curve:

$$C_p = 28e^{-0.63t} + 10.5e^{-0.46t} + 14e^{-0.077t}$$

Note: When feathering curves by hand, a minimum of three points should be used to determine the line. Moreover, the rate constants and *y* intercepts may vary according to the individual's skill. Therefore, values for C_p should be checked by substitution of various times for *t*, using the derived equation. The theoretical curve should fit the observed data.

3. $C_p = 11.14 \ \mu g/mL$.

4. The initial decline in the plasma drug concentration is due mainly to uptake of drug into tissues. During the initial distribution of drug, some drug elimination also takes place. After the drug has equilibrated with the tissues, the drug declines at a slower rate because of drug elimination.

5. A third compartment may indicate that the drug has a slow elimination component. If the drug is eliminated by a very slow elimination component, then drug accumulation may occur with multiple drug doses or long IV drug infusions. Depending on the blood sampling, a third compartment may be missed. However, some data may fit both a two- and a three-compartment model. In this case, if the fit for each compartment model is very close statistically, the more simple compartment model should be used.

6. Because of the heterogeneity of the tissues, drug equilibrates into the tissues at different rates and the different drug concentrations are usually observed in the different tissues. The drug concentration in the "tissue" compartment represents an "average" drug concentration and does not represent the drug concentration in any specific tissue.

7. $C_p = Ae^{-at} + Be^{-bt}$

After substitution,

$$C_p = 4.62e^{-8.94t} + 0.64e^{-0.19t}$$

a. $V_p = \dfrac{D_0}{A + B} = \dfrac{75,000}{4.62 + 0.64} = 14,259 \text{ mL}$

b. $V_t = \dfrac{V_p k_{12}}{k_{21}} = \dfrac{(14,259)(6.52)}{(1.25)} = 74,375 \text{ mL}$

c. $k_{12} = \dfrac{AB(b - a)^2}{(A + B)(Ab + Ba)}$

$$k_{12} = \frac{(4.62)\,(0.64)\,(0.19 - 8.94)^2}{(4.62 + 0.64)\,[\,(4.62)\,(0.19) + (0.64)\,(8.94)\,]}$$

$$k_{12} = 6.52 \text{ hr}^{-1}$$

$$k_{21} = \frac{Ab + Ba}{A + B} = \frac{(4.62)\,(0.19) + (0.64)\,(8.94)}{4.62 + 0.64}$$

$$k_{21} = 1.25 \text{ hr}^{-1}$$

d. $k = \dfrac{ab(A + B)}{Ab - Ba} = \dfrac{(8.94)\,(0.19)\,(4.62 + 0.64)}{(4.62)\,(0.19) + (0.64)\,(8.94)}$

$$= 1.35 \text{ hr}^{-1}$$

8. The tissue compartments may not be sampled directly to obtain the drug concentration. Theoretical concentration, C_t, represents the average concentration in all the tissues outside the central compartment. The amount of drug in the tissue, D_t, represents the total amount of drug outside the central or plasma compartment. Occasionally C_t may be equal to a particular tissue drug concentration in an organ. However, this C_t may be equivalent by chance only.

9. The data were analyzed using computer software called RSTRIP, and found to fit a two-compartment model:

$A(1) = 2.0049$ $A(2) = 6.0057$ (two preexponential values)

$k(1) = 0.15053$ $k(2) = 7.0217$ (two exponential values)

The equation that describes the data is

$$C_p = 2.0049e^{-0.15053t} + 6.0057e^{-7.0217t}$$

The coefficient of correlation $= 0.999$ (very good fit).

The model selection criterion $= 11.27$ (good model).

The sum of squared deviations $= 9.3 \times 10^{-5}$ (there is little deviation between the observed data and the theoretical value).

Alpha $= 7.0217$ hr^{-1}, beta $= 0.15053$ hr^{-1}.

10. **a.** Late-time samples were taken in some patients, yielding data that resulted in a monoexponential elimination profile. It is also possible that a patient's illness contributes to impaired drug distribution.

   b. The range of distribution half-lives is 30–45 minutes.

   c. None. Tissue concentrations are not generally well predicted from the two-compartment model. Only the amount of drug in the tissue compartment may be predicted.

   d. No. At steady state, the rate in and the rate out of the tissues is the same, but the drug concentrations are not necessarily the same. The plasma and each tissue may have different drug binding.

   e. None. Only the pooled tissue is simulated by the tissue compartment.

CHAPTER 5

FREQUENTLY ASKED QUESTIONS

1. Slow IV infusion may be used to avoid side effects due to rapid drug administration. For example, intravenous immune globulin (human) may cause a rapid fall in blood pressure and possible anaphylactic shock in some patients when infused rapidly. Some antisense drugs also cause a rapid fall in blood pressure when injected rapidly IV into the body. The rate of infusion is particularly important in administering antiarrythmic agents in patients. The rapid IV bolus injection of many drugs (eg, lidocaine) that follow the pharmacokinetics of multiple-compartment models may cause an adverse response due to the initial high drug concentration in the central (plasma) compartment before slow equilibration with the tissues.

2. The loading drug dose is used to rapidly attain the target drug concentration, which is approximately the steady-state drug concentration. However, the loading dose will not maintain the steady-state level unless an appropriate IV drug infusion rate or maintenance dose is also used. If a larger IV drug infusion rate or maintenance dose is given, the resulting steady-state drug concentration will be much higher and will remain sustained at the higher level. A higher infusion rate may be administered if the initial steady-state drug level is inadequate for the patient.

3. The common complications associated with intravenous infusion include phlebitis and infections at the infusion site caused by poor intravenous techniques or indwelling catheters.

LEARNING QUESTIONS

1. a. To reach 95% of C_{SS}:

$$4.32t_{1/2} = (4.32)(7) = 30.2 \text{ hr}$$

b. $D_L = C_{SS}V_D = (10)(0.231)(65,000) = 150 \text{ mg}$

c. $R = C_{ss}V_Dk = (10)(15,000)(0.099) = 14.85$ mg/hr

d. $Cl_T = V_Dk = (15,000)(0.099) = 1485$ mL/hr

e. To establish a new C_{ss} will still take $4.32t_{1/2}$. However, the $t_{1/2}$ will be longer in renal failure.

f. If Cl_T is decreased by 50%, then the infusion rate R should be decreased proportionately:

$$R = 10(0.50)(1485) = 7.425 \text{ mg/hr}$$

2. a. The steady-state level can be found by plotting the IV infusion data. The plasma drug–time curves plateau at 10 μg/mL. Alternatively, V_D and k can be found from the single IV dose data:

$$V_D = 100 \text{ mL/kg} \qquad k = 0.2 \text{ hr}^{-1}$$

b. Using equations developed in Example 2 in the first set of examples in Chapter 5:

$$0.95\frac{R}{V_Dk} = \frac{R}{V_Dk}(1 - e^{-kt})$$

$$0.95 = 1 - e^{-0.2t}$$

$$0.05 = e^{-0.2t}$$

$$t_{95\%ss} = \frac{\ln 0.05}{-0.2} = 15 \text{ hr}$$

c. $Cl_T = V_dk$ $\qquad\qquad$ $V_D = \dfrac{D_0}{C_p^0}$

$\quad Cl_T = 100 \times 0.2$ $\qquad\qquad$ $V_D = \dfrac{1000}{10} = \dfrac{100 \text{ mL}}{\text{kg}}$

$\quad Cl_T = 20 \text{ mL/kg hr}$

d. The drug level 4 hours after stopping the IV infusion can be found by considering the drug concentration at the termination of infusion as C_p^0. At the termination of the infusion, the drug level will decline by a first-order process.

$$C_p = C_p^0 e^{-kt}$$

$$C_p = 9.9e^{-(0.2)(4)}$$

$$C_p = 4.5 \text{ }\mu\text{g/mL}$$

e. The infusion rate to produce a C_{ss} of 10 μg/mL is 0.2 mg/kg per hour. Therefore, the infusion rate needed for this patient is

$$0.2 \text{ mg/kg hr} \times 75 \text{ kg} = 15 \text{ mg/hr}$$

f. From the data shown, at 4 hours after the start of the IV infusion, the drug concentration is 5.5 μg/mL; the drug concentration after an IV bolus of

1 mg/kg is 4.5 μg/mL. Therefore, if a 1-mg dose was given and the drug is then infused at 0.2 mg/kg per hour, the plasma drug concentration will be 4.5 + 5.5 = 10 μg/mL.

3. Infusion rate R for a 75-kg patient:

$$R = (1 \text{ mg/kg hr})(75 \text{ kg}) = 75 \text{ mg/hr}$$

Sterile drug solution contains 25 mg/mL. Therefore, 3 mL contains (3 mL) × (25 mg/mL), or 75 mg. The patient should receive 3 mL (75 mg)/hr by IV infusion.

4. $C_{SS} = \dfrac{R}{V_D k}$ $R = C_{SS} V_D k$

$$R = (20 \text{ mg/L})(0.5 \text{ L/kg})(75 \text{ kg})\left(\frac{0.693}{3 \text{ hr}}\right) = 173.25 \text{ mg/hr}$$

Drug is supplied as 125 mg/mL. Therefore,

$$125 \text{ mg/mL} = \frac{173.25 \text{ mg}}{X} \qquad X = 1.386 \text{ mL}$$

$$R = 1.386 \text{ mL/hr}$$

$$D_L = C_{SS} V_D = (20 \text{ mg/L})(0.5 \text{ L/kg})(75 \text{ kg}) = 750 \text{ mg}$$

5. $C_{SS} = \dfrac{R}{k V_D} = \dfrac{R}{Cl_T}$

a. $Cl_T = \dfrac{R}{C_{SS}} = \dfrac{5.3 \text{ mg/kg hr} \times 71.71 \text{ kg}}{17 \text{ mg/L}} = 22.4 \text{ L/hr}$

b. At the end of IV infusion, $C_p = 17 \mu$g/mL. Assuming first-order elimination kinetics:

$$C_p = C_p^0 e^{-kt}$$

$$1.5 = 17 e^{-k(2.5)}$$

$$0.0882 = e^{-2.5k}$$

$$\ln 0.0882 = -2.5\ k$$

$$-2.43 = -2.5\ k$$

$$k = 0.971 \text{ hr}^{-1}$$

$$t_{1/2} = \frac{0.693}{0.971} = 0.714 \text{ hr}$$

c. $Cl_T = k V_D$ $V_D = \dfrac{Cl_T}{k}$

$$V_D = \frac{22.4}{0.971} = 23.1 \text{ L}$$

d. Probenecid blocks active tubular secretion of cephradine.

6. At steady state, the rate of elimination should equal the rate of absorption. Therefore, the rate of elimination would be 30 mg/hr. The C_{SS} is directly proportional to the rate of infusion R, as shown by

$$C_{SS} = \frac{R}{kV_D} \qquad kV_D = \frac{R}{C_{SS}}$$

$$\frac{R_{old}}{C_{SS,old}} = \frac{R_{new}}{C_{SS,new}}$$

$$\frac{30 \text{ mg/hr}}{20 \text{ } \mu g/mL} = \frac{40 \text{ mg/hr}}{C_{SS,new}}$$

$$C_{SS,new} = 26.7 \text{ } \mu g/mL$$

The new elimination rate will be 40 mg/hr.

7. a. $R = C_{SS}kV_D$

$R = (20 \text{ mg/L}) (0.693/8 \text{ hr}) (1.5 \text{ L/kg}) (75 \text{ kg}) = 194.9 \text{ mg/hr}$

$R \approx 195 \text{ mg/hr}$

b. $D_L = C_{SS}V_D = (20)(1.5)(75) = 2250$ mg given by IV bolus injection

c. The loading dose is given to obtain steady-state drug concentrations as rapidly as possible.

d. 15 mL of the antibiotic solution contains 225 mg of drug. Thus, an IV infusion rate of 15 mL/hr is equivalent to 225 mg/hr. The C_{SS} achieved by the manufacturer's recommendation is

$$C_{SS} = \frac{R}{kV_D} = \frac{225}{(0.0866)(112.5)} = 23.1 \text{ mg/L}$$

The theoretical C_{SS} of 23.1 mg/L is close to the desired C_{SS} of 20 mg/L. Assuming a reasonable therapeutic window, the manufacturer's suggested starting infusion rate is satisfactory.

CHAPTER 6

 FREQUENTLY ASKED QUESTIONS

1. Elimination half-life, $t_{1/2}$, is a concise and informative term that describes the time needed for half the dose to be removed from the body. Alternatively, the elimination half-life indicates the time for the plasma drug concentration to decline to one-half from whatever concentration it started at. Classical pharmacokinetic models are based on $t_{1/2}$ (or k) and V_D. Some pharmacokineticists prefer Cl and V_D, and regard $t_{1/2}$ as a derived parameter.

2. A *parameter* is a model-based numerical constant estimated statistically from the data. Model parameters are used generally to make predictions about the behavior of the real process. A parameter is termed independent if the parameter is not dependent on other parameters of the model. In the classical one-compartment model, k and V_D are independent model parameters, and $t_{1/2}$ and Cl are regarded as derived parameters. In the physiologic model, Cl and V_D are regarded as independent model parameters, while k is a dependent parameter since k depends on Cl/V_D. In practice, both Cl and k are dependent on various physiologic factors, such as blood flow, drug metabolism, renal secretion, and drug reabsorption. Most biologic events are the result of many events that are described more aptly as mutually interacting rather than acting independently. Thus, the underlying elimination process may be adequately described as fraction of drug removed per minute (k) or as volume of fluid removed per minute (Cl).

3. With most drugs, total body clearance (often termed "clearance") is the sum of renal and nonrenal clearances. Creatinine is an endogenous marker that accumulates in the blood when renal function is impaired. Creatinine is excreted by glomerular filtration and is not reabsorbed. Creatinine clearance is a measure of glomerular filtration rate. Renal clearance is therefore proportional to creatinine clearance but not equal to it, since most drugs are reabsorbed to some extent, and some drugs are actively secreted.

LEARNING QUESTIONS

3. **a.**
$$Cl_T = V_D k = V_D \frac{0.693}{t_{1/2}}$$

$$\text{Average } Cl_T = \frac{(30)\,(0.693)}{3.4} = 6.11 \text{ L/hr}$$

$$\text{Upper } Cl_T \text{ limit} = \frac{(30)\,(0.693)}{1.8} = 11.55 \text{ L/hr}$$

$$\text{Lower } Cl_T \text{ limit} = \frac{(30)\,(0.693)}{6.8} = 3.06 \text{ L/hr}$$

b. $Cl_R = k_e V_D = 0.36 \text{ L/hr}$

$$k_e = \frac{0.36}{30} = 0.012 \text{ hr}^{-1}$$

$$Cl_{nr} = Cl_T - Cl_r$$

$$Cl_{nr} = 6.11 - 0.36 = 5.75 \text{ L/hr}$$

$$Cl_{nr} = k_m V_D$$

$$k_m = \frac{5.75}{30} = 0.192 \text{ hr}^{-1}$$

4. a. Apparent $V_D = (0.21)(78,000 \text{ mL})$

$$= 16,380 \text{ mL}$$

$$Cl_T = kV_D$$

$$Cl_T = \left(\frac{0.693}{2}\right)(16,380)$$

$$Cl_T = 5676 \text{ mL/hr} = 94.6 \text{ mL/min}$$

b. $k_e = 70\%$ of the elimination constant

$$k_e = (0.7)\left(\frac{0.693}{2}\right) = 0.243 \text{ hr}^{-1}$$

$$Cl_R = k_e V_D$$

$$Cl_R = (0.243)(16,380) = 3980 \text{ mL/hr} = 66.3 \text{ mL/min}$$

c. Normal GFR = creatinine clearance = 122 mL/min

$$Cl_R \text{ of drug} = 66.3 \text{ mL}$$

Because the Cl_R of the drug is less than the creatinine clearance, the drug is filtered at the glomerulus and is partially reabsorbed.

5. a. During intravenous infusion, the drug levels will reach more than 99% of the plasma steady-state concentration after seven half-lives of the drug.

$$Cl_T = \frac{R}{C_{SS}}$$

$$= \frac{300,000 \; \mu g/hr}{11 \; \mu g/mL} = 27,272 \text{ mL/hr}$$

b. $Cl_T = kV_D$

$$V_D = \frac{27,272}{0.693} = 39,354 \text{ mL}$$

c. Since $k_m = 0 \qquad k_e \approx k$

$$Cl_T = Cl_R = 27,272 \text{ mL/hr}$$

d. $Cl_R = 27,272 \text{ mL/hr} = 454 \text{ mL/min}$

Normal GFR is 100–130 mL/min. The drug is probably filtered and actively secreted in the kidney.

6. $Cl_R = \dfrac{\text{excretion rate}}{C_p} = \dfrac{200 \text{ mg/2 hr}}{2.5 \text{ mg/100 mL}}$

$Cl_R = 4000 \text{ mL/hr}$

7. $Cl_T = \dfrac{R}{C_{SS}}$

$Cl_T = \dfrac{5.3 \text{ mg/kg hr}}{17 \text{ mg/L}} = 0.312 \text{ L/kg hr}$

For a 71.7-kg adult,

$$Cl_T = (0.312 \text{ L/kg hr})(71.7 \text{ kg}) = 22.4 \text{ L/hr}$$

11. From the data, determine urinary rate of drug excretion per time period by multiplying urinary volume by the urinary concentration for each point. Average C_p for each period by taking the mean of two consecutive points. Plot dD_u/dt versus C_p to determine renal clearance from slope. The renal clearance from slope is 1493.4 mL/hr (Fig. C-5).

Time (hr)	Plasma Concentration (μg/mL)	Urinary Volume (mL)	Urinary Concentration (μg/mL)	Urinary Rate, dD_u/dt (μg/hr)	Average C_p
0	250.00	100.00	0.00	0.00	
1	198.63	125.00	2,680.00	334,999.56	224.32
2	157.82	140.00	1,901.20	266,168.41	178.23
3	125.39	100.00	2,114.80	211,479.74	141.61
4	99.63	80.00	2,100.35	168,027.76	112.51
5	79.16	250.00	534.01	133,503.70	89.39
6	62.89	170.00	623.96	106,073.18	71.03
7	49.97	160.00	526.74	84,278.70	56.43
8	39.70	90.00	744.03	66,962.26	44.84
9	31.55	400.00	133.01	53,203.77	35.63

Figure C-5

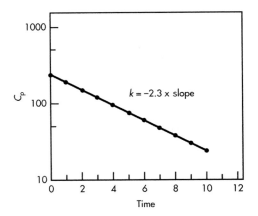

Figure C-6

To determine the total body clearance by the area method, the area under the plasma concentration curve [AUC] must be calculated and summed. The tailpiece is extrapolated because the data are not taken to the end. A plot of log C_p versus t (Fig. C-6) yields a slope of $k = 0.23$ hr^{-1}. The tailpiece of area is extrapolated using the last data point divided by k or $31.55/0.23 = 137.17$ μg/mL per hour.

Subtotal area	(0–9 hr)	953.97
Tailpiece	(9–∞ hr)	137.17
Total area	(0–∞)	1091.14

$$\text{Total clearance} = Cl_T = \frac{FD_0}{[\text{AUC}]_0^\infty} = \frac{2{,}500{,}000}{1091.14} = 2{,}291.2 \text{ mL/hr}$$

Because total body clearance is much larger than renal clearance, the drug is probably also excreted by a nonrenal route.

Nonrenal clearance = 2291.2 − 1493.4 = 797.8 mL/hr

The easiest way to determine clearance by a compartmental approach is to estimate k and V_D from the graph. V_D is 10 L and k is 0.23 hr^{-1}. Total clearance is 2300 mL/min (a slightly different value when compared with the area method).

CHAPTER 7

FREQUENTLY ASKED QUESTIONS

1. For drugs absorbed by a first-order process, the absorption half-life is $0.693/k_a$. Although drug absorption involves many stochastic (system based random) steps, the overall rate process is often approximated by a first-order process, especially with oral solutions and immediate-release drug products such as compressed tablets or capsules. The determination of the absorption rate constant, k_a, is most often calculated by the Wagner–Nelson method for drugs, which follow a one-compartment model with first-order absorption and first-order elimination.

2. The fraction of drug absorbed, F, and the absorption rate constant, k_a, are independent parameters. A drug in an oral solution may have a more rapid rate of absorption compared to a solid drug product. If the drug is released from the drug product slowly or is formulated so that the drug is absorbed slowly, the drug may be subjected to first-pass effects, degraded in the gastrointestinal tract, or eliminated in the feces so that less drug (smaller F) may be absorbed systemically compared to the same drug formulated to be absorbed more rapidly from the drug product.

3. A drug with a rate of absorption slower than its rate of elimination will not be able to obtain optimal systemic drug concentrations to achieve efficacy. Such drugs are generally not developed into products.

4. Drug clearance is generally not affected by drug absorption from most absorption sites. In the gastrointestinal tract, a drug is absorbed via the hepatic portal vein to the liver and may be subject to hepatic clearance.

5. The fraction of drug absorbed may be less than 1 (ie, 100% bioavailable) after oral administration.

LEARNING QUESTIONS

1. **a.** The elimination rate constant is $0.1\ \text{hr}^{-1} (t_{1/2} = 6.93\ \text{hours})$.

   b. The absorption rate constant, k_a, is $0.3\ \text{hr}^{-1}$ (absorption half-life $= 2.31$ hours).

   The calculated $t_{max} = \dfrac{\ln(k_a/k)}{k_a - k} = 5.49\ \text{hr}$

c. The y intercept was observed to be 60 ng/mL. Therefore the equation that fits the observed data is

$$C_p = 60\left(e^{-0.1t} - e^{-0.3t}\right)$$

Note: Answers obtained by "hand" feathering the data on semilog graph paper may vary somewhat depending on graphing skills and skill in reading data from a graph.

2. By direct observation of the data, the t_{max} is 6 hours and the C_{max} is 23.01 ng/mL. The apparent volume of distribution, V_D, is obtained from the intercept, I, of the terminal elimination phase, and substituting $F = 0.8$, $D = 10,000,000$ ng, $k_a = 0.3$ hr^{-1}, $k = 0.1$ hr^{-1}:

$$I = \frac{Fk_a D_0}{V_D(k_a - k)} \qquad 60 = \frac{(0.8)\,(0.3)\,(10,000,000)}{V_D(0.3 - 0.1)}$$

$$V_D = 200 \text{ L}$$

3. The percent-of-drug-unabsorbed method is applicable to any model with first-order elimination, regardless of the process of drug input. If the drug is given by IV injection, the elimination rate constant, k, may be determined accurately. If the drug is administered orally, k and k_a may *flip-flop*, resulting in an error unless IV data are available to determine k. For a drug that follows a two-compartment model, an IV bolus injection is used to determine the rate constants for distribution and elimination.

4. After an IV bolus injection, a drug such as theophylline follows a two-compartment model with a rapid distribution phase. During oral absorption, the drug is distributed during the absorption phase, and no distribution phase is observed. Pharmacokinetic analysis of the plasma drug concentration data obtained after oral drug administration will show that the drug follows a one-compartment model.

5. The equations for a drug that follows the kinetics of a one-compartment model with first-order absorption and elimination are

$$C_p = \frac{FD_0}{V_D(k_a - k)}\left(e^{kt} - e^{-k_a t}\right) \qquad t_{max} = \frac{\ln(k_a / k)}{k_a - k}$$

As shown by these equations:

a. t_{max} is influenced by k_a and k and not by F, D_0, or V_D.

b. C_p is influenced by F, D_0, V_D, k_a, and k.

6. A drug product that might provide a zero-order input is an oral controlled-release tablet or a transdermal drug delivery system (patch). An IV drug infusion will also provide a zero-order drug input.

7. The general equation for a one-compartment open model with oral absorption is

$$C_p = \frac{FD_0}{V_D(k_a - k)}\left(e^{-kt} - e^{-k_a t}\right)$$

From $C_p = 45(e^{-0.17t} - e^{-1.5t})$,

$$\frac{FD_0 k_a}{V_D(k_a - k)} = 45$$

$$k = 0.17 \text{ hr}^{-1}$$

$$k_a = 1.5 \text{ hr}^{-1}$$

a. $t_{max} = \dfrac{\ln(k_a/k)}{k_a - k} = \dfrac{\ln(1.5/0.17)}{1.5 - 0.17} = 1.64 \text{ hr}$

b. $C_{max} = 45(e^{-(0.17)(1.64)} - e^{-(1.5)(1.64)})$

$\qquad = 30.2 \ \mu\text{g/mL}$

c. $t_{1/2} = \dfrac{0.693}{k} = \dfrac{0.693}{0.17} = 4.08 \text{ hr}$

8 a. Drug A $\qquad t_{max} = \dfrac{\ln(1.0/0.2)}{1.0 - 0.2} = 2.01 \text{ hr}$

$\qquad$ Drug B $\qquad t_{max} = \dfrac{\ln(0.2/1.0)}{0.2 - 1.0} = 2.01 \text{ hr}$

b. $\qquad\qquad\qquad C_{max} = \dfrac{FD_0 k_a}{V_D(k_a - k)}(e^{-kt_{max}} - e^{-k_a t_{max}})$

$\qquad$ Drug A $\qquad C_{max} = \dfrac{(1)(500)(1)}{(10)(1 - 0.2)}(e^{-(0.2)(2)} - e^{-(1)(2)})$

$\qquad\qquad\qquad\qquad C_{max} = 33.4 \ \mu\text{g/mL}$

$\qquad$ Drug B $\qquad C_{max} = \dfrac{(1)(500)(0.2)}{(20)(0.2 - 1.0)}(e^{-1(2)} - e^{-(0.2)(2)})$

$\qquad\qquad\qquad\qquad C_{max} = 3.34 \ \mu\text{g/mL}$

9. a. The method of residuals using manual graphing methods may give somewhat different answers depending on personal skill and the quality of the graph paper. Values obtained by the computer program ESTRIP gave the following estimates:

$$k_a = 2.84 \text{ hr}^{-1} \qquad k = 0.186 \text{ hr}^{-1} \qquad t_{1/2} = 3.73 \text{ hr}$$

b. A drug in an aqueous solution is in the most absorbable form compared to other oral dosage forms. The assumption that $k_a > k$ is generally true for drug solutions and immediate-release oral dosage forms such as compressed tablets and capsules. Drug absorption from extended-release dosage forms may have $k_a < k$. To demonstrate unequivocally which slope represents the true k, the drug must be given by IV bolus or IV infusion, and the slope of the elimination curve obtained.

c. The Loo–Riegelman method requires IV data. Therefore, only the method of Wagner and Nelson may be used on these data.

d. Observed t_{max} and C_{max} values are taken directly from the experimental data. In this example, C_{max} is 85.11 ng/mL, which occurred at a t_{max} of 1.0 hour. The theoretical t_{max} and C_{max} are obtained as follows:

$$t_{max} = \frac{2.3 \log(k_a/k)}{k_a - k} = \frac{2.3 \log(2.84/0.186)}{2.84 - 0.186} = 1.03 \text{ hr}$$

$$C_{max} = \frac{FD_0 k_a}{V_D(k_a - k)}(e^{-kt_{max}} - e^{-k_a t_{max}})$$

where $FD_0 k_a/V_D(k_a - k)$ is the y intercept equal to 110 ng/mL and $t_{max} = 1.03$ hours.

$$C_{max} = (110)(e^{-(0.186)(1.0)} - e^{-(2.84)(1.03)})$$

$$C_{max} = 85 \text{ ng/mL}$$

e. A more complete model-fitting program, such as WIN NONLIN, is needed to fit the data statistically to a one-compartment model.

CHAPTER 8

FREQUENTLY ASKED QUESTIONS

1. Some of the advantages of administering a drug by constant IV infusion include, the following. (1) A drug may be infused continuously for many hours without disturbing the patient. (2) Constant infusion provides a stable blood drug level for drugs that have a narrow therapeutic index. (3) Some drugs are better tolerated when infused slowly. (4) Some drugs may be infused simultaneously with electrolytes or other infusion media in an acute-care setting. Disadvantages of administering a drug by constant IV infusion include the following. (1) Some drugs are more suitable to be administered as a bolus IV injection. For example, some reports show that an aminoglycoside given once daily resulted in fewer side effects compared with dividing the dose into two or three doses daily. Due to drug accumulation in the kidney and adverse toxicity, aminoglycosides are generally not given by prolonged IV infusions. In contrast, a prolonged period of low drug level for penicillins and tetracyclines may not be as efficacious and may result in a longer cure time for an infection. The pharmacodynamics of the individual drug must be studied to determine the best course of action. (2) Drugs such as nitroglycerin are less likely to produce tolerance when administered intermittently versus continuously.

2. A loading or priming dose is used to rapidly raise the plasma drug concentration to therapeutic drug levels to obtain a more rapid pharmacodynamic response. In addition, the loading dose along with the maintenance dose allows the drug to reach steady state concentration quickly, particularly for drugs with long elimination half-lives.

    An alternative way of explaining the loading dose is based on clearance. After multiple IV dosing, the maintenance dose required is based on Cl, C_{SS}, and τ:

$$C_{SS} = \frac{\text{Dose}}{\tau\, Cl}$$
$$\text{Dose} = C_{SS}\tau\, Cl$$

    If C_{SS} and τ are fixed, a drug with a smaller clearance requires a smaller maintenance dose. In practice, the dosing interval is adjustable and may be longer for drugs with a small Cl if the drug does not need to be dosed frequently. The steady-state drug level is generally determined by the desired therapeutic drug.

3. *Accumulation index, R,* is a ratio that indicates steady-state drug concentration to the drug concentration after the first dose. The accumulation index does not measure the absolute size of overdosing; it measures the amount of drug cumulation that can occur due to frequent drug administration. Factors that affect R are the elimination rate constant, k, and the dosing interval, τ. If the first dose is not chosen appropriately, the steady-state level may still be incorrect. Therefore, the first dose and the dosing interval must be determined correctly to avoid any significant drug accumulation. The accumulation index is a good indication of accumulation due to frequent drug dosing, applicable to any drug, regardless of whether the drug is bound to tissues.

4. The loading dose will affect only the initial drug concentrations in the body. Steady-state drug levels are obtained after several elimination half lives (eg, 4.32 $t_{1/2}$ for 95% steady-state level). Only 5% of the drug contributed by the loading dose will remain at 95% steady state. At 99% steady-state level, only 1% of the loading dose will remain.

5. Two possible examples are digoxin and amitriptyline.

6. After an IV bolus drug injection, the drug is well distributed within a few minutes. In practice, however, an IV bolus dose may be administered slowly over several minutes or the drug may have a slow distribution phase. Therefore, clinicians often prefer to take a blood sample 15 minutes or 30 minutes after IV bolus injection and refer to that drug concentration as the peak concentration. In some cases, a blood sample is taken an hour later to avoid the fluctuating concentration in the distributive phase. The error due to changing sampling time can be large for a drug with a short elimination half-life.

LEARNING QUESTIONS

1. $V_D = 0.20\,(50 \text{ kg}) = 10{,}000 \text{ mL}$

a. $D_{max} = \dfrac{D_0}{1 - f} = \dfrac{50 \text{ mg}}{1 - e^{-(0.693/2)\,(8)}} = 53.3 \text{ mg}$

$C_{max} = \dfrac{D_{max}}{V_D} = \dfrac{53.3 \text{ mg}}{10{,}000 \text{ ml}} = 5.33 \ \mu\text{g/mL}$

b. $D_{min} = 53.3 - 50 = 3.3 \text{ mg}$

$C_{min} = \dfrac{3.3 \text{ mg}}{10{,}000 \text{ mL}} = 0.33 \ \mu\text{g/mL}$

c. $C_{av}^{\infty} = \dfrac{F D_0 1.44 t_{1/2}}{V_D \tau} = \dfrac{(50)\,(1.44)\,(2)}{(10{,}000)\,(8)} = 1.8 \ \mu\text{g/mL}$

2. a. $D_0 = \dfrac{C_{av}^{\infty} V_D \tau}{1.44 t_{1/2}}$

$= \dfrac{(10)\,(40{,}000)\,(6)}{(1.44)\,(5)} = 333 \text{ mg every 6 hours}$

b. $\tau = \dfrac{F D_0 1.44 t_{1/2}}{V_D C_{av}^{\infty}}$

$= \dfrac{(225{,}000)\,(1.44)\,(5)}{(40{,}000)\,(10)} = 4.05 \text{ hr}$

6. Dose the patient with 200 mg every 3 hours.

$D_L = \dfrac{D_0}{1 - e^{-k\tau}} = \dfrac{200}{1 - e^{-(0.23)\,(3)}} = 400 \text{ mg}$

Notice that D_L is twice the maintenance dose, because the drug is given at a dosage interval equal approximately to the $t_{1/2}$ of 3 hours.

8. The plasma drug concentration, C_p, may be calculated at any time after n doses by Equation 8.21 and proper substitution.

$C_p = \dfrac{D_0}{V_D} \left(\dfrac{1 - e^{-nk\tau}}{1 - e^{-k\tau}} \right) e^{-kt}$

$C_p = \dfrac{200}{40} \left(\dfrac{1 - e^{-(3)\,(0.347)\,(4)}}{1 - e^{-(0.347)\,(4)}} \right) e^{-(0.347)\,(1)} = 4.63 \text{ mg/L}$

Alternatively, one may conclude that for a drug whose elimination $t_{1/2}$ is 2 hours, the predicted plasma drug concentration is approximately at steady state after 3 doses or 12 hours. Therefore, the above calculation may be simplified to the following:

$$C_p = \frac{D_0}{V_D} = \left(\frac{1}{1 - e^{-k\tau}}\right) e^{-k\tau}$$

$$C_p = \left(\frac{200}{40}\right) \left(\frac{1}{1 - e^{-(0.347)(4)}}\right) e^{-(0.347)(1)} = 4.71 \text{ mg/L}$$

9. $C_{max}^\infty = \dfrac{D_0/V_D}{1 - e^{-k\tau}}$

where

$$V_D = 20\% \text{ of } 82 \text{ kg} = (0.2)(82) = 16.4 \text{ L}$$

$$k = (0.693/3) = 0.231 \text{ hr}^{-1}$$

$$D_0 = V_D C_{max}^\infty (1 - e^{-k\tau}) = (16.4)(10)(1 - e^{-(0.231)(8)})$$

a. $D_0 = 138.16$ mg to be given every 8 hours

b. $C_{min}^\infty = C_{max}^\infty(e^{-k\tau}) = (10)(e^{-(0.231)(8)}) = 1.58 \text{ mg/L}$

c. $C_{av}^\infty = \dfrac{D_0}{kV_D\tau} = \dfrac{138.16}{(0.231)(16.4)(8)} = 4.56 \text{ mg/L}$

d. In the above dosage regimen, the C_{min}^∞ of 1.59 mg/L is below the desired C_{min}^∞ of 2 mg/L. Alternatively, the dosage interval, τ, could be changed to 6 hours.

$$D_0 = V_D C_{max}^\infty (1 - e^{-k\tau}) = (16.4)(10)(1 - e^{-(0.231)(6)})$$

$$D_0 = 123 \text{ mg to be given every 6 hours}$$

$$C_{min}^\infty = C_{max}^\infty(e^{-k\tau}) = (10)(e^{-(0.231)(6)}) = 2.5 \text{ mg/L}$$

$$C_{av}^\infty = \frac{D_0}{kV_D\tau} = \frac{123}{(0.231)(16.4)(6)} = 5.41 \text{ mg/L}$$

10. a. $C_{av}^\infty = \dfrac{FD_0}{kV_D\tau}$

Let $C_{av}^\infty = 27.5$ mg/L

$$D_0 = \frac{C_{av}^\infty kV_D\tau}{F} = \frac{(27.5)(0.693/10.6)(0.5)(78)(6)}{0.77} = 546.3 \text{ mg}$$

$$D_0 = 546.3 \text{ mg every 6 hours}$$

b. If a 500-mg capsule is given every 6 hours,

$$C_{av}^\infty = \frac{FD_0}{kV_D\tau} = \frac{(0.77)(500)}{(0.693/10.6)(0.5)(78)(6)} = 25.2 \text{ mg/L}$$

c. $D_L = \dfrac{D_M}{1 - e^{-k\tau}} = \dfrac{500}{1 - e^{-(0.654)(6)}} = 1543 \text{ mg}$

$$D_L = 3 \times 500 \text{ mg capsules} = 1500 \text{ mg}$$

CHAPTER 9

 FREQUENTLY ASKED QUESTIONS

1. A patient with concomitant hepatic disease may have decreased biotransformation enzyme activity. Infants and young subjects may have immature hepatic enzyme systems. Alcoholics may have liver cirrhosis and lack certain coenzymes. Other patients may experience enzyme saturation at normal doses due to genetic polymorphism. Pharmacokinetics provides a simple way to identify nonlinear kinetics in these patients and to estimate an appropriate dose. Finally, concomitant use of other drugs may cause nonlinear pharmacokinetics at lower drug doses due to enzyme inhibition.

2. A drug that follows linear pharmacokinetics generally has a constant elimination half-life and a constant clearance with an increase in the dose. The steady-state drug concentrations and AUC are proportional to the size of the dose. Nonlinear pharmacokinetics results in dose-dependent Cl, $t_{1/2}$, and AUC. Nonlinear pharmacokinetics are often described in terms of V_{max} and K_M.

3. The physiologic model based on organ drug clearance describes nonlinear drug metabolism in terms of blood flow and intrinsic hepatic clearance (Chapter 11). Drugs are extracted by the liver as they are presented by blood flow. The physiologic model accounts for the sigmoid profile with changing blood flow and extraction, whereas the Michaelis–Menten model simulates the metabolic profile based on V_{max} and K_M. The Michaelis–Menten model was applied mostly to describe *in-vitro* enzymatic reactions. When V_{max} and K_M are estimated in patients, blood flow is not explicitly considered. This semiempirical method was found by many clinicians to be useful in dosing phenytoin. The organ clearance model was more useful in explaining clearance change due to impaired blood flow. In practice, the physiologic model has limited use in dosing patients because blood flow data for patients are not available.

4. *Chronopharmacokinetics* is the main cause of nonlinear pharmacokinetics that is not dose related. The time dependent or temporal process of drug elimination can be the result of rhythmic changes in the body. For example, nortriptyline and theophylline levels are higher when administered between 7 and 9 AM compared to between 7 and 9 PM after the same dose. Biological rhythmic differences in clearance cause a lower elimination rate in the morning compared to the evening. Other factors that cause nonlinear pharmacokinetics may result from enzyme induction (eg, carbamazepine) or enzyme inhibition after multiple doses of the drug. Furthermore, the drug or a metabolite may accumulate following multiple dosing and affect the metabolism or renal elimination of the drug.

LEARNING QUESTIONS

2. Capacity-limited processes for drugs include:
- Absorption
    Active transport
    Intestinal metabolism by microflora
- Distribution
    Protein binding
- Elimination
    Hepatic elimination
    Biotransformation
    Active biliary secretion
- Renal excretion
    Active tubular secretion
    Active tubular reabsorption

4. $C_p^0 = \dfrac{\text{dose}}{V_D} = \dfrac{10{,}000\ \mu g}{20{,}000\ mL} = 0.5\ \mu g/mL$

From Equation 9.1,

$$\text{Elimination rate} = -\frac{dC_p}{dt} = \frac{V_{max}\,C_p}{K_M + C_p}$$

Because $K_M = 50\ \mu g/mL$, $C_p \ll K_M$ and the reaction rate is first order. Thus, the above equation reduces to Equation 9.3.

$$-\frac{dC_p}{dt} = \frac{V_{max}\,C_p}{K_M} = k'\,C_p$$

$$k' = \frac{V_{max}}{K_M} = \frac{20\ \mu g/hr}{50\ \mu g} = 0.4\ hr^{-1}$$

For first-order reactions,

$$t_{1/2} = \frac{0.693}{k'} = \frac{0.693}{0.4} = 1.73\ hr$$

The drug will be 50% metabolized in 1.73 hours.

7. When INH is coadminstered, plasma phenytoin concentration is increased due to a reduction in metabolic rate v. Equation 9.1 shows that v and K_M are inversely related (K_M in denominator). An increase in K_M will be accompanied by an increase in plasma drug concentration. Figure 9-4 shows that an increase in K_M is accompanied by an increase in amount of drug in the body at any time t. Equation 9.4 relates drug concentration to K_M, and it can be seen that the two are proportionally related, although they are not linearly proportional to each other due to the complexity of the equation. An actual study in the literature shows that k is increased severalfold in the presence of INH in the body.

8. The K_M has the unit of concentration. In laboratory studies, K_M is expressed in moles per liter, or micromoles per milliliter, because reactions are expressed in moles and not milligrams. In dosing, drugs are given in milligram and plasma drug concentrations are expressed as milligrams per liter or micrograms per milliliter. The units of K_M for pharmacokinetic models are estimated from *in-vivo* data. They are therefore commonly expressed as milligrams per liter, which is preferred over micrograms per milliliter because dose is usually expressed in milligrams. The two terms may be shown to be equivalent and convertible. Occasionally, when simulating amount of drug metabolized in the body as a function of time, the amount of drug in the body has been assumed to follow Michaelis–Menten kinetics, and K_M assumes the unit of D_0 (eg, mg). In this case, K_M takes on a very different meaning.

CHAPTER 10

 FREQUENTLY ASKED QUESTIONS

1. No. For some drugs, protein binding does not affect the overall distribution of other drugs. Typically, if a drug is highly bound, there is an increased chance of a significant change in the fraction of free drug when binding is altered.

2. Albumin, α_1-acid glycoprotein, and lipoprotein. For some drugs and hormones, there may be a specific binding protein.

3. Most drugs are assumed to be *restrictively bound,* and binding reduces drug clearance and elimination. However, some *nonrestrictively bound* drugs may be cleared easily. Changes in binding do not affect the rate of elimination of these drugs. Some drugs, such as some semisynthetic penicillins that are bound to plasma protein, may be actively secreted in the kidney. The elimination rates of these drugs are not affected by protein binding.

4. *Partitioning* refers to the relative distribution of a drug in the lipid and aqueous phases. Generally, a high partition coefficient ($P_{oil/water}$) favors tissue distribution and leads to a larger volume of distribution. Partitioning is a major factor that, along with protein binding of a drug, determines drug distribution.

5. It is important to examine why albumin level is reduced in the patient. For example, is the reduced albumin level due to uremia or hepatic dysfunction? In general, reduced protein binding will increase free drug concentration. Any change in drug clearance should be considered before reducing the dose, since the volume of distribution may be increased, partially offsetting the increase in free drug concentration.

6. In general, the early phase after an IV bolus dose is the distributive phase. The elimination phase occurs in the later phase, although distribution may continue for some drugs, especially for a drug with a long elimination half-life. The elimination phase is generally more gradual, since some drug may be returned to the blood from the tissues as drug is eliminated from the body.

7. Generally, the long distribution half-life is caused by a tissue/organ that has a high drug concentration, due either to intracellular drug binding or high affinity for tissue distribution. Alternatively, the drug may be metabolized slowly within the tissue.

8. The distribution half-life determines the time it takes for a tissue organ to be equilibrated. It takes 4.32 distribution half-lives for the tissue organ to be 95% equilibrated and one distribution half-life for the drug to be 50% equilibrated. The concept is analogous to reaching steady-state during drug infusion (see Chapter 5).

9. The answer is **False**. The free drug concentrations in the tissue and plasma are the same after equilibration, but the total drug concentration in the tissue is not the same as the total drug concentration in the plasma. The bound drug concentration may vary depending on local tissue binding or the lipid solubility of the drug. Many drugs have a long distributive phase due to tissue drug binding or lipid solubility. Drugs may equilibrate slowly into these tissues and then be slowly eliminated. Drugs with limited tissue affinity are easily equilibrated. Some examples of drugs with a long distributive phase are discussed in relation to the two-compartment model (Chapter 4).

10. The ratio, r, is defined as the ratio of the number of moles of drug bound to the number of moles of protein in the system. For a simple case of one binding site, r reflects the proportion of binding sites occupied; r is affected by (1) the association binding constant, (2) the free drug concentration, and (3) the number of binding sites per mole of protein. When $[D]$, or free drug concentration, is equal to 1 (or the dissociation constant K), the protein is 50% occupied for a drug with 1:1 binding according to Equation 10.19. (This can be verified easily by substituting for $[D]$ into the right side the equation and determining r.) For a drug with n similar binding sites, binding occurs at the extent of 1:2 of bound drug:protein when $[D] = 1/[K_a(2n-1)]$. This equation, however, reflects binding *in vitro* when drug concentration is not changing; therefore, its conclusions are somewhat limited.

LEARNING QUESTIONS

1. The zone of inhibition for the antibiotic in serum is smaller due to drug–protein binding.

2. Calculate $r/(D)$ versus r, then graph the results on rectangular coordinates.

r	$r/(D \times 10^4)$
0.4	1.21
0.8	0.90
1.2	0.60
1.6	0.30

The y intercept $= nK_a = 1.5 \times 10^4$
The x intercept $= n = 2$

Therefore,

$$K_a = 1.5 \times 10^4/2 = 0.75 \times 10^4$$

K_a may also be found from the slope.

8. The liver is important for the synthesis of plasma proteins. In chronic alcoholic liver disease or cirrhosis, fewer plasma proteins are synthesized in the liver, resulting in a lower plasma protein concentration. Thus, for a given dose of naproxen, less drug is bound to the plasma proteins, and the total plasma drug concentration is smaller.

10. Protein binding may become saturated at any drug concentration in patients with defective proteins or when binding sites are occupied by metabolic wastes generated during disease states (eg, renal disease). Diazoxide is an example of nonlinear binding at therapeutic dose.

11. The answer is **False**. The percent bound refers to the percent of total drug that is bound. The percent bound may be ≥99% bound for some drugs. Saturation may be better estimated using the Scatchard plot approach and by examining "r," which is the number of moles of drug bound divided by the number of moles of protein. When r is 0.99, most of the binding sites are occupied. The f_b, or fraction of bound drug, is useful for determining f_u, $f_u = 1 - f_b$.

12. Adenosine is extensively taken up by cells including the blood elements and the vascular endothelium. Adenosine is rapidly metabolized by deamination and/or is used as AMP in phosphorylation. Consequently, adenosine has a short elimination half-life.

CHAPTER 11

FREQUENTLY ASKED QUESTIONS

1. Hepatic drug clearance describes drug metabolism in the liver and accounts for both the effect of blood flow and the intrinsic ability of the liver to metabolize a drug. Hepatic drug clearance is added to renal clearance and other clearances to obtain total (body) clearance, which is important in determining the maintenance dose of a drug. Hepatic drug clearance is often considered nonrenal clearance when it is measured as the difference between total clearance and renal clearance.

2. Most orally administered drugs pass through the liver prior to systemic absorption. The rate of blood flow can greatly affect the extent of drug that reaches the systemic circulation. Also, intrinsic metabolism may differ among individuals and may be genetically determined. These factors may cause drug levels to be more erratic for drugs that undergo extensive metabolism compared to drugs that are excreted renally.

3. Protein synthesis may be altered by liver dysfunction. In general, when drug protein binding is reduced, the free drug may be metabolized more easily. However, some drugs may be metabolized regardless of whether the drug is bound or free (for discussion of nonrestrictive binding, see Chapter 10). In such cases, there is little change in pharmacodynamic activity due to changes in drug protein binding.

4. Erythromycin, morphine, propranolol, various steroids, and other drugs have large metabolic clearance. In hepatic disease, highly potent drugs that have a narrow therapeutic index should be monitored carefully. Troglitazone (Rezulin), for example, is a drug that can cause severe side effects in patients with liver dysfunction; liver transaminase should be monitored in diabetic patients.

LEARNING QUESTIONS

1. **a.** $k = k_m + k_e + k_b = 0.20 + 0.25 + 0.15 = 0.60 \text{ hr}^{-1}$

$$t_{1/2} = \frac{0.693}{k} = \frac{0.693}{0.60} = 1.16 \text{ hr}$$

b. $k = k_{\mathrm{m}} + k_{\mathrm{e}} = 0.45\ \mathrm{hr}^{-1}$

$t_{1/2} = 1.54\ \mathrm{hr}$

c. $k = 0.35\ \mathrm{hr}^{-1}$

$t_{1/2} = 1.98\ \mathrm{hr}$

d. $k = 0.80\ \mathrm{hr}^{-1}$

$t_{1/2} = 0.87\ \mathrm{hr}$

2. a. $k = 0.347\ \mathrm{hr}^{-1}$

$k_{\mathrm{e}} = (0.9)(0.347) = 0.312\ \mathrm{hr}^{-1}$

b. Renal excretion, 90% of the drug is excreted unchanged.

5. Normal hepatic clearance, Cl_{H}:

$$Cl_{\mathrm{H}} = Q\left(\frac{Cl_{\mathrm{int}}}{Q + Cl_{\mathrm{int}}}\right) \qquad Q = 1.5\ \mathrm{L/min} \qquad Cl_{\mathrm{int}} = 0.040\ \mathrm{L/min}$$

$$Cl_{\mathrm{H}} = 1.5\left(\frac{0.040}{1.5 + 0.040}\right) = 0.039\ \mathrm{L/min}$$

a. Congestive heart failure:

$$Cl_{\mathrm{H}} = 1.0\left(\frac{0.040}{1.0 + 0.040}\right) = 0.038\ \mathrm{L/min}$$

b. Enzyme induction:

$$Cl_{\mathrm{H}} = 1.5\left(\frac{0.090}{1.5 + 0.090}\right) = 0.085\ \mathrm{L/min}$$

Note: A change in blood flow, Q, did not markedly affect Cl_{H} for a drug with low Cl_{int}.

6. Normal hepatic clearance:

$$Cl_{\mathrm{H}} = 1.5\left(\frac{12}{1.5 + 12}\right) = 1.33\ \mathrm{L/min}$$

Congestive heart failure (CHF):

$$Cl_{\mathrm{H}} = 1.0\left(\frac{12}{1.0 + 12}\right) = 0.923\ \mathrm{L/min}$$

a. $$Cl_{\mathrm{H}} = Q(\mathrm{ER}) = Q\left(\frac{Cl_{\mathrm{int}}}{Q + Cl_{\mathrm{int}}}\right)$$

$$\mathrm{ER} = \frac{Cl_{\mathrm{int}}}{Q + Cl_{\mathrm{int}}}$$

$$\mathrm{Normal\ ER} = \frac{12}{1.5 + 12} = 0.89\ \mathrm{L/min}$$

$$\text{CHF ER} = \frac{12}{1.0 + 12} = 0.92 \text{ L/min}$$

b. $F = 1 - \text{ER} = 1 - 0.89$
$F = 0.11 \text{ or } 11\%$

10. a. Because <0.5% of the unchanged drug is excreted in the urine, hepatic clearance nearly approximates total body clearance.

$$Cl_H \approx Cl_T = kV_D = \left(\frac{0.693}{3.9}\right)(4.3)\,(80) = 61.1 \text{ L/hr}$$

b. $Cl_H = Q\,\text{ER}$ $Q = (1.5 \text{ L/min})\,(60 \text{ min}) = 90 \text{ L/hr}$
$\text{ER} = 61.1/90 = 0.68.$

11. a. $Cl_T = kV_D = \left(\frac{0.693}{1.6}\right)(0.78)\,(81) = 27.4 \text{ L/hr}$

b. $Cl_R = k_e V_D$

$$k_e = 0.12k = (0.12)\left(\frac{0.693}{1.6}\right) = 0.052 \text{ hr}^{-1}$$

$Cl_R = (0.052)\,(0.78)\,(81) = 3.29 \text{ L/hr}$

Alternatively,

$Cl_R = f_e Cl_T$
$Cl_R = 0.12 \, Cl_T = (0.12)\,(27.4) = 3.29 \text{ L/hr}$

c. $Cl_H = Cl_T - Cl_R = 27.4 - 3.29 = 24.11 \text{ L/hr}$

CHAPTER 13

FREQUENTLY ASKED QUESTIONS

1. An *absorption window* refers to the segment of the gastrointestinal tract from which the drug is well absorbed and beyond which the drug is either poorly absorbed or not absorbed at all. After oral administration, most drugs are well absorbed in the duodenum and to a lesser extent in the jejunum. A small amount of drug absorption may occur from the ileum.

2. Food, particularly food with a high fat content, stimulates the production of bile, which is released into the duodenum. The bile helps to solubilize a lipid-soluble drug, thereby increasing drug absorption. Fatty food also slows gastrointestinal motility, resulting in a longer *residence time* for the drug to be absorbed from the small intestine.

3. After oral administration, the drug in solution may precipitate in the gastrointestinal tract. The precipitated drug needs to redissolve before it can be absorbed. Some drug solutions are prepared with a co-solvent, such as alcohol or glycerin, and form coarse crystals on precipitation that dissolve slowly, whereas other drugs precipitate into fine crystals that redissolve rapidly. The type of precipitate is influenced by the solvent, by the degree of agitation, and by the physical environment. *In-vitro* mixing and dilution of the drug solution in artificial gastric juice, artificial intestinal juice, or in other pH buffers may predict the type of drug precipitate that is formed.

In addition, drugs dissolved in a highly viscous solution (eg, simple syrup) may have slower absorption because of the viscosity of the solution. Furthermore, drugs that are readily absorbed across the gastrointestinal membrane may not be completely bioavailable (ie, 100% systemic absorption) due to *first-pass effects* (discussed in Chapter 11).

4. The major biologic factor that delays gastrointestinal drug absorption is a delay in gastric emptying time. Any factor that delays stomach emptying time, such as fatty food, will delay the drug entering into the duodenum from the stomach and, thereby, delay drug absorption.

LEARNING QUESTIONS

1. In the presence of food, undissolved aspirin granules larger than 1 mm are retained up to several hours longer in the stomach. In the absence of food, aspirin granules are emptied from the stomach within 1–2 hours. When the aspirin granules empty into the duodenum slowly, drug absorption will be as slow as with a sustained-release drug product. Enteric-coated aspirin granules taken with an evening meal may provide relief of pain for arthritic patients late into the night.

2. The answer is b. A basic drug formulated as a suspension will depend on stomach acid for dissolution as the basic drug forms a hydrochloric acid (HCl) salt. If the drug is poorly soluble, adding milk may neutralize some acid so that the drug may not be completely dissolved. Making a HCl salt rather than a suspension of the base ensures that the drug is soluble without being dependent on stomach HCl for dissolution.

3. Protein drugs are generally digested by proteolytic enzymes present in the GI tract and therefore are not adequately absorbed by the oral route. Protein drugs

are most commonly given parenterally. Other routes of administration, such as intranasal and rectal administration, have had some success or are under current investigation for the systemic absorption of protein drugs.

4. The answer is c. Raising the pH of an acid drug above its pK_a will increase the dissociation of the drug, thereby increasing its aqueous solubility.

5. The large intestine is most heavily populated by bacteria, yeasts, and other microflora. Some drugs which are not well absorbed in the small intestine are metabolized by the microflora to products that are absorbed in the large bowel. For example, drugs with an azo link (eg, sulfasalazine) are cleaved by bacteria in the bowel and the cleaved products (eg, 5-aminosalicylic acid and sulfapyridine) are absorbed. Other drugs, such as antibiotics (eg, tetracyclines), may destroy the bacteria in the large intestine, resulting in an overgrowth of yeast (eg, *Candida albicans*) and leading to a yeast infection. Destruction of the microflora in the lower bowel can also lead to cramps and diarrhea.

6. First-pass effects are discussed more fully in Chapter 11. Alternative routes of drug administration such as buccal, inhalation, sublingual, intranasal, and parenteral will bypass the first-pass effects observed after oral drug administration.

7. Although antacid statistically decreased the extent of systemic drug absorption ($p < 0.05$) as shown by an $AUC_{0-4\,hr}$ of 349 ± 108 pg hr/mL, compared to the control (fasting) $AUC_{0-4\,hr}$ value of 417 ± 135 pg hr/mL, the effect of antacid is not clinically significant. A high-fat diet decreased the rate of systemic drug absorption, as shown by a longer t_{max} value (64 minutes) and lower C_{max} value (303 pg/mL).

CHAPTER 14

FREQUENTLY ASKED QUESTIONS

1. **a.** For optimal drug absorption after oral administration, the drug should be water soluble and highly permeable so it can be absorbed throughout the gastrointestinal tract. Ideally, the drug should not change into a polymorphic form that could affect its solubility. The drug should be stable in both gastric and intestinal pH and preferably should not be hygroscopic.

   b. For parenteral administration, the drug should be water soluble and stable in solution, preferably at autoclave temperature. The drug should be nonhydroscopic and preferably should not change into another polymorphic form.

2. A lipid-soluble drug may be prepared in an oil-in-water (o/w) emulsion or dissolved in a nonaqueous solution in a soft gelatin capsule. A co-solvent may improve the solubility and dissolution of the drug.

3. The rate of hydrolysis (decomposition) of the ester drug may be reduced by formulating the drug in a co-solvent solution. A reduction in the percent of the aqueous vehicle will decrease the rate of hydrolysis. In addition, the drug should be formulated at the pH in which the drug is most stable.

4. Excipients are needed in a formulation to solubilize the drug, increase the dissolution rate, decrease gastrointestinal transit time, or improve oral absorption by complexation. Excipients can also decrease the rate of oral absorption in the gastrointestinal tract by reducing drug solubility, decreasing the dissolution rate, or forming a less soluble complex.

LEARNING QUESTIONS

1. The rate-limiting steps in the oral absorption of a solid drug product are the rate of drug dissolution within the gastrointestinal tract and the rate of permeation of the drug molecules across the intestinal mucosal cells. Generally, disintegration of the drug product is rapid and not rate limiting. Water-soluble drugs dissolve rapidly in the aqueous environment of the gastrointestinal tract, so the permeation of the intestinal mucosal cells may be the rate-limiting step. The drug absorption rate may be altered by a variety of methods, all of which depend on knowledge of the biopharmaceutic properties of the drug and the drug product and on the physiology of the gastrointestinal tract. Drug examples are described in detail in this chapter and in Chapter 13.

2. Most drugs are absorbed by passive diffusion. The duodenum area provides a large surface area and blood supply that maintains a large drug concentration gradient favorable for drug absorption from the duodenum into the systemic circulation.

3. If the initial drug absorption rate, dD_A/dt, was slower than the drug elimination rate, dD_E/dt, then therapeutic drug concentrations in the body would not be achieved. It should be noted that the rate of absorption is generally first order, $dD_A/dt = D_0 k_a$, where, D_0 is the drug dose which is great initially. Even if $k_a < k$, the initial drug absorption rate may be greater than the drug elimination rate. After the drug is absorbed from the absorption site, $dD_A/dt \leq dD_E/dt$.

4. A drug prepared as an oral aqueous drug solution is generally the most bioavailable. However, the same drug prepared as a well-designed immediate-release tablet or capsule may have similar bioavailability. In the case of an oral drug solution, there is no dissolution step; the drug molecules come into contact with intestinal membrane, and the drug is rapidly absorbed. As a result of first-pass effects (discussed in Chapter 11), a drug given in an oral drug solution may not be 100% bioavailable. If the drug solution is formulated with a high solute concentration—such as sorbitol solution, which yields a high osmotic pressure—gastric motility may be slowed, thus slowing the rate of drug absorption.

5. Anticholinergic drugs prolong gastric emptying, which will delay the absorption of an enteric-coated drug product.

6. Erythromycin may be formulated as enteric-coated granules to protect the drug from degradation at the stomach pH. Enteric-coated granules are less affected by gastric emptying and food (which delays gastric emptying) compared to enteric-coated tablets.

CHAPTER 15

 FREQUENTLY ASKED QUESTIONS

1. Preclinical animal toxicology and clinical efficacy studies were performed on the marketed *brand* drug product as part of the New Drug Application (NDA) prior to FDA approval. These studies do not have to be repeated for the *generic* bio-equivalent drug product. The manufacturer of the generic drug product must submit an Abbreviated New Drug Application (ANDA) to the FDA, demonstrating that the generic drug product is a therapeutic equivalent (see definitions in Chapter 15) to the brand drug product.

2. The *sequence* is the order in which the drug products (ie, treatments) are given (eg, brand product followed by generic product or vice versa). Sequence is important to prevent any bias due to the order of the treatments in the study. The term *washout* refers to the time for total elimination of the dose. The time for washout is determined by the elimination half-life of the drug. *Period* refers to the drug-dosing day on which the drug is given to the subjects. For example, for Period One, half the subjects receive treatment A, brand product, and the other half of the subjects receive treatment B, generic product.

3. Manufacturers are required to perform a food-intervention bioavailability study on all drugs whose bioavailability is known to be affected by food. In addition, a food-intervention bioavailability study is required on all modified-release products since (1) the modified-release formulation (eg, enteric coating, sustained-release coating) may be affected by the presence of food and (2) modified-release products have a greater potential to be affected by food due to their longer residence time in the gastrointestinal tract and changes in gastrointestinal motility.

4. If the drug is not absorbed systemically from the drug product, a *surrogate marker* must be used as a measure of bioequivalence. This surrogate marker may be a pharmacodynamic effect or, as in the case of cholestyramine resin, the binding capacity for bile acids *in vitro*.

LEARNING QUESTIONS

3. a. Oral solution: the drug is in the most bioavailable form.

b. Oral solution: same reason as above.

c. Absolute bioavailability $= \dfrac{[AUC]\,\text{oral solution}/\text{dose}_{\text{soln}}}{[AUC]_{IV}/\text{dose}_{IV}} = \dfrac{145/10}{29/2} = 1.0$

d. Relative bioavailability $= \dfrac{[AUC]\,\text{tablet}/\text{dose}_{\text{tab}}}{[AUC]\,\text{solution}/\text{dose}_{\text{soln}}} = \dfrac{116/10}{145/10} = 0.80$

e. (1) $C_p^0 = 6.67\ \mu g/mL$ (by extrapolation of IV curve)

$$V_D = \frac{2000\ \mu g/kg}{6.67\ \mu g/mL} = 300\ mL/kg$$

(2) $t_{1/2} = 3.01\ hr$

(3) $k = 0.23\ hr^{-1}$

(4) $Cl_T = kV_D = 69\ mL/kg\ hr$

4. Plot the data on both rectangular and semilog graph paper. The following answers were obtained from estimates from the plotted plasma level–time curves. More exact answers may be obtained mathematically by substitution into the proper formulas.

a. 1.37 hr

b. 13.6 hr

c. 8.75 hr

d. 5 hr

e. 4.21 $\mu g/mL$

f. 77.98 $\mu g\ hr/mL$

5.

Subject	Drug Product		
	Period 1	**Period 2**	**Week 3**
1	A	B	C
2	B	C	A
3	C	A	B
4	A	C	B
5	C	B	A
6	B	A	C

6. a. Absolute bioavailability $= \dfrac{D_{u,\,PO}^{\infty}/\text{dose}_{PO}}{D_{u,\,IV}^{\infty}/\text{dose}_{IV}}$

$$= \frac{340/4}{20/0.2} = 0.85\ \text{or}\ 85\%$$

b. Relative bioavailability $= \dfrac{D_u^\infty \text{ cap/dose cap}}{D_u^\infty \text{ sol/dose sol}}$

$$= \frac{360/4}{380/4} = 0.947 \text{ or } 94.7\%$$

7. The fraction of drug absorbed systemically is the absolute bioavailability.

$$\text{Fraction of drug absorbed} = \frac{\% \text{ of dose excreted after PO}}{\% \text{ of dose excreted after IV}}$$

$$= \frac{48\%}{75\%} = 0.64$$

CHAPTER 16

 FREQUENTLY ASKED QUESTIONS

1. Specifications provide a test and a quantitative limit (acceptance criteria) to a test (eg, the total content must be within ±5% or the amount of impurities in the drug substance must not be more than [NMT] 1%). Thus, one batch of nominally 200-mg ibuprofen tablets may contain an average content of 198 mg, whereas the average content for another batch of 200-mg ibuprofen tablets may have an average content of 202 mg. Both batches meet a specification of ±5% and would be considered to meet the label claim of 200 mg of ibuprofen per tablet.

2. The manufacturer must consider whether the excipient is critical or not critical to drug release. If the excipient (eg, starch) is not critical to drug release (ie, a non-release-controlling excipient), then small changes in the starch concentration, generally less than 3% of the total target dosage form weight, is unlikely to affect the formulation quality and performance. A qualitative change in the excipient may affect drug release and thus will have significant effect on the formulation performance.

CHAPTER 17

FREQUENTLY ASKED QUESTIONS

1. Extended-release drug products have many advantages compared to immediate-release drug products, as discussed in Chapter 14. However, a extended-release drug product of a drug that has a long elimination half-life (eg, chlorpheniramine maleate, digoxin, levothyroxine) has no advantage over the same drug given in an immediate-release (conventional) drug product. For some drugs, the clinical rationale for an extended-release drug product that provides a long-sustained drug level is not established. Nitroglycerin, for example, is less likely to produce tolerance with intermittent dosing compared with dosing by a continuous-release product. For some antibiotics there is also a specific duration of postantibiotic effect, during which bactericidal activity continues even when the plasma drug level is depleted. Some drugs are better tolerated with a "pulse" type of drug input into the body.

2. A zero-order rate for drug absorption will give more constant plasma drug concentrations with minimal fluctuations between peak and trough levels compared to first-order drug absorption. Depending on the therapeutic window for the drug and the relationship between the pharmacokinetics and pharmacodynamics of the drug, zero-order drug absorption may not always be more efficacious than first-order absorption.

LEARNING QUESTIONS

1. **a.** For many drugs, the plasma drug concentration is proportional to the drug concentration at the receptor site and the pharmacodynamic effect. By maintaining a prolonged, constant plasma drug concentration, the pharmacodynamic effect is also maintained.

   b. A drug that releases at a zero-order rate and is absorbed at a zero-order rate provides a more constant plasma drug concentration compared to a first-order drug release.

2. **a.** Both *A* and *B* release drug at a zero-order rate (straight line). Curve *B* shows that 100% of drug is released in 12 hours, or about 8.3% per hour.

b. Product *C*.

c. Product *C* initially releases drug at a zero-order rate (first 3 hours).

d. Drug release usually slows down toward the end of dissolution because most tablets get smaller as dissolution proceeds, resulting in a smaller surface for water penetration inward and drug diffusion outward. Also, as drug dissolution occurs, the concentration gradient (Fick's law) gets progressively smaller due to the buildup of drug in the bulk solution.

e. As the surface drug of a sustained-release product is dissolved, the interior drug has to traverse a longer or a more tortuous path to reach the outside, resulting in the slowing rate of dissolution.

3. a. A drug given 10 mg 4 times daily would be equivalent to 40 mg/day or 20 mg/12 hr at the rate of 1.67 mg/hr.

b. 0.5 mL/hr should deliver 1.67 mg of drug. Therefore, the concentration should be

$$\frac{1.67 \text{ mg}}{0.5 \text{ mL}} = 3.34 \text{ mg/mL}$$

4. Using the infusion equation,

$$k = \frac{0.693}{3.5} = 0.198 \text{ hr}^{-1}$$

$$V_D = 10 \text{ L} \qquad C_p = 20 \text{ mg/L}$$

$$R = C_p V_D k = (20)(10)(0.198) = 39.6 \text{ mg/hr}$$

Total drug needed = $R \times 12$ hr = $(39.6)(12) = 475.2$ mg

CHAPTER 18

 FREQUENTLY ASKED QUESTIONS

1. The most frequent route of administration for biologic compounds is parenteral (eg, IM or IV). For example, β-interferon for multiple sclerosis is given IM to allow gradual drug release into the systemic circulation.

2. Glycosylation is the addition of a carbohydrate group to the molecule. For example, Betaseron (interferon beta-1A) is not glycosylated, whereas Avonex (interferon β-1B) is glycosylated. Glycosylation will increase the water solubility and the molecular weight of the drug. Although both drugs are β-interferons, glycosylation affects the pharmacokinetics, the stability, and the efficacy of these drugs.

3. The distribution of a biotechnology compound depends on its physicochemical characteristics. Many peptides, proteins, and nucleotides have polar chains so that a major portion of the drug is distributed in the extracellular fluid with a volume of 7–15 L. Drugs that easily penetrate into the cell have higher volumes of distribution, about 15–45 L, due to the larger volume of intracellular fluid.

LEARNING QUESTIONS

None

CHAPTER 19

FREQUENTLY ASKED QUESTIONS

1. Doubling a dose does not double the drug response (or the pharmacodynamic effect). The pharmacodynamic effect of a drug is proportional to the log of the plasma drug concentration—usually within 20% to 80% of the maximal response. Near the maximal pharmacodynamic effect, doubling the dose may only cause a very small increase in effect. No further increase in pharmacodynamic effect is achieved by an increase in dose once the maximum pharmacodynamic effect, E_{max}, is obtained.

2. For many drugs, the drug responses over time plotted versus plasma drug concentrations produces a loop-shaped (*hysteresis loop*) profile. The hysteresis loop shows that the plasma drug concentration is not always a good indicator of drug response. A *clockwise* hysteresis loop shows that response decreases with time and may be the result of drug tolerance or formation of an antagonistic metabolite.

3. The *effect compartment* is postulated to describe the pharmacodynamics of drugs that are not well described by drug concentration in the plasma compartment. The effect compartment is assumed to be the receptor site in the body for drug response. Drug concentration in this site is referred to as drug concentration in the effect compartment. The amount of drug in the effect compartment is relatively small and is insignificant compared to the amount of drug in other tissues. Drug elimination from the effect compartment is governed by k_{eo}, a first-order rate constant that is estimated from the pharmacodynamic data. Drug concentration in the effect compartment may be equilibrated with the central compartment when a steady-state plasma drug concentration is reached.

LEARNING QUESTIONS

1. a. True. Drug concentration is more precise because an identical dose may result in different plasma drug concentration in different subjects due to individual differences in pharmacokinetics.

   b. True. The kinetic relationship between drug response and drug concentration is such that the response is proportional to log concentration of the drug.

   c. True. The data show that after IV bolus dose, the response begins at the same point indicating that the initial plasma drug concentration is the same. In uremic patients, the volume of distribution may be affected by changes in protein binding and electrolyte levels, which may range from little or no effect to strongly affecting the V_D.

   d. False. The drug is likely to be excreted through the kidney, since the slope (elimination) is reduced in uremic patients.

   e. True. Assuming that the volume of distribution is unchanged, the starting pharmacologic response should be the same if the receptor sensitivity is unchanged. In a few cases, receptor sensitivity to the drug can be altered in uremic patients. For example, the effect of digoxin will be more intense if the serum potassium level is depleted.

2. These antibiotics inhibit β-lactamase by irreversible binding to the enzyme protein via an acylation reaction, similar to antibiotic binding to the protein in the cell wall. β-lactamase breaks the cyclic amide bond of the antibiotics.

3. Several answers are possible.

   a. Pharmacokinetic considerations: Subsequent doses induce the hepatic drug metabolizing enzymes (auto-induction), thereby decreasing the elimination half-life resulting in lower steady-state drug concentrations.

   b. Pharmacodynamic considerations: The patient develops tolerance to the drug, resulting in the need for a higher dose to produce the same effect.

5. CNS drugs.

6. An allergic response to a drug may be unpredictable and does not generally follow a dose–response relationship.

7. PAT (postantibiotic time) is the time for continued antibacterial activity even though the plasma antibiotic concentration has fallen below MEC, or minimum effective concentration.

8. AUC/MIC or AUIC is a pharmacokinetic parameter incorporating MIC together in order to provide better prediction of antibiotic response (cure percent). An example is ciprofloxacin. AUIC is a good predictor of percent cure in infection treated at various dose regimens.

CHAPTER 20

 ## FREQUENTLY ASKED QUESTIONS

1. Therapeutic drug monitoring (TDM) may be performed by sampling other biologic fluids, such as saliva or, when available, tissue or ear fluids. However, the sample must be correlated to blood or special tissue level. Urinary drug concentrations generally are not reliable. Saliva is considered an ultrafiltrate of plasma and does not contain significant albumin. Saliva drug concentrations represent free plasma drug levels and have been used with limited success to monitor some drugs.

   Pharmacodynamic end points such as prothrombin clotting time for warfarin, blood glucose concentrations for antidiabetic drugs, blood pressure for antihypertensive drugs, and other clinical observations are useful indications that the drug is dosed correctly.

2. Most pharmacokinetic models require well-controlled studies in which many blood samples are taken from each subject and the pharmacokinetic parameters estimated. In patient care situations, only a limited number of blood samples is collected, which does not allow for the complete determination of the drug's pharmacokinetic profile in the individual patient. However, the data from blood samples taken from a large demographic sector are more reflective of the disease states and pharmacogenetics of the patients treated. Population pharmacokinetics allow data from previous patients to be used in addition to the limited blood sample from the individual patient. The type of information obtained is less constrained and is sometimes dependent on the model and algorithm used for analysis. However, many successful examples have been reported in the literature.

3. The major considerations in TDM include the pathophysiology of the patient, the blood sample collection, and the data analysis. Clinical assessment of patient history, drug interaction, and demographic factors are all part of a successful program for therapeutic drug monitoring.

4. With the Bayesian approach, the estimates of patient parameters are constrained more narrowly, to allow easier parameter estimation based on information provided from the population. The information is then combined with one or more serum concentrations from the patient to obtain a set of final patient parameters (generally Cl and V_D). When no serum sample is taken, the Bayesian approach is reduced to an *a priori* model using only population parameters.

5. Pharmacokinetics provides a means of studying whether an unusual drug action is related to pharmacokinetic factors, such as drug disposition, distribution, or binding, or is related to pharmacodynamic interaction, such as a difference in receptor sensitivity, drug tolerance, or some other reason. Many drug interactions involving enzyme inhibition, stimulation, and protein binding were discovered as a result of pharmacokinetic, pharmacogenetic, and pharmacodynamic investigations.

LEARNING QUESTIONS

1. Steady-state drug concentrations are achieved in approximately 5 half-lives. For a drug with a half-life of 36 hours, steady-state drug concentrations are achieved in approximately 180 hours (or 7.5 days). Thus, dose adjustment in patients is difficult for drugs with very long half-lives. In contrast, steady-state drug concentrations are achieved in approximately 20–30 hours (or 1 day) for drugs whose half-lives are 4–6 hours.

2. $C_{\max}^{\infty} = \dfrac{D_0}{V_D}\left(\dfrac{1}{1 - e^{-k\tau}}\right)$

$C_{\max}^{\infty} = \dfrac{250{,}000}{42{,}000}\left(\dfrac{1}{1 - e^{-(6)(1.034)}}\right)$

$C_{\max}^{\infty} = \dfrac{250{,}000}{42{,}000}\left(\dfrac{1}{0.998}\right) = 5.96\ \mu g/mL$

At steady state, the peak concentration of penicillin G will be 5.96 $\mu g/mL$.

3. $C_{av}^{\infty} = \dfrac{D}{kV_D\tau} = \dfrac{250{,}000}{(0.99)(20{,}000)(6)} = 2.10\ \mu g/mL$

Free drug concentration at steady state = $2.10(1 - 0.97) = 0.063\ \mu g/mL$.

4. $C_{av}^{\infty} = \dfrac{1.44 D_0 F t_{1/2}}{V_D \tau}$

For the Normal Patient:

$V_D = (0.392)(1)(1000) = 392$ mL/kg

$C_{av}^{\infty} = \dfrac{(1.44)(D_0)(1)(1.49)}{(392)(6)} = 2\ \mu g/mL$

$D_0 = \dfrac{(392)(6)(2)}{(1.44)(1.49)} = 2192\ \mu g/kg = 2.2$ mg/kg

For the Uremic Patient:

$V_D = (23.75)(1)(1000) = 237.5$ mL/kg

$C_{av}^{\infty} = \dfrac{(1.44)(D_0)(1)(6.03)}{(237.5)(6)} = 2\ \mu g/mL$

$D_0 = \dfrac{(2)(237.5)(6)}{(1.44)(6.03)} = 328.2\ \mu g/kg = 0.3$ mg/kg

5. a. $V_D = 306{,}000$ mL

Dose $= 0.5 \times 10^6$ ng

$C_{av}^{\infty} = \dfrac{(1.44)(DF t_{1/2})}{V_D \tau} = \dfrac{(1.44)(0.5 \times 10^6)(0.56)(0.95)}{(306{,}000)(1)} = 1.25$ ng/mL

b. The patient is adequately dosed.

c. $F = 1$; using the above equation, the C_{av}^{∞} is 2.2 ng/mL; although still effective, the C_{av}^{∞} will be closer to the toxic serum concentration of 3 ng/mL.

6. The Cl_{Cr} for this patient shows normal kidney function.

$t_{1/2} = 2$ hr $k = 0.693/2 = 0.3465$ hr^{-1}

$V_D = 0.2$ L/kg $\times 80$ kg $= 16$ L

a. $C_{max}^{\infty} = \dfrac{D_0/V_D}{1 - e^{-k\tau}} = \dfrac{250/16}{1 - e^{-(0.3465)(8)}} = 16.68$ mg/L

$C_{min}^{\infty} = C_{max}^{\infty} e^{-k\tau} = 16.68 e^{-(0.3465)(8)} = 1.04$ mg/L

The dosage regimen of 250 mg every 8 hours gives a C_{max}^{∞} above 16 mg/L and a C_{min}^{∞} below 2 mg/L. Therefore, this dosage regimen is not correct.

b. Several trials might be necessary to obtain a more optimal dosing regimen. One approach is to change the dosage interval, τ, to 6 hours and to calculate the dose, D_0:

$D_0 = C_{max}^{\infty} V_D (1 - e^{-k\tau}) = (16)(14)(1 - e^{-(0.3465)(6)}) = 196$ mg

$C_{min}^{\infty} = C_{max}^{\infty} e^{-k\tau} = 16 e^{-(0.3465)(6)} = 2$ mg/L

A dose of 196 mg (approximately 200 mg) given every 6 hours should achieve the desired drug concentrations.

10. Assume desired $C_{av}^{\infty} = 0.0015$ $\mu g/mL$ and $\tau = 24$ hours.

$$C_{av}^{\infty} = \frac{FD_0 \, 1.44 t_{1/2}}{V_D \tau}$$

$$D_0 = \frac{C_{av}^{\infty} V_D \tau}{F \, 1.44 t_{1/2}}$$

$$D_0 = \frac{(0.0015)(4)(68)(24)}{(0.80)(1.44)(30)} = 0.283 \text{ mg}$$

Give 0.283 mg every 24 hours.

a. For a dosage regimen of one 0.30-mg tablet daily,

$$C_{av}^{\infty} = \frac{(0.80)(0.3)(1.44)(30)}{(4)(68)(24)} = 0.0016 \text{ } \mu g/mL$$

which is within the therapeutic window.

b. A dosage regimen of 0.15 mg every 12 hours would provide smaller fluctuations between C_{max}^{∞} and C_{min}^{∞} compared to a dosage regimen of 0.30 mg every 24 hours.

c. Since the elimination half-life is long (30 hours), a loading dose is advisable.

$$D_L = D_m \left(\frac{1}{1 - e^{-k\tau}} \right)$$

$$D_L = 0.30 \left(\frac{1}{1 - e^{-(0.693/30)(24)}} \right) = 0.70 \text{ mg}$$

For cardiotonic drugs related to the digitalis glycosides, it is recommended that the loading dose be administered in several portions with approximately half the total as the first dose. Additional fractions may be given at 6- to 8-hour intervals, with careful assessment of the clinical response before each additional dose.

d. There is no rationale for a controlled-release drug product because of the long elimination half-life of 30 hours inherent in the drug.

11. a. $C_{av}^{\infty} = \dfrac{FD_0 \, 1.44 t_{1/2}}{V_D \tau}$

$$C_{av}^{\infty} = \frac{(1500)(1.44)(6)}{(1.3)(63)(4)} = 39.6 \text{ } \mu g/mL$$

b. $D_L = D_M \left(\dfrac{1}{1 - e^{-k\tau}} \right)$

c. A D_L of 4.05 g is needed, which is equivalent to 8 tablets containing 0.5 g each.

d. The time to achieve 95–99% of steady state is, approximately, $5 t_{1/2}$ without a loading dose. Therefore,

$$5 \times 6 = 30 \text{ hr}$$

12. a. $C_{ss} = \dfrac{R}{kV_D}$ $R = C_{ss}kV_D$

$$R = (5)\left(\frac{0.693}{2}\right)(0.173)(75) = 22.479 \text{ mg/hr}$$

$$D_L = C_{ss}V_D = (5)(0.173)(75) = 64.875 \text{ mg}$$

b. $\dfrac{R_{old}}{C_{SS,old}} = \dfrac{R_{new}}{C_{SS,new}}$

$$\frac{22.479}{2} = \frac{R_{new}}{5}   R_{new} = 56.2 \text{ mg/hr}$$

c. $4.32 t_{1/2} = 4.32(2) = 8.64 \text{ hr}$

13. $t_{1/2} = 8 \text{ hr}$ $k = 0.693/8 = 0.0866 \text{ hr}^{-1}$

$V_D = (1.5 \text{ L/kg})(75 \text{ kg}) = 112.5 \text{ L}$ $C_{SS} = 20 \text{ } \mu g/mL$

a. $R = C_{SS}V_D = (20)(0.0866)(112.5) = 194.85 \text{ mg/hr}$

b. $D_L = C_{SS}V_D = (20)(112.5) = 2250 \text{ mg}$

Alternatively, $D_L = R/k = 194.85/0.0866 = 2250 \text{ mg}$

c. 0.2 mL of a 15-mg/mL solution contains 3 mg.

$$R = 3 \text{ mg/hr/kg} \times 75 \text{ kg} = 225 \text{ mg/hr}$$

$$C_{SS} = \frac{R}{kV_D} = \frac{225}{(0.0866)(112.5)} = 23.1 \text{ mg/L}$$

The proposed starting infusion rate given by the manufacturer should provide adequate drug concentrations.

CHAPTER 21

FREQUENTLY ASKED QUESTIONS

1. Renal disease can cause profound changes in the body that must be evaluated by assessing the patient's condition and medical history. Renal dysfunction is often accompanied by reduced protein drug binding and by reduced glomerular filtration rate in the kidney. Some changes in hepatic clearance may also occur. While there is no accurate method for predicting the resulting *in-vivo* changes, a decrease in albumin may increase f_u, or the fraction of free plasma drug

concentration in the body. The f_u is estimated from $f_u = 1 - f_b$, where f_b is the fraction of bound plasma drug. For the uremic patient, the fraction of drug bound f_b' is affected by a change in plasma protein: $f_b'/f_b = p'/4.4$, where p is the normal plasma protein concentration (4.4 g/dL assuming albumin is the protein involved) and p' is the uremic plasma protein concentration; f_b' is the fraction of drug bound in the uremic patient. Since f_u' or fraction of unbound drug, is increased in the uremic patient, the free drug concentration may be increased and sometimes lead to more frequent side effects. On the other hand, an increase in plasma free drug in the uremic patient is offset somewhat by a corresponding increase in the volume of distribution as plasma protein drug binding is reduced. Reduction in GFR is more definite; it is invariably accompanied by a reduction in drug clearance and by an increase in the elimination half-life of the drug.

2. Two approaches to dose adjustment in renal disease are the clearance method and the elimination rate constant method. The methods are based on estimating either the uremic Cl_R or uremic k_R after the creatinine clearance is obtained in the uremic patient.

3. Aminoglycosides are given as a larger dose spaced farther apart (once daily). Keeping the same total daily dose of the aminoglycoside improves the response (efficacy) and possibly lessens side effects in many patients. Model simulation shows reduced exposure (AUC) to the effect compartment (toxicity), while the activity is not altered. The higher drug dose produces a higher peak drug concentration. In the case of gentamicin, the marketed drug is chemically composed of three related, but distinctly different, chemical components, which may distribute differently in the body.

4. Hepatic disease may reduce albumin and α_1-acid glycoprotein (AAG) concentrations resulting in decreased drug protein binding. Blood flow to the liver may also be affected. Generally, for a drug with linear binding, f_u may be increased as discussed in FAQ #1. Consult Chapter 10 also for a discussion of restrictive clearance of drugs. Examples of binding to AAG are the protease inhibitors for AIDS.

5. Congestive heart failure (CHF) can reduce renal or hepatic blood flow and decrease hepatic and renal drug clearance. In CHF, less blood flow is available in the splanchnic circulation to the small intestine and may result in less systemic drug bioavailability after oral drug administration. Severe disturbances to blood flow will affect the pharmacokinetics of many drugs. Myocardiac infarction (MI) is a clinical example which often causes drug clearance to be greatly reduced, especially for drugs with large hepatic extraction.

LEARNING QUESTIONS

1. The normal dose of tetracycline is 250 mg PO every 6 hours. The dose of tetracycline for the uremic patient is determined by the k_u/k_N ratio, which is

determined by the kidney function, as in Figure 21–5. From line H in the figure, at Cl_{Cr} of 20 mL, $k_u/k_N = 40\%$. In order to maintain the average concentration of tetracycline at the same level as in normal patients, the dose of tetracycline must be reduced.

$$\frac{D_u}{D_N} = \frac{k_u}{k_N} = 40\%$$

$$D_u = (250)(0.40) = 100 \text{ mg}$$

Therefore, 100 mg of tetracycline should be given PO every 6 hours.

2. The drug in this patient is eliminated by the kidneys and the dialysis machine. Therefore,

Total drug clearance $= Cl_T + Cl_D$

Using Equation 21.33,

$$Cl_D = \frac{Q(C_a - C_v)}{C_a}$$

$$Cl_D = \frac{50(5 - 2.4)}{5} = 26 \text{ mL/min}$$

Total drug clearance $= 10 + 26 = 36$ mL/min

Since the drug clearance is increased from 10 to 36 mL/min, the dose should be increased if dialysis is going to continue. Since dose is directly proportional to clearance,

$$\frac{D_u}{D_N} = \frac{36}{10} = 3.6$$

The new dose should be 3.6 times the dose given before dialysis if the same level of antibiotics is to be maintained.

4. The creatinine clearance of a patient is determined experimentally by using Equation 21.11,

$$Cl_{Cr} = \frac{C_u V 100}{C_{Cr} 1440}$$

$$Cl_{Cr} = \frac{(0.1)(1800)(100)}{(2.2)(1440)} = 5.68 \text{ mL/min}$$

Assuming that the normal Cl_{Cr} in this patient is 100 mL/min, the uremic dose should be 5.7% of the normal dose, since kidney function is drastically reduced:

$$(0.057)(20 \text{ mg/kg}) = 1.14 \text{ mg/kg given every 6 hours}$$

5. From Figure 21.5, line F, at a Cl_{Cr} of 5 mL/min,

$$\frac{k_u}{k_N} = 45\%$$

a. The dose given should be as follows:

$$(0.45)(600 \text{ mg}) = 270 \text{ mg every 12 hours}$$

b. Alternatively, the dose of 600 mg should be given every

$$12 \times \frac{100}{45} = 26.7 \text{ hr}$$

c. Since it may be desirable to give the drug once every 24 hours, both dose and dosing interval may be adjusted so that the patient will still maintain an average therapeutic blood level of the drug, which can then be given at a convenient time. Using the equation for C_{av}^{∞},

$$C_{av}^{\infty} = \frac{D_0}{kV_D\tau}$$

$$D_0 = 600 \text{ mg}$$

$$\tau = 26.7 \text{ hr}$$

$$C_{av}^{\infty} = \frac{600}{kV_D \times 26.7}$$

To maintain C_{av}^{∞} the same, calculate a new dose, D_N, with a new dosing interval, τ_N, of 24 hours.

$$C_{av}^{\infty} = \frac{D_N}{kV_D 24}$$

Thus,

$$\frac{600}{26.7} = \frac{D_N}{24}$$

Therefore,

$$D_N = \frac{24}{26.7} \times 600 = 539 \text{ mg}$$

The drug can also be given at 540 mg daily.

6. For females, use 85% of the Cl_{Cr} value obtained in males.

$$Cl_{Cr} = \frac{0.85[140 - \text{age (yr)}] \text{ body weight (kg)}}{72 \ (Cl_{Cr})}$$

$$Cl_{Cr} = \frac{0.85[140 - 38]62}{(72)(1.8)} = 41.5 \text{ mL/min}$$

9. Gentamycin is listed in group K (Table 21.4). From the nomogram in Figure 21-5,

$$Cl_{Cr} = 20 \text{ mL/min} \qquad \frac{k_u}{k_n} = 25\%$$

Uremic dose = 25% of normal dose = $(0.25) \ (1 \text{ mg/kg}) = 0.25 \text{ mg/kg}$

For a 72-kg Patient:

Uremic dose $= (0.25)(75) = 18.8$ mg

The patient should receive 18.8 mg every 8 hours by multiple IV bolus injections.

10. a. During the first 48 hours postdose, $t_{1/2} = 16$ hours. For IV bolus injection, assuming first-order elimination:

$$D_B = D_0 e^{-kt}$$

$$D_B = 1000 e^{-(0.693/16)(48)}$$

$$D_B = 125 \text{ mg remaining in body just before dialysis}$$

During dialysis, $t_{1/2} = 4$ hours, and

$$D_B = 125 e^{-(0.693/4)(8)} = 31.3 \text{ mg after dialysis}$$

b. $V_D = (0.5 \text{ L/kg})(75 \text{ kg}) = 37.5 \text{ L}$

Drug concentration just before dialysis:

$$C_p = 125 \text{ mg}/37.5 \text{ L} = 3.33 \text{ mg/L}$$

Drug concentration just after dialysis:

$$C_p = 31.3 \text{ mg}/3.75 \text{ L} = 0.83 \text{ mg/L}$$

CHAPTER 22

 FREQUENTLY ASKED QUESTIONS

1. Differential equations are used to describe the rate of drug transfer between different tissues and the blood. Differential equations have the advantage of being very adaptable to computer simulation without a lot of mathematical manipulations.

2. After an IV bolus drug injection, a drug is diluted rapidly in the venous pool. The venous blood is oxygenated in the lung and becomes arterial blood. The arterial blood containing the diluted drug then perfuses all the body organs through the systemic circulation. Some drug diffuses into the tissue and others are eliminated. In cycling through the body, the blood leaving a tissue (venous) generally has a lower drug concentration than the perfusing blood (arterial). In practice, only venous blood is sampled and assayed. Drug concentration in the

venous blood rapidly equilibrates with the tissue and will become arterial blood in the next perfusion cycle (seconds later) through the body. In pharmacokinetics, the drug concentration is assumed to decline smoothly and continuously. The difference in drug concentration between arterial and venous blood reflects drug uptake by the tissue, and this difference may have important consequences in drug therapy, such as tumor treatment.

3. Statistical moment is adaptable to mean residence time calculation and is widely used in pharmacokinetics.

4. *Mean residence time* (MRT) represents the average staying time of the drug in a body organ or compartment as the molecules diffuse in and out. MRT is an alternative concept used to describe how long a drug stays in the body. The main advantage of MRT is that it is based on probability and is consistent with how drug molecules behave in the physical world.

LEARNING QUESTIONS

1. a. $\text{MRT} = \dfrac{[\text{AUMC}]_0^\infty}{[\text{AUC}]_0^\infty} = \dfrac{100 \ (\text{mg/L}) \ \text{hr}^2}{25 \ (\text{mg/L}) \ \text{hr}} = 4 \ \text{hr}$

b. $Cl_T = \dfrac{D_0}{[\text{AUC}]_0^\infty} = \dfrac{500 \ \text{mg}}{20 \ (\text{mg/L}) \ \text{hr}} = 25 \ \text{L/hr}$

c. V_{SS} may be calculated using Equation 22.49:

$$\text{MRT} = Cl_T/V_{SS}$$

Therefore,

$$V_{SS} = \frac{Cl_T}{\text{MRT}} = \frac{25}{4} = 6.25 \ \text{L}$$

2. MRT is not calculated directly based on its definition (AUC/C_0), because it is not possible to determine C_0 except with simple data involving a one-compartment model. Based on rigorous derivation, C_0 is not C_p^0 except in a one-compartment IV bolus dose; rather, it is the concentration D_0/V_D which is equal to $C_p = C_p^0$ in the simple IV bolus dose. With oral absorption data, it is not possible to determine D_0/V_D without using a model.

3. If the data in Problem 1 are fitted to obtain k, and $k = 0.25 \ \text{hr}^{-1}$,

$$\text{MRT} = \frac{1}{k} = \frac{1}{0.25} = 4 \ \text{hr}$$

Although the answer agrees with the result calculated above using a noncompartmental approach, the calculation now uses an equation with assumptions of the one-compartment model for IV bolus.

4. The principal considerations in interspecies scaling are size, protein–drug binding, and maximum lifespan potential (MLP) of the species.

5. The model assumptions should be consistent with known information about the system. The number of model parameters should not exceed the available data, and an adequate degree of freedom should be present to test for lack of fit. The law of parsimony should apply at all times.

APPENDIX D

GUIDING PRINCIPLES FOR HUMAN AND ANIMAL RESEARCH*

ETHICAL PRINCIPLES FOR MEDICAL RESEARCH INVOLVING HUMAN SUBJECTS

The *Declaration of Helsinki,* first published in 1964 by the World Medical Association, established recommendations guiding medical doctors in biomedical research involving human subjects (www.wma.net/e/policy/b3.htm). The Declaration governs international research ethics and defines rules for "research combined with clinical care" and "non-therapeutic research." The Declaration of Helsinki has been revised periodically and is the basis of Good Clinical Practices used today. A copy of the latest revision is reproduced in this Appendix. The Declaration of Helsinki addressed the following issues:

- "Medical research is subject to ethical standards that promote respect for all human beings and protect their health and rights."
- Research protocols should be clearly formulated into an experimental protocol and reviewed by an independent committee prior to initiation.
- Informed consent from all research participants is necessary.
- Research should be conducted by medically/scientifically qualified individuals.
- Risks should not exceed benefits.

The *Belmont Report,* Ethical Principles and Guidelines for the Protection of Human Subjects of Research, was published by the National Commission for the Protection of Human Subjects of Biomedical and Behavioral Research on April 18, 1979 (http://ohsr.od.nih.gov/mpa/belmont.php3). The Belmont Report identifies

*From *Guide for the Care and Use of Laboratory Animals,* DHEW publ. no. (NIH) 80-23, revised 1978, reprinted 1980. Bethesda, MD, Office of Science and Health Reports, DDR/NIH.

857

three principles, or general prescriptive judgments, that are relevant to research involving human subjects.

A. Boundaries between Practice and Research

1. *Practice* refers to interventions that are designed solely to enhance the well-being of an individual patient or client and that have a reasonable expectation of success. The purpose of medical or behavioral practice is to provide diagnosis, preventive treatment, or therapy to particular individuals.

2. *Research* designates an activity designed to test an hypothesis, permit conclusions to be drawn, and thereby to develop or contribute to generalizable knowledge (expressed, for example, in theories, principles, and statements of relationships). Research is usually described in a formal protocol that sets forth an objective and a set of procedures designed to reach that objective.

3. *Experimental* is when a clinician departs in a significant way from standard or accepted practice. The fact that a procedure is "experimental," in the sense of new, untested, or different, does not automatically place it in the category of research.

B. Basic Ethical Principles

1. Respect for Persons
2. Beneficence
3. Justice

C. Applications

1. Informed Consent
2. Assessment of Risks and Benefits
3. Selection of Subjects

The United States' *Code of Federal Regulations* (CFR) publishes regulations for the protection of human subjects. Title 45 Code of Federal Regulations Part 46 (45CFR46) contains federal regulations which directly apply to most of human research done in the United States and are intended to protect all human subjects. 45CFR46 does the following:

- Defines activities that are subject to regulation
- Details the composition and function of an Institutional Review Board (IRB)
- Describes expedited review procedures
- Lists the criteria for review of research
- Provides a detailed description of the informed concent process, including waivers
- Describes the process for documenting consent, including waivers
- There are three subparts of the regulations that include additional protections for vulnerable populations:
  Pregnant women, fetuses, and neonates
  Prisoners
  Children

Various resources concerning ethics involving human subjects research and Institutional Review Boards (IRBs) have been collected by the National Institutes of Health (www.nih.gov/sigs/bioethics/IRB.html).

GUIDING PRINCIPLES IN THE CARE AND USE OF ANIMALS

Animal experiments are to be undertaken only with the purpose of advancing knowledge. Consideration should be given to the appropriateness of experimental procedures, species of animals used, and number of animals required.

Only animals that are lawfully acquired shall be used in the laboratory, and their retention and use shall be in every case in compliance with federal, state, and local laws and regulations and in accordance with the NIH Guide.

Animals in the laboratory must receive every consideration for their comfort; they must be properly housed, fed, and their surroundings kept in a sanitary condition.

Appropriate anesthetics must be used to eliminate sensibility to pain during all surgical procedures. Where recovery from anesthesia is necessary during the study, acceptable technique to minimize pain must be followed. Muscle relaxants or paralytics are not anesthetics and they should not be used alone for surgical restraint. They may be used for surgery in conjunction with drugs known to produce adequate analgesia. Where use of anesthetics would negate the results of the experiment, such procedures should be carried out in strict accordance with the NIH Guide. If the study requires the death of the animal, the animal must be killed in a humane manner at the conclusion of the observations.

The postoperative care of animals shall be such as to minimize discomfort and pain, and in any case shall be equivalent to accepted practices in schools of veterinary medicine.

When animals are used by students for their education or the advancement of science, such work shall be under the direct supervision of an experienced teacher or investigator. The rules for the care of such animals must be the same as for animals used for research.

World Medical Association Declaration of Helsinki

Ethical Principles for Medical Research Involving Human Subjects

Adopted by the 18th WMA General Assembly, Helsinki, Finland, June 1964; amended by the 29th WMA General Assembly, Tokyo, Japan, October 1975; 35th WMA General Assembly, Venice, Italy, October 1983; 41st WMA General Assembly, Hong Kong, September 1989; 48th WMA General Assembly, Somerset West, Republic of South Africa, October 1996, and the 52nd WMA General Assembly, Edinburgh, Scotland, October 2000

A.   Introduction

1.   The World Medical Association has developed the Declaration of Helsinki as a statement of ethical principles to provide guidance to physicians and other participants in medical research involving human subjects. Medical research involving human subjects includes research on identifiable human material or identifiable data.

2.   It is the duty of the physician to promote and safeguard the health of the people. The physician's knowledge and conscience are dedicated to the fulfillment of this duty.

3.   The Declaration of Geneva of the World Medical Association binds the physician with the words, "The health of my patient will be my first consideration," and the International Code of Medical Ethics declares that, "A physician shall act only in the patient's interest when providing medical care which might have the effect of weakening the physical and mental condition of the patient."

4.   Medical progress is based on research which ultimately must rest in part on experimentation involving human subjects.

5.   In medical research on human subjects, considerations related to the well-being of the human subject should take precedence over the interests of science and society.

6.   The primary purpose of medical research involving human subjects is to improve prophylactic, diagnostic and therapeutic procedures and the understanding of the aetiology and pathogenesis of disease. Even the best proven prophylactic, diagnostic, and therapeutic methods must continuously be challenged through research for their effectiveness, efficiency, accessibility and quality.

7.   In current medical practice and in medical research, most prophylactic, diagnostic and therapeutic procedures involve risks and burdens.

8.   Medical research is subject to ethical standards that promote respect for all human beings and protect their health and rights. Some research populations are vulnerable and need special protection. The particular needs of the economically and medically disadvantaged must be recognized. Special attention is also required for those who cannot give or refuse consent for themselves, for those who may be subject to giving consent under duress, for those who will not benefit personally from the research and for those for whom the research is combined with care.

9.   Research Investigators should be aware of the ethical, legal and regulatory requirements for research on human subjects in their own countries as well as applicable international requirements. No national ethical, legal or regulatory requirement should be allowed to reduce or eliminate any of the protections for human subjects set forth in this Declaration.

B.   Basic principles for all medical research

10.   It is the duty of the physician in medical research to protect the life, health, privacy, and dignity of the human subject.

11.   Medical research involving human subjects must conform to generally accepted scientific principles, be based on a thorough knowledge of the scientific literature, other relevant sources of information, and on adequate laboratory and, where appropriate, animal experimentation.

12.   Appropriate caution must be exercised in the conduct of research which may affect the environment, and the welfare of animals used for research must be respected.

13.   The design and performance of each experimental procedure involving human subjects should be clearly formulated in an experimental protocol. This protocol should be submitted for consideration, comment, guidance, and where appropriate, approval to a specially appointed ethical review committee, which must be independent of the investigator, the sponsor or any other kind of undue influence. This independent committee should be in conformity with the laws and regulations of the country in which the research experiment is performed. The committee has the right to monitor ongoing trials. The researcher has the obligation to provide monitoring information to the committee, especially any serious adverse events. The researcher should also submit to the committee, for review, information regarding funding, sponsors, institutional affiliations, other potential conflicts of interest and incentives for subjects.

14.   The research protocol should always contain a statement of the ethical considerations involved and should indicate that there is compliance with the principles enunciated in this Declaration.

15.   Medical research involving human subjects should be conducted only by scientifically qualified persons and under the supervision of a clinically competent medical person. The responsibility for the human subject must always rest with a medically qualified person and never rest on the subject of the research, even though the subject has given consent.

16. Every medical research project involving human subjects should be preceded by careful assessment of predictable risks and burdens in comparison with foreseeable benefits to the subject or to others. This does not preclude the participation of healthy volunteers in medical research. The design of all studies should be publicly available.

17. Physicians should abstain from engaging in research projects involving human subjects unless they are confident that the risks involved have been adequately assessed and can be satisfactorily managed. Physicians should cease any investigation if the risks are found to outweigh the potential benefits or if there is conclusive proof of positive and beneficial results.

18. Medical research involving human subjects should only be conducted if the importance of the objective outweighs the inherent risks and burdens to the subject. This is especially important when the human subjects are healthy volunteers.

19. Medical research is only justified if there is a reasonable likelihood that the populations in which the research is carried out stand to benefit from the results of the research.

20. The subjects must be volunteers and informed participants in the research project.

21. The right of research subjects to safeguard their integrity must always be respected. Every precaution should be taken to respect the privacy of the subject, the confidentiality of the patient's information and to minimize the impact of the study on the subject's physical and mental integrity and on the personality of the subject.

22. In any research on human beings, each potential subject must be adequately informed of the aims, methods, sources of funding, any possible conflicts of interest, institutional affiliations of the researcher, the anticipated benefits and potential risks of the study and the discomfort it may entail. The subject should be informed of the right to abstain from participation in the study or to withdraw consent to participate at any time without reprisal. After ensuring that the subject has understood the information, the physician should then obtain the subject's freely-given informed consent, preferably in writing. If the consent cannot be obtained in writing, the non-written consent must be formally documented and witnessed.

23. When obtaining informed consent for the research project the physician should be particularly cautious if the subject is in a dependent relationship with the physician or may consent under duress. In that case the informed consent should be obtained by a well-informed physician who is not engaged in the investigation and who is completely independent of this relationship.

24. For a research subject who is legally incompetent, physically or mentally incapable of giving consent or is a legally incompetent minor, the investigator must obtain informed consent from the legally authorized representative in accordance with applicable law. These groups should not be included in research unless the research is necessary to promote the health of the population represented and this research cannot instead be performed on legally competent persons.

25. When a subject deemed legally incompetent, such as a minor child, is able to give assent to decisions about participation in research, the investigator must obtain that assent in addition to the consent of the legally authorized representative.

26. Research on individuals from whom it is not possible to obtain consent, including proxy or advance consent, should be done only if the physical/mental condition that prevents obtaining informed consent is a necessary characteristic of the research population. The specific reasons for involving research subjects with a condition that renders them unable to give informed consent should be stated in the experimental protocol for consideration and approval of the review committee. The protocol should state that consent to remain in the research should be obtained as soon as possible from the individual or a legally authorized surrogate.

27. Both authors and publishers have ethical obligations. In publication of the results of research, the investigators are obliged to preserve the accuracy of the results. Negative as well as positive results should be published or otherwise publicly available. Sources of funding, institutional affiliations and any possible conflicts of interest should be declared in the publication. Reports of experimentation not in accordance with the principles laid down in this Declaration should not be accepted for publication.

C. Additional principles for medical research combined with medical care

28. The physician may combine medical research with medical care, only to the extent that the research is justified by its potential prophylactic, diagnostic or therapeutic value. When medical research is combined with medical care, additional standards apply to protect the patients who are research subjects.

29. The benefits, risks, burdens and effectiveness of a new method should be tested against those of the best current prophylactic, diagnostic, and therapeutic methods. This does not exclude the use of placebo, or no treatment, in studies where no proven prophylactic, diagnostic or therapeutic method exists.

30. At the conclusion of the study, every patient entered into the study should be assured of access to the best proven prophylactic, diagnostic and therapeutic methods identified by the study.

31. The physician should fully inform the patient which aspects of the care are related to the research. The refusal of a patient to participate in a study must never interfere with the patient–physician relationship.

32. In the treatment of a patient, where proven prophylactic, diagnostic and therapeutic methods do not exist or have been ineffective, the physician, with informed consent from the patient, must be free to use unproven or new prophylactic, diagnostic and therapeutic measures, if in the physician's judgement it offers hope of saving life, reestablishing health or alleviating suffering. Where possible, these measures should be made the object of research, designed to evaluate their safety and efficacy. In all cases, new information should be recorded and, where appropriate, published. The other relevant guidelines of this Declaration should be followed. ∎

APPENDIX E

POPULAR DRUGS AND PHARMACOKINETIC PARAMETERS

TABLE E.1 Pharmacokinetic and Pharmacodynamic Parameters for Selected Drugs[1]

DRUG	ORAL AVAILABILITY (%)	URINARY EXCRETION (%)	BOUND IN PLASMA (%)	CLEARANCE[2] (mL/min)	VOLUME OF DISTRIBUTION (L)	HALF-LIFE (hr)	EFFECTIVE[3] CONCENTRATIONS	TOXIC[3] CONCENTRATIONS
Acetaminophen	88 ± 15	3 ± 1	0	350 ± 100	67 ± 8	2.0 ± 0.4	10–20 µg/mL	>300 µg/mL
Acyclovir	15–30	75 ± 10	15 ± 4	330 ± 80	48 ± 13	2.4 ± 0.7		
Alendrenate	0.59 (0.58–0.98)					very long (related to bone turnover)		
Alprazolam	88 ± 16	20	71 ± 3	0.74 ± 0.14 ml/min/kg	0.72 ± 0.12 L/Kg	12 ± 2	20–40 ng/mL	
Alteplase (TPA)	—	LOW	—	10 ± 4 ml/min/kg	0.1 ± 0.01 L/Kg	0.08 ± 0.04		
Amikacin		98	4	91 ± 42	19 ± 4	2.3 ± 0.4		
Amoxicillin	93 ± 10	86 ± 8	18	180 ± 28	15 ± 2	1.7 ± 0.3		
Amphotericin B		2–5	>90	32 ± 14	53 ± 36	18 ± 7		
Ampicillin	62 ± 17	82 ± 10	18 ± 2	270 ± 50	20 ± 5	1.3 ± 0.2		
Aspirin[4]	68 ± 3	1.4 ± 1.2	49	650 ± 80	11 ± 2	0.25 ± 0.3	See Salicyclic acid	
Atenolol	56 ± 30	94 ± 8	<5	170 ± 14	67 ± 11	6.1 ± 2.0	1 µg/mL	
Atropine	50	57 ± 8	14–22	410 ± 250	120 ± 49	4.3 ± 1.7		
Captopril	65	38 ± 11	30 ± 6	840 ± 100	57 ± 13	2.2 ± 0.5	50 ng/mL	
Carbamazepine[4]	>70	<1	74 ± 3	89 ± 37	98 ± 26	15 ± 5	6.5 ± 3 µg/mL	>9 µg/mL
Cephalexin	90 ± 9	91 ± 18	14 ± 3	300 ± 80	18 ± 2	0.90 ± 0.18		
Cephalothin		52	71 ± 3	470 ± 120	18 ± 8	0.57 ± 0.32		
Chloramphenicol	75–90	25 ± 15	53 ± 5	170 ± 14	66 ± 4	2.7 ± 0.8		
Chlordiazepoxide[4]	100	<1	96.5 ± 1.8	38 ± 34	21 ± 2	10 ± 3	>0.7 µg/mL	
Chloroquine[4]	89 ± 16	61 ± 4	61 ± 9	750 ± 120	13,000 ± 4600	8.9 ± 3.1 days	15–30 ng/mL	0.25 µg/mL
Chlorpropamide	>90	20 ± 18	96 ± 1	2.1 ± 0.4	6.8 ± 0.8	33 ± 6		
Cimetidine	62 ± 6	62 ± 20	19	540 ± 130	70 ± 14	1.9 ± 0.3	0.8 µg/mL	
Ciprofloxacin	60 ± 12	65 ± 12	40	420 ± 84	130 ± 28	4.1 ± 0.9		
Clonidine	95	62 ± 11	20	210 ± 84	150 ± 30	12 ± 7	0.2–2 ng/mL	
Cyclosporine	23.7	<1	93 ± 2	410 ± 70	85 ± 15	5.6 ± 2	100–400 ng/mL	>400 ng/mL

Drug							
Diazepam[4]	100	<1	98.7 ± 0.2	27 ± 4	77 ± 20	43 ± 13	300–400 ng/mL	
Digitoxin	>90	32 ± 15	97 ± 1	3.9 ± 1.3	38 ± 10	6.7 ± 1.7 days	>10 ng/mL	>35 ng/mL
Digoxin	70 ± 13	60 ± 11	25 ± 5	130 ± 67	440 ± 150	39 ± 13	>0.8 ng/mL	>2 ng/mL
Diltiazem[4]	44 ± 10	<4	78 ± 3	840 ± 280	220 ± 85	3.7 ± 1.2		
Diflunisal	90	6 ± 3	99.9 ± 0.01	0.1 ± 0.02 mL/min/kg	0.1 ± 0.02 L/kg	11 ± 2		
Dirithromycin	10% (6–14) abs bio (urinary data)	17–25	10–30	226–1040 mL/min	800 L (504–1041)	44 (16–65)		
Disopyramide	83 ± 11	55 ± 6	Dose-dependent	84 ± 28	41 ± 11	6.0 ± 1.0	3 ± 1 μg/mL	>8 μg/mL
Erythromycin	35 ± 25	12 ± 7	84 ± 3	640 ± 290	55 ± 31	1.6 ± 0.7		
Erythropoietin				7.88 mL/min	3.70 L per 1.73 m^2	4.92		
Ethambutol	77 ± 8	79 ± 3	<5	600 ± 60	110 ± 14	3.1 ± 0.4		>10 μg/mL
Ethosuximide	—	25 ± 15	0	0.19 ± 0.04 mL/min/kg	0.72 ± 0.16 L/kg	45 ± 8	40–100 μg/mL	
Famciclovir	77 ± 8	74 ± 9	<20	8.0 ± 1.5 mL/min/kg	0.98 ± 0.13 L/kg	2.3 ± 0.4		
Famotidine	45 ± 14	67 ± 15	17 ± 7	7.1 ± 1.7 mL/min/kg	1.3 ± 0.2 L/kg	2.6 ± 1.0	13 ng/ml	
Fluoxetine	>60	<2.5	94	9.6 ± 6.9 mL/min/kg	35 ± 21 L/kg	53 ± 41	<500 ng/mL	
Furosemide	61 ± 17	66 ± 7	98.8 ± 0.2	140 ± 30	7.7 ± 1.4	1.5 ± 0.1		25 μg/mL
Ganciclovir	3	73 ± 31	1–2	4.6 ± 1.8 mL/min/kg	1.1 ± 0.3 L/kg	4.3 ± 1.6		
Gentamicin		>90	<10	90 ± 25	18 ± 6	2–3		
Hydralazine	20–60	1–15	87	3900 ± 900	105 ± 70	1.0 ± 0.3	100 ng/mL	
Imipramine[4]	40 ± 12	<2	90.1 ± 1.4	1050 ± 280	1600 ± 600	18 ± 7	100–300 ng/mL	>1 μg/mL
Indinavir						~3		
Indomethacin	98	15 ± 8	90	140 ± 30	18 ± 5	2.4 ± 0.4	0.3–3 μg/mL	>5 μg/mL
Labetalol	18 ± 5	<5	50	1750 ± 700	660 ± 240	4.9 ± 2.0	0.13 μg/mL	
Lidocaine	35 ± 11	2 ± 1	70 ± 5	640 ± 170	77 ± 28	1.8 ± 0.4	1.5–6 μg/mL	>6 μg/mL
Lithium	100	95 ± 15	0	25 ± 8	55 ± 24	22 ± 8	0.5–1.25 meq/L	>2 meq/L
Lomefloxacin	97 ± 2	65 ± 9	10	3.3 ± 0.5 mL/min/kg	2.3 ± 0.3 L/kg	8.0 ± 1.4		

(Continued)

TABLE E.1 Pharmacokinetic and Pharmacodynamic Parameters for Selected Drugs[1] (Continued)

DRUG	ORAL AVAILABILITY (%)	URINARY EXCRETION (%)	BOUND IN PLASMA (%)	CLEARANCE[2] (mL/min)	VOLUME OF DISTRIBUTION (L)	HALF-LIFE (hr)	EFFECTIVE[3] CONCENTRATIONS	TOXIC[3] CONCENTRATIONS
Lovastatin	<5	negligible	95	4–18 mL/min/kg	—	1.1–1.7 hr	—	
Meperidine	52 ± 3	1–25	58 ± 9	1200 ± 350	310 ± 60	3.2 ± 0.8	0.4–0.7 µg/mL	
Methotrexate	70 ± 27	48 ± 18	34 ± 8	150 ± 60	39 ± 13	7.2 ± 2.1		10 µM
Metoprolol	38 ± 14	10 ± 3	11 ± 1	1050 ± 210	290 ± 50	3.2 ± 0.2	25 ng/mL	
Metronidazole[4]	99 ± 8	10 ± 2	10	90 ± 20	52 ± 7	8.5 ± 2.9	3–6 µg/mL	
Mexiletine	87 ± 13	4–15	63 ± 3	6.3 ± 2.7 mL/min/kg	4.9 ± 0.5 L/kg	9.2 ± 2.1 hr	0.5–2.0 µg/mL	>2.0 µg/mL
Midazolam	44 ± 17	56 ± 26	95 ± 2	460 ± 130	77 ± 42	1.9 ± 0.6		
Morphine	24 ± 12	6–10	35 ± 2	1600 ± 700	230 ± 60	1.9 ± 0.5	65 ng/mL	
Moxalactam	—	76 ± 12	50	120 ± 30	19 ± 6	2.1 ± 0.7		
Notilmicin	—	80–90	<10	1.3 ± 0.2 mL/min/kg	0.2 ± 0.02 L/kg	2.3 ± 0.7 hr		
Nifedipine	50 ± 13	0	96 ± 1	490 ± 130	55 ± 15	1.8 ± 0.4	47 ± 20 ng/mL	
Nortriptyline[4]	51 ± 5	2 ± 1	92 ± 2	500 ± 130	1300 ± 300	31 ± 13	50–140 ng/mL	>500 ng/mL
Phenobarbital	100 ± 11	24 ± 5	51 ± 3	4.3 ± 0.9	38 ± 2	4.1 ± 0.8 days	10–25 µg/mL	>30 µg/mL
Phenytoin	90 ± 3	2	89 ± 23	Dose-dependent	45 ± 3	Dose-dependent	>10 µg/mL	>20 µg/mL
Pravastatin	18 ± 8	47 ± 7	43–48	3.5 ± 2.4 mL/min/kg	0.46 ± 0.04 L/kg	1.8 ± 0.8 hr		
Prazosin	68 ± 17	<1	95 ± 1	210 ± 20	42 ± 9	2.9 ± 0.8		
Procainamide[4]	83 ± 16	67 ± 8	16 ± 5	350–840	130 ± 20	3.0 ± 0.6	3–14 µg/mL	>14 µg/mL
Propranolol[4]	26 ± 10	<0.5	87 ± 6	840 ± 210	270 ± 40	3.9 ± 0.4	20 ng/mL	
Pyridostigmine	14 ± 3	80–90		600 ± 120	77 ± 21	1.9 ± 0.2	50–100 ng/mL	
Quinidine[4]	80 ± 15	18 ± 5	87 ± 3	330 ± 130	190 ± 80	6.2 ± 1.8	2–6 µg/mL	>8 µg/mL
Ranitidine	52 ± 11	69 ± 6	15 ± 3	730 ± 80	91 ± 28	2.1 ± 0.2	100 ng/mL	
Ribavirin	45 ± 5	35 ± 8	0	5 ± 1.0 mL/min/kg	9.3 ± 1.5 L/kg	28 ± 7 hr		
Rifampin[4]		7 ± 3	89 ± 1 high (AAG)	240 ± 110	68 ± 25	3.5 ± 0.8		
Ritonavir	<5					~3 hr		
Saquinavir	<5		high (AAG)	*<989 L/hr	*<1503 L	7–12 hr (beta) (1.38 hr)		

Drug							
Salicylic acid	100	2–30	80–90[5]	14[5]	12 ± 2	10–15[5]	150–300 µg/mL	>200 µg/mL
Simvastatin	<5	negligible	94	7.6 ml/min/kg	—	1.9 hr	—	—
Sotalol	90–100	>75	0	2.6 ± 0.5 ml/min/kg	2.0 ± 0.4 L/kg	12 ± 3 hr		
Sulfamethoxazole	100	14 ± 2	62 ± 5	22 ± 3	15 ± 1.4	10 ± 5		
Sulfisoxazole	96 ± 14	49 ± 8	91 ± 1	23 ± 3.5	10.5 ± 1.4	6.6 ± 0.7		
Sumatriptan	14 ± 5 (oral) 97 ± 16 (SQ)	22 ± 4	14–21	16 ± 2 ml/min/kg	0.65 ± 0.1 L/kg	1.9 ± 0.3 hr		
Tamoxifen	—	<1	>98	1.4 ml/min/kg	50–60 L/kg	4–11 days	2.3 ± 1.8 ng/mL	
Terbutaline	14 ± 2	56 ± 4	20	240 ± 40	125 ± 15	14 ± 2		
Tetracycline	77	58 ± 8	65 ± 3	120 ± 20	105 ± 6	11 ± 1.5		
Theophylline	96 ± 8	18 ± 3	56 ± 4	48 ± 21	35 ± 11	8.1 ± 2.4	10–20 µg/mL	>20 µg/mL
Tobramycin		90	<10	77	18 ± 6	2.2 ± 0.1		
Tocainide	89 ± 5	38 ± 7	10 ± 15	180 ± 35	210 ± 15	14 ± 2	6–15 µg/mL	
Tolbutamide	93 ± 10	0	96 ± 1	17 ± 3	7 ± 1	5.9 ± 1.4	80–240 µg/mL	
Trimethoprim	100	69 ± 17	44	150 ± 40	130 ± 15	11 ± 1.4		
Tubocurarine		63 ± 35	50 ± 8	135 ± 42	27 ± 8	2.0 ± 1.1	0.6 ± 0.2 µg/mL	
Valproic acid	100 ± 10	1.8 ± 2.4	93 ± 1	7.7 ± 1.4	9.1 ± 2.8	14 ± 3	30–100 µg/mL	>150 µg/mL
Vancomycin		79 ± 11	30 ± 10	98 ± 7	27 ± 4	5.6 ± 1.8	120 ± 20 ng/mL	
Verapamil	22 ± 8 (oral) 35 ± 13 (Sublingual)	<3	90 ± 2	15 ± 6 ml/min/kg	5.0 ± 2.1 L/kg	4.0 ± 1.5 hr		
Warfarin	93 ± 8	<2	99 ± 1	3.2 ± 1.7	9.8 ± 4.2	37 ± 15	2.2 ± 0.4 µg/mL	
Zidovudine	63 ± 13	18 ± 5	<25	26 ± 6 ml/min/kg	1.4 ± 0.4 L/kg	1.1 ± 0.2 hr		
Zalcitabine	88 ± 17	65 ± 17	<4	4.1 ± 1.2 ml/min/kg	0.53 ± 0.13 L/kg	2.0 ± 0.8 hr		

See footnotes on next page.

(Continued)

TABLE E.1 Pharmacokinetic and Pharmacodynamic Parameters for Selected Drugs[1] *(Continued)*

[1]The values in this table represent the parameters determined when the drug is administered to healthy normal volunteers or to patients who are generally free from disease except for the condition for which the drug is being prescribed. The values presented here are adapted, with permission, from Hardman JG: Design and optimization of dosage regimens: Pharmacokinetic data. In: *Goodman and Gilman's The Pharmacological Basis of Therapeutics.* 9th ed. Gilman AG et al (editors). McGraw-Hill, 1995. This source must be consulted for the effects of disease states on the pertinent pharmacokinetic parameters.

[2]For a standard 70-kg person.

[3]No pharmacodynamic values are given for antibiotics since these vary depending upon the infecting organism.

[4]One or more metabolites are active. Clearance given for aspirin is for conversion to the active metabolite, salicylic acid; see that compound for further clearance data.

[5]The values are within the therapeutic range for drugs exhibiting dose-dependent pharmacokinetics.

[6]Volume of distribution and clearance determined orally (when F is unknown, Cl/F, or V_D/F) are listed as less than actual since F may be less than 1.

[7]Effective levels for antibiotics are variable depending on the susceptibility of the microorganisms.

[8]Generally, the beta half-life is listed, but it may be essential to consult the alpha half-life if the effective concentration is high or the distributive phase is long.

[9]The percent of urinary drug excretion is 100. fe is the fraction of drug excreted unchanged."100–100 fe" yields the percent of drug eliminated by other routes, often assumed to be metabolism. It is worth noting that in some cases the mass balance may be off, and sometimes biliary excretion is significant.

[10]For simplicity, most PK parameters are listed on a per kilogram basis, whereas others are parameters based on average BW or body surface reported in the study.

[11]Some parameters are listed without consideration of the curvilinear phase which is present for most drugs.

From Katzung BG: Basic & Clinical Pharmacology. 7th ed. Norwalk, CT, Appleton & Lange, 1998.

Physician's Desk Reference, 1997

Dirithromycin:
Sides GD et al, Anti Micr. Chem. 31; Supp C: P65–75, 1993

Erythropoetin:
Jensen-JD et al: J-Am-Soc-Nephrol. 1994 Aug; 5(2):177–85

Indinavir:
Lin JH et al: Drug Metab Dispos 1996 Oct;24(10):1111–1120

Alendronate:
Gertz BJ, Holland SD, Kline WF, Matuszewski BK, Freeman A, Quan H, Lasseter KC, Mucklow JC, Porras: Clin Pharmacol Ther, 1995 Sep (3);288–298

Protease inhibitors:
Barry M, Gibbons S, Back D, Mulcahy F: Clin Pharmacokinet 1997 Mar;32(3):194–209

Zidovudine, zalcitabine, and saquinavir:
Vanhove GF, Kastrissios H, Gries JM, Verotta D, Park K, Collier AC, Squires K, Sheiner LB, Blaschke: Antimicrob Agents Chemother 1997 Nov;2428–2432

INDEX

Page numbers followed by "t" denote tables; those followed by "f" denote figures.